WORLD HEALTH ORGANIZATION
INTERNATIONAL AGENCY FOR RESEARCH ON CANCER

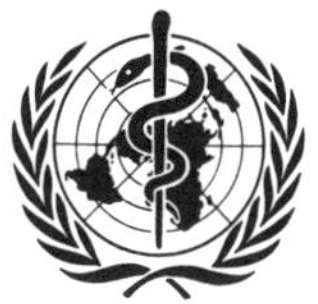

IARC Monographs on the Evaluation of Carcinogenic Risks to Humans

VOLUME 87

Inorganic and Organic Lead Compounds

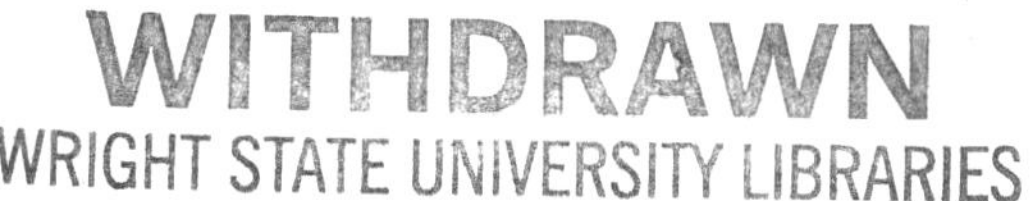

This publication represents the views and expert opinions of an IARC Working Group on the Evaluation of Carcinogenic Risks to Humans, which met in Lyon,

10–17 February 2004

2006

IARC MONOGRAPHS

In 1969, the International Agency for Research on Cancer (IARC) initiated a programme on the evaluation of the carcinogenic risk of chemicals to humans involving the production of critically evaluated monographs on individual chemicals. The programme was subsequently expanded to include evaluations of carcinogenic risks associated with exposures to complex mixtures, life-style factors and biological and physical agents, as well as those in specific occupations.

The objective of the programme is to elaborate and publish in the form of monographs critical reviews of data on carcinogenicity for agents to which humans are known to be exposed and on specific exposure situations; to evaluate these data in terms of human risk with the help of international working groups of experts in chemical carcinogenesis and related fields; and to indicate where additional research efforts are needed.

The lists of IARC evaluations are regularly updated and are available on Internet: http://monographs.iarc.fr/

This programme has been supported by Cooperative Agreement 5 UO1 CA33193 awarded since 1982 by the United States National Cancer Institute, Department of Health and Human Services. Additional support has been provided since 1986 by the European Commission, Directorate-General EMPL (Employment, and Social Affairs), Health, Safety and Hygiene at Work Unit, and since 1992 by the United States National Institute of Environmental Health Sciences.

This publication was made possible, in part, by a Cooperative Agreement between the United States Environmental Protection Agency, Office of Research and Development (USEPA-ORD) and the International Agency for Research on Cancer (IARC) and does not necessarily express the views of USEPA-ORD.

Published by the International Agency for Research on Cancer,
150 cours Albert Thomas, 69372 Lyon Cedex 08, France

Distributed by WHO Press, World Health Organization, 20 Avenue Appia, 1211 Geneva 27, Switzerland (tel.: +41 22 791 3264; fax: +41 22 791 4857; e-mail: bookorders@who.int).

IARC Library Cataloguing in Publication Data

Inorganic and Organic Lead Compounds/IARC Working Group on the Evaluation of Carcinogenic Risks to Humans (2004 : Lyon, France)
(IARC monographs on the evaluation of carcinogenic risks to humans ; v. 87)
1. Carcinogens – congresses 2. Lead – adverse effects 3. Lead – toxicity
I. IARC Working Group on the Evaluation of Carcinogenic Risks to Humans II. Series

ISBN 92 832 1287 8 (NLM Classification: W1)
ISSN 1017-1606

PRINTED IN FRANCE

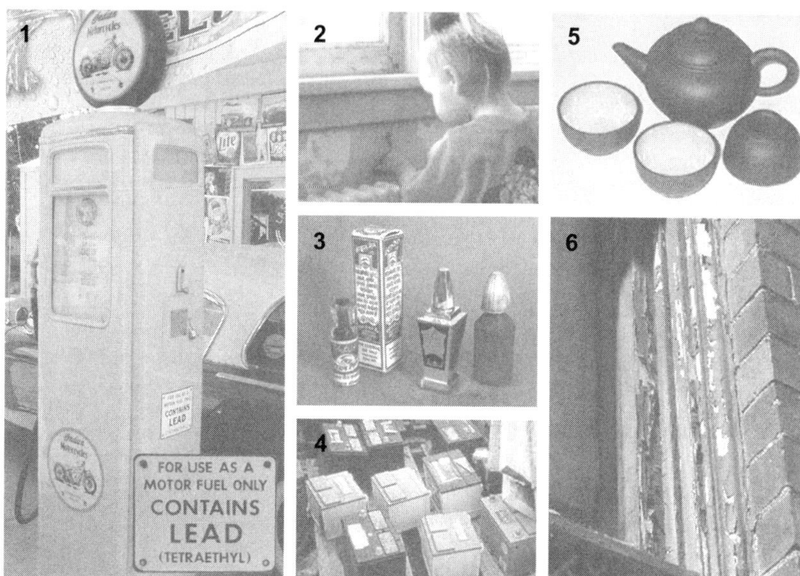

1 Leaded gasoline: tetraethyl lead has been used as an additive in gasoline for decades.

2 Exposure to lead-based paint in older homes: a major source of lead exposure for children

3 Products like surma and kohl, used in some cultures for cosmetic purposes and in traditional medicine, often contain large amounts of lead.

4 Lead-acid batteries: the largest single application of lead world-wide

5 Lead-glazed tableware: the bluish-grey crackled glaze of these teacups may leach considerable amounts of lead.

6 Lead-based paint in older homes

Cover design: Georges Mollon, IARC

CONTENTS

NOTE TO THE READER

The term 'carcinogenic risk' in the *IARC Monographs* series is taken to mean the probability that exposure to an agent will lead to cancer in humans.

Inclusion of an agent in the *Monographs* does not imply that it is a carcinogen, only that the published data have been examined. Equally, the fact that an agent has not yet been evaluated in a monograph does not mean that it is not carcinogenic.

The evaluations of carcinogenic risk are made by international working groups of independent scientists and are qualitative in nature. No recommendation is given for regulation or legislation.

Anyone who is aware of published data that may alter the evaluation of the carcinogenic risk of an agent to humans is encouraged to make this information available to the Carcinogen Identification and Evaluation Group, International Agency for Research on Cancer, 150 cours Albert Thomas, 69372 Lyon Cedex 08, France, in order that the agent may be considered for re-evaluation by a future Working Group.

Although every effort is made to prepare the monographs as accurately as possible, mistakes may occur. Readers are requested to communicate any errors to the Carcinogen Identification and Evaluation Group, so that corrections can be reported in future volumes.

IARC WORKING GROUP ON THE EVALUATION OF CARCINOGENIC RISKS TO HUMANS: INORGANIC AND ORGANIC LEAD COMPOUNDS

Lyon, 10–17 February 2004

LIST OF PARTICIPANTS

Members

Ahti Anttila, Finnish Cancer Registry, Institute for Statistical and Epidemiological Cancer Research, Liisankatu 21 B, 00170 Helsinki, Finland

Pietro Apostoli, Institute of Occupational Health and Industrial Hygiene, University of Brescia, P. le Spedali Civili 1, 25123 Brescia, Italy (*unable to attend*)

James A. Bond, Editor-in-Chief, Chemico-Biological Interactions, 25 Rabbitbrush Road, Santa Fe, NM 87506, USA (*Subgroup Chair, Other Relevant Data*)

Lars Gerhardsson, Department of Occupational and Environmental Medicine, Sahlgrenska University Hospital, St. Sigfridsgatan 85, 412 66 Göteborg, Sweden

Brian L. Gulson, Graduate School of the Environment, Macquarie University, Sydney, NSW 2109, Australia

Andrea Hartwig, Institute of Food Technology and Food Chemistry, Technical University Berlin, Gustav-Meyer-Allee 25, D-13355 Berlin, Germany

Perrine Hoet, Unit of Industrial Toxicology and Occupational Medicine, Faculty of Medicine, Catholic University of Louvain, Clos Chapelle-aux-Champs 30-54, 1200 Brussels, Belgium

Masayuki Ikeda, Kyoto Industrial Health Association, 67 Nishinokyo-Kitatsuboicho, Nakagyo-ku, Kyoto 604-8472, Japan

Eileen K. Jaffe, Biomolecular Structure and Function Group, Fox Chase Cancer Center, 333 Cottman Avenue, Philadelphia, PA 19111, USA (*Subgroup Chair, Exposure Data*)

Philip J. Landrigan, Department of Community and Preventive Medicine, Mount Sinai School of Medicine, 10 East 101 Street, Box 1057, New York, NY 10029-6574, USA (*unable to attend*)

Len Levy, Institute of Environment and Health, Cranfield University, Silsoe, Bedfordshire MK45 4DT, United Kingdom (*Overall Chair*)

Herbert L. Needleman, Lead Research Group, University of Pennsylvania, 310 Keystone Bldg, 3520 Fifth Avenue, Pittsburgh, PA 15213, USA

Ellen J. O'Flaherty, Department of Environmental Health, College of Medicine, University of Cincinnati, Cincinnati, OH 45219, USA (*retired*)

Steve Olin, ILSI Risk Science Institute, One Thomas Circle, NW, 9th Floor, Washington, DC 20005-5802, USA

Jørgen H. Olsen, Danish Cancer society, Institute of Cancer Epidemiology, Strandboulevarden 49, 2100 Copenhagen, Denmark (*Subgroup Chair, Cancer in Humans*)

Toby G. Rossman, Nelson Institute of Environmental Medicine, New York University School of Medicine, 57 Old Forge Road, Tuxedo, NY 10987, USA

Tadashi Sakai, Occupational Poisoning Center, Tokyo Rosai Hospital 13-21, Omorimi-nami-4, Ota-ku, Tokyo, 143-0013, Japan (*deceased*)

Xiaoming Shen, Research Center for Childhood Lead Poisoning Prevention, Shanghai Second Medical University, 1665 Kong Jiang Road, Shanghai 200092, People's Republic of China (*unable to attend*)

Tom Sorahan, Institute of Occupational and Environmental Medicine, University of Birmingham, University Road West, Edgbaston, Birmingham B15 2TT, United Kingdom

Kyle Steenland, Rollins School of Public Health, Department of Environmental and Occupational Health, Emory University, 1518 Clifton Road, Atlanta, GA 30322, USA

F. William Sunderman, Jr, Department of Laboratory Medicine, University of Connecticut Medical School, Farmington, CT, Department of Chemistry and Biochemistry, Middlebury College, Middlebury, VT 05753, USA (*retired*)

Tania M. Tavares, Laboratório de Química Analítica Ambiental, Instituto de Química, Universidade Federal da Bahia, R. Barão de Geremoabo n 147, 4o andar, s/405, Campus Universitário de Ondina, 40.170-290 Salvador, Bahia, Brazil

Rudra D. Tripathi, Ecotoxicology and Bioremediation Laboratory, National Botanical Research Institute, Rana Pratap Marg, Lucknow-226001 (UP), India

Michael P. Waalkes, Inorganic Carcinogenesis Section, Laboratory of Comparative Carcinogenesis, National Cancer Institute at the National Institute of Environmental Health Sciences, 111 Alexander Drive, P.O. Box 12233, MD F0-09 (South Campus (101/F095A), Research Triangle Park, NC 27709, USA (*Subgroup Chair, Cancer in Experimental Animals*)

Invited Specialist

Ted Junghans, Technical Resources International Inc., 6500 Rock Spring Drive, Suite 650, Bethesda, MD 20817-1197, USA

Representative

Representative of the US National Institute of Environmental Health Sciences

C. William Jameson, National Toxicology Program, National Institute of Environmental Health Sciences, 79 Alexander Drive, Research Triangle Park, NC 27709, USA

Observers

Observer for the International Lead Zinc Research Organization, Inc.[1]

Craig J. Boreiko, Manager, Environment and Health, International Lead Zinc Research Organization, P.O. Box 12036, Research Triangle Park, NC 27709-2036, USA

Observer for the Lead Development Association International[2]

Vagn Englyst, Rönnskär Smelter, Department of Occupational Health, 932 81 Skelleftehamn, Sweden

IARC Secretariat

Robert A. Baan, Carcinogen Identification and Evaluation (*Responsible Officer, Rapporteur, Subgroup on Other Relevant Data*)
Véronique Bouvard, Carcinogen Identification and Evaluation
Vincent J. Cogliano, Carcinogen Identification and Evaluation (*Head of Programme*)
Catherine Cohet, Carcinogen Identification and Evaluation
Fatiha El Ghissassi, Carcinogen Identification and Evaluation (*Co-Rapporteur, Subgroup on Other Relevant Data*)
Tony Fletcher, Visiting Scientist, Environmental Cancer Epidemiology
Marlin Friesen, Nutrition and Cancer
Yann Grosse, Carcinogen Identification and Evaluation (*Rapporteur, Subgroup on Cancer in Experimental Animals*)
Jay Hunt, Visiting Scientist, Environmental Cancer Epidemiology
Douglas McGregor, Carcinogen Identification and Evaluation
Dave McLean, Special Training Awardee, Radiation and Cancer
Garnett P. McMillan, Post-doctoral Fellow, Epidemiology for Cancer Prevention
Nikolai Napalkov, Carcinogen Identification and Evaluation
Béatrice Secretan, Carcinogen Identification and Evaluation (*Rapporteur, Subgroup on Exposure Data*)
Kurt Straif, Carcinogen Identification and Evaluation (*Rapporteur, Subgroup on Cancer in Humans*)
Olga Van der Hel, Post-doctoral Fellow, Environmental Cancer Epidemiology
Rosamund Williams (*Editor*)

Administrative assistance

Sandrine Egraz, Carcinogen Identification and Evaluation
Michel Javin, Administrative Services
Martine Lézère, Carcinogen Identification and Evaluation

---

[1]A non-profit research foundation for the purpose of conducting research on behalf of the international community of lead and zinc miners and smelters.

[2]Representative organization for the lead-producing and lead-using industries at the European and global levels.

Jane Mitchell, Carcinogen Identification and Evaluation
Georges Mollon, Communications
Elspeth Perez, Carcinogen Identification and Evaluation

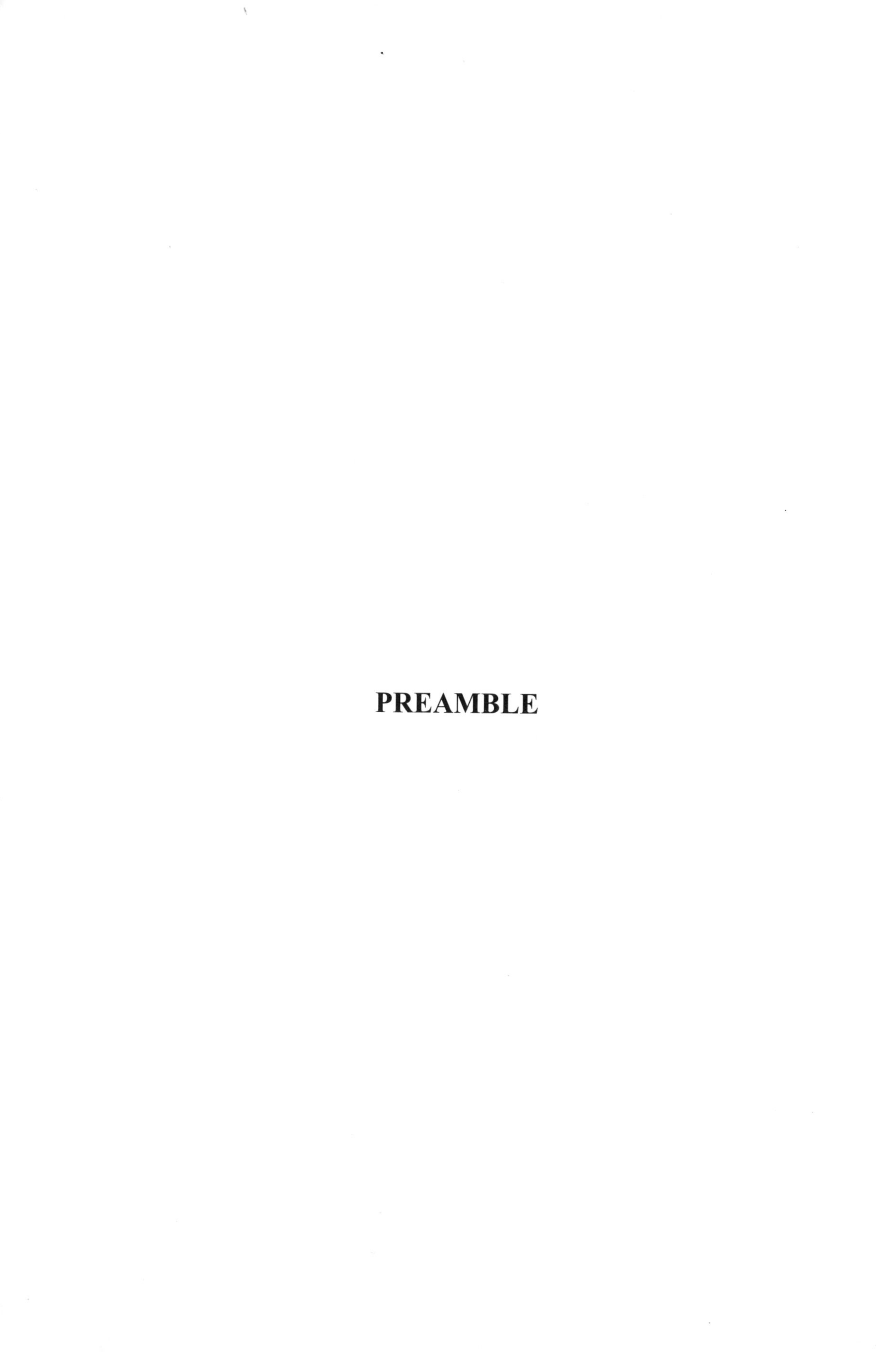

PREAMBLE

IARC MONOGRAPHS PROGRAMME ON THE EVALUATION OF CARCINOGENIC RISKS TO HUMANS

PREAMBLE

1. BACKGROUND

In 1969, the International Agency for Research on Cancer (IARC) initiated a programme to evaluate the carcinogenic risk of chemicals to humans and to produce monographs on individual chemicals. The *Monographs* programme has since been expanded to include consideration of exposures to complex mixtures of chemicals (which occur, for example, in some occupations and as a result of human habits) and of exposures to other agents, such as radiation and viruses. With Supplement 6 (IARC, 1987a), the title of the series was modified from *IARC Monographs on the Evaluation of the Carcinogenic Risk of Chemicals to Humans* to *IARC Monographs on the Evaluation of Carcinogenic Risks to Humans*, in order to reflect the widened scope of the programme.

The criteria established in 1971 to evaluate carcinogenic risk to humans were adopted by the working groups whose deliberations resulted in the first 16 volumes of the *IARC Monographs series*. Those criteria were subsequently updated by further ad-hoc working groups (IARC, 1977, 1978, 1979, 1982, 1983, 1987b, 1988, 1991a; Vainio *et al.*, 1992).

2. OBJECTIVE AND SCOPE

The objective of the programme is to prepare, with the help of international working groups of experts, and to publish in the form of monographs, critical reviews and evaluations of evidence on the carcinogenicity of a wide range of human exposures. The *Monographs* may also indicate where additional research efforts are needed.

The *Monographs* represent the first step in carcinogenic risk assessment, which involves examination of all relevant information in order to assess the strength of the available evidence that certain exposures could alter the incidence of cancer in humans. The second step is quantitative risk estimation. Detailed, quantitative evaluations of epidemiological data may be made in the *Monographs*, but without extrapolation beyond the range of the data available. Quantitative extrapolation from experimental data to the human situation is not undertaken.

The term 'carcinogen' is used in these monographs to denote an exposure that is capable of increasing the incidence of malignant neoplasms; the induction of benign neoplasms may in some circumstances (see p. 19) contribute to the judgement that the exposure is carcinogenic. The terms 'neoplasm' and 'tumour' are used interchangeably.

Some epidemiological and experimental studies indicate that different agents may act at different stages in the carcinogenic process, and several mechanisms may be involved. The aim of the *Monographs* has been, from their inception, to evaluate evidence of carcinogenicity at any stage in the carcinogenesis process, independently of the underlying mechanisms. Information on mechanisms may, however, be used in making the overall evaluation (IARC, 1991a; Vainio *et al.*, 1992; see also pp. 25–27).

The *Monographs* may assist national and international authorities in making risk assessments and in formulating decisions concerning any necessary preventive measures. The evaluations of IARC working groups are scientific, qualitative judgements about the evidence for or against carcinogenicity provided by the available data. These evaluations represent only one part of the body of information on which regulatory measures may be based. Other components of regulatory decisions vary from one situation to another and from country to country, responding to different socioeconomic and national priorities. **Therefore, no recommendation is given with regard to regulation or legislation, which are the responsibility of individual governments and/or other international organizations.**

The *IARC Monographs* are recognized as an authoritative source of information on the carcinogenicity of a wide range of human exposures. A survey of users in 1988 indicated that the *Monographs* are consulted by various agencies in 57 countries. About 2500 copies of each volume are printed, for distribution to governments, regulatory bodies and interested scientists. The Monographs are also available from IARC*Press* in Lyon and via the Marketing and Dissemination (MDI) of the World Health Organization in Geneva.

3. SELECTION OF TOPICS FOR MONOGRAPHS

Topics are selected on the basis of two main criteria: (a) there is evidence of human exposure, and (b) there is some evidence or suspicion of carcinogenicity. The term 'agent' is used to include individual chemical compounds, groups of related chemical compounds, physical agents (such as radiation) and biological factors (such as viruses). Exposures to mixtures of agents may occur in occupational exposures and as a result of personal and cultural habits (like smoking and dietary practices). Chemical analogues and compounds with biological or physical characteristics similar to those of suspected carcinogens may also be considered, even in the absence of data on a possible carcinogenic effect in humans or experimental animals.

The scientific literature is surveyed for published data relevant to an assessment of carcinogenicity. The IARC information bulletins on agents being tested for carcinogenicity (IARC, 1973–1996) and directories of on-going research in cancer epidemiology (IARC, 1976–1996) often indicate exposures that may be scheduled for future meetings. Ad-hoc working groups convened by IARC in 1984, 1989, 1991, 1993 and

1998 gave recommendations as to which agents should be evaluated in the IARC Monographs series (IARC, 1984, 1989, 1991b, 1993, 1998a,b).

As significant new data on subjects on which monographs have already been prepared become available, re-evaluations are made at subsequent meetings, and revised monographs are published.

4. DATA FOR MONOGRAPHS

The *Monographs* do not necessarily cite all the literature concerning the subject of an evaluation. Only those data considered by the Working Group to be relevant to making the evaluation are included.

With regard to biological and epidemiological data, only reports that have been published or accepted for publication in the openly available scientific literature are reviewed by the working groups. In certain instances, government agency reports that have undergone peer review and are widely available are considered. Exceptions may be made on an ad-hoc basis to include unpublished reports that are in their final form and publicly available, if their inclusion is considered pertinent to making a final evaluation (see pp. 25–27). In the sections on chemical and physical properties, on analysis, on production and use and on occurrence, unpublished sources of information may be used.

5. THE WORKING GROUP

Reviews and evaluations are formulated by a working group of experts. The tasks of the group are: (i) to ascertain that all appropriate data have been collected; (ii) to select the data relevant for the evaluation on the basis of scientific merit; (iii) to prepare accurate summaries of the data to enable the reader to follow the reasoning of the Working Group; (iv) to evaluate the results of epidemiological and experimental studies on cancer; (v) to evaluate data relevant to the understanding of mechanism of action; and (vi) to make an overall evaluation of the carcinogenicity of the exposure to humans.

Working Group participants who contributed to the considerations and evaluations within a particular volume are listed, with their addresses, at the beginning of each publication. Each participant who is a member of a working group serves as an individual scientist and not as a representative of any organization, government or industry. In addition, nominees of national and international agencies and industrial associations may be invited as observers.

6. WORKING PROCEDURES

Approximately one year in advance of a meeting of a working group, the topics of the monographs are announced and participants are selected by IARC staff in consultation with other experts. Subsequently, relevant biological and epidemiological data are collected by the Carcinogen Identification and Evaluation Unit of IARC from recognized sources of information on carcinogenesis, including data storage and retrieval systems such as MEDLINE and TOXLINE.

For chemicals and some complex mixtures, the major collection of data and the preparation of first drafts of the sections on chemical and physical properties, on analysis, on production and use and on occurrence are carried out under a separate contract funded by the United States National Cancer Institute. Representatives from industrial associations may assist in the preparation of sections on production and use. Information on production and trade is obtained from governmental and trade publications and, in some cases, by direct contact with industries. Separate production data on some agents may not be available because their publication could disclose confidential information. Information on uses may be obtained from published sources but is often complemented by direct contact with manufacturers. Efforts are made to supplement this information with data from other national and international sources.

Six months before the meeting, the material obtained is sent to meeting participants, or is used by IARC staff, to prepare sections for the first drafts of monographs. The first drafts are compiled by IARC staff and sent before the meeting to all participants of the Working Group for review.

The Working Group meets in Lyon for seven to eight days to discuss and finalize the texts of the monographs and to formulate the evaluations. After the meeting, the master copy of each monograph is verified by consulting the original literature, edited and prepared for publication. The aim is to publish monographs within six months of the Working Group meeting.

The available studies are summarized by the Working Group, with particular regard to the qualitative aspects discussed below. In general, numerical findings are indicated as they appear in the original report; units are converted when necessary for easier comparison. The Working Group may conduct additional analyses of the published data and use them in their assessment of the evidence; the results of such supplementary analyses are given in square brackets. When an important aspect of a study, directly impinging on its interpretation, should be brought to the attention of the reader, a comment is given in square brackets.

7. EXPOSURE DATA

Sections that indicate the extent of past and present human exposure, the sources of exposure, the people most likely to be exposed and the factors that contribute to the exposure are included at the beginning of each monograph.

Most monographs on individual chemicals, groups of chemicals or complex mixtures include sections on chemical and physical data, on analysis, on production and use and on occurrence. In monographs on, for example, physical agents, occupational exposures and cultural habits, other sections may be included, such as: historical perspectives, description of an industry or habit, chemistry of the complex mixture or taxonomy. Monographs on biological agents have sections on structure and biology, methods of detection, epidemiology of infection and clinical disease other than cancer.

For chemical exposures, the Chemical Abstracts Services Registry Number, the latest Chemical Abstracts primary name and the IUPAC systematic name are recorded; other synonyms are given, but the list is not necessarily comprehensive. For biological agents, taxonomy and structure are described, and the degree of variability is given, when applicable.

Information on chemical and physical properties and, in particular, data relevant to identification, occurrence and biological activity are included. For biological agents, mode of replication, life cycle, target cells, persistence and latency and host response are given. A description of technical products of chemicals includes trade names, relevant specifications and available information on composition and impurities. Some of the trade names given may be those of mixtures in which the agent being evaluated is only one of the ingredients.

The purpose of the section on analysis or detection is to give the reader an overview of current methods, with emphasis on those widely used for regulatory purposes. Methods for monitoring human exposure are also given, when available. No critical evaluation or recommendation of any of the methods is meant or implied. The IARC published a series of volumes, *Environmental Carcinogens: Methods of Analysis and Exposure Measurement* (IARC, 1978–93), that describe validated methods for analysing a wide variety of chemicals and mixtures. For biological agents, methods of detection and exposure assessment are described, including their sensitivity, specificity and reproducibility.

The dates of first synthesis and of first commercial production of a chemical or mixture are provided; for agents which do not occur naturally, this information may allow a reasonable estimate to be made of the date before which no human exposure to the agent could have occurred. The dates of first reported occurrence of an exposure are also provided. In addition, methods of synthesis used in past and present commercial production and different methods of production which may give rise to different impurities are described.

Data on production, international trade and uses are obtained for representative regions, which usually include Europe, Japan and the United States of America. It should not, however, be inferred that those areas or nations are necessarily the sole or major sources or users of the agent. Some identified uses may not be current or major applications, and the coverage is not necessarily comprehensive. In the case of drugs, mention of their therapeutic uses does not necessarily represent current practice, nor does it imply judgement as to their therapeutic efficacy.

Information on the occurrence of an agent or mixture in the environment is obtained from data derived from the monitoring and surveillance of levels in occupational environments, air, water, soil, foods and animal and human tissues. When available, data on the generation, persistence and bioaccumulation of the agent are also included. In the case of mixtures, industries, occupations or processes, information is given about all agents present. For processes, industries and occupations, a historical description is also given, noting variations in chemical composition, physical properties and levels of occupational exposure with time and place. For biological agents, the epidemiology of infection is described.

Statements concerning regulations and guidelines (e.g., pesticide registrations, maximal levels permitted in foods, occupational exposure limits) are included for some countries as indications of potential exposures, but they may not reflect the most recent situation, since such limits are continuously reviewed and modified. The absence of information on regulatory status for a country should not be taken to imply that that country does not have regulations with regard to the exposure. For biological agents, legislation and control, including vaccines and therapy, are described.

8. STUDIES OF CANCER IN HUMANS

(*a*) *Types of studies considered*

Three types of epidemiological studies of cancer contribute to the assessment of carcinogenicity in humans — cohort studies, case–control studies and correlation (or ecological) studies. Rarely, results from randomized trials may be available. Case series and case reports of cancer in humans may also be reviewed.

Cohort and case–control studies relate the exposures under study to the occurrence of cancer in individuals and provide an estimate of relative risk (ratio of incidence or mortality in those exposed to incidence or mortality in those not exposed) as the main measure of association.

In correlation studies, the units of investigation are usually whole populations (e.g. in particular geographical areas or at particular times), and cancer frequency is related to a summary measure of the exposure of the population to the agent, mixture or exposure circumstance under study. Because individual exposure is not documented, however, a causal relationship is less easy to infer from correlation studies than from cohort and case–control studies. Case reports generally arise from a suspicion, based on clinical experience, that the concurrence of two events — that is, a particular exposure and occurrence of a cancer — has happened rather more frequently than would be expected by chance. Case reports usually lack complete ascertainment of cases in any population, definition or enumeration of the population at risk and estimation of the expected number of cases in the absence of exposure. The uncertainties surrounding interpretation of case reports and correlation studies make them inadequate, except in rare instances, to form the sole basis for inferring a causal relationship. When taken together with case–control and cohort studies, however, relevant case reports or correlation studies may add materially to the judgement that a causal relationship is present.

Epidemiological studies of benign neoplasms, presumed preneoplastic lesions and other end-points thought to be relevant to cancer are also reviewed by working groups. They may, in some instances, strengthen inferences drawn from studies of cancer itself.

(*b*) *Quality of studies considered*

The Monographs are not intended to summarize all published studies. Those that are judged to be inadequate or irrelevant to the evaluation are generally omitted. They may be mentioned briefly, particularly when the information is considered to be a useful supplement to that in other reports or when they provide the only data available. Their inclusion does not imply acceptance of the adequacy of the study design or of the analysis and interpretation of the results, and limitations are clearly outlined in square brackets at the end of the study description.

It is necessary to take into account the possible roles of bias, confounding and chance in the interpretation of epidemiological studies. By 'bias' is meant the operation of factors in study design or execution that lead erroneously to a stronger or weaker association than in fact exists between disease and an agent, mixture or exposure circumstance. By 'confounding' is meant a situation in which the relationship with disease is made to appear stronger or weaker than it truly is as a result of an association between the apparent causal factor and another factor that is associated with either an increase or decrease in the incidence of the disease. In evaluating the extent to which these factors have been minimized in an individual study, working groups consider a number of aspects of design and analysis as described in the report of the study. Most of these considerations apply equally to case–control, cohort and correlation studies. Lack of clarity of any of these aspects in the reporting of a study can decrease its credibility and the weight given to it in the final evaluation of the exposure.

Firstly, the study population, disease (or diseases) and exposure should have been well defined by the authors. Cases of disease in the study population should have been identified in a way that was independent of the exposure of interest, and exposure should have been assessed in a way that was not related to disease status.

Secondly, the authors should have taken account in the study design and analysis of other variables that can influence the risk of disease and may have been related to the exposure of interest. Potential confounding by such variables should have been dealt with either in the design of the study, such as by matching, or in the analysis, by statistical adjustment. In cohort studies, comparisons with local rates of disease may be more appropriate than those with national rates. Internal comparisons of disease frequency among individuals at different levels of exposure should also have been made in the study.

Thirdly, the authors should have reported the basic data on which the conclusions are founded, even if sophisticated statistical analyses were employed. At the very least, they should have given the numbers of exposed and unexposed cases and controls in a case–control study and the numbers of cases observed and expected in a cohort study. Further tabulations by time since exposure began and other temporal factors are also important. In a cohort study, data on all cancer sites and all causes of death should have been given, to reveal the possibility of reporting bias. In a case–control study, the effects of investigated factors other than the exposure of interest should have been reported.

Finally, the statistical methods used to obtain estimates of relative risk, absolute rates of cancer, confidence intervals and significance tests, and to adjust for confounding should have been clearly stated by the authors. The methods used should preferably have been the generally accepted techniques that have been refined since the mid-1970s. These methods have been reviewed for case–control studies (Breslow & Day, 1980) and for cohort studies (Breslow & Day, 1987).

(*c*) *Inferences about mechanism of action*

Detailed analyses of both relative and absolute risks in relation to temporal variables, such as age at first exposure, time since first exposure, duration of exposure, cumulative exposure and time since exposure ceased, are reviewed and summarized when available. The analysis of temporal relationships can be useful in formulating models of carcinogenesis. In particular, such analyses may suggest whether a carcinogen acts early or late in the process of carcinogenesis, although at best they allow only indirect inferences about the mechanism of action. Special attention is given to measurements of biological markers of carcinogen exposure or action, such as DNA or protein adducts, as well as markers of early steps in the carcinogenic process, such as proto-oncogene mutation, when these are incorporated into epidemiological studies focused on cancer incidence or mortality. Such measurements may allow inferences to be made about putative mechanisms of action (IARC, 1991a; Vainio *et al.*, 1992).

(*d*) *Criteria for causality*

After the individual epidemiological studies of cancer have been summarized and the quality assessed, a judgement is made concerning the strength of evidence that the agent, mixture or exposure circumstance in question is carcinogenic for humans. In making its judgement, the Working Group considers several criteria for causality. A strong association (a large relative risk) is more likely to indicate causality than a weak association, although it is recognized that relative risks of small magnitude do not imply lack of causality and may be important if the disease is common. Associations that are replicated in several studies of the same design or using different epidemiological approaches or under different circumstances of exposure are more likely to represent a causal relationship than isolated observations from single studies. If there are inconsistent results among investigations, possible reasons are sought (such as differences in amount of exposure), and results of studies judged to be of high quality are given more weight than those of studies judged to be methodologically less sound. When suspicion of carcinogenicity arises largely from a single study, these data are not combined with those from later studies in any subsequent reassessment of the strength of the evidence.

If the risk of the disease in question increases with the amount of exposure, this is considered to be a strong indication of causality, although absence of a graded response is not necessarily evidence against a causal relationship. Demonstration of a decline in risk after cessation of or reduction in exposure in individuals or in whole populations also supports a causal interpretation of the findings.

Although a carcinogen may act upon more than one target, the specificity of an association (an increased occurrence of cancer at one anatomical site or of one morphological type) adds plausibility to a causal relationship, particularly when excess cancer occurrence is limited to one morphological type within the same organ.

Although rarely available, results from randomized trials showing different rates among exposed and unexposed individuals provide particularly strong evidence for causality.

When several epidemiological studies show little or no indication of an association between an exposure and cancer, the judgement may be made that, in the aggregate, they show evidence of lack of carcinogenicity. Such a judgement requires first of all that the studies giving rise to it meet, to a sufficient degree, the standards of design and analysis described above. Specifically, the possibility that bias, confounding or misclassification of exposure or outcome could explain the observed results should be considered and excluded with reasonable certainty. In addition, all studies that are judged to be methodologically sound should be consistent with a relative risk of unity for any observed level of exposure and, when considered together, should provide a pooled estimate of relative risk which is at or near unity and has a narrow confidence interval, due to sufficient population size. Moreover, no individual study nor the pooled results of all the studies should show any consistent tendency for the relative risk of cancer to increase with increasing level of exposure. It is important to note that evidence of lack of carcinogenicity obtained in this way from several epidemiological studies can apply only to the type(s) of cancer studied and to dose levels and intervals between first exposure and observation of disease that are the same as or less than those observed in all the studies. Experience with human cancer indicates that, in some cases, the period from first exposure to the development of clinical cancer is seldom less than 20 years; studies with latent periods substantially shorter than 30 years cannot provide evidence for lack of carcinogenicity.

9. STUDIES OF CANCER IN EXPERIMENTAL ANIMALS

All known human carcinogens that have been studied adequately in experimental animals have produced positive results in one or more animal species (Wilbourn *et al.*, 1986; Tomatis *et al.*, 1989). For several agents (aflatoxins, 4-aminobiphenyl, azathioprine, betel quid with tobacco, bischloromethyl ether and chloromethyl methyl ether (technical grade), chlorambucil, chlornaphazine, ciclosporin, coal-tar pitches, coal-tars, combined oral contraceptives, cyclophosphamide, diethylstilboestrol, melphalan, 8-methoxypsoralen plus ultraviolet A radiation, mustard gas, myleran, 2-naphthylamine, nonsteroidal estrogens, estrogen replacement therapy/steroidal estrogens, solar radiation, thiotepa and vinyl chloride), carcinogenicity in experimental animals was established or highly suspected before epidemiological studies confirmed their carcinogenicity in humans (Vainio *et al.*, 1995). Although this association cannot establish that all agents and mixtures that cause cancer in experimental animals also cause cancer in humans, nevertheless, **in the absence of adequate data on humans, it is biologically plausible and prudent to regard agents and mixtures for which there is *sufficient evidence* (see p. 24) of carcinogenicity in experimental animals as if they presented a carcinogenic risk to humans**. The possibility that a given agent may cause cancer through a species-specific mechanism which does not operate in humans (see p. 27) should also be taken into consideration.

The nature and extent of impurities or contaminants present in the chemical or mixture being evaluated are given when available. Animal strain, sex, numbers per group, age at start of treatment and survival are reported.

Other types of studies summarized include: experiments in which the agent or mixture was administered in conjunction with known carcinogens or factors that modify carcinogenic effects; studies in which the end-point was not cancer but a defined precancerous lesion; and experiments on the carcinogenicity of known metabolites and derivatives.

For experimental studies of mixtures, consideration is given to the possibility of changes in the physicochemical properties of the test substance during collection, storage, extraction, concentration and delivery. Chemical and toxicological interactions of the components of mixtures may result in nonlinear dose–response relationships.

An assessment is made as to the relevance to human exposure of samples tested in experimental animals, which may involve consideration of: (i) physical and chemical characteristics, (ii) constituent substances that indicate the presence of a class of substances, (iii) the results of tests for genetic and related effects, including studies on DNA adduct formation, proto-oncogene mutation and expression and suppressor gene inactivation. The relevance of results obtained, for example, with animal viruses analogous to the virus being evaluated in the monograph must also be considered. They may provide biological and mechanistic information relevant to the understanding of the process of carcinogenesis in humans and may strengthen the plausibility of a conclusion that the biological agent under evaluation is carcinogenic in humans.

(*a*) *Qualitative aspects*

An assessment of carcinogenicity involves several considerations of qualitative importance, including (i) the experimental conditions under which the test was performed, including route and schedule of exposure, species, strain, sex, age, duration of follow-up; (ii) the consistency of the results, for example, across species and target organ(s); (iii) the spectrum of neoplastic response, from preneoplastic lesions and benign tumours to malignant neoplasms; and (iv) the possible role of modifying factors.

As mentioned earlier (p. 11), the *Monographs* are not intended to summarize all published studies. Those studies in experimental animals that are inadequate (e.g., too short a duration, too few animals, poor survival; see below) or are judged irrelevant to the evaluation are generally omitted. Guidelines for conducting adequate long-term carcinogenicity experiments have been outlined (e.g. Montesano *et al.*, 1986).

Considerations of importance to the Working Group in the interpretation and evaluation of a particular study include: (i) how clearly the agent was defined and, in the case of mixtures, how adequately the sample characterization was reported; (ii) whether the dose was adequately monitored, particularly in inhalation experiments; (iii) whether the doses and duration of treatment were appropriate and whether the survival of treated animals was similar to that of controls; (iv) whether there were adequate numbers of animals per group; (v) whether animals of each sex were used; (vi) whether animals were allocated randomly to groups; (vii) whether the duration of observation was adequate; and (viii) whether the data were adequately reported. If available, recent data on the incidence of specific tumours in historical controls, as well as in concurrent controls, should be taken into account in the evaluation of tumour response.

When benign tumours occur together with and originate from the same cell type in an organ or tissue as malignant tumours in a particular study and appear to represent a stage in the progression to malignancy, it may be valid to combine them in assessing tumour incidence (Huff *et al.*, 1989). The occurrence of lesions presumed to be preneoplastic may in certain instances aid in assessing the biological plausibility of any neoplastic response observed. If an agent or mixture induces only benign neoplasms that appear to be end-points that do not readily progress to malignancy, it should nevertheless be suspected of being a carcinogen and requires further investigation.

(*b*) *Quantitative aspects*

The probability that tumours will occur may depend on the species, sex, strain and age of the animal, the dose of the carcinogen and the route and length of exposure. Evidence of an increased incidence of neoplasms with increased level of exposure strengthens the inference of a causal association between the exposure and the development of neoplasms.

The form of the dose–response relationship can vary widely, depending on the particular agent under study and the target organ. Both DNA damage and increased cell division are important aspects of carcinogenesis, and cell proliferation is a strong determinant of dose–response relationships for some carcinogens (Cohen & Ellwein, 1990). Since many chemicals require metabolic activation before being converted into their reactive intermediates, both metabolic and pharmacokinetic aspects are important in determining the dose–response pattern. Saturation of steps such as absorption, activation, inactivation and elimination may produce nonlinearity in the dose–response relationship, as could saturation of processes such as DNA repair (Hoel *et al.*, 1983; Gart *et al.*, 1986).

(c) *Statistical analysis of long-term experiments in animals*

Factors considered by the Working Group include the adequacy of the information given for each treatment group: (i) the number of animals studied and the number examined histologically, (ii) the number of animals with a given tumour type and (iii) length of survival. The statistical methods used should be clearly stated and should be the generally accepted techniques refined for this purpose (Peto *et al.*, 1980; Gart *et al.*, 1986). When there is no difference in survival between control and treatment groups, the Working Group usually compares the proportions of animals developing each tumour type in each of the groups. Otherwise, consideration is given as to whether or not appropriate adjustments have been made for differences in survival. These adjustments can include: comparisons of the proportions of tumour-bearing animals among the effective number of animals (alive at the time the first tumour is discovered), in the case where most differences in survival occur before tumours appear; life-table methods, when tumours are visible or when they may be considered 'fatal' because mortality rapidly follows tumour development; and the Mantel-Haenszel test or logistic regression, when occult tumours do not affect the animals' risk of dying but are 'incidental' findings at autopsy.

In practice, classifying tumours as fatal or incidental may be difficult. Several survival-adjusted methods have been developed that do not require this distinction (Gart *et al.*, 1986), although they have not been fully evaluated.

10. OTHER DATA RELEVANT TO AN EVALUATION OF CARCINOGENICITY AND ITS MECHANISMS

In coming to an overall evaluation of carcinogenicity in humans (see pp. 25–27), the Working Group also considers related data. The nature of the information selected for the summary depends on the agent being considered.

For chemicals and complex mixtures of chemicals such as those in some occupational situations or involving cultural habits (e.g. tobacco smoking), the other data considered to be relevant are divided into those on absorption, distribution, metabolism and excretion; toxic effects; reproductive and developmental effects; and genetic and related effects.

Concise information is given on absorption, distribution (including placental transfer) and excretion in both humans and experimental animals. Kinetic factors that may affect the dose–response relationship, such as saturation of uptake, protein binding, metabolic activation, detoxification and DNA repair processes, are mentioned. Studies that indicate the metabolic fate of the agent in humans and in experimental animals are summarized briefly, and comparisons of data on humans and on animals are made when possible. Comparative information on the relationship between exposure and the dose that reaches the target site may be of particular importance for extrapolation between species. Data are given on acute and chronic toxic effects (other than cancer), such as organ toxicity, increased cell proliferation, immunotoxicity and endocrine effects. The presence and toxicological significance of cellular receptors is described. Effects on reproduction, teratogenicity, fetotoxicity and embryotoxicity are also summarized briefly.

Tests of genetic and related effects are described in view of the relevance of gene mutation and chromosomal damage to carcinogenesis (Vainio *et al.*, 1992; McGregor *et al.*, 1999). The adequacy of the reporting of sample characterization is considered and, where necessary, commented upon; with regard to complex mixtures, such comments are similar to those described for animal carcinogenicity tests on p. 18. The available data are interpreted critically by phylogenetic group according to the end-points detected, which may include DNA damage, gene mutation, sister chromatid exchange, micronucleus formation, chromosomal aberrations, aneuploidy and cell transformation. The concentrations employed are given, and mention is made of whether use of an exogenous metabolic system *in vitro* affected the test result. These data are given as listings of test systems, data and references. The data on genetic and related effects presented in the *Monographs* are also available in the form of genetic activity profiles (GAP) prepared in collaboration with the United States Environmental Protection Agency (EPA) (see also Waters *et al.*, 1987) using software for personal computers that are Microsoft Windows® compatible. The EPA/IARC GAP software and database may be downloaded free of charge from *www.epa.gov/gapdb.*

Positive results in tests using prokaryotes, lower eukaryotes, plants, insects and cultured mammalian cells suggest that genetic and related effects could occur in mammals. Results from such tests may also give information about the types of genetic effect produced and about the involvement of metabolic activation. Some end-points described are clearly genetic in nature (e.g., gene mutations and chromosomal aberrations), while others are to a greater or lesser degree associated with genetic effects (e.g. unscheduled DNA synthesis). In-vitro tests for tumour-promoting activity and for cell transformation may be sensitive to changes that are not necessarily the result of genetic alterations but that may have specific relevance to the process of carcinogenesis. A critical appraisal of these tests has been published (Montesano *et al.*, 1986).

Genetic or other activity detected in experimental mammals and humans is regarded as being of greater relevance than that in other organisms. The demonstration that an agent or mixture can induce gene and chromosomal mutations in whole mammals indicates that it may have carcinogenic activity, although this activity may not be detectably expressed in any or all species. Relative potency in tests for mutagenicity and related effects is not a reliable indicator of carcinogenic potency. Negative results in tests for mutagenicity in selected tissues from animals treated *in vivo* provide less weight, partly because they do not exclude the possibility of an effect in tissues other than those examined. Moreover, negative results in short-term tests with genetic end-points cannot be considered to provide evidence to rule out carcinogenicity of agents or mixtures that act through other mechanisms (e.g. receptor-mediated effects, cellular toxicity with regenerative proliferation, peroxisome proliferation) (Vainio *et al.*, 1992). Factors that may lead to misleading results in short-term tests have been discussed in detail elsewhere (Montesano *et al.*, 1986).

When available, data relevant to mechanisms of carcinogenesis that do not involve structural changes at the level of the gene are also described.

The adequacy of epidemiological studies of reproductive outcome and genetic and related effects in humans is evaluated by the same criteria as are applied to epidemiological studies of cancer.

Structure–activity relationships that may be relevant to an evaluation of the carcinogenicity of an agent are also described.

For biological agents — viruses, bacteria and parasites — other data relevant to carcinogenicity include descriptions of the pathology of infection, molecular biology (integration and expression of viruses, and any genetic alterations seen in human tumours) and other observations, which might include cellular and tissue responses to infection, immune response and the presence of tumour markers.

11. SUMMARY OF DATA REPORTED

In this section, the relevant epidemiological and experimental data are summarized. Only reports, other than in abstract form, that meet the criteria outlined on p. 11 are considered for evaluating carcinogenicity. Inadequate studies are generally not summarized: such studies are usually identified by a square-bracketed comment in the preceding text.

(*a*) *Exposure*

Human exposure to chemicals and complex mixtures is summarized on the basis of elements such as production, use, occurrence in the environment and determinations in human tissues and body fluids. Quantitative data are given when available. Exposure to biological agents is described in terms of transmission and prevalence of infection.

(*b*) *Carcinogenicity in humans*

Results of epidemiological studies that are considered to be pertinent to an assessment of human carcinogenicity are summarized. When relevant, case reports and correlation studies are also summarized.

(*c*) *Carcinogenicity in experimental animals*

Data relevant to an evaluation of carcinogenicity in animals are summarized. For each animal species and route of administration, it is stated whether an increased incidence of neoplasms or preneoplastic lesions was observed, and the tumour sites are indicated. If the agent or mixture produced tumours after prenatal exposure or in single-dose experiments, this is also indicated. Negative findings are also summarized. Dose–response and other quantitative data may be given when available.

(*d*) *Other data relevant to an evaluation of carcinogenicity and its mechanisms*

Data on biological effects in humans that are of particular relevance are summarized. These may include toxicological, kinetic and metabolic considerations and evidence of DNA binding, persistence of DNA lesions or genetic damage in exposed humans. Toxicological information, such as that on cytotoxicity and regeneration, receptor binding and hormonal and immunological effects, and data on kinetics and metabolism in experimental animals are given when considered relevant to the possible mechanism of the carcinogenic action of the agent. The results of tests for genetic and related effects are summarized for whole mammals, cultured mammalian cells and nonmammalian systems.

When available, comparisons of such data for humans and for animals, and particularly animals that have developed cancer, are described.

Structure–activity relationships are mentioned when relevant.

For the agent, mixture or exposure circumstance being evaluated, the available data on end-points or other phenomena relevant to mechanisms of carcinogenesis from studies in humans, experimental animals and tissue and cell test systems are summarized within one or more of the following descriptive dimensions:

(i) Evidence of genotoxicity (structural changes at the level of the gene): for example, structure–activity considerations, adduct formation, mutagenicity (effect on specific genes), chromosomal mutation/aneuploidy

(ii) Evidence of effects on the expression of relevant genes (functional changes at the intracellular level): for example, alterations to the structure or quantity of the product of a proto-oncogene or tumour-suppressor gene, alterations to metabolic activation/inactivation/DNA repair

(iii) Evidence of relevant effects on cell behaviour (morphological or behavioural changes at the cellular or tissue level): for example, induction of mitogenesis, compensatory cell proliferation, preneoplasia and hyperplasia, survival of premalignant or malignant cells (immortalization, immunosuppression), effects on metastatic potential

(iv) Evidence from dose and time relationships of carcinogenic effects and interactions between agents: for example, early/late stage, as inferred from epidemiological studies; initiation/promotion/progression/malignant conversion, as defined in animal carcinogenicity experiments; toxicokinetics

These dimensions are not mutually exclusive, and an agent may fall within more than one of them. Thus, for example, the action of an agent on the expression of relevant genes could be summarized under both the first and second dimensions, even if it were known with reasonable certainty that those effects resulted from genotoxicity.

12. EVALUATION

Evaluations of the strength of the evidence for carcinogenicity arising from human and experimental animal data are made, using standard terms.

It is recognized that the criteria for these evaluations, described below, cannot encompass all of the factors that may be relevant to an evaluation of carcinogenicity. In considering all of the relevant scientific data, the Working Group may assign the agent, mixture or exposure circumstance to a higher or lower category than a strict interpretation of these criteria would indicate.

(*a*) *Degrees of evidence for carcinogenicity in humans and in experimental animals and supporting evidence*

These categories refer only to the strength of the evidence that an exposure is carcinogenic and not to the extent of its carcinogenic activity (potency) nor to the mechanisms involved. A classification may change as new information becomes available.

An evaluation of degree of evidence, whether for a single agent or a mixture, is limited to the materials tested, as defined physically, chemically or biologically. When the agents evaluated are considered by the Working Group to be sufficiently closely related, they may be grouped together for the purpose of a single evaluation of degree of evidence.

(i) *Carcinogenicity in humans*

The applicability of an evaluation of the carcinogenicity of a mixture, process, occupation or industry on the basis of evidence from epidemiological studies depends on the variability over time and place of the mixtures, processes, occupations and industries. The Working Group seeks to identify the specific exposure, process or activity which is considered most likely to be responsible for any excess risk. The evaluation is focused as narrowly as the available data on exposure and other aspects permit.

The evidence relevant to carcinogenicity from studies in humans is classified into one of the following categories:

Sufficient evidence of carcinogenicity: The Working Group considers that a causal relationship has been established between exposure to the agent, mixture or exposure circumstance and human cancer. That is, a positive relationship has been observed between the exposure and cancer in studies in which chance, bias and confounding could be ruled out with reasonable confidence.

Limited evidence of carcinogenicity: A positive association has been observed between exposure to the agent, mixture or exposure circumstance and cancer for which a causal interpretation is considered by the Working Group to be credible, but chance, bias or confounding could not be ruled out with reasonable confidence.

Inadequate evidence of carcinogenicity: The available studies are of insufficient quality, consistency or statistical power to permit a conclusion regarding the presence or absence of a causal association between exposure and cancer, or no data on cancer in humans are available.

Evidence suggesting lack of carcinogenicity: There are several adequate studies covering the full range of levels of exposure that human beings are known to encounter, which are mutually consistent in not showing a positive association between exposure to the agent, mixture or exposure circumstance and any studied cancer at any observed level of exposure. A conclusion of 'evidence suggesting lack of carcinogenicity' is inevitably limited to the cancer sites, conditions and levels of exposure and length of observation covered by the available studies. In addition, the possibility of a very small risk at the levels of exposure studied can never be excluded.

In some instances, the above categories may be used to classify the degree of evidence related to carcinogenicity in specific organs or tissues.

(ii) *Carcinogenicity in experimental animals*

The evidence relevant to carcinogenicity in experimental animals is classified into one of the following categories:

Sufficient evidence of carcinogenicity: The Working Group considers that a causal relationship has been established between the agent or mixture and an increased incidence of malignant neoplasms or of an appropriate combination of benign and malignant neoplasms in (a) two or more species of animals or (b) in two or more independent studies in one species carried out at different times or in different laboratories or under different protocols.

Exceptionally, a single study in one species might be considered to provide sufficient evidence of carcinogenicity when malignant neoplasms occur to an unusual degree with regard to incidence, site, type of tumour or age at onset.

Limited evidence of carcinogenicity: The data suggest a carcinogenic effect but are limited for making a definitive evaluation because, e.g. (a) the evidence of carcinogenicity is restricted to a single experiment; or (b) there are unresolved questions regarding the adequacy of the design, conduct or interpretation of the study; or (c) the agent or mixture increases the incidence only of benign neoplasms or lesions of uncertain neoplastic potential, or of certain neoplasms which may occur spontaneously in high incidences in certain strains.

Inadequate evidence of carcinogenicity: The studies cannot be interpreted as showing either the presence or absence of a carcinogenic effect because of major qualitative or quantitative limitations, or no data on cancer in experimental animals are available.

Evidence suggesting lack of carcinogenicity: Adequate studies involving at least two species are available which show that, within the limits of the tests used, the agent or mixture is not carcinogenic. A conclusion of evidence suggesting lack of carcinogenicity is inevitably limited to the species, tumour sites and levels of exposure studied.

(*b*) *Other data relevant to the evaluation of carcinogenicity and its mechanisms*

Other evidence judged to be relevant to an evaluation of carcinogenicity and of sufficient importance to affect the overall evaluation is then described. This may include data on preneoplastic lesions, tumour pathology, genetic and related effects, structure–activity relationships, metabolism and pharmacokinetics, physicochemical parameters and analogous biological agents.

Data relevant to mechanisms of the carcinogenic action are also evaluated. The strength of the evidence that any carcinogenic effect observed is due to a particular mechanism is assessed, using terms such as weak, moderate or strong. Then, the Working Group assesses if that particular mechanism is likely to be operative in humans. The strongest indications that a particular mechanism operates in humans come from data on humans or biological specimens obtained from exposed humans. The data may be considered to be especially relevant if they show that the agent in question has caused changes in exposed humans that are on the causal pathway to carcinogenesis. Such data may, however, never become available, because it is at least conceivable that certain compounds may be kept from human use solely on the basis of evidence of their toxicity and/or carcinogenicity in experimental systems.

For complex exposures, including occupational and industrial exposures, the chemical composition and the potential contribution of carcinogens known to be present are considered by the Working Group in its overall evaluation of human carcinogenicity. The Working Group also determines the extent to which the materials tested in experimental systems are related to those to which humans are exposed.

(*c*) *Overall evaluation*

Finally, the body of evidence is considered as a whole, in order to reach an overall evaluation of the carcinogenicity to humans of an agent, mixture or circumstance of exposure.

An evaluation may be made for a group of chemical compounds that have been evaluated by the Working Group. In addition, when supporting data indicate that other, related compounds for which there is no direct evidence of capacity to induce cancer in humans or in animals may also be carcinogenic, a statement describing the rationale for this conclusion is added to the evaluation narrative; an additional evaluation may be made for this broader group of compounds if the strength of the evidence warrants it.

The agent, mixture or exposure circumstance is described according to the wording of one of the following categories, and the designated group is given. The categorization of an agent, mixture or exposure circumstance is a matter of scientific judgement, reflecting the strength of the evidence derived from studies in humans and in experimental animals and from other relevant data.

Group 1 — The agent (mixture) is carcinogenic to humans.
The exposure circumstance entails exposures that are carcinogenic to humans.

This category is used when there is *sufficient evidence* of carcinogenicity in humans. Exceptionally, an agent (mixture) may be placed in this category when evidence of carcinogenicity in humans is less than sufficient but there is *sufficient evidence* of carcinogenicity in experimental animals and strong evidence in exposed humans that the agent (mixture) acts through a relevant mechanism of carcinogenicity.

Group 2

This category includes agents, mixtures and exposure circumstances for which, at one extreme, the degree of evidence of carcinogenicity in humans is almost sufficient, as well as those for which, at the other extreme, there are no human data but for which there is evidence of carcinogenicity in experimental animals. Agents, mixtures and exposure circumstances are assigned to either group 2A (probably carcinogenic to humans) or group 2B (possibly carcinogenic to humans) on the basis of epidemiological and experimental evidence of carcinogenicity and other relevant data.

Group 2A — The agent (mixture) is probably carcinogenic to humans.
The exposure circumstance entails exposures that are probably carcinogenic to humans.

This category is used when there is *limited evidence* of carcinogenicity in humans and *sufficient evidence* of carcinogenicity in experimental animals. In some cases, an agent (mixture) may be classified in this category when there is *inadequate evidence* of carcinogenicity in humans, *sufficient evidence* of carcinogenicity in experimental animals and strong evidence that the carcinogenesis is mediated by a mechanism that also operates in humans. Exceptionally, an agent, mixture or exposure circumstance may be classified in this category solely on the basis of *limited evidence* of carcinogenicity in humans.

Group 2B — The agent (mixture) is possibly carcinogenic to humans.
The exposure circumstance entails exposures that are possibly carcinogenic to humans.

This category is used for agents, mixtures and exposure circumstances for which there is *limited evidence* of carcinogenicity in humans and less than *sufficient evidence* of carcinogenicity in experimental animals. It may also be used when there is *inadequate evidence* of carcinogenicity in humans but there is *sufficient evidence* of carcinogenicity in experimental animals. In some instances, an agent, mixture or exposure circumstance for which there is *inadequate evidence* of carcinogenicity in humans but *limited evidence* of carcinogenicity in experimental animals together with supporting evidence from other relevant data may be placed in this group.

Group 3 — The agent (mixture or exposure circumstance) is not classifiable as to its carcinogenicity to humans.

This category is used most commonly for agents, mixtures and exposure circumstances for which the *evidence of carcinogenicity* is *inadequate* in humans and *inadequate* or *limited* in experimental animals.

Exceptionally, agents (mixtures) for which the *evidence of carcinogenicity* is *inadequate* in humans but *sufficient* in experimental animals may be placed in this category when there is strong evidence that the mechanism of carcinogenicity in experimental animals does not operate in humans.

Agents, mixtures and exposure circumstances that do not fall into any other group are also placed in this category.

Group 4 — The agent (mixture) is probably not carcinogenic to humans.

This category is used for agents or mixtures for which there is *evidence suggesting lack of carcinogenicity* in humans and in experimental animals. In some instances, agents or mixtures for which there is *inadequate evidence* of carcinogenicity in humans but *evidence suggesting lack of carcinogenicity* in experimental animals, consistently and strongly supported by a broad range of other relevant data, may be classified in this group.

13. REFERENCES

Breslow, N.E. & Day, N.E. (1980) *Statistical Methods in Cancer Research*, Vol. 1, *The Analysis of Case–Control Studies* (IARC Scientific Publications No. 32), Lyon, IARC*Press*

Breslow, N.E. & Day, N.E. (1987) *Statistical Methods in Cancer Research*, Vol. 2, *The Design and Analysis of Cohort Studies* (IARC Scientific Publications No. 82), Lyon, IARC*Press*

Cohen, S.M. & Ellwein, L.B. (1990) Cell proliferation in carcinogenesis. *Science*, **249**, 1007–1011

Gart, J.J., Krewski, D., Lee, P.N., Tarone, R.E. & Wahrendorf, J. (1986) *Statistical Methods in Cancer Research*, Vol. 3, *The Design and Analysis of Long-term Animal Experiments* (IARC Scientific Publications No. 79), Lyon, IARC*Press*

Hoel, D.G., Kaplan, N.L. & Anderson, M.W. (1983) Implication of nonlinear kinetics on risk estimation in carcinogenesis. *Science*, **219**, 1032–1037

Huff, J.E., Eustis, S.L. & Haseman, J.K. (1989) Occurrence and relevance of chemically induced benign neoplasms in long-term carcinogenicity studies. *Cancer Metastasis Rev.*, **8**, 1–21

IARC (1973–1996) *Information Bulletin on the Survey of Chemicals Being Tested for Carcinogenicity/Directory of Agents Being Tested for Carcinogenicity*, Numbers 1–17, Lyon, IARC*Press*

IARC (1976–1996), Lyon, IARC*Press*

Directory of On-going Research in Cancer Epidemiology 1976. Edited by C.S. Muir & G. Wagner

Directory of On-going Research in Cancer Epidemiology 1977 (IARC Scientific Publications No. 17). Edited by C.S. Muir & G. Wagner

Directory of On-going Research in Cancer Epidemiology 1978 (IARC Scientific Publications No. 26). Edited by C.S. Muir & G. Wagner

Directory of On-going Research in Cancer Epidemiology 1979 (IARC Scientific Publications No. 28). Edited by C.S. Muir & G. Wagner

Directory of On-going Research in Cancer Epidemiology 1980 (IARC Scientific Publications No. 35). Edited by C.S. Muir & G. Wagner

Directory of On-going Research in Cancer Epidemiology 1981 (IARC Scientific Publications No. 38). Edited by C.S. Muir & G. Wagner

Directory of On-going Research in Cancer Epidemiology 1982 (IARC Scientific Publications No. 46). Edited by C.S. Muir & G. Wagner
Directory of On-going Research in Cancer Epidemiology 1983 (IARC Scientific Publications No. 50). Edited by C.S. Muir & G. Wagner
Directory of On-going Research in Cancer Epidemiology 1984 (IARC Scientific Publications No. 62). Edited by C.S. Muir & G. Wagner
Directory of On-going Research in Cancer Epidemiology 1985 (IARC Scientific Publications No. 69). Edited by C.S. Muir & G. Wagner
Directory of On-going Research in Cancer Epidemiology 1986 (IARC Scientific Publications No. 80). Edited by C.S. Muir & G. Wagner
Directory of On-going Research in Cancer Epidemiology 1987 (IARC Scientific Publications No. 86). Edited by D.M. Parkin & J. Wahrendorf
Directory of On-going Research in Cancer Epidemiology 1988 (IARC Scientific Publications No. 93). Edited by M. Coleman & J. Wahrendorf
Directory of On-going Research in Cancer Epidemiology 1989/90 (IARC Scientific Publications No. 101). Edited by M. Coleman & J. Wahrendorf
Directory of On-going Research in Cancer Epidemiology 1991 (IARC Scientific Publications No.110). Edited by M. Coleman & J. Wahrendorf
Directory of On-going Research in Cancer Epidemiology 1992 (IARC Scientific Publications No. 117). Edited by M. Coleman, J. Wahrendorf & E. Démaret
Directory of On-going Research in Cancer Epidemiology 1994 (IARC Scientific Publications No. 130). Edited by R. Sankaranarayanan, J. Wahrendorf & E. Démaret
Directory of On-going Research in Cancer Epidemiology 1996 (IARC Scientific Publications No. 137). Edited by R. Sankaranarayanan, J. Wahrendorf & E. Démaret

IARC (1977) *IARC Monographs Programme on the Evaluation of the Carcinogenic Risk of Chemicals to Humans*. Preamble (IARC intern. tech. Rep. No. 77/002)

IARC (1978) *Chemicals with* Sufficient Evidence *of Carcinogenicity in Experimental Animals* — IARC Monographs *Volumes 1–17* (IARC intern. tech. Rep. No. 78/003)

IARC (1978–1993) *Environmental Carcinogens. Methods of Analysis and Exposure Measurement*, Lyon, IARC*Press*
Vol. 1. Analysis of Volatile Nitrosamines in Food (IARC Scientific Publications No. 18). Edited by R. Preussmann, M. Castegnaro, E.A. Walker & A.E. Wasserman (1978)
Vol. 2. Methods for the Measurement of Vinyl Chloride in Poly(vinyl chloride), Air, Water and Foodstuffs (IARC Scientific Publications No. 22). Edited by D.C.M. Squirrell & W. Thain (1978)
Vol. 3. Analysis of Polycyclic Aromatic Hydrocarbons in Environmental Samples (IARC Scientific Publications No. 29). Edited by M. Castegnaro, P. Bogovski, H. Kunte & E.A. Walker (1979)
Vol. 4. Some Aromatic Amines and Azo Dyes in the General and Industrial Environment (IARC Scientific Publications No. 40). Edited by L. Fishbein, M. Castegnaro, I.K. O'Neill & H. Bartsch (1981)
Vol. 5. Some Mycotoxins (IARC Scientific Publications No. 44). Edited by L. Stoloff, M. Castegnaro, P. Scott, I.K. O'Neill & H. Bartsch (1983)
Vol. 6. N-Nitroso Compounds (IARC Scientific Publications No. 45). Edited by R. Preussmann, I.K. O'Neill, G. Eisenbrand, B. Spiegelhalder & H. Bartsch (1983)

Vol. 7. Some Volatile Halogenated Hydrocarbons (IARC Scientific Publications No. 68). Edited by L. Fishbein & I.K. O'Neill (1985)

Vol. 8. Some Metals: As, Be, Cd, Cr, Ni, Pb, Se, Zn (IARC Scientific Publications No. 71). Edited by I.K. O'Neill, P. Schuller & L. Fishbein (1986)

Vol. 9. Passive Smoking (IARC Scientific Publications No. 81). Edited by I.K. O'Neill, K.D. Brunnemann, B. Dodet & D. Hoffmann (1987)

*Vol. 10. Benzene and Alkylated Benzenes (*IARC Scientific Publications No. 85). Edited by L. Fishbein & I.K. O'Neill (1988)

Vol. 11. Polychlorinated Dioxins and Dibenzofurans (IARC Scientific Publications No. 108). Edited by C. Rappe, H.R. Buser, B. Dodet & I.K. O'Neill (1991)

Vol. 12. Indoor Air (IARC Scientific Publications No. 109). Edited by B. Seifert, H. van de Wiel, B. Dodet & I.K. O'Neill (1993)

IARC (1979) *Criteria to Select Chemicals for* IARC Monographs (IARC intern. tech. Rep. No. 79/003)

IARC (1982) *IARC Monographs on the Evaluation of the Carcinogenic Risk of Chemicals to Humans*, Supplement 4, *Chemicals, Industrial Processes and Industries Associated with Cancer in Humans* (IARC Monographs, Volumes 1 to 29), Lyon, IARC*Press*

IARC (1983) *Approaches to Classifying Chemical Carcinogens According to Mechanism of Action* (IARC intern. tech. Rep. No. 83/001)

IARC (1984) *Chemicals and Exposures to Complex Mixtures Recommended for Evaluation in IARC Monographs and Chemicals and Complex Mixtures Recommended for Long-term Carcinogenicity Testing* (IARC intern. tech. Rep. No. 84/002)

IARC (1987a) *IARC Monographs on the Evaluation of Carcinogenic Risks to Humans*, Supplement 6, *Genetic and Related Effects: An Updating of Selected* IARC Monographs *from Volumes 1 to 42*, Lyon, IARC*Press*

IARC (1987b) *IARC Monographs on the Evaluation of Carcinogenic Risks to Humans*, Supplement 7, *Overall Evaluations of Carcinogenicity: An Updating of* IARC Monographs *Volumes 1 to 42*, Lyon, IARC*Press*

IARC (1988) *Report of an IARC Working Group to Review the Approaches and Processes Used to Evaluate the Carcinogenicity of Mixtures and Groups of Chemicals* (IARC intern. tech. Rep. No. 88/002)

IARC (1989) *Chemicals, Groups of Chemicals, Mixtures and Exposure Circumstances to be Evaluated in Future IARC Monographs, Report of an ad hoc Working Group* (IARC intern. tech. Rep. No. 89/004)

IARC (1991a) *A Consensus Report of an IARC Monographs Working Group on the Use of Mechanisms of Carcinogenesis in Risk Identification* (IARC intern. tech. Rep. No. 91/002)

IARC (1991b) *Report of an ad-hoc* IARC Monographs *Advisory Group on Viruses and Other Biological Agents Such as Parasites* (IARC intern. tech. Rep. No. 91/001)

IARC (1993) *Chemicals, Groups of Chemicals, Complex Mixtures, Physical and Biological Agents and Exposure Circumstances to be Evaluated in Future* IARC Monographs, *Report of an ad-hoc Working Group* (IARC intern. Rep. No. 93/005)

IARC (1998a) *Report of an ad-hoc* IARC Monographs *Advisory Group on Physical Agents* (IARC Internal Report No. 98/002)

IARC (1998b) *Report of an ad-hoc* IARC Monographs *Advisory Group on Priorities for Future Evaluations* (IARC Internal Report No. 98/004)

McGregor, D.B., Rice, J.M. & Venitt, S., eds (1999) *The Use of Short and Medium-term Tests for Carcinogens and Data on Genetic Effects in Carcinogenic Hazard Evaluation* (IARC Scientific Publications No. 146), Lyon, IARC*Press*

Montesano, R., Bartsch, H., Vainio, H., Wilbourn, J. & Yamasaki, H., eds (1986) *Long-term and Short-term Assays for Carcinogenesis — A Critical Appraisal* (IARC Scientific Publications No. 83), Lyon, IARC*Press*

Peto, R., Pike, M.C., Day, N.E., Gray, R.G., Lee, P.N., Parish, S., Peto, J., Richards, S. & Wahrendorf, J. (1980) Guidelines for simple, sensitive significance tests for carcinogenic effects in long-term animal experiments. In: *IARC Monographs on the Evaluation of the Carcinogenic Risk of Chemicals to Humans*, Supplement 2, *Long-term and Short-term Screening Assays for Carcinogens: A Critical Appraisal*, Lyon, IARC*Press*, pp. 311–426

Tomatis, L., Aitio, A., Wilbourn, J. & Shuker, L. (1989) Human carcinogens so far identified. *Jpn. J. Cancer Res.*, **80**, 795–807

Vainio, H., Magee, P.N., McGregor, D.B. & McMichael, A.J., eds (1992) *Mechanisms of Carcinogenesis in Risk Identification* (IARC Scientific Publications No. 116), Lyon, IARC*Press*

Vainio, H., Wilbourn, J.D., Sasco, A.J., Partensky, C., Gaudin, N., Heseltine, E. & Eragne, I. (1995) Identification of human carcinogenic risk in IARC Monographs. *Bull. Cancer,* **82**, 339–348 (in French)

Waters, M.D., Stack, H.F., Brady, A.L., Lohman, P.H.M., Haroun, L. & Vainio, H. (1987) Appendix 1. Activity profiles for genetic and related tests. In: *IARC Monographs on the Evaluation of Carcinogenic Risks to Humans*, Suppl. 6, *Genetic and Related Effects: An Updating of Selected IARC Monographs from Volumes 1 to 42*, Lyon, IARC*Press*, pp. 687–696

Wilbourn, J., Haroun, L., Heseltine, E., Kaldor, J., Partensky, C. & Vainio, H. (1986) Response of experimental animals to human carcinogens: an analysis based upon the IARC Monographs Programme. *Carcinogenesis*, **7**, 1853–1863

GENERAL REMARKS ON THE SUBSTANCES CONSIDERED

This eighty-seventh volume of *IARC Monographs* contains evaluations of inorganic and organic lead compounds. Lead salts and organic lead compounds were considered by the first *IARC Monographs* Working Groups (Volumes 1 and 2; IARC, 1972, 1973) and they have been reviewed in Volume 23 (IARC, 1980) and updated in Supplement 7 (IARC, 1987). Since 1987, new epidemiological and experimental studies have become available. An *IARC Monographs* Advisory Group recommended lead compounds as a high and urgent priority for re-evaluation (IARC, 2003).

Lead is found at low concentrations in the earth's crust, predominantly as lead sulfide, but the widespread occurrence of lead in the environment is largely the result of anthropogenic activity. As a result, human exposure to lead is universal, and all humans carry a body burden of lead. Lead has long been of concern for its adverse health effects other than cancer, in particular its neuro-developmental effects on the fetus, infants, and children. These health effects are discussed in this Volume in some detail. Nonetheless, the main focus of this Monograph is on the epidemiological studies and experimental investigations attempting to determine whether exposure to lead is associated with the development of some forms of cancer. In this database, however, there are several limitations that complicate the analysis and evaluation of the carcinogenic potential of lead compounds. Some of these limitations are discussed below.

In occupational studies on lead-exposed workers, exposure assessment is complicated by the historical fact that workers with high exposure often were removed from the job, either temporarily or permanently. This may introduce exposure misclassification, making it difficult to discern dose–response relationships using conventional measures such as cumulative exposure or duration of exposure to lead. It should be noted also that the presence of disease can influence the toxicokinetics of lead and, consequently, the reported concentration of lead in blood. Such effects may well affect the findings of clinical studies based on lead measurements made after diagnosis of disease.

Although inhalation is an important route of human exposure to lead, the Working Group noted that there was only one long-term inhalation study in experimental animals available for evaluation, and data on inhalation toxicokinetics in humans are very limited. To make inferences about human exposure to lead by inhalation, the Working Group considered information on the toxicokinetics of lead by the inhalation and ingestion routes in experimental animals. Likewise, because of the limited data in humans on mechanistic aspects of lead carcinogenicity, the Working Group considered mechanistic data in experimental systems, in order to make inferences regarding mechanisms of lead carcinogenicity in humans. However, definitive conclusions regarding the mechanism of carcinogenesis of lead in humans could not be drawn.

In view of the magnitude of human exposure to organic lead, in particular tetraethyl lead, the Working Group found it remarkable that only a single, inadequately conducted study in experimental animals was available for evaluation, and that there are no studies for other organic lead compounds. In addition, in the epidemiological studies of tetraethyl lead it is not possible to separate with certainty the populations exposed to organic, but not inorganic, lead. On the other hand, various studies indicate that organic lead compounds are metabolized *in vivo*, at least in part, to ionic lead. To the extent to which ionic lead, generated from organic lead compounds, is present in the body, it will be expected to exert the toxicities associated with inorganic lead.

Despite these limitations and the resulting complexities in the analysis, several aspects of the database stand out, as discussed below.

- Among the many neurological effects of lead, there appears to be an unusual propensity for lead to induce brain gliomas in rats. There are also some suggestions from the epidemiological studies that this type of brain tumour may be associated with lead exposure in humans.
- Both water-soluble and water-insoluble lead compounds are capable of causing tumours in animals at sites distant from their administration. This indicates that biologically effective amounts of lead can be mobilized even from insoluble lead compounds. In humans, the observation that lead poisoning can occur from indwelling metallic lead shot indicates that toxicologically relevant amounts of lead can be mobilized *in vivo* from metallic lead.
- Unlike several other metals (for example, beryllium, cadmium, chromium, and nickel), lead compounds have repeatedly been shown to be carcinogenic in experimental animals by the oral route.
- The evidence indicating that various lead compounds cause renal tumours in male and female mice and rats cannot be accounted for by a male-rat-specific mechanism of renal carcinogenesis.
- The extensive data on lead in experimental systems support the concept that one expression of lead toxicity is genetic toxicity. Important mechanisms of lead genetic toxicity include increases in reactive oxygen species and interaction with proteins, including those involved in DNA repair.

Studies in experimental animals support the concept that the lead component of lead compounds is critical to the carcinogenic process. For compounds such as lead arsenate and lead chromate, whose non-lead moieties have been determined to be *carcinogenic to humans* (IARC 1990, 2004), a full characterization of the cancer risk must reflect the carcinogenic activity of both the lead and the non-lead moieties.

References

IARC (1972) *IARC Monographs on the Evaluation of Carcinogenic Risk of Chemicals to Man*, Vol 1, *Some Inorganic Substances, Chlorinated Hydrocarbons, Aromatic Amines,* N-*Nitroso Compounds, and Natural Products*, Lyon

IARC (1973) *IARC Monographs on the Evaluation of Carcinogenic Risk of Chemicals to Man*, Vol 2, *Some Inorganic and Organometallic Compounds*, Lyon

IARC (1980) *IARC Monographs on the Evaluation of the Carcinogenic Risk of Chemicals to Humans*, Vol 23, *Some Metals and Metallic Compounds*, Lyon

IARC (1987) *IARC Monographs on the Evaluation of Carcinogenic Risks to Humans*, Suppl 7, *Overall Evaluations of Carcinogenicity: An Updating of* IARC Monographs *Volumes 1 to 42*, Lyon

IARC (1990) *IARC Monographs on the Evaluation of Carcinogenic Risks to Humans*, Vol 49, *Chromium, Nickel and Welding*, Lyon

IARC (2003) *Report of an Ad-Hoc IARC Monographs Advisory Group on Priorities for Future Evaluations* (IARC Internal Report 03/001), Lyon

IARC (2004) *IARC Monographs on the Evaluation of Carcinogenic Risks to Humans*, Vol 84, *Some Drinking-water Disinfectants and Contaminants, including Arsenic*, Lyon

MONOGRAPH ON INORGANIC AND ORGANIC LEAD COMPOUNDS

INORGANIC AND ORGANIC LEAD COMPOUNDS

Metallic lead and several inorganic and organic lead compounds have been considered by previous working groups convened by IARC (IARC, 1972, 1973, 1976, 1980, 1987). New data have since become available, and these are included in the present monograph and have been taken into consideration in the evaluation. The agents considered in this monograph are some inorganic and organic lead compounds.

1. Exposure Data

1.1 Chemical and physical data

1.1.1 *Nomenclature, synonyms, trade names, molecular formulae, chemical and physical properties*

Synonyms, trade names and molecular formulae for lead and some inorganic and organic lead compounds are presented in Table 1. The lead compounds shown are those for which data on carcinogenicity or mutagenicity are available or which are commercially most important. The list is not exhaustive.

Selected chemical and physical properties of the lead compounds listed in Table 1 are presented in Table 2.

Lead (atomic number, 82; relative atomic mass, 207.2) has a valence +2 or +4. The alchemists believed lead to be the oldest metal and associated it with the planet Saturn. Lead is a bluish-white metal of bright lustre, is very soft, highly malleable, ductile and a poor conductor of electricity. It is very resistant to corrosion; lead pipes bearing the insignia of Roman emperors, used as drains from the baths, are still in service (Lide, 2003). Natural lead is a mixture of four stable isotopes: ^{204}Pb (1.4%), ^{206}Pb (25.2%), ^{207}Pb (21.7%) and ^{208}Pb (51.7%) (O'Neil, 2003). Lead isotopes are the end-products of each of the three series of naturally occurring radioactive elements: ^{206}Pb for the uranium series, ^{207}Pb for the actinium series and ^{208}Pb for the thorium series. Forty-three other isotopes of lead, all of which are radioactive, are recognized (Lide, 2003).

Table 1. Synonyms and trade names, registry numbers, molecular formulae, and molecular weights for lead and lead compounds

Chemical name	Synonyms and trade names (Chemical Abstracts Service name in italics)	CAS registry number[a]	Molecular formula	Molecular weight[b]
Calcium plumbate	Pigment Brown 10	12013-69-3	Ca_2PbO_4	[351.4]
Lead, lead powder	C.I. 77575; C.I. Pigment Metal 4; Lead element; Lead Flake; Lead S 2; Pb-S 100; SSO 1	7439-92-1	Pb[c]	207.2[c]
Lead acetate	*Acetic acid, lead(2+) salt*; acetic acid lead salt (2:1); dibasic lead acetate; lead bis(acetate); lead diacetate; lead dibasic acetate; lead(2+) acetate; lead(II) acetate; neutral lead acetate; normal lead acetate; plumbous acetate; salt of Saturn; sugar of lead	301-04-2	$Pb(C_2H_3O_2)_2$	325.3
Lead acetate trihydrate	*Acetic acid, lead(2+) salt, trihydrate*; lead diacetate trihydrate; lead(II) acetate trihydrate; plumbous acetate trihydrate; sugar of lead	6080-56-4	$Pb(C_2H_3O_2)_2 \cdot 3H_2O$	379.3
Lead arsenate	*Arsenic acid (H_3AsO_4), lead(2+) salt (2:3)*; lead(2+) orthoarsenate ($Pb_3(AsO_4)_2$); Nu Rexform; trilead diarsenate	3687-31-8	$Pb_3(AsO_4)_2$	899.4
Lead azide	*Lead azide ($Pb(N_3)_2$)*; lead azide (PbN_6); lead diazide; lead(2+) azide; RD 1333	13424-46-9 [85941-57-7]	$Pb(N_3)_2$	291.2
Lead bromide	*Lead bromide ($PbBr_2$)*; lead dibromide	10031-22-8	$PbBr_2$	367.0
Lead carbonate	*Carbonic acid, lead(2+) salt (1:1)*; lead carbonate ($PbCO_3$); basic lead carbonate; dibasic lead carbonate; lead(2+) carbonate; plumbous carbonate; cerussite; white lead	598-63-0	$PbCO_3$	267.2
Lead chloride	*Lead chloride ($PbCl_2$)*; lead dichloride; lead(2+) chloride; lead(II) chloride; plumbous chloride; natural cotunite	7758-95-4	$PbCl_2$	278.1
Lead chromate	*Chromic acid (H_2CrO_4), lead(2+) salt (1:1)*; lead chromate(VI); lead chromate ($PbCrO_4$); lead chromium oxide ($PbCrO_4$); plumbous chromate; Royal Yellow 6000; chrome yellow	7758-97-6 [8049-64-7]	$PbCrO_4$	323.2
Lead fluoride	*Lead fluoride (PbF_2)*; lead difluoride; lead difluoride (PbF_2); lead(2+) fluoride; plumbous fluoride	7783-46-2 [106496-44-0]	PbF_2	245.2

Table 1 (contd)

Chemical name	Synonyms and trade names (Chemical Abstracts Service name in italics)	CAS registry number[a]	Molecular formula	Molecular weight[b]
Lead fluoroborate	Borate(1-), tetrafluoro-, lead(2+) salt (2:1); borate(1-), tetrafluoro-, lead(2+); lead fluoborate; lead tetrafluoroborate; lead boron fluoride; lead fluoroborate ($Pb(BF_4)_2$); lead(II) tetrafluoroborate	13814-96-5 [35254-34-3]	$Pb(BF_4)_2$	380.8
Lead hydrogen arsenate	*Arsenic acid (H_3AsO_4), lead(2+) salt (1:1)*; lead arsenate ($PbHAsO_4$); acid lead arsenate; arsenic acid lead salt; lead acid arsenate; lead arsenate; lead hydrogen arsenate ($PbHAsO_4$); lead(2+) monohydrogen arsenate	7784-40-9 [14034-76-5; 37196-28-4]	$PbHAsO_4$	347.1
Lead iodide	*Lead iodide (PbI_2)*; C.I. 77613; *lead diiodide*; lead(II) iodide; plumbous iodide	10101-63-0 [82669-93-0]	PbI_2	461.0
Lead naphthenate	*Naphthenic acids, lead salts*; lead naphthenates; naphthenic acid, lead salt; Naphthex Pb; Trokyd Lead	61790-14-5	Unspecified	
Lead nitrate	*Nitric acid, lead(2+) salt*; lead dinitrate; lead nitrate ($Pb(NO_3)_2$); lead(2+) bis(nitrate); lead(2+) nitrate; lead(II) nitrate; plumbous nitrate	10099-74-8 [18256-98-9]	$Pb(NO_3)_2$	331.2
Lead dioxide	*Lead oxide (PbO_2)*; C.I. 77580; lead brown; lead oxide brown; lead peroxide; lead superoxide; lead(IV) oxide; plumbic oxide; Thiolead A	1309-60-0 [60525-54-4]	PbO_2	239.2
Lead monoxide	*Lead oxide (PbO)*; C.I. 77577; C.I. Pigment Yellow 46; *lead monooxide*; lead oxide yellow; lead protoxide; lead(2+) oxide; lead(II) oxide; litharge; Litharge S; Litharge Yellow L-28; plumbous oxide; yellow lead ochre	1317-36-8 [1309-59-7; 12359-23-8]	PbO	223.2
Lead trioxide	*Lead trioxide (Pb_2O_3)*; C.I. 77579; *lead sesquioxide*; lead sesquioxide (Pb_2O_3); plumbous plumbate	1314-27-8	Pb_2O_3	462.4
Lead phosphate	*Phosphoric acid, lead(2+) salt (2:3)*; lead phosphate ($Pb_3P_2O_8$); C.I. 77622; C.I. Pigment White 30; lead diphosphate; *lead orthophosphate*; lead phosphate (3:2); lead(2+) phosphate ($Pb_3(PO_4)_2$); lead(II) phosphate (3:2); Perlex Paste 500; Perlex Paste 600A; Trilead phosphate; lead phosphate dibasic	7446-27-7	$Pb_3(PO_4)_2$	811.5

Table 1 (contd)

Chemical name	Synonyms and trade names (Chemical Abstracts Service name in italics)	CAS registry number[a]	Molecular formula	Molecular weight[b]
Lead phosphite, dibasic	Dibasic lead phosphite; lead dibasic phosphite; dibasic lead metaphosphate; C.I. 77620; lead oxide phosphonate, hemihydrate	1344-40-7	$2PbO \cdot PbHPO_3 \cdot 1/2H_2O$	[743]
Lead molybdate	Lead molybdate(VI); lead molybdate oxide ($PbMoO_4$)	10190-55-3	$PbMoO_4$	367.1
Lead stearate	*Octadecanoic acid, lead(2+) salt*; 5002G; lead distearate; lead(2+) octadecanoate; lead(2+) stearate; lead(II) octadecanoate; lead(II) stearate; Listab 28ND; Pbst; SL 1000 (stabilizer); SLG; Stabinex NC18; stearic acid, lead(2+) salt	1072-35-1 [11097-78-2; 37223-82-8]	$Pb(C_{18}H_{35}O_2)_2$	774.1
Lead stearate, dibasic	Dibasic lead stearate; Listab 51; lead, bis(octadecanoato)dioxodi-; stearic acid, lead salt, dibasic	56189-09-4	$2PbO \cdot Pb(C_{17}H_{35}COO)_2$	1220
Lead styphnate	*1,3-Benzenediol, 2,4,6-trinitro-, lead(2+) salt (1:1)*; 2,4-dioxa-3-plumbabicyclo[3.3.1]nona-1(9),5,7-triene, 3,3-didehydro-6,8,9-trinitro-; lead, [styphnato(2-)]-; lead tricinate; lead trinitroresorcinate; Tricinat; 2,4,6-trinitroresorcinol, lead(2+) salt (1:1)	15245-44-0 [4219-19-6; 6594-85-0; 59286-40-7; 63918-97-8]	$Pb(C_6H_3N_3O_8)$	[452.3]
Lead subacetate	*Lead, bis(acetato-êO)tetrahydroxytri-*; lead acetate ($Pb_3(AcO)_2(OH)_4$); lead, bis(acetato)-tetrahydroxytri-; lead, bis(acetato-O)tetra-hydroxytri-; bis(acetato)dihydroxytrilead; lead acetate hydroxide ($Pb_3(OAc)_2(OH)_4$); lead acetate, basic; monobasic lead acetate	1335-32-6	$Pb(CH_3COO)_2 \cdot 2Pb(OH)_2$	807.7
Lead sulfate	*Sulfuric acid, lead(2+) salt (1:1)*; Anglislite; C.I. 77630; C.I. Pigment White 3; Fast White; Freemans White Lead; HB 2000; Lead Bottoms; lead monosulfate; lead(II) sulfate (1:1); lead(2+) sulfate; lead(II) sulfate; Milk White; Mulhouse White; TS 100; TS 100 (sulfate); TS-E; sublimed white lead	7446-14-2 [37251-28-8]	$PbSO_4$	303.3
Lead sulfide	*Lead sulfide (PbS)*; C.I. 77640; lead monosulfide; lead sulfide (1:1); lead(2+) sulfide; lead(II) sulfide; natural lead sulfide; P 128; P 37; plumbous sulfide	1314-87-0 [51682-73-6]	PbS	239.3

Table 1 (contd)

Chemical name	Synonyms and trade names (Chemical Abstracts Service name in italics)	CAS registry number[a]	Molecular formula	Molecular weight[b]
Lead tetraoxide	*Lead oxide (Pb_3O_4)*; Azarcon; C.I. 77578; C.I. Pigment Red 105; Entan; Gold Satinobre; Heuconin 5; lead orthoplumbate; lead oxide (3:4); *lead oxide red*; lead tetroxide; Mennige; Mineral Orange; Mineral red; Minium; Minium Non-Setting RL 95; Minium red; Orange Lead; Paris Red; *red lead*; red lead oxide; Sandix; Saturn Red; trilead tetraoxide; trilead tetroxide; plumboplumbic oxide	1314-41-6 [12684-34-3]	Pb_3O_4	685.6
Lead thiocyanate	Thiocyanic acid, lead(2+) salt; lead bis(thiocyanate); lead dithiocyanate; lead(2+) thiocyanate; lead(II) thiocyanate	592-87-0 [10382-36-2]	$Pb(SCN)_2$	323.4
Tetraethyl lead	*Plumbane, tetraethyl-*; lead, tetraethyl-; TEL; tetraethyllead; tetraethylplumbane	78-00-2	$Pb(C_2H_5)_4$	323.5
Tetramethyl lead	*Plumbane, tetramethyl-*; lead, tetramethyl-; tetramethyllead; tetramethylplumbane; TML	75-74-1	$Pb(CH_3)_4$	267.3

From IARC (1980); Lide (2003); National Library of Medicine (2003); O'Neil (2003); STN International (2003)

[a] Deleted Chemical Abstracts Service numbers shown in square brackets

[b] Values in square brackets were calculated from the molecular formula.

[c] Atomic formula; atomic weight

Table 2. Physical and chemical properties of lead and lead compounds

Chemical name	Physical form	Melting-point (°C)	Boiling-point (°C)	Density (g/cm^3)	Solubility (per 100 g H_2O)
Lead, lead powder	Soft silvery-gray metal; cubic	327.5	1749	11.3	Insol. in water; sol. in conc. acid
Lead acetate	White crystal	280	Dec.	3.25	44.3 g at 20 °C; sl. sol. in ethanol
Lead acetate trihydrate	Colourless crystal	75 (dec)	–	2.55	45.6 g at 15 °C; sl. sol. in ethanol
Lead arsenate	White crystal	1042 (dec)	–	5.8	Insol. in water; sol. in nitric acid
Lead azide	Colourless orthorhombic needle	~350 (expl)	–	4.7	23 mg at 18 °C; v. sol. in acetic acid
Lead bromide	White orthorhombic crystal	371	892	6.69	975 mg at 25 °C; insol. in ethanol
Lead carbonate	Colourless orthorhombic crystal	~315 (dec)	–	6.6	Insol. in water; sol. in acid and alkaline solutions
Lead chloride	White orthorhombic needle or powder	501	951	5.98	1.08 g at 25 °C; sol. in alkaline solutions; insol. in ethanol
Lead chromate	Yellow-orange monoclinic crystals	844	–	6.12	17 µg at 20 °C; sol. in dilute acids
Lead fluoride	White orthorhombic crystal	830	1293	8.44	67 mg at 25 °C
Lead fluoroborate	Stable only in aqueous solution	–	–	–	Sol. in water
Lead hydrogen arsenate	White monoclinic crystal	280 (dec)		5.94	Insol. in water; sol. in nitric acid and alkaline solutions
Lead iodide	Yellow hexagonal crystal or powder	410	872 (dec)	6.16	76 mg at 25 °C; insol. in ethanol
Lead molybdate	Yellow tertiary crystal	~1060	–	6.7	Insol. in water; sol. in nitric acid and sodium hydroxide
Lead naphthenate	No data available				
Lead nitrate	Colourless cubic crystal	470	–	4.53	59.7 g at 25 °C; sl. sol. in ethanol

Table 2 (contd)

Chemical name	Physical form	Melting-point (°C)	Boiling-point (°C)	Density (g/cm^3)	Solubility (per 100 g H_2O)
Lead monoxide (PbO); litharge	Red tetrahedral crystal	Transforms to massicot at 489 °C	–	9.35	Insol. in water and ethanol; sol. in dilute nitric acid
Massicot	Yellow orthorhombic crystal	897	–	9.64	Insol. in water and ethanol; sol. in dilute nitric acid
Lead trioxide (Pb_2O_3)	Black monoclinic crystal or red amorphous powder	530 (dec)	–	10.05	Insol. in water; sol. in alkaline solutions
Lead phosphate	White hexagonal crystal	1014	–	7.01	Insol. in water and ethanol; sol. in alkali and nitric acid
Lead phosphite, dibasic	Pale yellow powder			6.1	
Lead stearate	White powder	~100	–	1.4	Insol. in water; sol. in hot ethanol
Lead styphnate	No data available				
Lead subacetate	White powder	Dec.	–	–	6.3 g at 0 °C; 25 g at 100 °C
Lead sulfate	Orthorhombic crystal	1087	–	6.29	4.4 mg at 25 °C; sl. sol. in alkaline solutions; insol. in acids
Lead sulfide	Black powder or silvery cubic crystal	1113	–	7.60	Insol. in water; sol. in acids
Lead tetraoxide	Red tetrahedral crystals	830	–	8.92	Insol. in water and ethanol; sol. in hot hydrochloric acid
Lead thiocyanate	White to yellowish powder	–	–	3.82	50 mg at 20 °C
Tetraethyl lead	Liquid	–136	200 (dec)	1.653 at 20 °C	Insol. in water; sol. in benzene; sl. sol. in ethanol and diethyl ether
Tetramethyl lead	Liquid	–30.2	110	1.995 at 20 °C	Insol. in water; sol. in benzene, ethanol and diethyl ether

From IARC (1980); Lide (2003); Physical and Theoretical Chemistry Laboratory (2004)
Abbreviations: conc., concentrated; insol., insoluble; sl. sol., slightly soluble; sol., soluble; v. sol., very soluble; dec, decomposes; expl., explodes

1.1.2 *Technical products and impurities*

Lead is produced in purity greater than 99.97% in many countries. Lead oxides and mixtures of lead and lead oxides are also widely available. Tables 3 and 4 show the specifications for metallic lead and some lead compounds, respectively, from selected countries.

Table 3. Specifications for metallic lead from selected countries

Country	% Pb (min.)	Contaminants with limits (% max.[a])	Reference
Argentina	99.97	Fe, 0.002; Sb, 0.004; Zn, 0.001; Cu, 0.002; Ag, 0.0095; Bi, 0.035; Cd, 0.001; Ni, 0.001	Industrias Deriplom SA (2003)
Australia	99.97–99.99	Ag, 0.001; As, 0.001; Bi, 0.005–0.029; Cu, 0.001; Sb, 0.001; Zn, 0.001; Cd, 0.001	Pasminco Metals (1998)
Belgium	99.9–99.95	(ppm) Bi, 90–250; Ag, 10–15; Cu, 5–10; As, 5; Sb, 3; Sn, 3; As+Sb+Sn, 8; Zn, 3–5; Fe, 3; Cd, 3–10; Ni, 2–3	Umicore Precious Metals (2002)
Bulgaria	99.97–99.99	Ag, 0.001–0.005; Cu, 0.0005–0.003; Zn, 0.0002–0.0015; Fe, 0.001; Cd, 0.0002–0.001; Ni, 0.0005–0.001; As, 0.0005–0.002; Sb, 0.0005–0.005; Sn, 0.0005–0.001; Bi, 0.005–0.03	KCM SA (2003)
Canada	99.97–99.99	NR	Noranda (2003); Teck Cominco (2003)
Kazakhstan	99.95–99.9996	NR	Southpolymetal (2003)
Mexico	99.97–99.99	Ag, 0.0015; Cu, 0.0005; Zn, 0.0005; Fe, 0.0010; Bi, 0.0250; Sb, 0.0005; As, 0.0005; Sn, 0.0005; Ni, 0.0002; Te, 0.0001	Penoles (2003)
Republic of Korea	99.995	Ag, 0.0003; Cu, 0.0003; As, 0.0003; Sb, 0.0003; Zn, 0.0003; Fe, 0.0003; Bi, 0.0015; Sn, 0.0003	Korea Zinc Co. (2003)
USA	99.995–99.9999	(ppm) Sb, 1; As, 1–5; Bi, 0.2–4; Cu, 1–4; Ag, < 0.1–2; Tl, 1–2; Sn, 0.3–1; Fe, < 0.1–0.3; Ca, 0.1–0.4; Mg, 0.1–0.3	ESPI Corp. (2002)

NR, not reported
[a] Unless otherwise specified

Table 4. Specifications for some lead compounds from selected countries

Country	Compound	Contaminants with limits (% max.)	Grade[a]	Reference
Argentina	Lead oxide	Fe, 0.003; Sb, 0.001–0.004; Zn, 0.0005–0.001; Cu, 0.0005–0.002; Ag, 0.001–0.0095; Bi, 0.003–0.035; Cd, 0.0008–0.001; Ni, 0.0008–0.001	5 grades of red lead ($Pb_3O_4 + PbO_2 + PbO$); 3 grades of yellow litharge (PbO, 99.65–99.96%; free Pb, 0.03–0.30%; Pb_3O_4, 0.0048–0.05%); 1 grade of green powder (PbO + Pb, 80%+20% or 62%+38%)	Industrias Deriplom SA (2003)
Australia	Lead oxide	Bi, 0.05–0.06; Ag, 0.001; Cu, 0.001; Sn, 0.0005–0.001; Sb, 0.0001–0.0002; As, 0.0001; Se, 0.0001; S, 0.0007; Cd, 0.0005; Ni, 0.0002–0.0003; Zn, 0.0005; Fe, 0.0002–0.0005; Mn, 0.0003–0.0005; Te, 0.00003–0.0001; Co, 0.0001–0.0002; Cr, 0.0002; Ba, 0.0005; V, 0.0004; Mo, 0.0003–0.0005	VRLA-refined™ and MF-refined™	Pasminco Metals (2000)
USA	Lead acetate	NR	5N	ESPI Corp. (2002)
	Lead bromide		3N and 5N	
	Lead chloride		3N and 5N	
	Lead fluoride		3N	
	Lead iodide		3N and 5N	
	Lead molybdate		3N	
	Lead monoxide		3N and 5N	
	Lead tetraoxide		3N	
	Lead sulfide		3N and 5N	

VRLA, valve-regulated lead acid; MF, maintenance-free; NR, not reported
[a] 3N, 99.9%; 5N, 99.999%

1.2 Production

Commercial lead metal is described as being either primary or secondary. Primary lead is produced directly from mined lead ore. Secondary lead is produced from scrap lead products which have been recycled.

1.2.1 *The ores and their preparation*

The most important lead ore is *galena* (lead sulfide). Other important ores such as *cerussite* (lead carbonate) and *anglesite* (lead sulfate) may be regarded as weathered products of *galena* and are usually found nearer to the surface of the earth's crust. Lead and zinc ores often occur together and, in most extraction methods, have to be separated. The most common separation technique is selective froth flotation. The ore is first processed to a fine suspension in water by grinding in ball or rod mills — preferably to a particle size of < 0.25 mm. Air is then bubbled through this pulp contained in a cell or tank and, following the addition of various chemicals and proper agitation, the required mineral particles become attached to the air bubbles and are carried to the surface to form a stable mineral containing froth which is skimmed off. The unwanted or gangue particles are unaffected and remain in the pulp. For example, with lead–zinc sulfide ores, zinc sulfate, sodium cyanide or sodium sulfite can be used to depress the zinc sulfide, while the lead sulfide is floated off to form a concentrate. The zinc sulfide is then activated by copper sulfate and floated off as a second concentrate (Lead Development Association International, 2003a).

Around 3 million tonnes of lead are mined in the world each year. Lead is found all over the world but the countries with the largest mines are Australia, China and the United States of America, which together account for more than 50% of primary production. The most common lead ore is *galena* (lead sulfide). Other elements frequently associated with lead include zinc and silver. In fact, lead ores constitute the main sources of silver, contributing substantially towards the world's total silver output (Lead Development Association International, 2003b). Table 5 shows mine production of lead concentrate by country in the year 2000. Table 6 shows the trends in lead mine production by geographic region from 1960 to 2003.

1.2.2 *Smelting*

(*a*) *Two-stage processes*

The first stage in smelting consists of removing most of the sulfur from the lead concentrate. This is achieved by a continuous roasting process (sintering) in which the lead sulfide is largely converted to lead oxide and broken down to a size convenient for use in a blast furnace — the next stage in the process. The sinter plant gases containing sulfur are converted to sulfuric acid (Lead Development Association International, 2003a).

Table 5. Mine production of lead concentrate in 2000[a]

Country	Production (tonnes)	Country	Production (tonnes)
Algeria	818	Mexico	137 975
Argentina	14 115	Morocco	81 208[c]
Australia	739 000	Myanmar	1 200[b]
Bolivia	9 523	Namibia	11 114[c]
Bosnia and Herzegovina	200[b]	Peru	270 576
Brazil	8 832	Poland	51 200[c]
Bulgaria	10 500	Republic of Korea	2 724
Canada	152 765	Romania	18 750[c]
Chile	785[c]	Russian Federation	13 300
China	660 000[b]	Serbia and Montenegro	9 000
Colombia	226	South Africa	75 262
Democratic People's Republic of Korea	60 000[b,c]	Spain	40 300
		Sweden	106 584[c]
Ecuador	200[b]	Tajikistan	800[b]
Georgia	200[b]	Thailand	15 600
Greece	18 235[b]	The former Yugoslav Republic of Macedonia	25 000[b]
Honduras	4 805		
India	28 900	Tunisia	6 602
Iran	15 000[b]	Turkey	17 270
Ireland	57 825	United Kingdom	1 000[b]
Italy	2 000	USA	465 000
Japan	8 835	Viet Nam	1 000[b]
Kazakhstan	40 000	World total[d]	3 180 000[c]

From Smith (2002)

In addition to the countries listed, lead is also produced in Nigeria, but information is inadequate to estimate output.

[a] Data available at 1 July 2003

[b] Estimated

[c] Revised

[d] Data from the USA and estimated data are rounded to no more than three significant digits, so that values may not add to total shown.

The graded sinter (lead oxide) is mixed with coke and flux, such as limestone, and fed into the top of the blast furnace, where it is smelted using an air blast (sometimes pre-heated) introduced near the bottom. The chemical processes that take place in the furnace at about 1200 °C result in the production of lead bullion (lead containing only metallic impurities) which is tapped off from the bottom of the furnace and either cast into ingots or collected molten in ladles for transfer to the refining process. In the Imperial Smelting Furnace process, a very similar procedure is used for the simultaneous production of zinc and lead.

These traditional two-stage processes largely favour the release of hazardous dusts and fumes. They necessitate the use of extensive exhaust ventilation and result in large volumes

Table 6. Trends in lead mine production worldwide

Year	Production (thousand tonnes) by geographical region[a]						
	A[b]	B	C	D[b]	E	F[b]	Total
1960	370	207	822	84	306	583	2372
1965	366	250	984	99	361	724	2784
1970	476	210	1341	120	441	855	3443
1975	435	165	1340	140	395	1085	3560
1980	482	278	1298	112	382	1030	3582
1985	412	261	1197	155	474	1076	3575
1990	727	175	1184	545	556	NRS	3187
1995	382	186	1047	715	424	NRS	2753
2000	360	178	1053	805	650	NRS	3046
2003	218	123	1043	770	666	NRS	2821

From International Lead and Zinc Study Group (1990, 2004)
NRS, not reported separately
[a] Data from following countries:
A, Austria, Denmark, Finland, France, Germany (the Federal Republic of Germany before reunification), Greece, Ireland, Italy, Norway, Portugal, Spain, Sweden, United Kingdom and former Yugoslavia
B, Algeria, Congo, Morocco, Namibia, South Africa, Tunisia and Zambia
C, Argentina, Bolivia, Brazil, Canada, Chile, Colombia, Guatemala, Honduras, Mexico, Nicaragua, Peru and USA
D, Myanmar, India, Iran, Japan, Philippines, Republic of Korea, Thailand and Turkey
E, Australia
F, Bulgaria, China, former Czechoslovakia, Hungary, People's Democratic Republic of Korea, Poland, Romania and the former Soviet Union; values for the latter four countries are estimates.
[b] From 1990 onwards, data from region F are included in region A (for Belarus, Bulgaria, Czech Republic, Estonia, Hungary, Latvia, Lithuania, Poland, Romania, the Russian Federation, Slovakia and Ukraine) or region D (for all former Soviet Republics, China and People's Democratic Republic of Korea); lead mine production for 1991 in the former Soviet Union is split as follows: Europe, 19%; Asia, 81%.

of lead-laden exhaust gases which are usually cleaned before they are discharged into the atmosphere. The collected dusts are returned to the smelting process (Lead Development Association International, 2003a).

(*b*) *Direct smelting processes*

The environmental problems and inefficient use of energy associated with the sinter/blast furnace and Imperial Smelting Furnace processes have led to a considerable amount of research into more economical and less polluting methods for the production of lead. Most of this research has been aimed at devising processes in which lead is converted directly from the sulfide to the metal without producing lead oxide. As a result, a number of direct smelting processes now exist, although at varying stages of development (Lead Development Association International, 2003a).

Direct smelting processes offer several significant advantages over conventional methods. The first and most obvious advantage is that sintering is no longer necessary. As a result, the creation of dust, a major occupational and environmental problem, is avoided. Moreover, the heat evolved during sintering (for the oxidation of the ore) is no longer wasted but is used in the smelting operation, thus providing a considerable saving of fuel. The volumes of gas that require filtering are largely reduced and, at the same time, the sulfur dioxide concentration of the off-gases is greater and these are therefore more suitable for the manufacture of sulfuric acid. The major difficulty in all direct smelting processes lies in obtaining both a lead bullion with an acceptably low sulfur content and a slag with a sufficiently low lead content for it to be safely and economically discarded. In several cases, further treatment of the crude bullion or the slag or both is required in a separate operation. There are several direct smelting processes which come close to meeting the desired criteria — the Russian Kivcet, the QSL (Queneau–Schuhmann–Lurgi), the Isasmelt and the Outokumpu processes are examples. The use of these newer processes will probably increase.

At present, the relative importance of the different smelting methods in terms of amounts of metal produced is as follows: conventional blast furnace, 80%; Imperial Smelting Furnace process, 10%; and direct processes, 10% (Lead Development Association International, 2003a).

1.2.3 *Hydrometallurgical processes*

With the prospect of even tighter environmental controls, the possibilities of utilizing hydrometallurgical techniques for the treatment of primary and secondary sources of lead are being investigated. Several processes have been described in the literature, but most are still in the developmental stage and probably not yet economically viable in comparison with the pyrometallurgical (smelting) processes. The goal of the hydrometallurgical processes in most cases is to fix the sulfur as a harmless sulfate and to put the lead into a solution suitable for electrolytic recovery. Most of these processes recirculate leach solutions and produce lead of high purity. For example, the Ledchlor process can be used on primary materials; other methods such as Rameshni SO_2 Reduction (RSR) and the processes developed by Engitec (CX-EW) and Ginatta (Maja *et al.*, 1989) are more concerned with recovery of lead from secondary sources, in particular from battery scrap (Lead Development Association International, 2003a).

1.2.4 *Primary lead refining*

Apart from gold and silver, lead bullion contains many other metallic impurities including antimony, arsenic, copper, tin and zinc. Copper is the first of the impurities to be removed. The lead bullion is melted at about 300–600 °C and held just above its melting-point when solid copper rises to the surface and is skimmed off. Sulfur is stirred into the melt to facilitate the operation by producing a dry powdery dross which is more readily removed. Once copper has been removed, there are a number of processes available for the extraction of the other impurities from the bullion. These include pyro-metallurgical techniques, in which elements are removed one or more at a time in several stages, and electrolytic processes that remove most of the impurities in one operation. Although electrolytic methods are used in large-scale production, pyrometallurgical techniques account for the larger portion of the world's refined lead production (Lead Development Association International, 2003c). Table 7 shows the trends in production of refined lead by geographic region from 1960 to 2003.

Table 7. Trends in refined lead production worldwide

Year	Production (thousand tonnes) by geographical region[a]						
	A[b]	B	C	D[b]	E	F[b]	Total
1960	950	70	1114	164	211	718	3227
1965	1046	124	1296	202	223	823	3714
1970	1412	147	1619	301	217	992	4688
1975	1354	124	1661	296	198	1195	4828
1980	1514	156	1776	397	241	1331	5415
1985	1613	159	1708	539	220	1416	5655
1990	2323	150	1900	924	229	NRS	5525
1995	1796	141	2102	1474	243	NRS	5756
2000	1882	125	2216	2163	263	NRS	6650
2003	1606	144	2043	2499	311	NRS	6603

From International Lead and Zinc Study Group (1990, 2004)
NRS, not reported separately
[a] Data from the following countries:
A, Austria, Belgium, Denmark, Finland, France, Germany (the Federal Republic of Germany before reunification), Greece, Ireland, Italy, Netherlands, Norway, Portugal, Spain, Sweden, Switzerland, United Kingdom and former Yugoslavia
B, Algeria, Morocco, Namibia, South Africa, Tunisia and Zambia
C, Argentina, Brazil, Canada, Mexico, Peru, USA and Venezuela
D, Myanmar, India, Indonesia, Japan, Malaysia, Philippines, Republic of Korea, China (Province of Taiwan), Thailand, and Turkey
E, Australia and New Zealand
F, Bulgaria, China, former Czechoslovakia, Germany (former Democratic Republic of), Hungary, People's Democratic Republic of Korea, Poland, Romania and former Soviet Union; values for Bulgaria, former German Democratic Republic, Romania, former Soviet Union, China and People's Democratic Republic of Korea are estimates.
[b] From 1990 onwards, data from region F are included in region A (Belarus, Bulgaria, Czech Republic, Estonia, Germany (former German Democratic Republic), Hungary, Latvia, Lithuania, Poland, Romania, Russian Federation and Ukraine) or in region D (China, all other former Soviet Republics and People's Democratic Republic of Korea); refined lead production in the former Soviet Union for 1991 is split as follows: Europe, 24%; Asia, 76%.

(*a*) *Pyrometallurgical processes*

(i) *Removal of antimony, arsenic and tin*

After the removal of copper, the next step is to remove antimony, arsenic and tin. There are two methods available — the softening process (so-called since these elements are standard hardeners for lead) and the Harris process. In the softening process, the lead bullion is melted and agitated with an air blast, causing preferential oxidation of the impurities which are then skimmed off as a molten slag. In the Harris process, the molten bullion is stirred with a flux of molten sodium hydroxide and sodium nitrate or another suitable oxidizing agent. The oxidized impurities are suspended in the alkali flux in the form of sodium antimonate, arsenate and stannate, and any zinc is removed in the form of zinc oxide (Lead Development Association International, 2003c).

(ii) *Removal of silver and gold*

After the removal of antimony, arsenic and tin, the softened lead may still contain silver and gold, and sometimes bismuth. The removal of the precious metals by the Parkes process is based on the fact that they are more soluble in zinc than in lead. In this process, the lead is melted and mixed with zinc at 480 °C. The temperature of the melt is gradually lowered to below 419.5 °C, at which point the zinc (now containing nearly all the silver and gold) begins to solidify as a crust on the surface of the lead and can be skimmed off. An alternative procedure, the Port Pirie process, used at the Port Pirie refinery in Australia, is based on similar metallurgical principles (Lead Development Association International, 2003c).

(iii) *Removal of zinc*

The removal of the precious metals leaves zinc as the main contaminant of the lead. It is removed either by oxidation with gaseous chlorine or by vacuum distillation. The latter process involves melting the lead in a large kettle covered with a water-cooled lid under vacuum. The zinc distils from the lead under the combined influence of temperature and reduced pressure and condenses on the underside of the cold lid (Lead Development Association International, 2003c).

(iv) *Removal of bismuth*

After removal of zinc, the only remaining impurity is bismuth, although it is not always present in lead ore. It is easily removed by electrolysis and this accounts for the favouring of electrolytic methods in Canada (see below), where bismuth is a frequent impurity. When pyrometallurgical methods of refining are used, bismuth is removed by adding a calcium–magnesium alloy to the molten lead, causing a quaternary alloy of lead–calcium–magnesium–bismuth to rise to the top of the melt where it can be skimmed off (Lead Development Association International, 2003c).

(*b*) *Electrolytic processes*

In the Betts process, massive cast anodes of lead bullion are used in a cell containing an electrolyte of acid lead fluorosilicate and thin cathode 'starter sheets' of high-purity lead. The lead deposited on the cathodes still contains tin and sometimes a small amount of antimony, and these impurities must be removed by melting and selective oxidation. For many years, the Betts process was the only process to remove bismuth efficiently. A more recent electrolytic process, first used in the 1950s in Italy, employs a sulfamate electrolyte. It is claimed to be an equally efficient refining method, with the advantage that the electrolyte is easier to prepare (Lead Development Association International, 2003c).

By combining the processes described above to build up a complete refining scheme, it is possible to produce lead of very high purity. Most major refiners will supply bulk quantities of lead of 99.99% purity and, for very specific purposes, it is possible to reach 99.9999% purity by additional processing (Lead Development Association International, 2003c).

1.2.5 *Secondary lead production*

Much of the secondary lead comes from lead batteries, with the remainder originating from other sources such as lead pipe and sheet. Lead scrap from pipes and sheet is 'clean' and can be melted and refined without the need for a smelting stage. With batteries, the lead can only be obtained by breaking the case open. This is commonly done using a battery breaking machine which, in addition to crushing the case, separates out the different components of the battery and collects them in hoppers. Thus, the pastes (oxide and sulfate), grids, separators and fragmented cases are all separated from one another. The battery acid is drained and neutralized, and the other components are either recycled or discarded (Lead Development Association International, 2003d).

Table 8 shows trends in recovery of secondary lead by geographic region from 1970 to 1988. Three million tonnes of lead are produced from secondary sources each year, by recycling scrap lead products. At least three-quarters of all lead is used in products which are suitable for recycling and hence lead has the highest recycling rate of all the common non-ferrous metals (Lead Development Association International, 2003a). Almost 50% of the 1.6 million tonnes of lead produced in Europe each year has been recycled. In the United Kingdom, the figure is nearer 60% (Lead Development Association International, 2003d).

(*a*) *Secondary lead smelting*

The workhorse of the secondary lead production industry used to be the blast furnace. Conversion from blast to rotary-furnace technology in Europe began in the 1960s and was largely complete by the 1990s, driven by the high price of metallurgical coke and the relative difficulty of preventing the escape of dust and fume. The blast furnace was used to provide a low-grade antimonial lead, which was softened. The high-antimony slags were accumulated for a subsequent blast furnace campaign to produce a high-antimony bullion

Table 8. Trends in recovery of secondary lead (refined lead and lead alloys produced from secondary materials)

Year	Recovery (thousand tonnes) by geographical region[a]					
	A	B	C	D	E	Total
1970	619	21	532	78	37	1287
1975	617	29	610	115	39	1410
1980	742	44	798	192	39	1815
1985	766	44	747	258	20	1835
1988	800	48	921	310	23	2102

From International Lead and Zinc Study Group (1990)
[a] Data from the following countries:
A, Austria, Belgium, Denmark, Finland, France, Germany (the Federal Republic of Germany before reunification), Greece, Ireland, Italy, Netherlands, Portugal, Spain, Sweden, Switzerland, United Kingdom and former Yugoslavia
B, Algeria, Morocco and South Africa
C, Argentina, Brazil, Canada, Mexico, USA and Venezuela
D, India, Japan and China (Province of Taiwan)
E, Australia and New Zealand

for blending into lead alloys. Although a few secondary smelters today still use furnaces based on blast furnace technology, most companies now use rotary furnaces in which the charge can be tailored to give a lead of approximately the desired composition. Alternatively, a two-stage smelting procedure can be employed, which yields crude soft lead and crude antimonial lead. In the latter process, for example, battery plates are first melted and crude soft lead is tapped off after a few hours while the antimonial slag and lead oxide and sulfate are retained in the furnace. Further plates are charged and more soft lead is withdrawn until sufficient slag has accumulated for the slag reduction stage. Then, coke or anthracite fines and soda ash are added, lead and antimony oxides and lead sulfate are reduced and the cycle ends with the furnace being emptied of antimonial lead and of slag for discarding. As with primary smelting, large volumes of gas are produced, carrying substantial quantities of dust. On leaving the smelter, the gases are cooled from about 900 °C to about 100 °C using air and/or water cooling, and pass into a baghouse where the dust is collected and eventually fed back into the smelter. The gases subsequently are released into the atmosphere. In the course of processing one tonne of lead, as much as 100 tonnes of air have to be cleaned in this way (Lead Development Association International, 2003d).

In the semi-continuous Isasmelt furnace process used for secondary lead production, the furnace is fed with a lead carbonate paste containing 1% sulfur. This is obtained as a result of the battery paste having gone through a desulfurizing process after battery breaking. Over the following 36 h, wet lead carbonate paste and coal as a reductant are continuously fed into the furnace. The soft lead that is produced is tapped every 3 h and contains 99.9% lead. After 36 h, the paste feed is stopped and the slag is reduced to produce antimonial lead alloy. As with the two-stage process described above, off-gases from the furnace are first cooled and then passed into a baghouse for fume and dust control (Lead Development Association International, 2003d).

(*b*) *Secondary lead refining*

The principal impurities that are removed in secondary lead refining are copper, tin, antimony and arsenic. Zinc, iron, nickel, bismuth, silver and other impurities may also be present. These impurities are generally removed using the same basic techniques as described above (Lead Development Association International, 2003d).

1.2.6 *Lead production by compound and country*

Table 9 summarizes the available information on the number of companies in various countries producing metallic lead and some lead compounds in 2002.

1.3 Use

Over the centuries the unique properties of lead have resulted in its use in many different applications. These properties are mainly its high resistance to corrosion, its softness and low melting-point, its high density and its relatively low conductivity (Lead Development Association International, 2003b).

Large quantities of lead, both as the metal and as the dioxide, are used in storage batteries. Lead is also used for cable covering, plumbing and ammunition. The metal is very effective as a sound absorber and as a radiation shield around X-ray equipment and nuclear reactors. It is also used to absorb vibration. Lead, alloyed with tin, is used in making organ pipes. Lead carbonate ($PbCO_3$), lead sulfate ($PbSO_4$), lead chromate ($PbCrO_4$), lead tetraoxide (Pb_3O_4) and other lead compounds (see Table 1 for synonyms) have been applied extensively in paints, although in recent years this use has been curtailed to reduce health hazards. Lead oxide (usually lead monoxide) is used in the production of fine 'crystal glass' and 'flint glass' with a high index of refraction for achromatic lenses. Lead nitrate and acetate are soluble salts that serve as intermediates and in specialty applications. Lead salts such as lead arsenate have been used as insecticides, but in recent years this use has been almost eliminated (Lide, 2003).

In most countries, lead is predominantly used as the metal and it may be alloyed with other materials depending on the application. Lead alloys are made by the controlled addition of other elements. The term 'unalloyed lead' implies that no alloying elements have been added intentionally; this may mean that the lead is of high purity, but the term also covers less pure lead containing incidental impurities (Lead Development Association International, 2003e).

Table 9. Lead production by compound and country

Compound	No. of companies	Countries
Metallic lead	10	Japan
	6	USA
	5	China, Mexico
	4	Belgium, Canada
	3	Brazil, Germany, Peru, Russian Federation
	2	Kazakhstan
	1	Argentina, Australia, Bolivia, Bulgaria, China (Province of Taiwan), Egypt, India, Ireland, Italy, Netherlands, Republic of Korea, Spain, Sweden, Turkey
Lead acetate	10	China
	8	India
	7	Mexico
	6	USA
	5	Brazil, Japan
	3	Spain
	2	Germany, Italy
	1	Australia, China (Province of Taiwan), France, Romania, Russian Federation
Lead arsenate	3	Japan
	1	Peru
Lead azide	2	Brazil
	1	Japan
Lead bromide	1	Germany, India, Japan, United Kingdom, USA
Lead carbonate	6	India
	2	China, China (Province of Taiwan), Germany, USA
	1	Argentina, Australia, Italy, Japan, Mexico, Republic of Korea, Romania, Ukraine and United Kingdom
Lead chloride	5	India
	4	USA
	1	Australia, Belgium, China, China (Province of Taiwan), Germany, Japan, Mexico, Romania, Spain
Lead chromate (Pigment Yellow 34)	22	China
	8	India
	6	USA
	5	China (Province of Taiwan), Japan, Spain
	3	Germany, Italy
	2	Brazil, Republic of Korea, Netherlands, United Kingdom
	1	Argentina, Austria, Belgium, Canada, Colombia, France, Mexico, Peru, Romania, Russian Federation, Turkey, Venezuela
Lead fluoride	4	China
	3	India, Japan, USA
	1	Argentina, Canada, France, Germany

Table 9 (contd)

Compound	No. of companies	Countries
Lead fluoroborate	7	China, India
	5	USA
	3	Japan
	2	Australia, China (Province of Taiwan), France, Germany
	1	Argentina, Brazil, Russian Federation, Spain
Lead iodide	2	Japan, United Kingdom
	1	China, India, USA
Lead naphthenate	6	China
	5	Japan, Mexico
	3	Argentina, USA
	2	France, India, Peru, Spain
	1	Australia, Belgium, Brazil, Canada, China (Province of Taiwan), Germany, Italy, Romania, Thailand, Turkey
Lead nitrate	12	India
	8	China
	7	USA
	6	Japan
	4	Brazil, Mexico
	3	Spain
	2	Belgium, Germany
	1	Australia, Italy, Russian Federation, Tajikistan
Lead monoxide	24	China
	7	Japan
	6	India
	4	China (Province of Taiwan), Germany, Mexico, USA
	3	France, Spain
	2	Brazil, Italy, Peru, Republic of Korea, Russian Federation
	1	Argentina, Australia, Canada, Kazakhstan, Malaysia, Portugal, South Africa, Tajikistan, Turkey, United Kingdom
Lead dioxide	6	India
	4	Japan
	3	USA
	2	Germany
	1	Australia, Italy, South Africa, Spain, United Kingdom
Lead phosphate	6	China
	2	India
	1	Japan, Russian Federation
Lead stearate	25	China
	17	India
	9	China (Province of Taiwan)
	4	Japan
	3	Germany, Spain, Thailand
	2	Mexico, Peru, Philippines, Republic of Korea, USA
	1	Albania, Argentina, Belgium, Brazil, Indonesia, Italy, Portugal, Romania, South Africa, Turkey

Table 9 (contd)

Compound	No. of companies	Countries
Lead stearate, dibasic	15	India
	8	China
	5	China (Province of Taiwan)
	2	Japan, Philippines, Spain, Thailand, USA
	1	Belgium, Germany, Indonesia, Peru, Republic of Korea, South Africa, Turkey, United Kingdom
Lead styphnate	2	Brazil
	1	Japan
Lead subacetate	4	India
	3	Mexico
	2	China
	1	Australia, Brazil, China (Province of Taiwan), Romania, Spain, USA
Lead sulfate	6	India
	4	Mexico
	3	Germany
	2	Spain
	1	China, Japan, Romania, USA
Lead sulfide	4	India
	2	France, Japan
	1	Austria, China, Germany, USA
Lead tetraoxide	22	China
	5	India, Japan
	4	China (Province of Taiwan)
	3	Mexico, Spain
	2	Brazil, France, Germany, Italy, Russian Federation, USA
	1	Argentina, Kazakhstan, Peru, Poland, Portugal, Republic of Korea, South Africa, Tajikistan, Turkey, United Kingdom
Lead thiocyanate	2	USA
Lead trioxide	1	China
Tetraethyl lead	1	Germany, Italy
Tetramethyl lead	2	Russian Federation
	1	Italy

From Chemical Information Services (2003)

Trends in the reported consumption of lead by geographical region between 1960 and 2003 are shown in Table 10. Tables 11 and 12 show the trends in total lead consumption by country and by major use category, respectively, in selected countries between 1985 and 2001.

For six of the major lead-consuming countries (France, Germany, Italy, Japan, the United Kingdom, USA), detailed historical data are available from 1960 to 1990 (Tables 13–19). In this period, total consumption of lead reported by these countries rose from 2.06 to 2.94 million tonnes, an overall increase of 43% and an average annual increase of 1.2%. During those three decades, however, there were marked changes in the rates of lead consumption. These included: (1) the rapid expansion of consumption during the 1960s and early 1970s leading to peak levels in 1973 prior to the onset of the first world energy crisis; (2) the steep reduction in 1974–75 and the subsequent revival in 1977–79, with lead consumption recovering to its 1973 level; (3) the decrease in 1980–82 during the second energy crisis; and (4) the sustained growth from 1983 until 1990 in the industrialized world as a whole, supported by rapid advances in some of the newly-industrializing countries, but with much more restricted progress in the fully-industrialized countries where the rates of economic expansion and industrial activity slowed down compared with those previously achieved (International Lead and Zinc Study Group, 1992).

1.3.1 *Lead–acid batteries*

By far the largest single application of lead worldwide is in lead–acid batteries. The most common type of lead–acid battery consists of a heavy duty plastic box (normally polypropylene) containing grids made from a lead–antimony alloy (commonly containing 0.75–5% antimony) with minor additions of elements such as copper, arsenic, tin and selenium to improve grid properties. For the new generation of sealed, maintenance-free batteries, a range of lead–calcium–tin alloys is used. These contain up to 0.1% calcium and 0–0.5% tin. The tin-containing alloys are used in the positive grids to protect against corrosion. Grids are still manufactured in pairs on special casting machines, but production of grids in strip form by continuous casting or expansion of rolled sheet is becoming increasingly popular as it facilitates automation and minimizes the handling of plates. The spaces in the grids are filled with a paste consisting largely of lead dioxide. When immersed in sulfuric acid, these pasted grids (plates) form an electric cell that generates electricity from the chemical reactions that take place. The reactions require the presence of lead dioxide and lead metal and each cell produces a voltage of 2V. These reactions are reversible and the battery can therefore be recharged. A rechargeable cell is known as a secondary cell and provides a means of storing electricity. Lead is well suited for this application because of its specific conductivity and its resistance to corrosion. The addition of antimony or calcium gives the lead an increased hardness to resist the mechanical stresses within the battery caused, for example, by the natural vibration of road vehicles and by the chemical reactions taking place (Lead Development Association International, 2003e).

Table 10. Trends in total industrial consumption of refined lead

Year	Consumption (thousand tonnes) by geographical region[a]						
	A[b]	B	C	D[b]	E	F[b]	Total
1960	1152	19	986	204	65	654	3080
1965	1306	33	1229	270	70	762	3670
1970	1517	46	1488	360	72	1019	4502
1975	1403	76	1454	413	86	1310	4742
1980	1652	102	1476	600	85	1446	5361
1985	1614	98	1510	735	69	1470	5496
1990	2439	114	1648	1193	59	NRS	5454
1995	1948	112	2017	1718	84	NRS	5879
2000	2022	130	2332	1989	46	NRS	6519
2003	2030	154	2012	2471	45	NRS	6712

From International Lead and Zinc Study Group (1990, 2004)
NRS, not reported separately
[a] Data from the following countries:
A, Austria, Belgium, Denmark, Finland, France, Germany (the Federal Republic of Germany before reunification), Greece, Ireland, Italy, Netherlands, Norway, Portugal, Spain, Sweden, Switzerland, United Kingdom and former Yugoslavia
B, Algeria, Egypt, Morocco, South Africa, Tunisia and Zambia
C, Argentina, Brazil, Canada, Mexico, Peru, USA and Venezuela
D, India, Iran, Japan, Malaysia, Philippines, Republic of Korea, China (Province of Taiwan), Thailand and Turkey
E, Australia and New Zealand
F, Albania, Bulgaria, China, Cuba, former Czechoslovakia, Germany (the former German Democratic Republic), Hungary, People's Democratic Republic of Korea; Poland, Romania, former Soviet Union; values for Albania, Cuba, China, Germany (the former German Democratic Republic), Peoples' Democratic Republic of Korea, Romania and former Soviet Union are estimates.
[b] From 1990 onwards, data from countries in region F are included in region A (Albania, Bulgaria, Czech Republic, Hungary, Poland, the former German Democratic Republic, Poland, Romania, Estonia, Latvia, Lithuania, Belarus, Russian Federation and Ukraine) or in region D (all other former Soviet Republics, China, Cuba and People's Democratic Republic of Korea). Lead metal consumption for 1991 in the former Soviet Union was split as follows: Europe, 86%, Asia, 14%.

The most common form of lead–acid battery is the so-called SLI battery (starting, lighting and ignition) used in road vehicles such as cars and trucks. Another form, the traction battery, is used to power vehicles such as golf carts and airport support vehicles. Other uses of lead power include larger stationary batteries for stand-by emergency power storage in hospitals and other critical facilities, and for some electricity utilities to help meet peak power demands and to maintain a stable electricity supply (Lead Development Association International, 2003e).

Table 11. Total industrial lead consumption

Country or region	Consumption (thousand tonnes) in year			
	1985	1990	1996	2001
Australia	49.5	45.9	67.0	41.0
Austria	58.0	65.5	58.0	59.0
Belgium	66.8	67.7	50.6	40.3
Brazil	79.6	75.0	110.0	112.0
Canada	104.5	71.7	93.4	71.8
China	NA	NA	470.1	700.0
Czech Republic	NA	NA	25.0	80.0
Finland	22.0	13.4	3.5	2.0
France[a]	234.3	261.6	273.8	282.5
Germany[a]	348.2	375.3	331.0	392.6
India	51.3	51.8	85.0	127.0
Italy[a]	235.0	259.0	268.0	283.0
Japan	397.4	417.0	329.9	284.7
Mexico	90.6	66.8	141.0	205.0
Netherlands	45.1	65.0	57.0	30.0
New Zealand	8.6	8.0	7.0	5.0
Republic of Korea	81.0	150.0	289.8	314.7
Romania	NA	NA	22.0	20.0
Scandinavia[b]	55.6	36.3	49.0	13.0
South Africa	48.2	65.9	63.1	59.1
South-East Asia[c]	125.2	185.0	413.0	427.0
Spain	125.3	126.7	144.0	246.0
Switzerland	10.5	8.7	10.5	12.6
United Kingdom[a]	303.2	334.0	309.2	266.5
USA[a]	1148.3	1288.4	1554.4	1587.3
Total	3688.2	4038.7	5225.3	5662.1

From International Lead and Zinc Study Group (1992, 2003)
NA, not available
[a] Data for these countries include total metal usage in all forms, i.e. refined lead and alloys (lead content), plus re-melted lead recovered from secondary materials. Data for other countries include refined lead and alloys only.
[b] Denmark, Norway and Sweden
[c] China, Hong Kong Special Administrative Region, China (Province of Taiwan), Indonesia, Malaysia, Philippines and Singapore

Since 1960 the manufacture of lead–acid batteries has remained the largest single use of lead in nearly all countries, accounting for an ever-increasing percentage of total lead consumption (see Tables 12, 14 and 15) (International Lead and Zinc Study Group, 1992).

Table 12. Trends in uses of lead in selected countries[a]

Use	Percentage of total usage in year			
	1985	1990	1996	2001
Batteries	57.7	63.0	72.5	76.7
Cable sheathing	5.6	4.5	2.1	1.4
Rolled and extruded products[b]	7.6	7.7	5.9	6.0
Shot/ammunition	2.8	2.8	2.3	2.1
Alloys	4.2	3.3	3.2	2.5
Pigments and other compounds	14.2	12.8	10.0	8.1
Gasoline additives	3.7	2.1	0.9	0.4
Miscellaneous	4.2	3.8	3.3	2.8
Total	100.0	100.0	100.0	100.0

From International Lead and Zinc Study Group (1992, 2003)
[a] Countries include: Australia, Austria, Belgium, Brazil, Canada, China (Hong Kong Special Administrative Region), China (Province of Taiwan), Denmark, Finland, France, Germany, India, Indonesia, Italy, Japan, Malaysia, Mexico, Netherlands, New Zealand, Norway, Philippines, Republic of Korea, Singapore, South Africa, Spain, Sweden, Switzerland, United Kingdom and USA.
[b] Including lead sheet

Table 13. Trends in total lead consumption in six major consuming countries

Country	Consumption (thousand tonnes) in year			
	1960	1973	1979	1990
France	196	240	233	262
Germany	281	342	342	375
Italy	108	259	280	259
Japan	162	347	368	417
United Kingdom	385	364	336	334
USA	926	1398	1358	1288
Total	2058	2950	2917	2935

From International Lead and Zinc Study Group (1992)
The data include refined metal and direct use of lead in scrap form.

Table 14. Trends in principal uses of lead in six major consuming countries[a]

Use	Percentage of total use in year		
	1960	1979	1990
Batteries	27.7	50.8	64.4
Cable sheathing	17.9	5.9	3.8
Rolled/extruded products	18.0	7.7	7.8
Shot/ammunition	3.2	3.2	3.8
Alloys	10.5	6.7	3.5
Pigment/compounds	9.9	12.3	10.9
Gasoline additives	9.1	9.8	2.7
Miscellaneous	3.7	3.6	3.1
Total	100.0	100.0	100.0

From International Lead and Zinc Study Group (1992)
[a] France, Germany, Italy, Japan, United Kingdom and USA

Table 15. Trends in consumption of lead for batteries in six major consuming countries

Country	Consumption (thousand tonnes) in year			
	1960	1973	1979	1990
France	45.0	90.0	110.7	163.5
Germany[a]	73.2	132.9	158.3	195.2
Italy	25.5	68.0	93.0	113.2
Japan	30.0	163.1	191.8	294.6
United Kingdom	76.2	106.5	113.9	103.7
USA	320.4	698.0	814.4	1019.6
Total	570.3	1258.5	1481.2	1889.8

From International Lead and Zinc Study Group (1992)
[a] Excludes consumption by some independent producers of lead oxides for batteries.

Table 16. Trends in consumption of lead for rolled/ extruded products in six major consuming countries

Country	Consumption (thousand tonnes) in year			
	1960	1973	1979	1990
France	43.7	31.0	27.2	22.4
Germany	44.3	31.1	32.7	39.1
Italy	29.1	50.3	40.8	21.5
Japan	35.9	39.6	26.7	10.9
United Kingdom	88.0	57.7	48.9	98.6
USA	130.1	90.2	47.7	35.8
Total	371.1	299.9	224.0	228.3

From International Lead and Zinc Study Group (1992)

Table 17. Trend in consumption of lead for cable sheathing in six major consuming countries

Country	Consumption (thousand tonnes) in year			
	1960	1973	1979	1990
France	60.8	41.1	21.4	16.3
Germany	83.9	54.6	31.5	12.2
Italy	24.0	44.8	40.0	48.7
Japan	47.0	28.7	36.8	4.9
United Kingdom	97.0	45.8	26.6	10.4
USA	54.7	39.0	16.4	18.3
Total	367.4	254.0	172.7	110.8

From International Lead and Zinc Study Group (1992)

Table 18. Trends in consumption of lead for alloys in six major consuming countries

Country	Consumption (thousand tonnes) in year			
	1960	1973	1979	1990
France	17.3	14.8	9.3	3.2
Germany	22.7	22.8	16.5	9.0
Italy	6.0	6.0	5.7	3.5
Japan	7.1	24.2	18.3	18.7
United Kingdom	37.0	35.0	24.5	22.0
USA	125.3	128.8	120.0	46.4
Total	215.4	231.6	194.3	102.8

From International Lead and Zinc Study Group (1992)

Table 19. Trends in consumption of lead for pigments and compounds in six major consuming countries

Country	Consumption (thousand tonnes) in year			
	1960	1973	1979	1990
France	11.9	34.5	33.0	29.4
Germany	38.4	69.6	76.8	100.3
Italy	10.1	45.2	60.4	40.0
Japan	17.2	64.2	62.4	64.0
United Kingdom	35.9	38.8	34.1	28.6
USA	89.3	98.7	90.8	56.5
Total	202.8	351.0	357.5	318.8

From International Lead and Zinc Study Group (1992)

1.3.2 *Lead sheet*

The use of lead sheet has increased dramatically over recent years, particularly for the building industry. Lead sheet has been produced for decades by traditional wide lead mills in which lead slabs are fed through large drum-like rollers, sometimes several times, to produce lead sheets of the desired thickness. The traditional wide lead mill is being replaced by more sophisticated rolling mills producing coils of lead 1.2–1.5 m wide. Most lead sheets in building applications are between 1.3 and 2.2 mm thick, but sheets of 2.6–3.6 mm are used for roofing prestige buildings. Thick sheet alloys are rolled for applications such as anodes for electrowinning and thin foils are used for sound attenuation. A manufacturing technique other than milling is continuous casting in which a rotating, water-cooled drum is partly immersed in a bath of molten lead. The drum picks up a solid layer of lead, which is removed over a knife edge adjacent to the drum as it rotates. The thickness is controlled by varying the speed of rotation and the temperature of the drum (Lead Development Association International, 2003e).

In the building industry, most of the lead sheet (or strip) is used as flashings or weatherings to prevent water from penetrating, the remainder being used for roofing and cladding. By virtue of its resistance to chemical corrosion, lead sheet is also used for the lining of chemical treatment baths, acid plants and storage vessels. The high density of lead sheet and its 'limpness' make it a very effective material for reducing the transmission of sound through partitions and doors of comparatively lightweight construction. Often the lead sheet is bonded adhesively to plywood or to other building boards for convenience of handling. A particular advantage of the high density of lead is that only relatively thin layers are needed to suppress the transmission of sound (Lead Development Association International, 2003e).

Lead sheet is the principal element in the product category 'rolled and extruded products'. In many countries, the demand for rolled and extruded lead products declined in the 1960s and 1970s, due in part to a rapid decline in the use of lead pipe (see Tables 14 and 16). Nevertheless, in a number of countries (see Table 12), lead sheet remains the third largest use of lead at about 6% of the total reported consumption (International Lead and Zinc Study Group, 1992, 2003).

1.3.3 *Lead pipes*

Lead piping, once a substantial use in the 'rolled and extruded products' category, has been replaced progressively by copper tubes for the transport of domestic water and the supply of gas and by plastic tubing for disposal of wastewater. Lead pipes have not been used in new supplies of domestic water for about 30 years. However, due to their corrosion-resistant properties, they are still used for transport of corrosive chemicals at chemical plants. Also, lead pipe of appropriate composition is extruded for cutting into short-length 'sleeves' used in the jointing of lead-sheathed cables (see below) (International Lead and Zinc Study, 1992; Lead Development Association International, 2003e).

1.3.4 *Cable sheathing*

Because of its corrosion resistance when in contact with a wide range of industrial and marine environments, soils and chemicals, lead was one of the first materials to be used to provide an impervious sheath on electric cables. Lead can be applied to the cable core in unlimited lengths by extrusion at temperatures that do not damage the most sensitive conductors (optical fibres) or insulating materials (paper or plastics). Lead is pliable and withstands the coiling, uncoiling, handling and bending operations involved in the manufacturing and installation of the cable. A lead sheath can be readily soldered at low temperatures when cables need to be jointed or new cables installed. With modern screw-type continuous extruders, unjointed submarine power cables as long as 100 km have been produced (Lead Development Association International, 2003e).

Until 1960 sheathing of electrical cables was the largest single use of lead in many countries including France, Germany, Japan and the United Kingdom, representing 25–30% of total lead consumption in these four countries. It was used much less extensively in the USA where, during the late 1950s, lead was replaced by alternative materials, generally plastics, as the sheathing material for telephone cables. Since the mid-1960s, however, there has been a gradual decline in the use of lead for cable sheathing in most countries (Table 17). By 1990, lead consumption for cable sheathing had fallen to 4.5% of total consumption and, by 2001, to 1.4% (Table 12) (International Lead and Zinc Study Group, 1992, 2003).

1.3.5 *Lead alloys*

(*a*) *Lead–antimony alloys*

By far the largest use of lead–antimony alloys is in batteries. At one time, antimony contents of ~10% were common, but the current generation of lead–acid batteries has a much lower antimony content. Alloys with 1–12% antimony are used widely in the chemical industry for pumps and valves, and in radiation shielding both for lining the walls of X-ray rooms and for bricks to house radioactive sources in the nuclear industry. The addition of antimony to lead increases the hardness of the lead, and therefore its resistance to physical damage, without greatly reducing its corrosion resistance (Lead Development Association International, 2003e).

(*b*) *Solders*

Soldering is a method of joining materials, in which a special metal (solder) is applied in the molten state to wet two solid surfaces and join them on solidification. Solders are classified according to their working temperatures. Soft solders, which have the lowest melting-points, are largely lead–tin alloys with or without antimony, while fusible alloys contain various combinations of lead, tin, bismuth, cadmium and other low melting-point metals. Depending on the application, lead–tin solders may contain from a few per cent to more than 60% tin.

A substantial proportion of solder is used in electrical or electronic assemblies. The advances made in the electronics industry have required the development of fast and highly-automated methods of soldering. Printed circuit assemblies can be soldered by passing them across a standing wave of continuously-circulating molten solder (Lead Development Association International, 2003e).

The use of lead solder in plumbing has declined with the replacement of lead piping by copper tubing and, more recently, as a result of concerns of potential leaching of lead into water supplies. Similarly, concerns of possible danger to health have restricted the use of lead solders in the canning industry, formerly an important market.

(*c*) *Lead for radiation shielding*

Lead and its alloys in metallic form, and lead compounds, are used in various forms of radiation shielding. The shielding of containers for radioactive materials is usually metallic lead (see above). Radioactive materials in laboratories and hospitals are usually handled by remote control from a position of safety behind a wall of lead bricks. X-ray machines are normally installed in rooms lined with lead sheet; lead compounds are constituents of the glass used in shielding partitions to permit safe viewing; and lead powder is incorporated into plastic and rubber sheeting materials used for protective clothing (Lead Development Association International, 2003e).

(*d*) *Other uses of lead alloys*

A variety of lead alloys are produced for a wide range of applications in various industries. In the 1990s, these alloys accounted for 130–150 000 tonnes of lead used in industrialized countries (Table 18). However, the trend in this sector had been one of steady decline during the previous three decades (Table 14), as some uses have been overtaken by technological changes or have been restricted by health and environmental regulations. The use of terne metal (a thin tin–lead alloy coating) for corrosion protection, and the addition of lead to brass and bronze to assist in free machining, and in bearing metals to reduce friction and wear in machinery, have declined slowly due to competition from alternative materials such as aluminum and plastics. The market for type metal in the printing industry has largely disappeared as hot metal printing has been replaced by new technology. In the USA, this use peaked at 30 000 tonnes in 1965 but had fallen to 1–2000 tonnes by the mid-1980s and is similarly low in other developed countries (International Lead and Zinc Study Group, 1992).

1.3.6 *Lead pigments and compounds*

The market for lead pigments and compounds constitutes the second largest use of lead after lead–acid batteries. The market peaked in the mid-1980s, when over 500 000 tonnes of lead were used in lead pigments and compounds, mainly by the plastics, glass and ceramics industries, and accounting for 14% of total lead consumption (Table 14). Since then these uses have been restricted by health and environmental concerns while still remaining the second largest use of lead (8% of total lead consumption) (Table 12).

Besides the six major consuming countries (Table 19), pigments and compounds are also the second most important use of lead in other countries including Brazil, Canada, the Republic of Korea, South Africa, Spain and countries of South-East Asia (International Lead and Zinc Study Group, 1992, 2003).

(*a*) *Lead pigments*

The use of lead in paints for domestic purposes and in some commercial and industrial applications is now severely restricted or banned in view of the potential health risks caused by exposure to weathered or flaking paint. However, lead tetraoxide (Pb_3O_4) still retains some of its traditional importance for rust-inhibiting priming paints applied directly to iron and steel in view of its anti-corrosion properties, but faces growing competition from zinc-rich paints containing zinc dust and zinc chromate. The use of lead carbonate (white lead) in decorative paints has been phased out. Calcium plumbate-based paints are effective on galvanized steel. Lead chromate (yellow) and lead molybdate (red orange) are still used in plastics and to a lesser extent in paints. Lead chromate is used extensively as the yellow pigment in road markings and signs, which are now commonplace in most European countries and in North America (Lead Development Association International, 2003e).

(*b*) *Lead stabilizers for polyvinyl chloride (PVC)*

Lead compounds are used in both rigid and plasticized PVC to extend the temperature range at which PVC can be processed without degradation. In the building industry, the widespread adoption of PVC materials for corrosion-resistant piping and guttering in industrial facilities, for potable water piping (lead content, < 1%), and for windows and door frames provides a major market for lead sulfate and lead carbonate as stabilizers to prevent degrading of PVC during processing and when exposed to ultraviolet light. However, concerns over potential health hazards are limiting the use of lead in PVC water piping in some countries. Dibasic lead phosphite also has the property of protecting materials from degradation by ultraviolet light. Normal and dibasic lead stearates are incorporated as lubricants. All these compounds are white pigments that cannot be used when clear or translucent articles are required (International Lead and Zinc Study Group, 1992; Lead Development Association International, 2003e). The levels of lead in 16 different PVC pipes used for water supplies in Bangladesh were found to be in the range of 1.1–6.5 mg/g (Hadi *et al.*, 1996).

(*c*) *Lead in glass*

Decorative lead crystal glass was developed in England in the seventeenth century. Normally added in the form of lead monoxide (PbO) at 24–36%, lead adds lustre, density and brilliance to the glass. Its attractiveness is further enhanced by decorative patterns that can be cut on the surface and by the characteristic ring associated with lead crystal. There is now a substantial market for a cheaper form of 'semi-crystal' containing 14–24% lead oxide, and such glasses are usually moulded with the decorative pattern rather than being hand-cut later. Lead is also used in optical glass (e.g. telescopes, binoculars), ophthalmic glass (e.g. spectacles), electrical glass (e.g. lamp tubing, cathode ray tubes) and radiation protection glass (e.g. for windows in remote-handling boxes, television tubes) (Lead Development Association International, 2003e).

(*d*) *Lead for ceramics*

Lead is used in a wide range of glaze formulations for items such as tableware (earthenware and china), wall and floor tiles, porcelain and sanitary-ware and electrical transistors and transducers. The lead compounds used are mainly lead monoxide (litharge, PbO), lead tetraoxide and lead silicates. The properties offered by lead compounds are low melting-points and wide softening ranges, low surface tension, good electrical properties and a hard-wearing and impervious finish. Lead compounds are also used in the formulation of enamels used on metals and glass.

Another important application for lead compounds is in a range of ceramics (other than the glazes) used in the electronics industry. Typical of these are piezoelectric materials such as the lead zirconate/lead titanate range of compositions known generally as PZI. These materials have a wide range of applications, such as spark generators, sensors, electrical filters, gramophone pick-ups and sound generators (International Lead and Zinc Study Group, 1992; Lead Development Association International, 2003e).

1.3.7 *Gasoline additives*

Tetraethyl and tetramethyl lead have been used as anti-knock additives in gasoline, at concentrations up to 0.84 g/L, as an economic method of raising the 'octane rating' to provide the grade of gasoline needed for the efficient operation of internal combustion engines of high compression ratio (Thomas *et al.*, 1999). However, increasing recognition of the potential health effects from exposure to lead has led to the reformulation of gasoline and the removal of lead additives. In addition, lead in gasoline is incompatible with the catalytic converters used in modern cars to control nitrogen oxides, hydrocarbons and other 'smog'-producing agents. The use of lead in gasoline in the USA has been phased out gradually since the mid-1970s, and moves to phase it out in the European Community began in the early 1980s. Since 1977 in the USA and 1991 in Europe, all new cars are required to run on unleaded gasoline. By the end of 1999, forty countries or regions had banned the use of lead in gasoline (Table 20), although it is still permitted in some of these countries for certain off-road and marine vehicles and for general aviation aircraft (Smith, 2002). Numerous other countries are planning the phase-out of lead in gasoline in the near future. About 79% of all gasoline sold in the world in the late 1990s was unleaded (International Lead Management Center, 1999). The market for tetraethyl and tetramethyl lead has declined considerably (Table 21) and will continue to do so (Lead Development

Table 20. Countries or regions that had phased out the use of lead in gasoline[a] by the end of 1999

Argentina	Finland	Netherlands
Austria	Germany	New Zealand
Bahamas	Guam	Nicaragua
Bangladesh	Guatemala	Norway
Belize	Haiti	Portugal
Bermuda	Honduras	Puerto Rico
Bolivia	Hong Kong SAR	Republic of Korea
Brazil	Hungary	Singapore
Canada	Iceland	Slovakia
Colombia	Japan	Sweden
Costa Rica	Luxembourg	Thailand
Denmark	Malaysia	USA
Dominican Republic	Mexico	US Virgin Islands
El Salvador		

From International Lead Management Center (1999)
[a] See Section 1.3.7 for permitted uses of leaded gasoline.

Table 21. Trends in consumption of lead for gasoline additives in five major consuming countries

Country	Consumption (thousand tonnes) in year			
	1960	1973	1979	1990
France	6.1	13.5	15.1	9.8
Germany	NA	9.4	10.8	NA
Italy	4.8	11.8	13.0	3.7
United Kingdom	27.1	54.4	58.9	45.1
USA	148.6	248.9	186.9	20.7
Total	186.6	338.0	284.7	79.3

From International Lead and Zinc Study Group (1992)
NA, not available

Association International, 2003e). In 2001, less than 0.5% of lead consumption was for gasoline additives (Table 12) (International Lead and Zinc Study Group, 2003).

1.3.8 *Miscellaneous uses*

About 150 000 tonnes of lead are employed each year in a variety of other uses, of which about 100 000 tonnes are consumed in the production of lead shot and ammunition in the major consuming countries (excluding Japan where this use is not reported separately). Globally, this use has remained relatively stable since the 1960s, at around 3–4% of total lead consumption (Tables 12 and 14).

Lead cames have long been a feature of stained-glass windows in churches and cathedrals. They consist of H-shaped sections of lead which hold together the individual pieces of glass. They are now being used more widely in modern homes both in the traditional way and in the form of self-adhesive strips stuck on to a larger piece of glass to simulate an integral came.

Lead weights for fishing have been largely phased out but lead stampings, pressings and castings are widely used for many weighting applications, for example curtain weights, wheel balance weights, weights for analytical instruments and yacht keels.

Lead wool is made by scratching fine strands from the surface of a lead disc. It is used for the caulking of joints in large pipes like gas mains and in some specialty batteries.

Lead-clad steel is a composite material manufactured by cold rolling lead sheet onto sheet steel that has been pretreated with a terne plate. A strong metallurgical bond is formed between the lead and the steel, which provides a material that combines the physical and chemical properties of lead with the mechanical properties of steel. Although primarily aimed at the sound-insulation market, lead-clad steel has also found use in radiation shielding and in the cladding of buildings.

Lead powder is incorporated into a plasticizer to form sheets of lead-loaded plastic. This material is used to make radiation-protective clothing and aprons for the medical, scientific and nuclear industries (see Section 1.4.5.c). It also has sound-insulating properties. Lead powder is also used as the basis for some corrosion-resistant paints (see Section 1.4.6).

Smaller amounts of lead are used in galvanizing, annealing and plating (International Lead and Zinc Study Group, 1992; Lead Development Association International, 2003e).

1.4 Occurrence

1.4.1 *Environmental occurrence*

Lead was one of the first metals used by man; there is evidence that it has been used for approximately 6000 years (Hunter, 1978). As a result, although both natural and anthropogenic processes are responsible for the distribution of lead throughout the environment, anthropogenic releases of lead are predominant. Industrial releases to soil from nonferrous smelters, battery plants, chemical plants, and disturbance of older structures containing lead-based paints are major contributors to total lead releases. Lead is transferred continuously between air, water, and soil by natural chemical and physical processes such as weathering, run-off, precipitation, dry deposition of dust, and stream/river flow; however, soil and sediments appear to be important sinks for lead. Lead is extremely persistent in both water and soil. Direct application of lead-contaminated sludge as fertilizers, and residues of lead arsenate used in agriculture, can also lead to the contamination of soil, sediments, surface water and ground water. In countries where leaded gasoline is still used, the major air emission of lead is from mobile and stationary sources of combustion. Besides environmental exposures, exposure to lead may arise from sources such as foods or beverages stored, cooked or served in lead-containing containers, food growing on contaminated soils, and traditional remedies, cosmetics and other lead-containing products.

The ubiquity of lead in the environment has resulted in present-day body burdens that are estimated to be 1000 times those found in humans uncontaminated by anthropogenic lead uses (Patterson *et al.*, 1991), but exposures have decreased substantially over the past 10–30 years in countries where control measures have been implemented.

The estimated contributions of the common sources and routes of lead exposure to total lead intake vary from country to country and over time. In 1990, the estimated daily intake of lead from consumption of food, water and beverages in the USA ranged from 2 to 9 µg/day for various age groups and was approximately 4 µg/day for children 2 years of age and younger (ATSDR, 1999). For many young children, the most important source of lead exposure is through ingestion of paint chips and leaded dusts and soils released from ageing painted surfaces or during renovation and remodeling (CDC, 1997a; Lanphear *et al.*, 1998). Compared with nonsmokers, smokers have an additional lead intake of approximately 6 µg/day, based on an estimated exposure of 14 µg/day and absorption of 30–50% of the inhaled lead into the bloodstream (IARC, 2004a).

Lead is absorbed into the body via inhalation and ingestion and, to a limited extent, through the skin. The uptake of inhaled or ingested lead is dependent on the type of lead compound involved, particle size, site of contact within the body, acidity of the body fluid at that site, and physiological status of the individual (see Section 4.1).

(*a*) *Natural occurrence*

Lead occurs naturally in the earth's crust in trace quantities at a concentration of approximately 8–20 mg/kg (Rudnick & Fountain, 1995; Taylor & McLennan, 1995). Metallic lead occurs in nature, but it is rare. The most important lead ore is *galena* (PbS). *Anglesite* ($PbSO_4$), *cerussite* ($PbCO_3$) and *minium* (Pb_3O_4) are other common lead minerals. Small amounts of lead reach the surface environment through natural weathering processes and volcanic emissions, thus giving a baseline environmental exposure. However, the abundant and widespread presence of lead in our current environment is largely a result of anthropogenic activity.

(*b*) *Air and dust*

Lead is released into the air by natural processes such as volcanic activity, forest fires, weathering of the earth's crust and radioactive decay from radon (WHO, 1995). However, these natural contributions are of relatively minor consequence. The vast majority of lead in the atmosphere results from human activity. Globally, the main source of lead in air has been exhaust from motor vehicles using leaded gasoline (see also Section 1.4.1(*f*)). Release of lead also occurs during lead smelting and refining, the manufacture of goods, and the incineration of municipal and medical wastes (ATSDR, 1999). Almost all lead in air is bound to fine particles of less than 1 µm diameter, although some may be solubilized in acid aerosol droplets. The size of these particles varies with the source and with the age of the particle from the time of emission (US EPA, 1986a; WHO, 1995).

Concentrations of lead in ambient air range from 76×10^{-6} μg/m³ in remote areas such as Antarctica (Maenhaut *et al.*, 1979), to 0.2 μg/m³ in rural areas in Chile (Frenz *et al.*, 1997) and to > 120 μg/m³ near stationary sources such as smelters (Nambi *et al.*, 1997). Tables 22–27 show examples of lead concentrations in air and dust worldwide by geographic region. A few studies are detailed below according to the main source of airborne lead.

Trends in emissions of lead in air in the USA have continued to fall since the late 1970s from both point sources (from 2.9 μg/m³ in 1979 to 0.4 μg/m³ in 1988) and urban sites (from 0.8 μg/m³ in 1979 to 0.1 μg/m³ in 1988). The large decrease in emissions from point sources resulted from the use of emission controls in industrial processes as well as automotive controls; the decrease in emissions from urban sites was primarily the result of the decreased use of leaded gasoline (ATSDR, 1999). Between 1976 and 1995, overall ambient air concentrations of lead in the USA declined by 97% (US EPA, 1996a). Lead concentrations in urban and suburban air in the USA (maximum quarterly mean concentrations) decreased between 1986 and 1995 from 0.18 μg/m³ to 0.04 μg/m³; rural air concentrations of lead during the same period were typically 3- to 5-fold lower (US EPA, 1996a). In remote sites, air lead concentrations as low as 0.001 μg/m³ have been reported (Eldred & Cahill, 1994).

Urban air lead concentrations are typically between 0.15 and 0.5 μg/m³ in most European cities (WHO, 2000a). In Bulgaria, the Czech Republic, Hungary, Poland, Romania, Slovakia and Slovenia, exposure to lead is primarily through airborne lead. It is estimated that in congested urban areas 90% of this is due to leaded gasoline. In 1998, there was a wide range in use of unleaded gasoline for automobiles, from 100% in Slovakia to 5–7% in Bulgaria and Romania. Table 22 illustrates improvements in air quality during the 1990s through a concerted effort by the countries to phase out the use of leaded gasoline (Regional Environmental Center for Central and Eastern Europe, 1998).

Lead concentration in the thoracic fraction of atmospheric particulate matter (PM_{10}) — that part of the inspirable fraction that penetrates into the respiratory tract below the larynx — in the ambient air of Delhi, India, in 1998, was reported to range from 0.1 to 2 μg/m³ (Table 26). Principal component analysis identified three major sources, namely vehicle emissions, industrial emissions and soil resuspension (Balachandran *et al.*, 2000). Samples collected from high-exposure areas of Mumbai, India, had higher lead concentrations than those collected in other high-exposure areas of the world including Beijing (China), Stockholm (Sweden) and Zagreb (Serbia and Montenegro) (Parikh *et al.*, 1999). A recent report of the Central Pollution Control Board (2001–2002) found concentrations of lead in air in Mumbai, India, to be on the decline. In fact, the introduction of unleaded petrol reduced lead concentrations in ambient air by about half in seven sites throughout India (Central Pollution Control Board, 1998–99).

In Semarang, Indonesia, mean urban airborne lead concentrations were found to be 0.35 μg/m³ in a highway zone, 0.95 μg/m³ in a residential zone (mainly due to solid-waste

Table 22. Lead concentrations in ambient air in central and eastern Europe

Country	Location	Mean concentration (µg/m³)[a] by year						
		1990	1991	1992	1993	1994	1995	1996
Bulgaria	Sofia	0.3	0.3	0.3	0.3	0.2	0.2	
	Pernik	0.5	0.4	0.4	0.2	0.2	0.4	
	Plovdiv	0.6	0.5	0.4	0.3	0.2	0.3	
	Kardjali	1.2	1.2	1.2	0.9	0.9	0.7	
Czech Republic[b]	Prague				0.06	0.04	0.01	
	Pribram				0.08	0.06	0.02	
	Usti n. Labem				0.06	0.04	0.03	
	Brno				0.07	0.08	0.05	
	Ostrava				0.05	0.08	0.05	
Hungary	Budapest				*0.20*	*0.22*	*0.22*	*0.19*
	Pecs				*0.42*	*0.44*	*0.25*	*0.21*
	Miskolc						*0.18*	*0.12*
	Debrecen				*0.56*	*0.30*	*0.27*	*0.28*
Poland[c]	Katowice	*0.73*	*0.90*	*1.16*	*0.68*	*0.68*	*0.78*	*0.58*
	Chorzuw	*2.69*	*0.85*	*0.76*	*0.44*	*0.44*	*0.81*	*1.00*
	Pszczyna	*0.64*	*0.55*	*0.45*	*0.49*	*0.49*	*0.62*	*0.16*
	Lodz		*1.16*	*1.48*	*0.87*	*0.87*	*1.85*	*0.55*
Romania	Copsa Mica	*30.30*	*21.30*	*16.07*	*42.20*	*18.91*	*12.70*	
	Bucuresti	*60.58*	*60.58*	*70.65*			*7.63*	
	Bala Mare	*5.45*	*8.20*	*97.50*	*15.07*	*16.12*	*13.34*	
	Medias	*10.15*	*21.80*	*7.20*	*4.18*	*9.99*	*14.70*	
	Zlatna	*22.72*	*27.10*	*10.00*	*14.00*	*9.44*	*11.46*	
Slovakia	Bratislava	0.11	0.09	0.11	0.10	0.05	0.06	
	B. Bystrica	0.11	0.09	0.08	0.05	0.03	0.03	
	Ruzomberok	0.14	0.05	0.06	0.03	0.04	0.02	
	Richnava	0.50	0.53	0.46	0.14	0.14	0.21	
Slovenia	Trbovlje		*0.90*	*0.70*	*0.30*			
	Zagorje		*1.50*	*0.70*	*0.30*			
	Hrastnik		*0.25*	*0.45*	*0.10*			

From Regional Environmental Center for Central and Eastern Europe (1998)
[a] Italicized text denotes short-term maximal concentration.
[b] Annual geometric means
[c] Maximum average daily concentration

Table 23. Lead concentration in outdoor air in Latin America and the Caribbean

Country	Location	Year of study	Period covered	Concentration ($\mu g/m^3$) mean or range of means	Reference
Bolivia	La Paz	NR	NR	1.1	Romieu *et al.* (1997)
Brazil	S. Paulo Osasco S. Caetano do Sul	1985 1985 1985	Annual average Annual average Annual average	0.39 0.16 0.31	Romieu *et al.* (1997)
	Santo Amaro, Bahia, near smelter	1989	4-day		Tavares (1990)
	at 526 m			2.8	
	at 955 m			0.13	
	S. Francisco Conde, Bahia (downwind of oil refinery)	July 1994[a] Jan. 1995	5-day	0.029 0.0051	Tavares (1996a)
	Lamarao de Passé, Bahia (downwind of petrochemical complex)	July 1994 Jan. 1995	5-day	0.0162 0.0054	
	Itacimirim/Praia do Forte, Bahia (Atlantic air masses)	July 1994 Jan. 1995	5-day	0.0015 0.00025	
Chile	San Felipe	1996	NR	0.19	Frenz *et al.* (1997)
	NS	1990	Annual average	1.1	Romieu *et al.* (1997)
Colombia	Bogota	1990	3-month average	3.0	Romieu *et al.* (1997)
Guatemala	Tegucigalpa NS	NR 1994	NR Annual average	0.18 0.17	Romieu *et al.* (1997)
Honduras	NS NS	1994 1994	Annual average 3-month average	1.11 1.83	Romieu *et al.* (1997)
Mexico	Mexico City	1988 1990 1994	3-month average	0.34–0.24 1.08–1.47 0.24–0.37	Romieu *et al.* (1997)
		1988 1990 1994	Annual average	1.95 1.23 0.28	
		1995	24-h average	0.54	

Table 23 (contd)

Country	Location	Year of study	Period covered	Concentration (µg/m[3]) mean or range of means	Reference
Peru	NS	1980	3-month average	1.8	Romieu *et al.* (1997)
		1985		1.9	
		1990		2.2	
		1994		2.1	
		1980	Annual average	1.7	
		1985		1.5	
		1990		1.6	
		1994		1.7	
Venezuela	Caracas	1982	Annual average	4.5	Romieu *et al.* (1997)
		1986		2.6	
		1990		1.9	
		1994		1.6	

NR, not reported; NS, not stated
[a] July is in wet season whereas January is during the dry season.

Table 24. Lead concentration in indoor dust in Latin America and the Caribbean

Country	Location	Year(s) of study	Source of contamination	Concentration (µg/g) mean ± SD or range of means	Reference
Mexico	Cd. Juarez, Chihuahua	1974	Lead smelter		Ordóñez *et al.* (2003)
			< 1.6 km	1322 ± 930	
			1.6–4 km	220	
	Villa de la Paz	NR	Mining	955 (range, 220–5190)	Yáñez *et al.* (2003)
	Mexico City	1983	Multiple urban	587 ± 303	Bruaux & Svartengren (1985)
Venezuela	Caracas (day-care centre)	1997–98	Urban	999–1707	Fernández *et al.* (2003)

NR, not reported; SD, standard deviation

Table 25. Lead concentrations in outdoor air and dust in Africa

Country	Location	Year(s) of study	Source of contamination	Concentration (µg/m³)[a] mean or range of means (range)	Reference
Egypt	Cairo	1983–84	Town centre	3.0	Ali *et al.* (1986)
			Residential/industrial	1.3	
			Residential district	1.4	
			Suburban district	0.6	
			Commercial	2.2	
	Cairo	NR	Industrial district	2	Hindy *et al.* (1987); Nriagu (1992)
Nigeria	Lagos	1981	Urban setting	770–1820 µg/g[b,c]	Ajayi & Kamson (1983)
		1991	Urban traffic	51–1180 µg/g[b]	Ogunsola *et al.* (1994a)
South Africa	Cape Town	NR	High traffic	1.5 (1.3–2.1)	von Schirnding *et al.* (1991a)
			Low traffic	0.8 (0.4–0.9)	
			High traffic	2900–3620[b]	
			Low traffic	410–2580[b]	
	KwaZulu/ Natal	1995	Industrial/highway	1.84	Nriagu *et al.* (1996a)
			Commercial	0.86	
			Park/beach	0.56	
			Residential	0.44	
			Rural	< 0.03	
	8 cities	1993–95	Urban setting	0.36–1.1	Nriagu *et al.* (1996b)
Zambia	Kasanda	1973–74	NR	10 (5–145)	Nriagu (1992)

Adapted from Nriagu (1992)
NR, not reported
[a] Unless specified otherwise
[b] Lead concentrations in dust
[c] Median values

Table 26. Lead concentrations in outdoor air and dust in Asia

Country	Location	Year(s) of study	Concentration (ng/m^3) mean or range of means (range)	Reference
China	Beijing and Shanghai	1984–97	60–980	Zhang, Z.-W. *et al.* (1998)[b]
	Provincial capitals		30–13 700	
	Other regions		8–2800	
	Beijing		21–318	Parikh *et al.* (1999)
	Taiyuan			Yang & Ma (1997)
	Winter		490–1125	
	Summer		115–504	
China (Province of Taiwan)	Tainan		180	[Environment Protection Administration ROC (1991)]
India	Delhi	1998	100–2000	Balachandran *et al.* (2000)
	Delhi	2000	590	Central Pollution Control Board (2001–2002)
		2001	550	
	Kolkata (road dust)[c]		536 μg/g	Chatterjee & Banerjee (1999)
	Mumbai		82–605 (31–1040)	Khandekar *et al.* (1984)
	Mumbai		30–440	Raghunath *et al.* (1997)
	Mumbai			Nambi *et al.* (1997)
	Industrial		500–120 000	
	Rural		110	
	Mumbai			Parikh *et al.* (1999)
	High-exposure area		432.4 (131–864)	
	Low-exposure area		268.2 (147–476)	
	Mumbai	1984–96		Tripathi *et al.* (2001)
	Urban		100–1120	
	Industrial		1180–4120	
	Nagpur	1996	42–65	Patel *et al.* (2001)
	7 cities	1980	60–310	Sadasivan *et al.* (1987)
	Whole country	1994	11 000	Gupta & Dogra (2002)
Indonesia	Semarang			Browne *et al.* (1999)
	Urban		350–990	
	Industrial		8410	
Japan	Tokyo and Kyoto	1996–97	15–81	Environment Agency, Japan (1997)

Table 26 (contd)

Country	Location	Year(s) of study	Concentration (ng/m^3) mean or range of means (range)	Reference
Korea	Pusan		902–1596	[Moon & Lee (1992)]
	Seoul	1984–93	100–1500[d]	Lee *et al.* (1994)
	Seoul	1986–94	22–1070	Reviewed by Moon & Ikeda (1996)
	Pusan	1990	1310 (210–2870)	Cho *et al.* (1992)
Malaysia	Kuala Lumpur		30–462	[Hisham & Pertanika (1995)]
	Kuala Lumpur (urban)		95	Hashim *et al.* (2000)
	Kemaman (semiurban)		27	
	Setiu (rural)		15	
Pakistan[c]	Karachi		7.9–101.8 μg/g	Rahbar *et al.* (2002)
Philippines	Whole country	1993	600–1300	Environmental Management Bureau (1996)
		1994	300–500	
	Manila	1994	300–1200[d]	
		1995	200–800[d]	
Saudi Arabia	Riyadh			Al-Saleh (1998)
	High traffic		3200	
	Residential		720	
Thailand	Bangkok		210–390	[Pollution Control Department (1996)]

Updated from Ikeda *et al.* (2000a)
[a] Unless specified otherwise
[b] Review of 15 reports published primarily in China between 1984 and 1997
[c] Lead concentration in dust
[d] Values read from graphs
References in square brackets could not be retrieved as original papers.

Table 27. Lead concentrations in outdoor air in Japan, 1996–97, as monitored in 16 monitoring stations

Statistical parameter	Monthly average concentration (ng/m^3)												
	1996									1997			
	Apr.	May	June	July	Aug.	Sept.	Oct.	Nov.	Dec.	Jan.	Feb.	March	Average[b]
AM[a]	54.9	56.3	51.1	40.3	34.9	44.2	52.4	62.2	73.5	56.5	49.5	55.3	51.3
ASD[a]	28.0	23.6	24.3	21.1	13.9	24.9	28.0	31.5	34.2	26.6	23.0	21.3	23.1
Min	16	< 10	< 10	< 10	< 10	11	12	16	20	14	15	19	13
Max	110	100	84	81	59	85	99	120	130	100	77	87	81
GM[a]													45.0
GSD[a]													1.78

From Environment Agency, Japan (1997)

AM, arithmetic mean; ASD, arithmetic standard deviation; min, minimum; max, maximum; GM, geometric mean; GSD, geometric standard deviation

[a] Values calculated by the Working Group; values < 10 were not included in the calculations.

[b] Mean, standard deviation, min. and max. of local annual arithmetic means among the 16 stations

burning) and 0.99 μg/m^3 in a commercial zone. Airborne lead concentrations of 8.41 μg/m^3 were recorded in an industrial area; values of this magnitude had not been reported previously in Indonesia (Browne *et al.*, 1999).

After leaded gasoline, lead mining and the smelting and refining of both primary and secondary lead are the next highest sources of lead emissions that can cause contamination of the nearby environment. The nature and extent of contamination depend on many factors, including the level of production, the effectiveness of emission controls, climate, topography and other local factors. Concentrations are usually highest within 3 km of the point source (US EPA, 1989, cited by WHO, 1995). For example, near a smelter in Santo Amaro, Bahia, Brazil, 4-day average values in 1989 of 2.8 ± 1.0 μg/m^3 (range, 1.8–3.9 μg/m^3) were reported 526 m from the smelter chimney in one direction and 0.13 ± 0.06 μg/m^3 (range, 0.08–0.22 μg/m^3) 955 m in the opposite direction (see Table 23; Tavares, 1990). A report from China found that lead concentrations in ambient air, plants and soil increased proportionally with proximity to a large primary smelter; air lead concentrations were 1.3 μg/m^3 at 1000 m from the source and 60 μg/m^3 at 50 m from the source (Wang, 1984). Some earlier studies have shown air pollution and soil contamination as far as 10 km from lead smelters (Djuric *et al.*, 1971; Landrigan *et al.*, 1975a).

A survey conducted in the vicinity of three lead industries in Maharashtra, India, showed the highest measured concentration of lead in air of 120 μg/m^3 in a residential area 200 m from one of the industries (see Table 26; Nambi *et al.,* 1997).

High concentrations of lead in household dust in the vicinity of lead smelters or mining activity, or from vehicles using leaded gasoline, have been reported (see Tables 24, 25 and 26). Lead concentrations in dust inside houses located in the vicinity of a lead smelter at Cd. Juarez, Chihuahua, Mexico, increased from 220 μg/g at 4 km to 1322 μg/g at less than 1.6 km from the smelter (Ordóñez *et al.*, 2003). An international study coordinated by WHO found a mean lead concentration (± standard deviation) in indoor dust in Mexico City of 587 ± 303 μg/g, compared with 440 ± 263 μg/g and 281 ± 500 μg/g in Sweden and Belgium, respectively (Bruaux & Svartengren, 1985). In 1997–98 lead concentrations of floor dust in day-care centres in Caracas, Venezuela, ranged from 999 to 1707 μg/g (Fernández *et al.*, 2003).

Data on lead in air in South America are scarce, and refer only to total lead in suspended particles. One study of lead concentrations in incoming Atlantic air masses reaching the north-eastern Brazilian coast in 1994–95 showed concentrations of 1.5 ng/m^3 during the rainy season (April–August) and of 0.25 ng/m^3 during the dry season (September–March) (see Table 23; Tavares, 1996a).

Biomass burning, which takes place during the dry season both for forest clearance and for agricultural purposes, can be an important source of lead in rural environments with otherwise low concentrations. Measurements in the Amazon forest during the wet season (September–March) showed lead concentrations of 0.33–0.61 ng/m^3 in particles smaller than 2.5 μm and 0.26–0.50 ng/m^3 in particles 2.5–10 μm in size; corresponding values during the dry season (June–September) were 0.73 ng/m^3 and 0.46 ng/m^3, respectively (Artaxo *et al.*, 1990).

Coal contains small amounts of lead, and fly ash from coal combustion and refuse incineration can leach substantial amounts of lead into ambient air (Wadge & Hutton, 1987). In an urban area of Taiwan, China, where the winter is cold, lead concentrations in air were reported to be about three times higher in winter (0.49–1.13 μg/m³) than in summer (0.12–0.50 μg/m³), due to use of lead-containing coal for heating (Yang & Ma, 1997). Surveys of lead in air in seven cities in India indicated concentrations ranging from 0.06 ± 0.02 μg/m³ in Coimbatore to 0.31 ± 0.10 μg/m³ in Kanpur (Sadasivan *et al.,* 1987). In addition to automobile exhaust, increased fuel burning in the winter and open burning of refuse were identified as sources of lead contamination (Table 26). In contrast, lead air concentrations in Japan in 1996–97 averaged 50 ng/m³ and little seasonal variation was observed (Table 27).

Lead concentrations in indoor air are affected by the presence of smokers, air conditioning and lead-painted surfaces. Two studies conducted in the Netherlands and the United Kingdom showed that air lead concentrations inside dwellings where there is no major internal lead source were highly correlated with those outside and averaged approximately 60% of those in the external air immediately outside the house (Diemel *et al.*, 1981; Davies *et al.*, 1987).

(*c*) *Water*

Lead enters groundwater from natural weathering of rocks and soil, indirectly from atmospheric fallout and directly from industrial sources. Lead can enter freshwater bodies from municipal sewage, from harbour activities and from lead storage sites and production plants, particularly mining and smelting. In local aquatic environments, pollution can also result from leaching of lead from lead shot, shotgun cartridges and fishing weights (WHO, 1995). The concentration of lead in surface water is highly variable depending upon the sources of pollution, the lead content of sediments and the characteristics of the system (pH, temperature). An additional and distinct hazard to the water supply is the use of lead piping or lead solder in plumbing systems. Water with low pH and low concentrations of dissolved salts (referred to as aggressive or corrosive water) can leach substantial quantities of lead from pipes, solder and fixtures (ASTDR, 1999). Lead-lined reservoirs, cisterns and water tanks can be a major source of lead contamination of drinking-water.

Lead concentrations in surface water, groundwater and tap-water in different geographical regions of the world are presented in Tables 28–31. A few examples are detailed below, according to the type of water analysed.

Seawater generally contains low levels of lead. It was estimated that lead concentrations in the ocean were 0.0005 μg/L in the pre-industrial era and around 0.005 μg/L in the late 1970s (US EPA, 1982).

Concentrations of lead in surface water and groundwater throughout the USA typically range between 5 and 30 μg/L and between 1 and 100 μg/L, respectively, although concentrations as high as 890 μg/L have been measured (US EPA, 1986a). The mean concentration of lead measured at nearly 40 000 surface-water stations throughout the

Table 28. Lead concentrations in water in Latin America and the Caribbean

Country	Location	Year of study	Source of contamination	Concentration (µg/L) mean (range)	Reference
Argentina	La Plata river, Buenos Aires		Industry, sewage, harbour activities		Verrengia Guerrero & Kesten (1994)
	Port	1989		28.1 (2.4–58.6)	
	Fishing Club	1989		11.3 (9.9–16.4)	
Bolivia	Pilcomayo river (at Potosi)	1999	Mine tailings	1399 (911–2111)	Smolders *et al.* (2003)
	Tarapaya river	1999	Mine tailings	2291 (1101–3980)	
	Cachi Mayu	1999	No specific source	1.0 (0.6–1.7)	
Brazil	Ribeira do Iguape river	1994	NR	< 20–70	Romieu *et al.* (1997)
	Sao Paulo State	1994	NR	2.8	
Chile	Antofagasta (household)	1998	Lead storage site	Max. 170	Sepúlveda *et al.* (2000)
Mexico	Drinking-water	1983	No specific source	2 ± 1 (1–3)	Bruaux & Svartengren (1985)
Uruguay	Tap-water	1992	Lead pipes	15 (0.2–230)	Schütz *et al.* (1997)

NR, not reported; max., maximum concentration (µg/L)

Table 29. Lead concentrations in fresh water, seawater and sediment in the Canary Islands, Egypt and Nigeria

Country	Location	Type of water/ sediment	Concentration mean or range of means (range)	Reference
Canary Islands (Spain)	Santa Cruz	Seawater	1.4–11.3 μg/L (0.42–116.9)	Díaz *et al.* (1990)
Egypt	Lake Nubia	Sediment	79 μg/g	Lasheen (1987)[a]
	Alexandria	Seawater	0.05–0.7 μg/L	Abdel-Moati & Atta (1991)
		Sediment	2–49 μg/g	
Nigeria	Agunpa river	River water	1.3–46 μg/L	Mombeshora *et al.* (1983)
		Sediment	62–75 μg/g	
	Ona river	River water	0.2–17 μg/L	
		Sediment	25–58 μg/g	

Adapted from Nriagu (1992)
[a] Original paper was not available

USA was 3.9 μg/L (Eckel & Jacob, 1988). Lead concentrations in surface water are typically higher in urban areas than in rural areas (US EPA, 1982).

Lead concentrations in the La Plata river at two sites in Buenos Aires, Argentina, ranged from 2.4 to 58.6 μg/L at the port area and from 9.9 to 16.4 μg/L at the Fishing Club (Table 28; Verrengia Guerrero & Kesten, 1994). The Ribeira do Iguape river, in South Brazil, receiving urban and industrial effluents, showed lead concentrations between < 20 and 70 μg/L in 1994 (Romieu *et al.*, 1997). Intensive mining and tailing releases to the Pilcomayo and Tarapaya rivers resulted in mean lead concentrations in the water of 1399 and 2291 μg/L, respectively, against 1.0 μg/L in Cachi Mayu, which had not been contaminated by specific lead sources (Smolders *et al.*, 2003).

Lead contamination of groundwater around the Hussain Sagar lake, Hyderabad, India, indicated that the source of pollution was the contaminated lake. Lead was detected at concentrations in the range of 1–28 μg/L in groundwater and 38.4–62.5 μg/L in the lake (Table 30). The concentrations were appreciably higher than those for uncontaminated fresh waters which are generally below 1 μg/L (Srikanth *et al.*, 1993). During a 2-year study of the Nainital lake, India, the average lead contamination levels in water and sediment were 600 μg/mL and 50.0 μg/g, respectively (Ali *et al.*, 1999). The lead content in various bodies of water in India ranged from 35 to 70 μg/L in the Eastern Ghats (Rai *et al.*, 1996), from 350 to 720 μg/L in various lakes in Lucknow, and from 510 to 1510 μg/L in Unnao (Chandra *et al.*, 1993). In the Gomti river, lead concentrations of 13–26 μg/L were reported (Singh, 1996) and in the Ganga river from 0.98 to 6.5 μg/L (Israili, 1991). The waters of Vasai Creek (Maharashtra, India) had concentrations of 10.5–29.5 μg/L, which was the result of contamination from 18 major industries that

Table 30. Lead concentrations in water and sediment in Asia

Country	Location	Type of water/ sediment	Concentration (µg/L)[a] mean or range of means (range)	Reference	Comments
India	Pilani	Tube well	88 (21–354)	Kaphalia *et al.* (1981)	pH of water, 7.5–9.1
	Lucknow	Tap-water	33 (0–67)		
		River	35 (8–58)		
	Cambay	Tank	6 (0–16)		
	Kanpur villages	Tube well	20 (0–40)		
	Company	Tube well	24 (0–80)		
	Mumbai	Drinking-water	12 ± 3	Khandekar *et al.* (1984)	
	Various cities along Ganga river	River	0.98–6.5	Israili (1991)	Highest concentration in water and sediment at Garsh Mukteshwara
		Sediment	1.2–16.0 µg/g		
	5 cities along Yamuna river	River (10 samples)	0.76–8.51	Israili & Khurshid (1991)	
	Koraput (Orissa)	Water stations	15 ± 1	Chandra *et al.* (1993)	
	Unnao (Uttar Pradesh)		510 ± 50 (summer)		
			1510 ± 150 (winter)		
	Various sites along Gomti river	River		Singh (1996)	Highest concentrations at Mohan Meakin, Sultampur and Pipraghat
		unfiltered	13–25		
		filtered	9–21		
	Hussain Sagar lake, Hyderabad	Lake	38.4–62.5	Srikanth *et al.* (1993)	
		Ground water			
		200–1000 m from lake	7–28		
		1000–2000 m from lake	1–9		

Table 30 (contd)

Country	Location	Type of water/ sediment	Concentration (µg/L)[a] mean or range of means (range)	Reference	Comments
India (contd)	Eastern Ghats (Koraput Orrisa)	Drinking-water facilities		Rai *et al.* (1996)	
		adequate	54 ± 5		
		primitive	35 ± 5		
		absent	70 ± 37		
	Nainital	Lake water	150–480	Ali *et al.* (1999)	
		Sediment	50.0 µg/g		
	Vasai Creek, Maharashtra	River/sea	10.5–29.5	Lokhande & Kelkar (1999)	
	Mumbai	Drinking-water		Parikh *et al.* (1999)	
	High exposure area		2.8 ± 0.8		
	Low exposure area		4.5 ± 1.7		
	Nagpur	Tap-water	2.82	Patel *et al.* (2001)	
		Well	3.30		
	Lucknow	Lake and ponds	350–720	Rai & Sinha (2001)	
	Darbhanga District, North-Bihar	9 ponds	[147–1056]	Rai *et al.* (2002)	Data for 1996–97; highest values for water and sediment in same pond
		Sediment	[72.21–240.95 µg/g]		
Indonesia	Central Kalimantan	6 rivers	0.41–5.23	Kurasaki *et al.* (2000)	Motor boats are an important mode of transport.
		3 channels	0.1–1.28		
		3 lakes	0.28–11.48		
		1 fish pond	0.51		
Malaysia	Klang river	1992[b]	28	APEC (1997)	
		1993	21		
		1994	18.6		
		1995	25.9		
		1996	8		
Pakistan	Karachi	Drinking-water from household	3.1–4.3	Rahbar *et al.* (2002)	

[a] Unless specified otherwise
[b] Year of sample collection

Table 31. Lead concentration in drinking-water, Japan, 2001

	Number [%] of samples with lead concentration (μg/L)				
	Total	< 5	5–< 10	10–< 15	≥ 15
Source water	5178	5110 [98.69]	53 [1.02]	5 [0.10]	10 [0.19]
Treated water[a]	5647	5536 [98.03]	84 [1.49]	14 [0.25]	13 [0.23]

From Ministry of Health, Labour and Welfare, Japan (2001)
[a] Concentrations measured at drinking-water treatment plants
Note: A drinking-water standard of < 10 μg/L lead was established in Japan as of 1 April, 2004 (Ministry of Health, Labour and Welfare, Japan, 2003).

collectively released about seven tonnes of lead per year into the creek (Lokhande & Kelkar, 1999).

Among six locations along four rivers in central Kalimantan, Indonesia, the highest lead concentrations were found in the Kahayan river (5.23 and 2.09 μg/L at two sampling sites), followed by Murung river (1.71 μg/L). Of various channel, lake and pond waters (7 locations), lake Tundai was found to be by far the most contaminated with lead (11.48 μg/L), followed by channel Dablabup (1.28 μg/L) (Kurasaki *et al.,* 2000).

Surveys in Canada and the USA showed that drinking-water supplies leaving treatment plants contain 2–8 μg/L lead (US EPA, 1986a; Dabeka *et al.*, 1987). EPA estimated that less than 1% of the public water systems in the USA have water entering the distribution system with lead concentrations above 5 μg/L. However, most lead contamination comes from corrosion by-products of lead pipes and lead-soldered joints (US EPA, 1991). A survey of 1245 drinking-water samples taken from various districts in the USA showed that average lead concentrations in water in copper, galvanized and plastic pipes were 9, 4.2 and 4.5 μg/L, respectively. These data show that even plumbing that did not use lead solder (e.g. plastic pipes) contained significant amounts of lead, primarily from the brass faucet fixtures which are used in almost all plumbing. The brass fixtures may account for approximately one-third of the lead in the first-draw water (Lee *et al.*, 1989).

Following an increased volcanic activity that resulted in the release of acid aerosols, Wiebe *et al.* (1991) analysed over 2000 water samples in Hawaii, USA, and found lead concentrations in drinking-water collected in catchment systems ranging from < 20 to 7000 μg/L.

The use of lead pipes in Uruguay resulted in tap-water concentrations of lead ranging between 0.2 and 230 μg/L (Schütz *et al.*, 1997). In 1983, lead concentrations in drinking-water from an underground source in Mexico City, Mexico, ranged between 1 and 3 μg/L, in spite of the past intensive use of lead in petrol (Bruaux & Svartengren, 1985). Storage of minerals near urban areas in Antofagasta, Chile, resulted in concentrations of lead in household water of up to 170 μg/L in 1998 (Sepúlveda *et al.*, 2000).

Water samples collected from tube wells, tanks and taps in India showed lead concentrations that varied between 0 and 354 μg/L (Kaphalia *et al.*, 1981). The lead concentration in drinking-water in Karachi, Pakistan, was found to be in the range of 3.08–4.32 μg/L as an arithmetic mean for each of five monitored areas (Rahbar *et al.*, 2002). Throughout Japan, more than 98% of the drinking-water samples had concentrations below 5 μg/L (Table 31; Ministry of Health, Labour & Welfare, 2001).

Gulson *et al.* (1997a) measured lead in household water throughout the day in an unoccupied test house in Australia. Lead concentrations in water ranged from 119 μg/L for the initial (first-draw) sample to 35–52 μg/L for hourly samples (125 mL) to 1.7 μg/L for a fully flushed sample.

(*d*) *Sediments*

Lead reaching surface waters is readily bound to suspended solids and sediments, and sediments from both freshwater and marine environments have been studied for their lead content. Sediments contain considerably higher concentrations of lead than corresponding surface waters, and provide a unique record of the history of global lead fluxes (WHO, 1995).

Concentrations of lead in sediments in Africa, Asia and Latin America are summarized in Tables 29, 30 and 32, respectively.

Average concentrations of lead in river sediments in the USA have been reported to be about 23 mg/kg (Fitchko & Hutchinson, 1975; US EPA, 1982). In coastal sediments a mean value of 87 mg/kg was measured (range, 1–912 mg/kg) (Nriagu, 1978; US EPA, 1982). Surface sediment concentrations of lead in Puget Sound, near Seattle, were found to range from 15 to 53 mg/kg (Bloom & Crecelius, 1987). An analysis of sediments taken from 10 lakes in Pennsylvania indicated that the lead does not principally originate from parent materials in the watershed (from the native rocks as a result of acid deposition), but rather from transport of anthropogenic lead through the atmosphere onto the soil surface and subsequent run-off of soil particulates into the lake (Case *et al.*, 1989).

The main reported sources of lead entering surface-water bodies in Latin America have been metallurgy, smelter and mining effluents, oil refineries and port activities. In Brazil, the All Saints bay showed values of 119 mg/kg in sediments at the river mouth downstream from a smelter; 176 mg/kg at the river mouth downstream from an oil refinery; and 618 mg/kg in the vicinity of metallurgical industries and an industrial port, compared with 35.7 mg/kg in an area with no specific source of lead, away from industries (Tavares, 1996a,b).

Mine tailings in Bolivia were responsible for an increase in lead concentrations from 7.4 mg/kg in Cachi mayu, where no specific source of lead contamination exists, to average values of 603 mg/kg (range, 292–991 mg/kg) and 902 mg/kg (range, 761–1236 mg/kg), in sediments from the Pilcomayo river at Potosi and from the Tarapaya river,

Table 32. Lead in sediments in Latin America and the Caribbean

Country	Location	Year(s) of study	Source of contamination	Concentration (µg/g) mean (range)	Reference
Brazil	All Saints bay, São Brás	1994	Downstream from lead smelter	119	Tavares (1996b)
	All Saints bay, Mataripe river mouth	1994	Oil refinery	176	
	All Saints bay, Aratu Port	1994	Metallurgies, industrial port	618	
	All Saints bay, Cabuçu	1994	No specific source	35.7	
	Ribeira do Iguape river	1994	NR	(3–240)	Romieu *et al.* (1997)
	Jacareí, São Paulo	1994	NR	(10–9100)	
Bolivia	Pilcomayo river, Potosi	1997–98	Mine tailings	603 (292–991)	Smolders *et al.* (2003)
	Tarapaya river	1997–98	Mine tailings	902 (761–1236)	
	Cachi mayu	1997–98	No specific source	7.4 (3.3–9.9)	
Honduras	Yojoa lake	NR	NR	371	Romieu *et al.* (1997)
Mexico	Gulf of Mexico coast	1983–87	NR	(0.29–90.15)	Albert & Badillo[a] (1991)
Uruguay	Montevideo	NR	NR	(20–160)	Romieu *et al.* (1997)

NR, not reported
[a] Review of 7 studies at 8 sites

respectively (Smolders *et al.*, 2003). Mean concentrations of lead in sediments from the Gulf of Mexico were found to range from 0.29 to 90.15 mg/kg (Albert & Badillo, 1991).

(*e*) *Soil*

Most of the lead released into the environment from emissions or as industrial waste is deposited in soil. Lead-containing wastes result from the processing of ores, the production of iron and steel, the various end-products and uses of lead, and the removal and remediation of lead paint (ATSDR, 1999). Lead in soil may be relatively insoluble (as a sulfate, carbonate or oxide), soluble, adsorbed onto clays, adsorbed and coprecipitated with sesquioxides, adsorbed onto colloidal organic matter or complexed with organic moieties present in soil (WHO, 1995). The soil pH, the content of humic and fulvic acids and the amount of organic matter influence the content and mobility of lead in soils. Since acidic conditions favour the solubilization and leaching of lead from the solid phase, acidic soils tend to have lower lead concentrations when analysed as dry soil. Acid rain promotes the release of lead into groundwater. Humic and fulvic acids can also mobilize lead, and certain complex organic molecules can act as chelators of lead (WHO, 1995).

Table 33 shows some sources and amounts of lead released in soils worldwide. Tables 34, 35 and 36 summarize data on lead concentration in soils in Latin America, Africa and Asia, respectively.

Background concentrations of lead in soil measured across the USA in the 1970s were estimated to be in the range of < 10–70 mg/kg (Boerngen & Shacklette, 1981). Soil samples taken at distances of 50–100 m from highways, outside the range of immediate impact from traffic emissions, usually show concentrations of lead below 40 mg/kg (WHO, 1995).

Studies carried out in Maryland and Minnesota indicate that within large light-industrial urban settings such as Baltimore, soil lead concentrations are generally highest in inner-city areas, especially where high traffic flows have long prevailed (Mielke *et al.*, 1983, 1989); the amount of lead in the soil is correlated with the size of the city, which in turn is related to traffic density (Mielke *et al.*, 1989; Mielke, 1991). It has been suggested that the higher lead concentrations in soil samples taken around houses in the inner city are the result of greater atmospheric lead content from the burning of leaded gasoline in cars and the washdown by rain of building surfaces to which the small lead particles adhere (Mielke *et al.*, 1989).

Table 33. Discharge of lead in soil worldwide

Source of lead	Amount released (tonnes/year)
Agricultural and food wastes	1500–27 000
Animal wastes, manure	3200–20 000
Logging and other wood wastes	6600–8200
Urban refuse	18 000–62 000
Municipal sewage sludge	2800–9700
Miscellaneous organic wastes, including excreta	20–1600
Solid wastes, metal manufacturing	4100–11 000
Coal fly ash, bottom fly ash	45 000–242 000
Fertilizer	420–2300
Peat (agricultural and fuel use)	450–2600
Wastage of commercial products	195 000–390 000
Atmospheric fallout	202 000–263 000
Mine tailings	130 000–390 000
Smelter slags and wastes	195 000–390 000
Total yearly discharge on land	803 090–1 818 800

From Nriagu and Pacyna (1988)
Many of these discharges remain localized due to the nature of the particulate matter.

Table 34. Lead concentrations in soils in Latin America and the Caribbean

Country	Location	Year(s) of study	Source of contamination	Concentration (mg/kg) mean ± SD (range)	Reference
Argentina	Buenos Aires	1975	NR	6–12	Romieu *et al.* (1997)
Brazil	Santo Amaro, Bahia[a]	1980	900 m from smelter, 12 m high chimney	10 601 ± 14 611 (32–107 268) 4415 ± 4.4[b]	Tavares (1990)
		1985	90 m high chimney	4812 ± 8523 (236–83 532) 2529 ± 2.9[b]	
	Jacareí, São Paolo	1994	NR	(51–338)	Romieu *et al.* (1997)
Chile	Antofagasta	1998	Storage of minerals	(81–3159)	Sepúlveda *et al.* (2000)
		1998	Upwind from storage site	(51–321)	
Ecuador	Andean village La Victoria	NR	Glazing of ceramics		Counter *et al.* (2000)
			At 1 m	29 213 ± 9458[a]	
			At 5 m	172 ± 26	
			At 10 m	81 ± 13	
			At 1 km	55 ± 2	
			At 2 km	19 ± 1	
			At 6 km	1.4 ± 0.1	
	Mambija, San Carlos and Esmeraldas		Control area	(2.3–21)	

Table 34 (contd)

Country	Location	Year(s) of study	Source of contamination	Concentration (mg/kg) mean ± SD (range)	Reference
Mexico	N and NE Mexico city irrigation districts	1980–81	Traffic fallout	5.3 ± 1.5	Albert & Badillo (1991)
	Mexico city airport	1979	Traffic fallout	(739–890)	
	Mexico city centre	1979	Traffic fallout	(6–107)	
	Mexico city Viaducto Piedad	1979	Traffic fallout	(43–578)	
	Mexico city Estadio Azteca	1979	Traffic fallout	(2.1–2.7)	
Venezuela	Caracas, Day-care centres	1997–98	Traffic (high flow)	Particle size, 44–62.5 µm: 113–375 Particle size, < 44 µm: 190–465	Fernández *et al.* (2003)
			Traffic (low flow)	Particle size, 44–62.5 µm: 106 ± 3 Particle size, < 44 µm: 142 ± 3	

NR, not reported; SD, standard deviation
[a] Leachable lead
[b] Geometric mean and standard deviation

Table 35. Lead concentrations in soil in Saudi Arabia and Africa

Country	Location	Source of contamination	Concentration (mg/kg) mean or range of means (range)	Reference
Saudi Arabia	NR	Heavy traffic	95.3	Al-Saleh
		Residential	34.5	(1998)
Kenya	Nairobi	City traffic	137–2196	Onyari *et al.*
		Industrial area	148–4088	(1991)
Zambia	Kasanda	2 km from lead smelter	100–> 2400	Nriagu (1992)
	Kabwe	5 km from lead smelter	(9862–2580)	Nwankwo &
	Lusaka	No specific	16 (11–40)	Elinder (1979)

NR, not reported

Lead-based paint can also be a major source of lead in soil. In the state of Maine, USA, 37% of soil samples taken within 1–2 feet (30–60 cm) of the foundation of a building more than 30 years of age had lead concentrations > 1000 mg/kg (Krueger & Duguay, 1989).

In a study of the association between the concentrations of lead in soil and in blood samples taken from children in urban and rural areas in Louisiana, USA, blood lead concentrations in children appeared to be closely associated with soil lead concentration (Mielke *et al.*, 1997a).

Three prospective studies were conducted in Boston, Baltimore and Cincinnati, USA, to determine whether abatement of lead in soil could reduce blood lead concentrations of children. No significant evidence was found that lead reduction had any direct impact on children's blood lead concentrations in either Baltimore or Cincinnati (US EPA, 1996b). In the Boston study, however, a median soil lead reduction from 2075 mg/kg to 50 mg/kg resulted in a mean decline of 2.47 μg/dL blood lead concentration 10 months after soil remediation (Weitzman *et al.*, 1993; Aschengrau *et al.*, 1994). A number of factors appear to be important in determining the influence of soil abatement on blood lead concentrations in children, including the site-specific exposure scenario, the extent of the remediation, and the magnitude of additional sources of lead exposure.

Children with pica — a serious eating disorder characterized by repetitive consumption of nonfood items — may be at increased risk for adverse effects through ingestion of large amounts of soil contaminated with lead. It has been estimated that an average child may ingest on average between 20 and 50 mg of soil per day through normal hand-to-mouth activity, whereas a child with pica may ingest up to 5000 mg of soil per day (LaGoy, 1987). This source can contribute an additional lead intake of 5 μg/day for a toddler engaging in normal hand-to-mouth activity, and significantly more for a child demonstrating pica behaviour (ATSDR, 1999).

Davis *et al.* (1992, 1994), using electron microprobe analysis of soil and waste rock from the mining district of Butte, Montana, USA, showed that the lead bioavailability of

Table 36. Lead concentrations in soil and plants in Asia

Country	Location	Source of contamination	Lead concentration in:		Reference	Comments
			Soil (mg/kg)	Plant (mg/kg)		
China	NR	Smelter			Wang (1984)	
		50 m	170	29.1		
		500 m	28	1.7		
India	Mumbai	Lead industries	200–3454	145–1048 (grass)	Nambi *et al.* (1997)	
		Control	8.6	1.42		
	Residential area of greater Kolkata	Lead factory	200–46 700	214 ± 17 (leaf)	Chatterjee & Banerjee (1999)	Soil contaminated at least up to 0.5 km
	Coimbatore	Sewage	Surface: 13.3–22.2 Subsurface: 10.26–19.3		Duraisamy *et al.* (2003)	The highest values were found in Nov.–Dec. and the lowest in March.
	Coimbatore	Fertilization with superphosphate and zinc sulfate	1992: 24–47.2 2000: 32.4–63.2		Kamaraj *et al.* (2003)	Fertilizer used during entire period
Mongolia		Urban	92		Burmaa *et al.* (2002)	
		Residential	44			
Philippines	Manila	Playground			Sharma & Reutergardh (2000)	
		contaminated	34.5–281.5			
		control	15			
Thailand	Grazing-land site	Highway	5.25–14.59	0.76–6.62 (grass)	Parkpian *et al.* (2003)	

these samples is constrained by alteration and encapsulation of the lead-bearing minerals (*galena*, *anglesite*, *cerussite* and *plumbojarosite*), which would limit the available lead-bearing surface area. The inherent chemical properties of soil-lead adsorption sites may reduce the bioavailability of soil lead compared with that of soluble lead salts and lead compounds ingested without soil and may explain the low blood lead concentrations observed in children in this mining community.

Davies (1983) calculated that uncontaminated soils in the United Kingdom have a (geometric) mean lead concentration of 42 mg/kg, with a maximum of 106 mg/kg.

A study conducted in Wales, United Kingdom, in an area where lead mining began 2000 years ago and ended in the middle of the 20th century, reported concentrations of lead in garden soils 14 times higher than in uncontaminated areas (Davies *et al.*, 1985).

In Port Pirie, Australia, a community with one of the world's largest and oldest primary lead smelters, lead concentrations in soils were found to be grossly elevated, ranging up to over 2000 mg/kg (McMichael *et al.*, 1985). The frequency of elevated lead concentrations in the blood of pregnant women and young children in this community was also increased above that found in other communities in Australia (Wilson *et al.*, 1986; McMichael *et al.*, 1988).

The main reported sources of lead in soil in Latin America have been from smelter activities, storage of minerals, glazing of ceramics, and leaded gasoline (Table 34). In Santo Amaro, Brazil, in 1980, lead concentrations as high as 107 268 mg/kg in soil have been found in orchards and homes around a smelter (arithmetic mean value for the area within 900 m from the smelter, 10 601 mg/kg), as a result of the use of dross as paving material around houses. At that time, the smelter had a 12-m high chimney. Five years later, after a 90-m high chimney was built, these values dropped to mean values of 4812 mg/kg (Tavares, 1990). In Antofagasta, in the north of Chile, storage of minerals resulted in lead concentrations up to 3159 mg/kg in soil around the site compared with values of 51–321 mg/kg upwind from the site (Sepúlveda *et al.*, 2000). Analysis of soil around ceramic glazing facilities in an Andean Equadorian village showed a significant fall in lead soil concentration with distance from the baking kilns; concentrations were 29 213 mg/kg at 1 m, 55 mg/kg at 1 km and 1.4 mg/kg at 6 km from the kilns (Counter *et al.*, 2000). In 1979, when tetraethyl lead was still added to gasoline, soil lead concentrations in Mexico City, Mexico, were determined near avenues in different parts of the city. Higher concentrations of lead were found in the north and north-west of the city, with the highest values found at the airport, ranging from 739 to 890 mg/kg. The centre of the city showed values between 6 and 107 mg/kg (Albert & Badillo, 1991). In 1980–81, agricultural soils north and north-east of the city, irrigated either directly from wastewaters or with clean water, were analysed for lead; there was no influence of irrigation on soil lead concentrations (Albert & Badillo, 1991). Soil lead concentrations in day-care centres near areas of high traffic flow in Caracas, Venezuela, ranged between 113 and 465 mg/kg, with higher values in soil particles $< 44\ \mu m$ (Fernández *et al.*, 2003). In Argentina, a study of phosphate fertilizers imported from different parts of the world showed lead concentrations between 5.1 and 30.7 mg/kg, which could potentially increase lead concentrations in soils undergoing continuous fertilization (Giuffré de López Camelo *et al.*, 1997).

A number of studies have reported soil lead concentrations in the proximity of smelters and mining areas. A report from China found that lead concentrations in ambient air, plants and soil increased proportionally with proximity to a primary smelter: lead concentration in soil was 28.0 mg/kg at 500 m and 170 mg/kg at 50 m distance from the smelter (Wang, 1984).

Concentrations of lead in soil have been found elevated in many locations in Asia (Table 36), such as in the vicinity of a lead refinery in Kolkata, India (Chatterjee & Banerjee, 1999), in sewage-affected soils (Duraisamy *et al.*, 2003), or on a playground in Manila, Philippines (Sharma & Reutergardh, 2000).

(*f*) *Lead in gasoline*

Globally, by far the largest source of lead emissions into air has been exhaust from motor vehicles using organic lead as an anti-knock agent in gasoline (see Section 1.3.7). In motor-vehicle exhaust from leaded gasoline, > 90% of the lead emission is inorganic lead (e.g. lead bromochloride) and < 10% is alkyl lead vapour. Furthermore, alkyl lead compounds decompose in the atmosphere to lead oxides through a combination of photolysis and oxidation reactions, over a period ranging from a few hours to a few days (ATSDR, 1999). Vehicle emissions increase lead concentrations in the surrounding air, and lead compounds adhere to dust particles that settle and increase the lead content of dusts and soils, thus constituting a major source of exposure of the general population. By comparing ratios of stable lead isotopes in remote areas with those characteristic of lead from industrial sources in various regions, investigators have shown that the lead found in pristine areas such as Greenland and Antarctica originated from motor vehicle exhaust from North America (Rosman *et al.*, 1994a) and South America (Rosman *et al.*, 1994b), respectively.

Nriagu and Pacyna (1988) estimated that in 1983 mobile sources worldwide contributed 248 000 tonnes of lead to the atmosphere. This compares with total estimated emissions to the atmosphere from all sources of 288 700–376 000 tonnes. By 1997, global emissions from leaded gasoline had been reduced to 40 000 tonnes and are still declining, as permissible lead contents of gasoline have been lowered and unleaded gasoline has replaced, or is replacing, leaded fuel in many countries (see Table 20). However, in a number of countries, leaded gasoline is still in use (see Section 1.3.7). Table 37 shows lead concentrations in gasoline over time in a number of countries worldwide.

In Japan, the use of lead in gasoline had been phased out since 1974 and reached almost zero in 1983 (Friberg & Vahter, 1983). The Central Pollution Control Board in India (1998–1999) reported a 50% reduction of lead concentration in air as unleaded gasoline came into use. Leaded gasoline has been banned in India with effect from February 2000. In Pakistan, the addition of lead to gasoline was reduced in 1998–99 from 0.42 to 0.34 g/L in regular gasoline and from 0.84 to 0.42 g/L in high-octane gasoline. In 2001, a directive

Table 37. Lead concentrations in gasoline, air and blood in adults and children worldwide

Country	Location	Population	Year(s) of study	Lead concentration in			Reference
				Gasoline (g/L)	Air[a] (μg/m^3)	Blood[a] (μg/dL)	
Belgium	NR	≥ 20 years	1979	0.45	1.05	17.0[b]	Ducoffre *et al.* (1990)
			1983	0.40	0.66	14.7[b]	
			1987	0.15	0.49	9.0[b]	
Canada	Ontario	3–6 years	1984	0.30	NR	11.9[c] (11.3–12.6)[d]	Loranger & Zayed (1994); Langlois *et al.* (1996)
			1988	0.09	NR	5.1[c] (4.8–5.4)[d]	
			1990	0.04	NR	3.6[c] (3.3–3.9)[d]	
			1992	0.00	NR	3.5[c] (3.1–3.8)[d]	
Finland	Helsinki	Children	1983	0.35	0.33	4.8 (2.1–8.3)	Pönkä *et al.* (1993); Pönkä (1998)
			1988	0.14	0.095	3.0 (2.1–4.1)	
			1996	0.00	0.007	2.6 (1.7–3.7)	
Greece	Athens	Adults	1979	0.80	3.2	NR	Chartsias *et al.* (1986); Kapaki *et al.* (1998)
			1982	0.40	1.76	16.0	
			1984	0.22	0.91	11.8	
			1988	0.15	0.7	8	
			1993	0.14	0.43	5.5	
Italy	Turin	≥ 18 years	1974	0.6	4.7	NR	Facchetti (1989); Bono *et al.* (1995)
			1980	0.6	3.1	21	
			1985	0.4	2.8	15.1 (± 3.9)[e]	
			1989	0.3	1.4	NR	
			1993	0.11	0.53	6.4 (± 1.7)[e]	
Japan	Rural	≥ 20 years	1977–80	0.00	NR	4.9[c] (± 0.15)[e] (men) 3.2[c] (± 0.15)[e] (women)	Watanabe *et al.* (1985)
Mexico	Mexico City	0.5–3 years	1988	0.2	NR	12.2	Octel Ltd (1982, 1988, 1990); Driscoll *et al.* (1992); Mexico City Commission for Prevention and Control of Pollution (1993); Rothenberg *et al.* (1998)
			1989	0.2	NR	14.6	
			1990	0.18	NR	9.8	
			1991	0.08	NR	8.6	
			1992	0.07	NR	9	
			1993	0.06	NR	7	

Table 37 (contd)

Country	Location	Population	Year(s) of study	Lead concentration in			Reference
				Gasoline (g/L)	Air[a] (µg/m^3)	Blood[a] (µg/dL)	
Nepal	Himalayas	Adults and children	NR	0.00	< 0.004[g]	3.4[c]	Piomelli *et al.* (1980)
New Zealand	Christchurch	Adults and children	1978–81	0.84	NR	15.2	Hinton *et al.* (1986); Walmsley *et al.* (1988, 1995)
			1982–83	0.84	NR	11.8	
			1984–85	0.84	NR	8.1	
			1989	0.45	NR	7.3	
			1994	0.2	NR	4.9	
South Africa	Cape Town	Adults	1984	0.84	NR	9.7 (3.0–16.0)	Maresky & Grobler (1993)
			1990	0.40	NR	7.2 (0.62–14.1)	
Spain	Barcelona	20–60 years	1984	0.60	1.03	18.6 (6.8–38.9)	Rodamilans *et al.* (1996)
		19–63 years	1994	0.15	0.24 (0.18–0.3)	8.8 (0.9–31.8)	
	Tarragona	16–65 years	1990	0.40	2.0 (0.97–3.26)	12.0[c] (± 1.8)[e]	Schuhmacher *et al.* (1996a)
			1995	0.13	0.23 (0.02–0.43)	6.3[c] (± 1.8)[e]	
Sweden	Trelleborg	3–19 years	1979	0.40	NA	5.6[c] (2.7–10.4)	[Stockholm Municipal Environment and Health Administration (1983)]; Strömberg *et al.* (1995)
			1983	0.15	NA	4.2[c] (1.9–8.1)	
			1993	0.00	NA	2.3[c] (1.0–6.7)	
	Stockholm	Adults	1980	0.40	1.20	7.7 (± 3.3)[e]	Elinder *et al.* (1986)
			1983	0.15	0.50	5.4 (± 3.3)[e]	
	Landskrona	3–19 years	1978	0.40	0.12–0.42	6.0[c] (1.8–25.0)	Skerfving *et al.* (1986); Schütz *et al.* (1989); Strömberg *et al.* (1995)
			1982	0.15	0.17	4.8[c] (1.5–10.0)	
			1984	0.15	NA	4.2[c] (1.4–12.9)	
			1988	0.00	NA	3.3[c] (1.5–7.1)	
			1994	0.00	NA	2.5[c] (1.2–12.3)	
Switzerland	Vaud, Fribourg	25–74 years	1984–85	0.15	NR	10.3[c] (8.0–17.2)[f]	Wietlisbach *et al.* (1995)
			1988–89	0.10	NR	7.3[c] (5.6–12.7)[f]	
			1992–93	0.05	NR	5.9[c] (4.4–10.2)[f]	

Table 37 (contd)

Country	Location	Population	Year(s) of study	Lead concentration in			Reference
				Gasoline (g/L)	Air[a] (µg/m³)	Blood[a] (µg/dL)	
United Kingdom	England	≥ 11 years	1979	0.42	NR	12.9[c]	Quinn (1985); Quinn & Delves, 1987, 1988, 1989; Delves *et al.* (1996)
			1981	0.38	NR	11.4[c]	
			1984	0.38	NR	8.0–10.9[c]	
			1985	0.38	0.48	9.5[c]	
			1986	0.14	0.24	8.4[c]	
			1995	0.055	NR	3.1[c]	
USA	Countrywide	1–74 years	1976	0.465	0.97	15.9	Annest *et al.* (1983); [US EPA (1985; 1992)]; Brody *et al.* (1994); Pirkle *et al.* (1994)
			1977	0.394		14.0	
			1978	0.349		14.6	
			1979	0.306	0.71	12.1	
			1980	0.30	0.49	9.5	
			1988–91	0.00	0.07 (0.05–0.12)[d]	2.8[c] (2.7–3.0)[d]	
Venezuela	Caracas	≥ 15 years	1986	0.62	1.9	17.4	Cedeño *et al.* (1990); Romero (1996)
			1989	0.45	1.3	15.2	
			1991	0.39	1.3	15.6	

From Thomas *et al.* (1999) with minor modifications
NR, not reported
References in square brackets could not be retrieved as original papers.
[a] Arithmetic mean (range), unless stated otherwise
[b] Median value
[c] Geometric mean
[d] 95% confidence interval
[e] Standard deviation
[f] 90% confidence interval
[g] Detection limit

by the Government of Pakistan established a permissible limit of 0.02 g/L; most of the petrol produced in Pakistan is now lead-free (Paul *et al.*, 2003).

By 1995, six countries in Latin America and the Caribbean (Antigua and Barbuda, Bermuda, Bolivia, Brazil, Columbia, and Guatemala) had removed all lead from gasoline (Pan American Health Organization, 1997). Brazil introduced the national alcohol programme [hydrated alcohol used as fuel in a mixture with gasoline] in 1975, leading to 100% of cars running on unleaded fuel by the beginning of the 1980s. This resulted in a decrease of annual atmospheric lead concentrations from an average of 1.11 μg/m^3 in 1980 to 0.27 μg/m^3 in 1990 in São Paulo. Similarly, by 1994, 80% of the cars in Guatemala and 46% in Mexico ran on unleaded gasoline, reducing the annual average concentration of lead in air to 0.17 and 0.28 μg/m^3, respectively. In Mexico City, the concentration was 1.95 μg/m^3 in 1988 and had decreased by 86% in 1994. Between 1982 and 1990, the city of Caracas, Venezuela, showed a decrease in the annual average atmospheric lead concentrations from 4.5 μg/m^3 to 1.9 μg/m^3 (57.8% decrease). However, this is still higher than the value of 1.5 μg/m^3 recommended by WHO and established as an air quality standard by US EPA. According to a survey carried out by the Pan American Center for Human Ecology and Health in Mexico in 1994, lead concentrations in gasoline in participating Latin American and Caribbean countries ranged from 1.32 g/L in Suriname to 0.03 g/L in Uruguay (Romieu & Lacasana, 1996; Romieu *et al.*, 1997).

Data on lead in gasoline, lead in air and blood lead concentrations of the local population in a number of countries worldwide are summarized in Table 37. An analysis of 17 published studies from five continents (Thomas *et al.*, 1999) found a strong linear correlation between blood lead concentrations in the population and the consumption-weighted average concentration of lead in gasoline, with a median correlation coefficient of 0.94. As the use of lead in gasoline was phased out, blood lead concentrations across study locations converged to a median of 3.1 ± 2.3 μg/dL, and air lead concentrations were reduced to ≤ 0.2 μg/m^3.

(*g*) *Lead in paint*

In the past, the use of lead pigments in paints was widespread, but it is now restricted in many countries. Dusting, flaking or peeling of paint from surfaces are major sources of lead contamination of surface dust and soil near houses, and contribute to the amount of lead in household dust. Exposure occurs not only through the direct ingestion of flaking and chalking paint but also through the inhalation of dust and soil contaminated with paint. Renovation and remodelling activities that disturb lead-based paints in homes can produce significant amounts of lead dust which can be inhaled or ingested. Removal of lead-based paint from surfaces by burning (gas torch or hot air gun), scraping or sanding can result, at least temporarily, in high levels of exposure for residents in these homes (ATSDR, 1999). Lead from paint can constitute the major source of lead exposure, in particular for young children, and can even make a significant contribution to blood lead concentrations in children living in areas that are highly contaminated with lead, e.g. around one of the largest lead mines in the world (Gulson *et al.*, 1994). Consumption of a single chip of paint with a lead concentration of 1–5 mg/cm^2 would provide greater short-term exposure than any other source of lead (US EPA, 1986a).

An estimated 40–50% of occupied housing in the USA in 1986 was thought to have lead-based paint on exposed surfaces (Chisolm, 1986). Intervention programmes to reduce exposures to lead in house dust have been reported (Lanphear *et al.*, 2000a; Galke *et al.*, 2001; Leighton *et al.*, 2003).

In a study by Schmitt *et al.* (1988) in the USA, soil samples taken from around the foundations of homes with wooden exteriors were found to have the highest lead concentrations (mean, 522 mg/kg) while concentrations around homes composed of brick were significantly lower (mean, 158 mg/kg). Lead concentrations up to 20 136 mg/kg were found in soil samples taken near house foundations adjacent to private dwellings with exterior lead-based paint. A state-wide study in Minnesota, USA, found that exterior lead-based paint was the major source of contamination in severely contaminated soils located near the foundations of private residences, while lead aerosols accounted for virtually all of the contamination of soils at some distance from the houses. Contamination due to lead-based paint was found to be highly concentrated over a limited area, while lead aerosols were less concentrated but more widespread (Minnesota Pollution Control Agency, 1987). (See also Section 1.4.1(*e*)).

Many countries have restricted the use of lead in paint. Leroyer *et al.* (2001) mention that lead in paint was banned in France in 1948. A lead concentration greater than 0.06% is not permitted in indoor paints sold in the USA (US DHUD, 1987). However, the lead content of paint remains unregulated in some countries (Nriagu *et al.*, 1996b). Ten per cent of lead metal used in India was reported to be used in the manufacture of paint, and wherever such paint is used there will be the potential for human exposure to lead (van Alphen, 1999). Results of a study of lead content of paint used in India are shown in Table 38. Of the 24 samples analysed, 17 had lead concentrations ≥ 0.5%, 13 had concentrations ≥ 1% and five had concentrations ≥ 10%. The lead in these paints was predominantly in the form of lead chromates (van Alphen, 1999).

(*h*) *Food*

A major source of lead for non-occupationally exposed adults is food and drink. The amount of lead intake from food is dependent on the concentration of lead in soil, air, water and other sources. Lead present in soils is taken up by food crops. Roots usually contain more lead than stems and leaves, while seeds and fruits have the lowest concentrations. In contrast, particulate lead present in air may adhere tenaciously to leafy vegetables. Leaves collected in or near urban areas have been shown to contain substantially elevated concentrations of lead. The use of leaded gasoline or the proximity of industries producing ambient emissions of lead can greatly influence lead concentrations in foodstuff. Therefore, caution is required with regard to concentrations of foodborne lead when extrapolating between regions and countries (WHO, 1995).

Typical lead concentrations in foodstuffs from some 30 countries are given in Table 39 (Galal-Gorchev, 1991a). Concentrations of lead in a variety of foodstuffs in the

Table 38. Lead content in some paints used in India

Paint colour[a]	Lead concentration (mg/kg)
Ultra white	< 1
White primer	< 1
White	< 1
Brown red	1
White	2
Phiroza	3
Oxford blue	3–6
Phorozi	5
Brown red	5
Brilliant white	6
Signal red	16
Bus green	32
New bus green	40
Deep green	50
Post office red	60–62
Mint green	61
Singal red	78
Tractor orange	114–130
Golden yellow	168–202

Adapted from van Alphen (1999)
[a] Paint samples from six companies in Bangalore and Chennai, India

USA, Canada, Latin America and the Caribbean, Africa, South Asia and Japan are shown in Tables 40–45, respectively. Lead concentrations of specific food items available in various countries are given in Tables 46–49. Studies from various countries on dietary lead intake by children and adults are listed in Tables 50–51. The section below presents a variety of specific sources of lead contamination in food.

(i) *Contamination of livestock*

Elevated concentrations of lead in the blood of cattle grazing near a lead smelter have been reported, although no inferences regarding lead in beef were made. Mean lead concentrations were highest in animals grazing near the smelter and decreased with increasing distance. Ingestion of soil along with the forage was thought to be the major source of lead (Neuman & Dollhopf, 1992).

Evidence has been shown for transfer of lead to milk and edible tissue in cattle poisoned by licking the remains of storage batteries which had been burned and left in a pasture (Oskarsson *et al.*, 1992). Concentrations of lead in muscle of eight acutely-sick cows that were slaughtered ranged from 0.14 to 0.50 mg/kg (wet weight basis). Normal lead concentrations in bovine meat from Sweden are < 0.005 mg/kg. Eight cows showing

Table 39. Representative concentrations of lead in foods[a]

Food category	Typical lead concentration (μg/kg)
Cereals	60
Roots and tubers	50
Fruit	50
Vegetables	50
Meat	50
Vegetable oils and fats	20
Fish	100
Pulses	40
Eggs	20
Nuts and oilseeds	40
Shellfish	200
Offal	200
Spices and herbs	300
Drinking-water	20
Canned beverages (lead-soldered cans)	200
Canned food (lead-soldered cans)	200

From Galal-Gorchev (1991a)
[a] Data collected from 30 countries in the Global Environmental Monitoring System/Food network

Table 40. Concentrations of lead in various foods in the USA

Food category	Concentration (μg/kg) range of mean
Dairy products	3–83
Meat, fish and poultry	2–83
Grain and cereal products	2–84
Vegetables	5–74
Fruit and fruit juices	5–53
Oils, fats and shortenings	2–28
Sugar and sweets, desserts	6–73
Canned food	16–649
Beverages	2–41

From US Environmental Protection Agency (1986a) Appendix 7D

Table 41. Concentrations of lead in various foods in Canada

Food category	Concentration (µg/kg) median (range)
Cereals, bread and toast (as prepared)	32.4 (11.5–78.3)
Water consumed directly	2.0 (0.25–71.2)
Coffee, tea, beer, liquor, sodas, etc. (as prepared)	8.8 (< 0.05–28.9)
Fruit juices, fruits (canned and fresh)	7.9 (1.5–109)
Dairy products and eggs	3.3 (1.21–81.9)
Starch vegetables, e.g. potatoes, rice	16.9 (5.5–83.7)
Other vegetables, vegetable juices and soups	31.7 (0.62–254)
Meat, fish, poultry, meat-based soups	31.3 (11–121)
Miscellaneous (pies, puddings, nuts, snack foods)	33.1 (13.6–1381)
Cheese (other than cottage cheese)	33.8 (27.7–6775)

From Dabeka *et al.* (1987)

no acute symptoms of poisoning were followed for 18 weeks. The mean lead concentration in milk 2 weeks after exposure was 0.08 ± 0.04 mg/kg; the highest concentration was 0.22 mg/kg. There was an initial rapid decrease in lead concentrations in milk during the first 6 weeks after exposure, after which the concentrations remained constant or increased slightly. Lead concentration in most milk samples was < 0.03 mg/kg 6 weeks after exposure. Two cows calved at 35 and 38 weeks post-exposure. The lead concentration in the blood of the cows at the time of delivery was high, which suggests mobilization of lead during the later stages of gestation and delivery. Lead concentrations in colostrum were increased compared to those in mature milk samples taken 18 weeks after exposure (i.e. during pregnancy), but decreased rapidly after delivery in mature milk to near the limit of detection.

Lead poisoning was observed in cattle and buffalo grazing near a primary lead–zinc smelter in India. Affected animals had a history of clinical signs characterized by head pressing, violent movement, blindness and salivation, and had high lead concentrations in blood (143 ± 1 µg/dL) and milk (0.75 ± 0.19 mg/L). Animals from the same pasture but without any history of clinical signs suggestive of lead poisoning had lower blood lead concentrations than the affected animals, but nonetheless higher than those reported for cattle in rural and urban areas of India (Dwivedi *et al.*, 2001).

Analysis of animal feed and meat from cattle, horse (an important food animal) and sheep in a metal-processing region (Oskemen) of eastern Kazakhstan revealed high lead concentrations in many feed and meat samples (horse > cattle > sheep). The highest concentrations of lead were found in the liver and kidney, and lower concentrations in muscle and lung. A lead concentration of 2.2 mg/kg was found in horse liver (Farmer & Farmer, 2000).

Recreational and subsistence hunters consume a wide range of species including birds and mammals, some of which represent significant exposure to toxic agents, including

Table 42. Lead concentrations in foods in Latin America and the Caribbean

Country	Location	Food item	Main source of lead	Concentration mean ± SD or range of means (range)	Year(s) of study	Reference
Argentina	Buenos Aires	Cultivated vegetables (leaves)	Traffic	2 mg/kg	1975	Romieu *et al.* (1997)
	Mixed	White wine	NR	55 ± 36 μg/L	NR	Roses *et al.* (1997)
		Red wine	NR	85 ± 55 μg/L		
Brazil	Santo Amaro, Bahia	Vegetables	Smelter	(0.01–215 mg/kg)[a]	1980	Tavares (1991)
	All Saints Bay	Mussels			1994	Tavares (1996b)
	Mataripe (N)		Oil refinery	(12.0–57.9 mg/kg)[a]		
	Såo Bras (NW)		Downstream smelter	(1.36–22.5 mg/kg)[a]		
	Baiacu (SW)		No specific source	5.30 mg/kg[a]		
	Paraiba valley, S. Paulo	Cow's milk	Smelter	0.05 (0.01–0.20 mg/L)	1994	Okada *et al.* (1997)
	Ribeira do Iguape	Fish	NR	0.03–12 mg/kg	1994	Romieu *et al.* (1997)
Chile	Antofagasta (pre-Andean region)	Vegetables	Rural areas, vulcanos	0.6–39.2 μg/kg[b]	NR	Queirolo *et al.* (2000)
		Potato skin		94 μg/kg[b]		
	Temucho Bay	Vegetables	NR	20 mg/kg	NR	Romieu *et al.* (1997)
Ecuador	Andean village: La Victoria		Glazing of ceramic		NR	Counter *et al.* (2000)
		Cherries		6.3 ± 2.0 mg/kg		
		Tomatoes		119 ± 1.2 mg/kg		
		Corn		61.7 mg/kg (9.86–118.68 mg/kg)		
		Wheat grain		23.9 mg/kg		
		Kernels of wheat		0.75 mg/kg		
Honduras	Lago Yojoa	Fish	NR	0.30 mg/kg	NR	Romieu *et al.* (1997)
Mexico	Vera Cruz, Campeche and Tabasco	4 crustaceae and 7 freshwater fish	Industrial region	0.03–5.62 mg/kg	1972	Albert & Badillo (1991)[c]

Table 42 (contd)

Country	Location	Food item	Main source of lead	Concentration mean ± SD or range of means (range)	Year(s) of study	Reference
	Gulf of Mexico	Oyster	NR	ND–3.0 mg/kg	1976–87	
	Coatzacoalcos river	Fish	NR	0.1–2.84 mg/kg	1983	
	Laguna de Terminos	Oyster	March–May June–October Dec–Feb	2.4 (0.7–4.1)[a] mg/kg 5.5 (5.1–5.9)[a] mg/kg 9.5 (8.5–10.5)[a] mg/kg	1985–86	
	N and NE Mexico districts	Alfalfa Beans	NR NR	(0.4–2.5 mg/kg) (0.3–3.5 mg/kg)	1980–81	
	Commercially available	Milk in different forms	NR	5–88 µg/L	1982	
	Commercially available	Canned products (fish, fruits and vegetables)	NR	(ND–2.35 mg/kg)	1988	
	Commercially available	Canned fruits	NR	0.6–1.6 mg/kg	NR	Tamayo *et al.* (1984)
Trinidad and Tobago	Imported	Iodized salt	NR	6.4 mg/kg	NR	Romieu *et al.* (1997)
Uruguay	Seashore	Bivalve shell fish	NR	6–32 mg/kg	1992	Romieu *et al.* (1997)
Venezuela	States of Guarico and Portuguesa	Rice (commercially available)	NR	0.024–0.21 mg/kg	NR	Buscema *et al.* (1997)

SD, standard deviation; NR, not reported; ND, not detectable
[a] Dry weight
[b] Fresh weight
[c] Review including mainly reports and literature not easily accessible

Table 43. Lead concentrations in food in Africa (Nigeria)

Food item	Lead concentration (mg/kg)
Condensed or powdered milk	0.25–0.83
Beef	1.3
Plantains	0.2
Melon seeds	0.43
Water and bitter leaf	0.25–0.3
Gari flour	0.11
Yam tubers	0.35

From Ukhun *et al.* (1990)

Table 44. Lead concentrations in foods in some Asian countries

Country	Place/location	Food item	Concentration (mg/kg)[a] mean or range of means (range)	Reference
India	Nine localities of Greater Mumbai (high to negligible vehicle traffic)	Cereals	0.23–0.56	Khandekar *et al.* (1984)
		Pulses	0.54–0.88	
		Leafy vegetables	0.47–1.12	
		Other vegetables	0.042–0.16	
		Meat	0.40–0.46	
		Fruit	0.032–0.044	
		Milk	0.16	
	Commercially available	Five brands of beer	10.4–15.7 μg/L (8.0–18.0)	Srikanth *et al.* (1995a)
	Commercially available	Rice and other cereal products	0.189–0.332 (0.128–0.371)	Srikanth *et al.* (1995b)
	Rajasthan	Milk from cattle and buffalo	0.21–1.47 μg/L	Dwivedi *et al.* (2001)
	Nagpur	Milk		Patel *et al.* (2001)
		Infant formula	4.13 μg/L	
		Dairy	4.75 μg/L	
		Human	2.73 μg/L	
Kazakhstan	4 districts around a metal production center	Muscle, liver, kidney, lung	0.49–1.03 (horse) 0.86–2.22 (cattle) 0.06–1.16 (sheep)	Farmer & Farmer (2000)
Pakistan	Karachi	Cooked food	1.25–3.90	Rahbar *et al.* (2002)
South Asia	14 regions of south Asia	181 rice samples	0.0048–0.090[b] (ND–0.269)	Watanabe *et al.* (1989)
Thailand	Grazing land site near highway	Milk	14 μg/L	Parkpian *et al.* (2003)

ND, not detectable
[a] Unless specified otherwise
[b] Dry weight

Table 45. Estimated lead concentrations in foods and dietary lead intake in Japan, 2001

Food category	Lead intake		Food intake[a] (g/day)	Estimated lead concentration[b] (µg/kg)
	(µg/day)	(%)		
Rice	6.63	[28.4]	356.3	[18.6]
Other cereals and potatoes	3.42	[14.7]	162.6	[21.0]
Sugar and confectionary	0.55	[2.4]	90.7	[6.1]
Fat and oil	0.25	[1.1]	11.3	[22.1]
Pulses and pulse products	1.06	[4.5]	57.2	[18.5]
Fruits	1.64	[7.0]	132	[12.4]
Green yellow vegetables	1.23	[5.3]	93.6	[13.1]
Other vegetables and algae	2.09	[9.0]	175.7	[11.9]
Beverages	2.39	[10.3]	509.3	[4.7]
Fish and shellfish	1.62	[6.9]	94.0	[17.2]
Meats and eggs	1.25	[5.4]	113.1	[11.1]
Milk and dairy products	0.73	[3.1]	170.0	[4.3]
Prepared foods	0.34	[1.5]		
Drinking-water	0.11	[0.5]		
Total	23.31	[100.0]	2042	

From National Institute of Health Sciences, Japan (2000)
[a] From Ministry of Health, Labour and Welfare, Japan (2002)
[b] Lead intake divided by food intake

Table 46. Lead concentrations in cow's milk and infant formula

Product	Canada[a] 1986 median (range) (µg/kg)	Mexico[b] 1982 average (µg/kg)	USA[c] late 1980s average (µg/kg)
Fluid milk	1.19 (0.01–2.5)	5	
Evaporated milk			
Can	71.9 (27–106)	88	10
Cardboard container	–	9	
Infant formula		13	
Ready to use, lead-solder can	30.1 (1.1–122)		10
Ready to use, lead-free can	1.6 (1.5–2)		1
Powder formula	6.6 (3.7–19)		
Powdered milk[d]	–	21	

Table adapted from WHO (1995)
[a] From Dabeka & McKenzie (1987)
[b] From Olguín *et al.* (1982) cited by WHO (1995)
[c] From Bolger *et al.* (1991)
[d] The concentration of lead in milk consumed by the infant will be highly dependent on the concentration of lead in water used to dilute the powdered milk.

Table 47. Distribution of lead concentrations in table wines produced worldwide[a]

Range of lead concentrations (μg/L)	Number of samples (n = 432)	Percentage of total samples analysed
0–10	36	8.3
11–25	62	14.4
26–50	105	24.3
51–100	144	33.3
101–250	64	14.8
251–500	12	2.8
501–673	9	2.1

From US Department of the Treasury (1991)
[a] Wines produced in 28 different countries and commercially available in the USA

Table 48. Lead concentrations in rice consumed in various countries

Country/area	Lead content (μg/kg fresh weight)		
	N	GM	GSD
China	215	22.17	2.31
China (Province of Taiwan)	104	10.84	3.18
Colombia	22	8.09	2.80
Indonesia	24	39.07	2.26
Italy	15	6.97	3.28
Japan	788	5.06	2.64
Malaysia	97	9.31	2.61
Philippines	26	37.60	2.71
Republic of Korea	172	7.95	1.79
Saudi Arabia[a]	27	[57.5][b]	[2.34][b]
Thailand	13	8.75	2.28
USA	29	7.42	2.11

From Zhang *et al.* (1996), Al-Saleh & Shinwari (2001)
GM, geometric mean; GSD, geometric standard deviation; N, no. of samples
[a] Samples of rice imported from Australia (n = 2), Egypt (n = 2), India (n = 17), Thailand (n = 4) and USA (n = 2)
[b] Estimated from arithmetic mean and ± arithmetic SD of 134.8 ± 285.9 mg/kg by the moment method

Table 49. Lead concentrations in a variety of food items

Location	Source	Lead concentration	Reference
Canada	Apple juice stored in glazed earthenware	65/117 samples > 7 mg/L 19/147 samples 500–1000 mg/L	Klein *et al.* (1970)
Ontario, Canada	Water boiled in lead-soldered electric kettle	0.75–1.2 mg/L	Ng & Martin (1977)
New York, USA	Alcoholic beverages stored in crystal containers	0.01–21.5 mg/L	Graziano & Blum (1991)
South Carolina, USA	Mourning dove	Feathers, 465.7–2011.6 μg/kg dry wt Muscle, 81.7–142.9 μg/kg wet wt Liver, 188.3–806.1 μg/kg wet wt	Burger *et al.* (1997)
Kuwait	Seafood (fish, shrimp)	0.06–0.16 mg/kg wet wt	Bu-Olayan & Al-Yakoob (1998)
Iowa, USA	Mexican candy wrappers	810–16 000 mg/kg	Fuortes & Bauer (2000)

lead. Wild game may be contaminated through the environment or from lead bullets ingested by or embedded in the animal (Burger *et al.*, 1997, 1998).

(ii) *Contamination from food preparation, storage and tableware*

Lead present in food storage and serving vessels such as lead-soldered cans, ceramic dishes, cooking vessels, crystal glassware, and labels on food wrap and/or dishes can contaminate food. Acidic foods tend to leach more lead, but certain foods such as corn and beans are associated with greater release of lead than would be predicted from their acidity alone. Also, oxygen appears to accelerate the release of lead from food containers (WHO, 1995).

If food is stored in ceramic or pottery-ware that is lead-glazed and fired in a low-temperature kiln, lead can migrate from the glaze into the food. The glazing process uses a flux, a material that, at high temperatures, reacts with and helps dissolve the components of the glaze. Lead oxide is commonly used as flux. Factors determining whether, and to what extent, lead will migrate include the temperature and extent of firing of the pottery during the manufacturing process, the temperature and duration of food storage, the age of the pottery and the acidity of the food. It is extremely difficult to quantify the extent of such exposures in view of variations in manufacturing processes and quality control practised in the country of origin; however, exposure can be quite significant, particularly to infants (WHO, 1995). Gersberg *et al.* (1997) estimated that dietary exposure to lead from beans prepared in Mexican ceramic pottery may account for the major fraction of the blood lead in children whose families use such ceramic-ware.

Table 50. Estimated dietary lead intake in adults and children

Country	Population studied	Daily intake (µg/day)[a]		Reference
Adults				
Belgium[b]	Men and women	230	M	Fouassin & Fondu (1980)
Belgium[b]	Men and women	96[c]	D	Buchet *et al.* (1983)
Canada	Men and women	43[c]	D	Dabeka *et al.* (1987)
China	Women	46	D	Vahter *et al.* (1991a)
	Women	24.6		Ikeda *et al.* (2000a)
China (Province of Taiwan)	Women	19.5		Ikeda *et al.* (2000a)
Croatia	Women	15	D	Vahter *et al.* (1991a)
Finland	Men and women	66	M	Varo & Koivistoinen (1983)
Germany	Men and women	54–61		Kampe (1983)
India	Men and women	6.4–76.9		Parikh *et al.* (1999)
Italy	Men and women	140		[IAEA (1987)]
Japan	Women	31	D	Vahter *et al.* (1991a)
	Women	9.3		Ikeda *et al.* (2000a)
Malaysia	Women	7.0		Ikeda *et al.* (2000a)
New Zealand	Men and women	213	M	Pickston *et al.* (1985)
Philippines	Women	11.3		Ikeda *et al.* (2000a)
Republic of Korea	Women	21.5		Ikeda *et al.* (2000a)
Sweden	Men and women	27	M	Slorach *et al.* (1983)
	Women	26	D	Vahter *et al.* (1991a,b)
Thailand	Women	15.1		Ikeda *et al.* (2000a)
Turkey	Men and women	70		[IAEA (1987)]
United Kingdom	Men and women	110	M	Sherlock *et al.* (1983)
		71	D	Sherlock *et al.* (1983)
USA	Men and women	83	M	Gartrell *et al.* (1985a)
Children				
India	6–10 years	15.2–23.3		Raghunath *et al.* (1997)
	6–10 years	14.4–19.1		Raghunath *et al.* (1999)
Poland	0–1 year	225		Olejnik *et al.* (1985)
	1–3 years	259		
	7–18 years	316		
UK	Infant	1–2	breast milk or formula	Kovar *et al.* (1984)
USA	< 6 months	16–17	infant formula	Ryu *et al.* (1983)
	Infant	34	M	Gartrell *et al.* (1985b)
	Toddler	43	M	

Adapted from WHO (1995); Ikeda *et al.* (2000a)
References in square brackets could not be retrieved as original papers.
[a] M, market basket survey; D, duplicate diet study
[b] Populations studied from the same region
[c] Median value

Table 51. Estimated respiratory and dietary intakes of lead in various cities in Asia

Country, city	Route	Lead in air (ng/m^3)	Intake[a] (µg/day)	Uptake[b] (µg/day)	Total (µg/day)	Dietary/ total (%)
China, Beijing + Shanghai	Respiratory	60–540	2.70	1.35	2.50	46
	Dietary		23.1	1.16		
Japan, Tokyo + Kyoto	Respiratory	70–81	1.13	0.57	1.24	54
	Dietary		9.0	0.68		
Malaysia, Kuala Lumpur	Respiratory	30–462	3.69	1.85	2.37	22
	Dietary		7.0	0.53		
Philippines, Manila	Respiratory	648	9.72	4.86	5.69	15
	Dietary		11.1	0.63		
Thailand, Bangkok	Respiratory	210–390	4.29	2.15	3.28	34
	Dietary		15.1	1.13		

From Ikeda *et al.* (2000a,b); data are on adult women and were based on studies in 1990s.
[a] Respiration volume was assumed to be 15 m^3/day.
[b] Uptake rates are assumed to be 50% in the lungs and 5–10% in the gastrointestinal tract.

Several studies have shown contamination of foods and beverages from lead used in the manufacture or repair of metal vessels. Coating the inner surface of brass utensils with a mixture of lead and tin, described as ‘tinning’, is widely practised by artisans in India. The tin–lead alloy contains 55–70% lead. Water boiled with tamarind in a tinned brass vessel for 5 min was found to contain 400–500 µg/L lead (Vatsala & Ramakrishna, 1985). Zhu *et al.* (1984) described 344 cases of chronic lead poisoning in Jiansu Province, China, in people who had drunk rainwater boiled in tin kettles. After boiling, the water contained 0.79–5.34 mg/L lead. Lead concentrations have also been shown to increase when water is boiled in kettles that contain lead in their heating elements. A study in India showed that although lead leaching from pressure cookers occurs during cooking, especially from the rubber gasket and safety valve, it is only a minor source of lead in cooked food (Raghunath & Nambi, 1998).

Lead-contaminated water may also contribute to foodborne lead where large volumes of water are used in food preparation and cooking, e.g. in foods prepared in boiling water. Experiments have shown that vegetables and rice cooked in water containing lead may absorb up to 80% of the lead in the water (Little *et al.*, 1981).

Trace metals, including lead, have been detected in human breast milk, thus breast-feeding could deliver lead to an infant. The reader is referred to Section 4.1.1(*a*)(v) for information on lead mobilisation in bones and transfer to breast milk during pregnancy and lactation. In a study in Australia, the mean lead concentration (± standard deviation) in breast milk from 21 lactating mothers was 0.73 ± 0.70 µg/kg (Gulson *et al.*, 1998a). Analysis of 210 human milk samples taken across Canada showed a mean lead concentration of 1.04 μg/kg (range, < 0.05–15.8 μg/kg) (Dabeka *et al.*, 1988). The median lead concentration in breast milk from 41 volunteers in Sweden was 2 μg/kg (range, 0.5–9.0 μg/kg) (Larsson *et al.*, 1981), whereas the mean value for breast milk 5 days postpartum from urban residents in Germany in 1983 was 13.3 μg/L (Sternowsky & Wessolowski, 1985). The concentration in 3-day postpartum milk samples from 114 women in Malaysia averaged 47.8 μg/L (Ong *et al.*, 1985).

Concentrations of lead in human milk vary considerably depending on the mother's exposure and occupation. Lead concentrations in the milk of a mother who had worked in a battery factory until 7 weeks before delivery decreased gradually from 19–63 to 4–14 μg/L in samples taken soon after delivery and those taken up to 32 weeks later, respectively (Ryu *et al.*, 1978). Lead concentrations in breast milk of 96 mothers in three districts (urban, mining area and rural) of Hubei, China averaged 76, 101 and 90 μg/L (geometric mean; $n = 21$, 11 and 32, respectively). The concentrations were very similar in colostrum and mature milk, and correlated well with blood lead concentrations (Wang *et al.*, 2000).

Gulson *et al.* (1998a) measured lead isotope ratios ($^{207}Pb/^{206}Pb$ and $^{206}Pb/^{204}Pb$) in mothers' breast milk and in infants' blood and established that, for the first 60–90 days postpartum, the contribution from breast milk to blood lead in the infants varied from 36% to 80%. Maternal bone and diet appeared to be the major sources of lead in breast milk.

Lead has also been reported in home-prepared reconstituted infant formula (breast-milk substitute). Lead concentrations in cows' milk and infant formula analysed in Canada, Mexico and the USA are shown in Table 46. Two of forty samples of infant formula collected in a study in the Boston area of the USA had lead concentrations > 15 μg/L. In both cases, the reconstituted formula had been prepared using cold tap-water run for 5–30 sec, drawn from the plumbing of houses > 20 years old. It was concluded that three preparation practices for infant formula should be avoided: (1) excessive water boiling, (2) use of lead-containing vessels and (3) use of morning (first-draw) water (Baum & Shannon, 1997).

Canning foods in lead-soldered cans may increase concentrations of lead in foods 8–10-fold. In 1974, for example, the lead concentration in evaporated milk in lead-soldered cans was 0.12 μg/g; in 1986, after these cans had been phased out, the concentration dropped to 0.006 μg/g (Capar & Rigsby, 1989). The lead content in canned foods in the USA dropped from an overall mean of 0.31 μg/g in 1980 to 0.04 μg/g in 1988 (National Food Processors Association, 1992). The production and use of three-piece lead-soldered cans ceased in 1991 in the USA. However, older lead-soldered cans may still be present in some households (ATSDR, 1999). Dabeka and McKenzie (1987, 1988) found that the intake of lead by 0–1 year-old infants fed infant formula, evaporated milk and concentrated liquid formula stored in lead-soldered cans exceeded the provisional tolerable weekly intake (PTWI) of 25 μg/kg body weight (bw) lead set by the Joint FAO/WHO Expert Committee on Food Additives (JECFA) in 1993 (FAO/WHO, 1993). This value does not include lead in water used to prepare infant formula. Mean intakes far in excess of the PTWI were obtained in studies carried out in areas with high lead content in tap-water (Galal-Gorchev, 1991b).

Lozeena, a bright orange powder from Iraq used to colour rice and meat, can contain 7.8–8.9% lead (CDC, 1998).

Lead may leach from lead crystal decanters into the liquids they contain. Three samples of port wine with an initial concentration of 89 µg/L lead were found to have lead concentrations of 5331, 3061 and 2162 µg/L after storage for four months in crystal decanters containing 32%, 32% and 24% lead monoxide, respectively (Graziano & Blum, 1991). Lead was also found to elute from lead crystal wine glasses within minutes. Mean lead concentrations in wine contained in 12 glasses increased from 33 µg/L initially to 68, 81, 92 and 99 µg/L after 1, 2, 3 and 4 h, respectively (Graziano & Blum, 1991). [See comments on this article in de Leacy, 1991; Zuckerman, 1991].

(iii) *Alcoholic beverages*

In addition to contamination from lead crystal glass, contamination of alcoholic beverages with lead may occur in several ways. For example, from lead solder used to repair casks or kegs and tap lines, from lead capsules used as seals on wine bottles, or from residues of lead arsenate pesticides in soils. Alcoholic beverages tend to be acidic and there is the possibility for large amounts of lead to dissolve during preparation, storage or serving (WHO, 1995). Wai *et al.* (1979) showed that wine can react with the lead capsule to form lead carbonate, which may dissolve in the wine during storage and pouring. In one study, lead concentrations in wine on the Swedish market ranged between 16 and 170 µg/L (Jorhem *et al.*, 1988). The analysis of 432 table wines originating from many countries and sold in the USA is summarized in Table 47. In a study of the lead content of Argentinian wines, red wine was found to have 50% higher lead concentrations than white wine, average values being 85 and 55 µg/L, respectively (Roses *et al.*, 1997).

Sherlock *et al.* (1986) found that in the UK the majority of canned and bottled beer (90 and 86% respectively) contained less than 10 µg/L lead. Draught beers typically contained higher lead concentrations, with 45% having concentrations > 10 µg/L, 16% having concentrations > 20 µg/L and 4% having concentrations > 100 µg/L. The higher lead concentrations in draught beers are thought to be due to the draught-dispensing equipment which may contain brass or gunmetal, both of which contain low but significant amounts of lead.

The analysis of lead concentration in five different beer brands in India showed that all brands had a mean lead concentration > 10 µg/L, with an overall mean of 13.2 µg/L. Assuming the lead concentration in beer to be 13 µg/L, the uptake of lead from beer to be 20% and consumption by three types of consumer to be 1, 5 or 10 L/week, this would result in a lead uptake of 2.6, 13 and 25 µg/week, respectively (Srikanth *et al.,* 1995a).

Illicit 'moonshine' whiskey made in stills composed of lead-soldered parts (e.g. truck radiators) may contain high concentrations of lead. Lead was detected in 7/12 samples of Georgia (USA) moonshine whiskey, with a maximum concentration of 5300 µg/L (Gerhardt *et al.*, 1980). In a more recent study, regular consumers of moonshine whiskey (15/49 subjects) had blood lead concentrations > 50 μg/dL (Morgan *et al.*, 2001).

In general, alcoholic beverages do not appear to be a significant source of lead intake for the average person.

(iv) *Fish and seafood*

The uptake and accumulation of lead by aquatic organisms from water and sediment are influenced by various environmental factors such as temperature, salinity and pH, as well as humic and alginic acid content of the sediment. In contaminated aquatic systems, only a minor fraction of lead is dissolved in the water. Lead in fish is accumulated mostly in gill, liver, kidney and bone. In contrast to inorganic lead compounds, tetraalkyllead is rapidly taken up by fish and rapidly eliminated after the end of exposure (WHO, 1989).

The Fish and Wildlife Service in the USA reported on the concentration of selected metals in 315 composite samples of whole fish collected at 109 stations nationwide in 1984–85. For lead, the geometric mean was 0.11 mg/kg (wet weight), with a maximum of 4.88 mg/kg. Lead concentrations in fish declined steadily from 1976 to 1984, suggesting that reduction in use of leaded gasoline and controls on mining and industrial discharges have reduced lead concentrations in the aquatic environment (Schmitt & Brumbaugh, 1990).

Recreational and subsistence fishers consume larger quantities of fish and shellfish than the general population and frequently fish the same waterbodies routinely. Thus, these populations are at greater risk of exposure to lead and other chemical contaminants if the waters they fish are contaminated. Ingestion of lead is also a matter of concern in regular consumers of seafood produced near industrial areas such as in All Saints Bay and Ribeira do Iguape in Brazil (Tavares, 1996a,b), as well as in Uruguay (Romieu *et al.*, 1997).

(v) *Rice and cereals*

Rice is an important source of lead intake, particularly in east and south-east Asia where rice is a staple component of the diet. Lead concentrations in rice consumed in some areas in Asia, Australia, Europe and North America are summarized in Table 48. The data show a substantial variation from < 10 to about 40 μg/kg fresh weight (Zhang *et al.*, 1996; Al-Saleh & Shinwari, 2001a). In a study performed by Watanabe *et al.* (1989), rice samples were collected in 15 areas of Asia and Australia (192 samples), and in four areas in other parts of the world (15 samples). Lead concentrations were distributed log-normally, with a geometric mean ± geometric standard deviation of 15.7 ± 3.5 μg/kg and concentrations ranging from 5 μg/kg in Japan to 90 μg/kg in India.

Lead in rice has been estimated to represent 28% (National Institute of Health Sciences, Japan, 2000; see Table 45), 14% (Zhang *et al.*, 2000), 12% (Moon *et al.*, 1995) and < 5% (Zhang *et al.*, 1997a) of dietary lead intake in a series of studies in China, Japan and the Republic of Korea. In Japan, dietary lead intake has decreased on average from 33 μg/day in 1980 to 7 μg/day in 1990, partly as a result of a decrease in rice consumption (Watanabe *et al.*, 1996).

Cereals other than rice, e.g. millet and maize, may also be important sources of dietary lead. The lead concentration in these cereals (43–47 μg/kg) is higher than that in rice (20–21 μg/kg) or wheat (26–30 μg/kg) (Zhang *et al.*, 1997b). In one study in China, lead from all cereals accounted for 26% of total dietary lead intake (Watanabe *et al.*, 2000). Lead intake from rice in Japan was found to be 1.5 times that from wheat in 1998–2000 (Shimbo *et al.*, 2001).

The contribution of lead in rice and cereal products to the total dietary intake of lead in southern India varies among different socioeconomic groups, based on occupation and choice of consumption. It has been suggested that rice is the major source of lead among the rural and economically-deprived populations, but sources of dietary lead appeared to be more diverse in the urban middle-class and the economically-privileged (Srikanth *et al.*, 1995b).

(vi) *Daily intake through food*

Estimates of daily dietary intakes of lead by adults and children worldwide are presented in Table 50. The available data indicate a general decrease in those areas where the concentration of lead in gasoline has decreased and those where a concerted effort has been made to avoid lead-soldered cans for food storage (Bolger *et al.*, 1991; OECD, 1993). Similar decreases in other countries are expected to occur when similar actions to eliminate these sources of lead exposure are taken.

Dietary lead intake by adult women in several Asian cities, in comparison with amounts of lead inhaled, is presented in Table 51. The ratio of dietary to total lead intake varied primarily as a reverse function of the lead concentration in atmospheric air (Ikeda *et al.*, 2000a). In Mumbai, India, where atmospheric lead concentrations in different zones of the city varied between 82 and 605 ng/m^3, the daily lead uptake by a nonsmoker living in the city area was estimated to be 33 μg, of which 75% come from food. For a suburban resident, 85% of the lead intake was estimated to come from food (Khandekar *et al.*, 1984).

(*i*) *Plants and fertilizers*

Lead occurs naturally in plants both from deposition and uptake; there is a positive linear relationship between lead concentrations in soil and in plants. As with other environmental compartments, measurement of 'background' concentrations of lead in plants is complicated by the general contamination of the environment from centuries of lead use, which has included direct application of lead-containing chemicals in agriculture and contamination of fertilizers with lead (WHO, 1995).

Lead has been detected in a superphosphate fertilizer at concentrations as high as 92 mg/kg (WHO, 1995). Sewage sludge, used as a source of nutrients in agriculture, may contain concentrations of lead > 1000 mg/kg; concentrations as high as 26 g/kg have been measured in the USA (WHO, 1995). In a study of soil that had received heavy sludge applications over years in the United Kingdom, the lead concentration was found to be 425 mg/kg, compared with 47 mg/kg in untreated soil (Beckett *et al.*, 1979).

Lead concentrations in grass and water plants in Asia are shown in Table 52.

Table 52. Lead concentrations in terrestrial and aquatic plants in Asia

Country	Location	Year(s) of study	Source of contamination	Plant[a]	Concentration (mg/kg) mean ± SD or range of means	Reference
India	Koraput	NR	NR	*Ipomea aquatic*	83.3 ± 4.2	Chandra *et al.* (1993)
				Trapa natans	68.5 ± 2.1	
	Unnao		(summer)	*Trapa natans*	54.5 ± 2.0	
				Ipomea aquatica	46.6 ± 1.5	
			(winter)	*Trapa natans*	1030.0 ± 51.5	
				Ipomea aquatica	845.0 ± 40.0	
	Eastern Ghats (Koraput, Orrisa)	NR	Local industries	*Spirodela polyrrhiza*	27 ± 1.6	Rai *et al.* (1996)
				Pistia stratiotes	29 ± 0.8	
	Mumbai	NR	Lead industries	Grass	145–1048	Nambi *et al.* (1997)
				Control grass	1.42	
	Lake Nainital	1997	NR	*Microcystis aeruginosa*	46 ± 2.5	Ali *et al.* (1999)
				Spirogyra adnata	95 ± 4.2	
				Salix babylonica (root)	37 ± 2.7	
	Residential area of greater Kolkata	1996	Lead factory	Leaf samples	214 ± 17	Chatterjee & Banerjee (1999)
	4 lakes and pounds in Lucknow	1998	NR	*Trapa natans*	75–375	Rai & Sinha (2001)
	Pond in North-Bihar	1996–97	NR	*Euryale ferox* Salisb.	331.6–1256.6	Rai *et al.* (2002)
Kazakhstan	Six districts in the East	NR	Metal production centre	Hay & pasteur grasses	1.6 ± 0.01– 19.4 ± 6.2	Farmer & Farmer (2000)
Thailand	Tropical grazing land site	NR	NR	Grass	0.76– 6.62	Parkpian *et al.* (2003)

NR, not reported
[a] Names in italics are aquatic plants.

Phytoremediation

Currently, lead-contaminated soils are being remediated by a variety of engineered technologies such as isolation and containment, mechanical separation, pyrometallurgical separation, the use of permeable treatment walls, and by soil flushing and soil washing, but these methods are expensive and not feasible at all sites (Mulligan *et al.* 2001). Phytoremediation — the use of plants for removal of pollutants and restoration of the environment — is an emerging clean-up technology for which various reviews provide information on important aspects (Salt *et al.*, 1995; Cunningham & Ow, 1996; Chaney *et al.*, 1997; Salt *et al.*, 1998).

For lead remediation, phytoextraction is the more attractive and much better studied method. Phytoextraction is the uptake of metal by roots and its accumulation in the part of the plant above ground, i.e. the shoot. Plants that are capable of accumulating more metal than 0.1% of dry weight of shoot are considered to be suitable for phytoextraction. There are various reports concerning accumulation and phytoextraction of lead (Table 53).

The basic problems with lead phytoextraction are the low bioavailability of lead in soil and its poor translocation from root to shoot. Of all toxic heavy metals, lead is the least phytoavailable. Water-soluble and exchangeable lead that is readily available for uptake by plants constitutes only about 0.1% of total lead in most soils (Huang *et al.*, 1997). Soil properties influence its uptake and translocation. In addition, only a few higher plants are known to hyperaccumulate lead, mainly owing to the very low translocation of lead from the root to the shoot. Piechalak *et al.* (2002) demonstrated up to 95% lead accumulation in the roots of *Vicia faba, Pisum sativum* and *Phaseolus vulgaris* but only 5–10% was transported to parts above ground (see Table 53).

To overcome these problems, a chelate is used to increase uptake rate and to increase lead translocation from roots to shoots. Of the many chelates, EDTA has been found to be the most appropriate. EDTA solubilizes soil lead and increases its translocation from root to shoot. It has also been shown to increase rate of transpiration, an important factor in lead phytoextraction (Wu *et al.* 1999). However, there are concerns about side-effects associated with chelate application. Lead EDTA easily percolates through the soil profile and causes groundwater pollution.

A number of plants used in phytoremediation are crop plants (see Table 53) and thus there is a potential risk that plants grown as part of phytoremediation programmes will re-enter the food chain. Furthermore, a number of algae and other plant species accumulate lead. Such species, if ingested by fish, could also re-cycle lead into the food chain. Recently, a study presented the development of a plant genetically modified to accumulate lead, which seems promising for phyto-remediation (Gisbert *et al.*, 2003).

Phytoremediation does have its limitations. It is a slower process than the traditional methods. Plants remove or degrade only small amounts of contaminants each growing season, so it can take several decades to clean up a site adequately. There are limits to plant growth such as temperature, soil type and availability of water. Lastly, most plants are

Table 53. Lead accumulation/biosorption and detoxification by plants

Plant	Treatment	Lead accumulation/ phytoextraction[a]	Reference
Zea mays shoot	20–100 μM $Pb(NO_3)_2$ in nutrient solution	Accumulation: 400–500 mg/kg	Huang & Cunningham (1996)
	Lead concentration in soil, 2500 mg/kg; treatment with HEDTA at 2 g/kg for 7 days	Phytoextraction: 10 600 mg/kg dw	
Brassica juncea shoot	Lead concentration in soil, 1200–1800 mg/kg	Accumulation: 45–100 mg/kg	Blaylock *et al.* (1997)
	600 mg/kg Pb: 10 mmol/kg EDTA 0.5 mmol/kg EDTA	Phytoextraction: ~ 15 000 mg/kg 5000 mg/kg	
Zea mays, Pisum sativum shoots	Lead concentration in soil, 2500 mg/kg; treatment with HEDTA at 2 g/kg for 7 days	Phytoextraction: ~ 10 000 mg/kg	Huang *et al.* (1997)
Brassica juncea shoot	Lead concentration in soil, 0.5 mM; treatment with EDTA at 0.75 mM for 48 h	Phytoextraction: 11 000 mg/kg dw[b]	Vassil *et al.* (1998)
Helianthus annuus	1 mM $Pb(NO_3)_2$ in nutrient solution from emergence of 1st pair of leaves until growth of 3rd pair of leaves	Accumulation: shoot, 11 027 mg/kg dw roots, 17 149 mg/kg dw	Kastori *et al.* (1998)
Vicia faba	1 mM $Pb(NO_3)_2$ treatment for 96 h	46 mg/g dw (in root)	Piechalak *et al.* (2002)
Pisum sativum		50 mg/g dw (in root)	
Phaseolus vulgaris		75 mg/g dw (in root)	

[a] Accumulation refers to the natural lead uptake by the plant from soil or a nutrient solution; phytoextraction refers to lead uptake following addition of a synthetic chelating agent to the lead-contaminated soil to improve the bioavailability of the lead.
[b] The value was 400 times higher than in untreated controls.

unable to grow on heavily-contaminated soils, thus only lightly-contaminated soils can be phytoremediated.

(*j*) *Others*

Table 54 presents some data on lead concentrations in other sources of exposure.

(i) *Traditional medicine*

Some traditional medicines and customs have been found to result in exposure to high concentrations of lead, most of which cannot be quantified with any degree of accuracy. Rather than occurring as trace ingredients or trace contaminants, various lead compounds

Table 54. Lead concentrations in various sources of exposure

Location	Source	Lead concentration	Reference
Traditional remedies			
Arizona, USA	'Greta', 'azarcon'	77 000–941 000 mg/kg	Baer *et al.* (1989)
Zabreb, Croatia	Metal-mineral tonics	0.90–72 900 mg/kg	Prpic-Majic *et al.* (1996)
Cosmetics			
Morocco, UK, USA	Eye make-up (kohl) from Eastern Mediterranean countries	< 100–696 000 mg/kg	Parry & Eaton (1991)
Others			
Arizona, USA	Pool cue chalk	1–14 080 mg/kg	Miller *et al.* (1996)
Wisconsin, USA	Dental intraoral radiograph film storage boxes (lead oxide)	3352 μg (range, 262–34 000)[a]	CDC (2001)

[a] Average amount of lead present on wipe samples from eight film packets stored in lead lined boxes

are used as major ingredients in traditional medicines in numerous parts of the world (Trotter, 1990). Lead concentrations in some traditional and complementary medicines are shown in Table 55.

Leaded 'kohl', also called 'Al kohl', is traditionally applied to the raw umbilical stump of the newborn in the belief of a beneficial astringent action. Lead metal and lead sulfide are used for inhalation of the fumes ('Bokhoor') produced from heating on hot coals, in the belief that this will ward off the devil and calm irritable infants and children (Fernando *et al.*, 1981; Shaltout *et al.*, 1981). An Asian remedy for menstrual cramps known as Koo Sar was reported to contain lead in concentrations as high as 12 mg/kg (CDC, 1999). The source of lead was thought to be the red dye used to colour the pills. The Hindus use as a treatment for diabetes ground seeds and roots, which were found to contain 8000 mg/kg lead (Pontifex & Garg, 1985).

Latin-American countries also report the use of traditional medicines with high lead concentrations. For example, the Mexican traditional remedies 'azarcon' (lead tetroxide) and/or 'greta' (mixed lead oxides), distributed as finely ground powders, may contain more than 70% lead. They are used in the treatment of 'empacho', a gastrointestinal disorder considered to be due to a blockage of the intestine (Trotter, 1990).

Some Chinese herbal medicines have metallic lead added to them (up to 20 000 mg/kg) to increase their weight and sale price (Wu *et al.*, 1996). Lead contaminants also are present in some calcium supplements; 17 of 70 brands tested had lead concentrations leading to a daily intake greater than the provisional total tolerable daily intake of 6 μg (Bourgoin *et al.*, 1993).

Table 55. Lead concentrations in herbal and folk medicines

Medicine	Concentration (μg/g)[a]	Prescribed for (where indicated)
Saptamrut loh	5.12	
Keshar gugal	2.08	
Punarvadi gugal	1.99	
Trifla gugal	4.18	
Ghasard	16 000	
Bala goli	25	
Kandu	6.7	
Arogyavardhini	63.2	Liver disease
Sankhvati	13.0	
Brahmivati	27 500	
Chyavan prash	7.30	
Trivanga bhasma	261 200	Diabetes
Diabline bhasma	37 770	Diabetes
Hepatogaurd	0.4	Liver disease
Basant malti	276 to 42 573	
Pushap Dhanva Ras	79.3 mg/tablet	
Shakti	55.9 mg/tablet	
Solution	5.27 μg/mL	Leg abscess
Powders	2.6–105 200	Leg abscess
Tablets	1.0–2816.7	Leg abscess

From Dunbabin *et al.*, (1992); Nambi *et al.* (1997)
[a] Unless otherwise specified

Medicinal herbs may be a potential source of lead exposure; analysis of 28 species showed lead concentrations (arithmetic mean ± arithmetic standard deviation) of 2.6 ± 0.4 mg/kg to 32.8 ± 3.1 mg/kg fresh weight (Dwivedi & Dey, 2002).

(ii) *Cosmetics*

Hair dyes and some cosmetics may contain lead compounds. Commercial hair dyes typically contain 3000–4000 mg/kg lead (Cohen & Roe, 1991). A later survey reported hair dyes formulated with lead acetate, with lead concentrations of 2300–6000 mg/kg (Mielke *et al.*, 1997b). Lead acetate is soluble in water and easily transferred to hands and other surfaces during and following application of a hair dye product. Measurements of 150–700 μg of lead on each hand following such applications have been reported (Mielke *et al.*, 1997b). In addition, lead is transferred by hand to mouth of the person applying the product, and to any other surface (comb, hair dryer, outside of product container, counter top) that comes into contact with the product. A dry hand passed through dry hair dyed with a lead-containing cream has been shown to pick up about 280 μg lead (Mielke *et al.*, 1997b).

Some traditional eye cosmetics produced locally may contain lead compounds, and their application, also to children, may result in lead exposure. Sprinkle (1995) reported blood lead concentrations of 9–24 μg/dL in nine children aged 3 months–5 years receiving daily application of such cosmetics, whereas concentrations of 2–6 μg/dL were found in nine children aged 1–6 years who had no or unknown application. Patel *et al.* (2001) also reported elevated blood lead concentrations (20.2 ± 13.0 μg/dL) in 45 children aged 6 months–6 years in India who used eye cosmetics daily.

Cosmetics used by Chinese opera actors may also contain lead (Lai, 1972).

(iii) *Ammunition*

Use of lead ammunition may result in exposure to lead dust, generated during gun or rifle discharge, at concentrations up to 1000 μg/m^3 (Elias, 1985), from lead pellets ingested by or embedded in animals that are used as food source (Burger *et al.*, 1997), and from lead pellets embedded in humans from shooting incidents (Manton, 1994; IARC, 1999). Firing-range instructors and employees may be exposed to high concentrations of lead and may show elevated blood lead concentrations (see Section 1.4.3.e).

(iv) *Miscellaneous*

Cigarette tobacco contains 2–12 μg of lead per cigarette (IARC, 2004a); the mean concentration of lead in filter-tipped cigarettes produced between 1960 and 1980 was 2.4 mg/kg. Up to 6% of lead may be inhaled, while the remainder is present in the ash and sidestream smoke (IARC, 2004a). Smoking a pack of 20 cigarettes per day, with 12 μg lead per cigarette, and inhaling 6% of the smoke, would result in daily exposure to 14 μg lead.

So-called recreational drug users who 'sniff' leaded gasoline vapours are at risk of toxic effects from organolead compounds as well as the hydrocarbon components of gasoline (Edminster & Bayer, 1985).

A lead poisoning hazard for young children exists in certain vinyl miniblinds that have had lead added to stabilize the plastic. Over time, the plastic deteriorates to produce lead dust that can be ingested when the blinds are touched by children who then put their hands in their mouths (Consumer Product Safety Commission, 1996; Norman *et al.*, 1997; West, 1998).

(*k*) *Blood lead concentrations from specific sources of exposure*

Blood lead concentrations resulting from exposure to a variety of specific sources, reported mainly as case reports, are presented in Table 56.

1.4.2 *Exposure of the general population*

Blood lead concentration is the most commonly used estimate of exposure to lead in the general population. Numerous reports show blood lead concentrations declining over time in many parts of the world, thereby validating global efforts to reduce lead exposures.

Table 56. Blood lead concentrations from various sources of exposure

Location	Source	Blood lead[a] (µg/dL) individual values or range[a]	Reference
Air dust			
New York, USA	Burning of newspapers in fireplace	35	Perkins & Oski (1976)
New York, USA	Dust at home from workers' clothing	Mean, 41.6–73.3	Baker *et al.* (1977)
California, USA	Dust on clothes from occupational exposure	31–36	Gerson *et al.* (1996)
New York, USA	Dust from removal of lead-based paint	20–> 80	CDC (1997a)
La Victoria and El Tejar, Ecuador	Tile-glazing activities	Median, 60 (range, 12–106)	Vahter *et al.* (1997)
Food/food containers			
Hawaii, USA	Lead-bearing cocktail glasses	131–156	Dickinson *et al.* (1972)
Ontario, Canada	Water heated in lead-soldered electric kettles	35–145	Ng & Martin (1977)
Seattle, USA	Ceramics from southern Italy	74 and 144	Wallace *et al.* (1985)
Nablus district, Israel	Contaminated flour	Mean, 80–122 (range, 42–166)	Hershko *et al.* (1989)
Vancouver, Canada	Water heated in a lead-soldered electric kettle	147–154	Lockitch *et al.* (1991)
Hungary	Contaminated paprika (lead tetraoxide)	18.8–213	Kákosy *et al.* (1996)
Vermont, USA	Apple cider prepared in lead-soldered evaporator	33–40	Carney & Garbarino (1997)
California, USA	Tamarindo candy	26–59	CDC (1998)
Michigan, USA	Lozeena (powdered food colouring)	25–84	CDC (1998)
Georgia, USA	Moonshine whiskey	> 50[b]	Morgan *et al.* (2001)
California, USA	Tamarindo candy and/or folk remedies	22–88	CDC (2002)

Table 56 (contd)

Location	Source	Blood lead[a] (µg/dL) individual values or range[a]	Reference
Traditional remedies			
California, USA	Azarcon	27–45	CDC (1981)
Minnesota, USA	'Pay-loo-ah'	60	CDC (1983)
Saudi Arabia	Traditional remedies	134–277	Abu Melha *et al.* (1987)
Guadalajara, Mexico	Azarcon (lead tetraoxide)	Blood, 29.6; urine, 49.4 µg/L	Cueto *et al.* (1989)
California, USA	Indian herbal medicine	71–80	Smitherman & Harber (1991)
California, USA	Azarcon, greta	20–86	CDC (1993)
New York, USA	Contaminated *hai ge fen* (clamshell powder)	76	Markowitz *et al.* (1994); Hill & Hill (1995)
Zagreb, Croatia	Ayurvedic metal-mineral tonics	2.6–92.1	Prpic-Majic *et al.* (1996)
Connecticut, USA	'Koo Sar' pills (Asian remedy for menstrual cramps)	42–44	CDC (1999)
Australia	Herbal remedy	Mother, 108; newborn, 244	Tait *et al.* (2002)
Cosmetics			
Nottingham, United Kingdom	Surma	Mean, 34.2	Ali *et al.* (1978)
California, USA	Traditional eye cosmetics (surma, kohl, alkohl)	Mean, 12.9	Sprinkle (1995)
Ammunition			
Texas, USA	Old gunshot wound	353	Dillman *et al.* (1979)
Texas, USA	Retained projectiles (bullets, shrapnel, buckshot)	Blood, 40–525; urine, 55–720 µg/L	Linden *et al.* (1982)
Florida, USA	Ingestion of 206 bullets	391	McNutt *et al.* (2001)
Saskatchewan, Canada	Air rifle pellets	35–56	Treble & Thompson (2002)

Table 56 (contd)

Location	Source	Blood lead[a] (µg/dL) individual values or range[a]	Reference
Others			
Oregon, USA	Curtain weight	238	Blank & Howieson (1983)
Maningrida, Australia	Petrol sniffing	42–92	Eastwell *et al.* (1983); Watson (1985)
Australia	Petrol sniffing	105	Burns & Currie (1995)
New York, USA	Ornamental clothing accessory	144–150	Esernio-Jenssen *et al.* (1996)
Hospital nurseries in the USA	Blood transfusions	Mean, 3.5 (range, 2–7)	Bearer *et al.* (2000, 2003)

[a] Unless stated otherwise
[b] Blood lead concentration in 15/38 patients

Representative data on blood lead concentrations are presented by region in Tables 57–64, and in the text by population subgroup: adults, pregnant women and neonates, and children.

(*a*) *Adults*

The UNEP/WHO Global Study to assess exposure to lead and cadmium through biological monitoring was one of the first international reliable studies with quality assurance. The geometric mean concentration of lead in blood in different populations ranged from 6 µg/dL in Beijing (China) and Tokyo (Japan) to 22.5 µg/dL in Mexico City (Mexico). The values were below 10 µg/dL in Baltimore (USA), Jerusalem (Israel), Lima (Peru), Stockholm (Sweden) and Zagreb (Serbia and Montenegro), and between 10 and 20 µg/dL in Brussels (Belgium) and Ahmedabad, Bangalore and Kolkata (India) (Friberg & Vahter, 1983).

Data from central and eastern Europe show relatively high levels of background exposure to lead at the time of the dissolution of the former Soviet Union (Table 57). There have been concerted efforts to lower exposure by phasing out the use of leaded gasoline and by controlling emissions from industries (Regional Environmental Center for Central and Eastern Europe, 1998).

In the USA, the extent of recent exposures to lead in the general population has been estimated based on blood lead measurements from the National Health and Nutrition Examination Surveys (NHANES). Geometric mean blood concentrations in adults aged

Table 57. Lead concentrations in blood in adults and children in central and eastern European countries

Country	City or area	Year(s) of study	Population	Blood lead (µg/dL) mean or range
Bulgaria	Momchilgrad	1991	Children, 5–7 years old	11.4
	Momchilgrad	1991	Teenagers, 12–14 years old	11.6
	Krichim	1991	Children	9.2
	Kurtovo Konare	1991	Children and teenagers	17.0
	Haskovo	1995	Children, 5–7 years old	10.1
	Haskovo	1995	Teenagers, 11–12 years old	11.4
	Nationwide	1995–96	Adults (men+women)	15
Czech Republic	Pribram	1992–94	Children, 1–3 years old	14.66; 6.61; 4.95[a]
			Children, 4–7 years old	10.2; 4.95; 4.67
			Children, 8–11 years old	12.50; 5.37; 4.51
			Teenagers, 12–14 years old	7.21; 4.84; 4.69
Hungary	Budapest	1992	–	11.9
	Sopron	1993	–	11.6
	Local	1994	–	7.4
	National	1995	–	6.26
	Budapest	1996	–	6.5
Poland	Five towns with no industrial lead emitters	1992–94	Men	4.25–7.68
			Women	2.38–4.83
			Children	2.39–6.23
	Based in the vicinity of zinc and copper mills	1992–94	Men	9.85–15.90
			Women	4.94–10.50
			Children	7.37–11.40
Romania (six areas of Bucharest)	North Railway Station	1983–85	Children	17.1
	Balta Alba	1983–85	Children	18.40
	Center	1983–85	Children	20.20
	Giurgiuhu	1983–85	Children	21.93
	Militari	1983–85	Children	17.84
	Pantelimon	1983–85	Children	20.51
Slovakia	Bratislava	1993	Children	3.65
	Middle Slovakia	1995	Children	4.5
	North Slovakia	1996	Children	3.04

From the final report of the National Integrated Program on Environment and Health Project (1995), presented in Regional Environmental Center for Central and Eastern Europe (1998)
–, not stated
[a] Geometric mean values for subjects living at distances from the lead smelter of less than 3 km, 3–5 km, and over 5 km, respectively

Table 58. Lead concentrations in blood in adults and children in the USA

Years of survey	Population	No. of subjects	Average age (years)	Smokers	Blood lead (µg/dL)		Reference
					GM	95% CI	
1976–80	Men + women	5537	20–74	Included	13.1	12.7–13.7	Pirkle *et al.* (1994)
1988–91	Men + women	6922	20–74	Included	3.0	2.8–3.2	Pirkle *et al.* (1994)
1999–2000	Men + women	4207	≥ 20	Included	1.8	1.67–1.83	CDC (2003a)
1978–80	Children	2271	1–5	–	15.0	14.2–15.8	Pirkle *et al.* (1994)
1988–91	Children	2234	1–5	–	3.6	3.3–4.0	Pirkle *et al.* (1994)
1991–94	Children	2392	1–5	–	2.7	2.5–3.0	CDC (1997b)
1999–2000	Children	723	1–5	–	2.2	2.0–2.5	CDC (2003a)

[a] GM, geometric mean; CI, confidence interval

20 years or older have declined by 87% from 13.1 µg/dL in 1976–80 to 1.75 µg/dL in 1999–2000 (Table 58). Concentrations were higher in men than in women, and higher in Mexican-Americans and non-Hispanic blacks than in non-Hispanic whites. In general, blood lead concentrations in adults increase slowly with age (Pirkle *et al.*, 1994; CDC, 1997b, 2003a).

Lead concentrations in the general population in several countries in Africa are summarized in Table 59. Most values were > 10 µg/dL, except for two rural areas in South Africa (Grobler *et al.*, 1985; Nriagu *et al.*, 1997a).

Reports from several Asian countries of blood lead concentrations in adults with no known occupational exposure to lead and no exposure to heavy traffic are summarized in Table 60. The values were mostly < 10 µg/dL, and few were above 13 µg/dL, with the exception of one concentration of 24 µg/dL for a rural population in Pakistan (Khan *et al.*, 1995). One study used urinary lead concentrations to monitor lead exposure in Japan. A substantial decrease in urinary lead was reported over the last 13 years. The amounts of lead excreted (geometric means) in 24-h urine samples were 4.74, 2.67 and 1.37 µg for men in 1985, 1993 and 1998, respectively, and 3.21, 2.14 and 1.02 µg for women in the same years (Jin *et al.*, 2000).

Blood lead concentrations in adults in Australia are summarized in Table 61. As observed in other parts of the world, concentrations have declined in the general population over the past two decades.

Table 59. Lead concentrations in blood in the general population in some countries in Africa

Country	City/area	Population/ age range	No. of subjects	Blood lead (µg/dL) mean (range)	Reference
Egypt	Urban area Rural area	Adults	NR	17.0–36.0 14.0–25.0	Kamal *et al.* (1991)
	Cairo	No lead exposure	50	18.2	Kamal *et al.* (1991)
Nigeria	Ibadan	Men Women		11.4 12.3	Omokhodion (1984)
	NR	Adults	24	12.9 ± 7.0 (1.7–32.5)	Ogunsola *et al.* (1994b)
	Kaduna	1–6 years	87	10.6 (max. 39)	Nriagu *et al.* (1997b)
South Africa	Urban area Rural area	Children Children	NR NR	22 11	[von Schirnding & Fuggle (1984)]
	Remote area	14–16 years	30	3.4 ± 1.5 (0.5–7.5)	Grobler *et al.* (1985)
	Cape Town	1st year-grade	200	12 (white) 18 (mixed)	von Schirnding *et al.* (1991a)[c]
	Cape Town	1st year-grade	104	18[b]	von Schirnding *et al.* (1991b)[c]
	Cape Province Mining village Village 40 km from mining area	Children Children Children	NR NR NR	14–16 16 13	Nriagu *et al.* (1996b)
	Besters Valamehlo (rural)	3–5, 8–10 years	1200 660	10 3.8	Nriagu *et al.* (1997a)
	Johannesburg	6–9 years	433	11.9 (6–26)	Mathee *et al.* (2002)
	Urban areas	Children	NR	15	Harper *et al.* (2003)[a]

Updated from Nriagu *et al.* (1996b); reference in square brackets could not be retrieved as original papers.
NR, not reported
[a] Review of several published studies
[b] Median value
[c] [It was not clear to the Working Group whether the two articles presented data from the same study population.]

Table 60. Lead concentrations in blood in adults in the general population in Asia

Country	City/area	Years of study	Population	No. of subjects	Smoking status	Blood lead (µg/dL) arithmetic mean[a] (range)	Reference
China	Shanghai	1986–88	Women	165	NR	14.1	Jiang *et al.* (1992)
	3 areas	1993–97	Women	250	Nonsmoker	4.6[b]	Zhang *et al.* (1999)
	Hubei	NR	Women				Wang *et al.* (2000)
			urban	33	NR	6.7	
			mining area	28	NR	6.7	
			rural	44	NR	5.3	
	Province of	1991–94	≥ 15 years of age	8828	NR	7.7 (ND–69.1)	Liou *et al.* (1996)
	Taiwan	1993–94	Men	1471	Included	7.3	Chu *et al.* (1998)
			Women	1332	Included	5.7	
India	Ahmedabad	NR	Men + women	200	Included	13.8	Friberg & Vahter (1983)
	Bangalore			73	Included	17.9	
	Kolkata			100	Included	10.7	
	Slums of Lucknow	1994–95	Women	500	NR	14.3 (13.0–15.7)	Awasthi *et al.* (1996; 2002)
Indonesia	Bandung	1983	Rural men	20	NR	12	Suzuki (1990)
Iraq	Bassora	NR	Men	60	NR	14.6	Mehdi *et al.* (2000)
Japan	Kanagawa	1991	Adults	62	NR	1.0 (0.6–2.4)	Arai *et al.* (1994)
	NR	NR	Men	70	NR	11.0 (5.0–17.2)	Oishi *et al.* (1996a)
			Women	68	NR	6.4 (3.8–11.4)	
	Kyoto, Sendai & Tokyo	1991–93	Women	72	Nonsmoker	3.2[b]	Zhang *et al.* (1999)
	30 sites	1991–98	Women	607	Nonsmoker	1.9[b]	Shimbo *et al.* (2000)
	NR	NR	Women	70	NR	6.4 (3.8–11.4)	Nomiyama *et al.* (2002)
Jordan	Irbid City	NR	Men	21	NR	5.7b	Hunaiti *et al.* (1995)

Table 60 (contd)

Country	City/area	Years of study	Population	No. of subjects	Smoking status	Blood lead (µg/dL) arithmetic mean[a] (range)	Reference
Pakistan	Rural area	1994–95	Men	36	NR	24.1	Khan *et al.* (1995)
Philippines	Manila	1999	Men + women	50	NR	12.6	Suplido & Ong (2000)
Republic of Korea	NR	NR	NR	26	NR	10.8	Kim *et al.* (1995a)
	Chonan	1997–99	Men + women	135	87% current	5.3 (2–10)	Lee, S.-S. *et al.* (2001); Schwartz *et al.* (2001)
Thailand	Bangkok	1993	Women	500	NR	6.2	Phuapradit *et al.* (1994)
	NR	NR	Men	30	NR	6.0 (2.1–9.7)	Wananukul *et al.* (1998)
	Chaiyapoom	NR	Rural	29	Nonsmoker	6.6 (4.0–9.0)	Suwansaksri & Wiwanitkit (2001)
United Arab Emirates	Abu Dhabi	1999	Men	100	NR	19.8; 13.3[b]	Bener *et al.* (2001)

NR, not reported; ND, not detectable
[a] Unless specified otherwise
[b] GM, geometric mean

Table 61. Lead concentrations in blood in adults and children in Australia

Reference	Location	Period of study	Population	No. of subjects	Age (years)	Blood lead concentration (µg/dL)	AM (range)	Comments
Mencel & Thorp (1976)	Sydney, NSW	1974	Adults	133	NR	12.4	2.7–51.1	
Moore *et al.* (1976)	Tasmania	NR	Clerks and students	47	18–61	14.3	SE, 0.72	Capillary blood samples
de Silva & Donnan (1977)	Melbourne, Vic.	NR	Male office workers	20	42.8	10.9	SD, 2.8	Venous blood samples
de Silva & Donnan (1980)	Victoria, Vic.	1979	Children	446	School age	11.4	3–3.7	
Calder *et al.* (1986)	Adelaide, SA, industrial suburb	1984	Boys and girls	513	≤ 4 yrs	16.3	2.7% > 30 µg/dL	
Wilson *et al.* (1986)	Port Pirie, SA	1982	Boys and girls	1239	1–14	18.2	15.4% ≥ 25 µg/dL 95.4% ≥ 10 µg/dL	
Fett *et al.* (1992)	Central Sydney, NSW, inner urban areas	1991–92	Boys and girls	158	9–48 months	11.2	50.6% > 10 µg/dL	
Threlfall *et al.* (1993)	Perth, WA	1991	Boys and girls	123	0.2–17	6.9[a]	3.2–14.7	
Gulson *et al.* (1994)	Broken Hill, NSW	1991–92	Adults and children	146	NR	–	2.7–47.1	
Taylor *et al.* (1995)	Victoria, Vic.	1993	Children	252	0.3–14	5.4[a]	1.0–36.8	
Mira *et al.* (1996)	Central and southern Sydney, NSW	1992–94	Boys and girls	718	9–62 months	7.0	16.1% > 10 µg/dL	
Chiaradia *et al.* (1997)	Goulburn, NSW	NR	Children of employees Control children	8 10	2–5 2–5.5	5.7 4.1	SD, 1.7 SD, 1.4	Lead–zinc–copper mine employees
Maynard *et al.* (2003)	Port Pririe, SA (town with widespread contamination from lead smelter)	1993 1994 1995 1997 1998 1999	Boys and girls Boys and girls Boys and girls Boys and girls Boys and girls| Boys and girls	679 551 803 753 775 825	1–4	13.6 13.3 12.1 11.4 10.1 10.6	NR NR NR NR NR NR	Surveys evaluating interventions

AM, arithmetic mean; NR, not reported; SE, standard error; SD, standard deviation
[a] Geometric mean

Table 62. Lead concentrations in blood in children living near the Santo Amaro smelter in Bahia, Brazil

Year of study	No. of subjects	Age (years)	Blood lead (µg/dL) mean ± SD (range)	Other bioindicators mean ± SD (range)	Reference	Comments
1980	555	1–9	59.2 ± 25.0 (16.0–152.1)	ZPP: 95.3 ± 80.2 µg/dL (3.8–782.8)	Carvalho *et al.* (1984, 1985a); Silvany-Neto *et al.* (1985); Tavares (1990)	Initial survey
	263			Lead in hair: 558 ± 644 ppm	Carvalho *et al.* (1989)	
1985	250	1–9	36.9 ± 22.9 (2.9–150.0)	ZPP: 70.4 ± 43.9 µg/dL (10.3–522.7)	Silvany-Neto *et al.* (1989); Tavares (1990, 1992)	90-m chimney built; population within 300 m from smelter transferred; EDTA treatment for 31 children; discontinued donation of smelter dross and used filters to neighbours; installation of stack filters; provided working clothes to employees
1992	100	1–5		ZPP: 65.5 ± 1.7 µg/dL[b]	Silvany-Neto *et al.* (1996); Carvalho *et al.* (1996, 1997)	Higher values found in girls; children with darker-skinned racial background; smelter slag present in home; children with pica; children of smelter workers
1998	47	1–4	17.1 ± 7.3 (2.0–36.2)		Carvalho *et al.* (2003)	Smelter closed in 1993 Sources of exposure remaining; higher blood lead found in: children with pica; smelter slag present in home; malnutrition; lead intoxication family history; sewage tubing being placed with disturbance of slag previously used on streets

[a] ZPP, zinc protoporphyrin; SD, standard deviation
[b] Geometric mean

Table 63. Lead concentrations in blood in children in Latin America and the Carribean

Country	Location	Year(s) of study	Source of exposure	No. of subjects	Age (years)	Mean blood lead (µg/dL)	Reference
Chile	Antofagasta	1997–98	Lead storage site (railway)	432	0–7	8.7 ± 1.99[a]	Sepúlveda *et al.* (2000)
			Port area	54	0–7	6.9 ± 1.94[a]	
			No exposure	75	0–7	4.2 ± 1.54[a]	
Equador	La Victoria	NR	Ceramic glazing	166	0.3–15	40.0 (6.2–119.1)	Counter *et al.* (2000)
	Zamora Province	NR	No exposure	56	1–15	6.6 (2.0–18.0)	
Jamaica	NR	1994–95	Rural	242	3–11	9.2[b] (3–28.5)	Lalor *et al.* (2001)
			Urban	90	3–11	14.0[b] (4–34.7)	
			Former mining area	61	3–11	35[b] (18–> 60)	
Mexico	Mexico City	< 1992	Urban	782 girls	5–11	10–17	Olaiz *et al.* (1996)
				801 boys	5–11	14–16.7	
	Ciudad Juárez, Chihuahua	1974	Smelter		1–9		Ordóñez *et al.* (2003)
			< 1 mile	35		38.7	
			1–2.5 miles	113		31.6	
			2.6–4 miles	198		28.7	
			4.1–6 miles	200		28.5	
			6.1–8 miles	206		27.7	
			Total	752		29.3	

NR, not recorded
[a] Geometric mean
[b] Median value

Table 64. Lead concentrations in blood in children in Asia

Country	City/area	Year(s) of study	Population	No. of subjects	Age (years)	Blood lead (µg/dL)		Reference	Comments
						AM[a]	Range		
Bangladesh	Dhaka	2000	B+G	779	4–12	12.3–17.5[b]		Kaiser *et al.* (2001)	
China	Jiangsu	NR	B+G	27	6–9	8.8	5.9–14.8	Zhou & Chen (1988)[c]	Capillary samples
	Shanghai	NR	B+G	83	8–13	18.4	ND–55.0	[Wang (1988)[c]]	Capillary samples
	Beijing	1990	B+G	287	5–7	7.8–12.3[b]	3.9–24.8	[Zheng *et al.* (1993)[c]]	Capillary samples
	Multiple sites	NR	B+G	[3746]	1–15	6.6–96.8		Shen *et al.* (1996)	Review of 17 articles published between 1986 and 1994
	Shanghai	1997	B+G	1969	1–6	9.6	0.1–69.7	Shen *et al.* (1999)	After removal of lead from gasoline
		1998	B+G	1972	1–6	8.1	1–23.9		
	Rural area	1998–2001	B+G	959	5–12	49.6	19.5–89.3	Wu *et al.* (2002)	Children exposed to parental lead-recycling small industry
			B+G	207	5–9	12.6	4.6–24.8		Non-polluted area
	Rural area	NR	B+G	469	mean, 8.5	50.5	22.0–93.8	Zheng *et al.* (2002)	Rural area near smelter
	Shantou	1999	B+G	332	1–5	10.4	3.4–38.6	Luo *et al.* (2003)	After removal of lead from gasoline in 1998
		2001	B+G	457	1–5	7.9	1.1–29.5		
China (Province of Taiwan)	Kaohsiung	1998–99	B+G	934	8–12	5.5	0.2–25.5	Wang *et al.* (2002a)	
India	Delhi	NR	B+G	82	0.2–13	9.6		Gogte *et al.* (1991)	Control
						23			Pica
						11.6			Surma
						30.8			Pica + surma
	New Delhi	NR	B+G	75	3–5	14	4–40	Kaul (1999)	Finger-prick method
	Jammu	NR	B+G	50	3–5	15	4–37		
	3 sites	NR	B+G					Kumar & Kesaree (1999)	
	urban			25	5–15	32.0	25–43		
	semi-urban			75	5–15	25.0	20–31		
	rural			50	5–15	15.0	13–22		
	Mumbai	1986–94	NR	566	6–10	8.6–14.4[b]		Raghunath *et al.* (1999)	Middle-class families
	Mumbai	1984–96	[B+G]	560	6–10	8.6–69.2[b]		Tripathi *et al.* (2001)	Capillary samples
	Delhi	1998	B+G	190	4–6	7.8		Kalra *et al.* (2003)	Children with ZPP > 50 µg/dL

Table 64 (contd)

Country	City/area	Year(s) of study	Popula-tion	No. of subjects	Age (years)	Blood lead (µg/dL)		Reference	Comments
						AM[a]	Range		
Indonesia	Jakarta	< 2001	B+G	397	6–12	8.6[b]	2.6–24.1	Albalak *et al.* (2003)	Capillary samples
Malaysia	Urban	1997	B+G	179	7–11	5.3	0.9–18.5	Hashim *et al.* (2000)	Finger-prick method
	Semi-urban			112	7–11	2.8	0.1[c]–12.3		
	Rural			55	7–11	2.5	0.05–5.2		
Republic of Korea	Ulsan	1997	B+G	426	8–11	4.77[b]		Lee *et al.* (2002)	Lead in gasoline was reduced to 0.013 g/L in 1993.
		1999	B+G	250	8–11	5.11[b]			
		2001	B+G	242	8–11	5.21[b]			
Mongolia	6 sites	NR	NR	142	NR	0.34–1.75		Burmaa *et al.* (2002)	Highest in Ulaanbaatar
Pakistan	Karachi	NR	Boys	77	6–8	16.9		Rahman *et al.* (2002)	
		NR	Girls	61	6–8	15.12			
	5 districts in Karachi	2000	B+G	400	3–5	12.0–21.6		Rahbar *et al.* (2002)	
Saudi Arabia	Riyadh	NR	Girls	533	6–12	8.1	2.3–27.4	Al-Saleh *et al.* (2001)	
Thailand	Kanchanaburi, downstream lead refinery plant	1997	NR	48	mean, 3.4	27.8		Tantanasrikul *et al.* (2002)	Initial survey
		1998	NR	48		30.6			After environmental deleading
		1999	NR	48		30.3			Second survey

NR, not reported; B, boys; G, girls; ZPP, zinc protoporphyrin
[a] AM, arithmetic mean, unless stated otherwise
[b] Geometric mean
[c] Cited by Shen *et al.* (1996); references in square brackets could not be retrieved as original papers.

(b) *Pregnant women and neonates*

Lead concentrations were measured in maternal blood and umbilical cord blood from 50 parturient women at delivery in a hospital in Athens, Greece. Lead concentrations (mean ± standard deviation) for women living in industrial areas with high air pollution were 37.2 ± 4.7 µg/L in maternal blood and 20.0 ± 3.4 µg/L in umbilical cord blood (correlation coefficient, $r = 0.57$), while those for women living in agricultural areas with low air pollution were 20.5 ± 5.6 µg/L and 12.9 ± 3.6 µg/L, respectively (correlation coefficient, $r = 0.70$). The authors concluded that the placenta demonstrates a dynamic protective function that is amplified when maternal blood lead concentrations are increased (Dussias *et al.*, 1997).

Data from Kosovo (Serbia and Montenegro) showed that 86% of the pregnant women living in the vicinity of a lead smelter had blood lead concentrations ≥ 10 µg/dL, while in a comparable area not near a smelter, only 3.4% of pregnant women showed elevated concentrations (Graziano *et al.*, 1990).

Rabinowitz and Needleman (1982) reported an umbilical cord blood lead concentration of 6.6 µg/dL (arithmetic mean), with a range of 0–37 µg/dL, in over 11 000 samples collected between 1979 and 1981 in Boston, USA. A decrease in the blood lead concentration of approximately 14% per year was noted during the period of collection.

Concentrations of lead (expressed as mean ± standard deviation) in umbilical cord blood of two groups of women giving birth in a hospital in Boston, USA, in 1980 and 1990, were found to be 6.56 ± 3.19 µg/dL and 1.19 ± 1.32 µg/dL, respectively (Hu *et al.*, 1996a).

In a study conducted at a medical centre in South Central Los Angeles, one of the most economically-depressed regions in California, USA, maternal blood lead concentrations in the third trimester of pregnancy were significantly higher in a group of 1392 immigrant women (geometric mean, 2.3 µg/dL) than in a group of 489 non-immigrant women (geometric mean, 1.9 µg/dL). Years living in the USA was the most powerful predictor of blood lead concentration. Drinking coffee during pregnancy, a history of pica, and/or low calcium intake were all significantly associated with higher blood lead concentrations (Rothenberg *et al.*, 1999).

In a study conducted in the United Arab Emirates, blood samples were collected from 113 mothers of 23 different nationalities and from their neonates (cord blood). Mean maternal blood lead concentration was 14.9 ± 2.14 µg/dL (range, 6.6–27.8 µg/dL) and mean cord blood lead concentration was 13.3 ± 2.49 µg/dL (range, 6.0–30.3 µg/dL). Sixteen per cent of samples from the mothers and 9% of cord blood samples had lead concentrations > 20 µg/dL (Al Khayat *et al.*, 1997a).

There are several studies showing high blood lead concentrations in pregnant women in India (Saxena *et al.*, 1994; Awasthi *et al.*, 1996; Raghunath *et al.*, 2000). The mean blood lead concentration in a cohort of 500 pregnant women living in the slums of Lucknow, north India, was 14.3 µg/dL, and 19.2% of women had concentrations ≥ 20 µg/dL. Blood lead concentration was not associated with age, height, weight, gestation, or history of abortion, although it was higher with higher parity. Women living in inner-city neighbourhoods with heavy vehicular traffic had mean blood lead concentrations significantly higher than those living in other neighbourhoods (Awasthi *et al.,* 1996). In another study conducted in Lucknow, India, the mean maternal blood lead concentration was significantly higher in cases of abnormal delivery (22.5 µg/dL) compared with normal deliveries (19.4 µg/dL). No significant difference in placental blood, cord blood and fetal membrane lead concentrations was observed between cases of normal and abnormal deliveries (Saxena *et al.,* 1994).

(*c*) *Children*

Data on blood lead concentrations in children are presented in Tables 57–59 and 61–64.

Between 1978 and 1988, decreases of 25–45% in average blood lead concentrations in children have been reported in Belgium, Canada, Germany, New Zealand, Sweden and the United Kingdom (OECD, 1993).

Blood lead concentrations were measured in 286 children aged 0–7 years living in the three largest cities of Finland (n = 172), in rural areas (n = 54) and near a lead smelter (n = 60) (Taskinen *et al.*, 1981). Mean blood lead concentrations among children in the urban, rural and lead-smelter areas varied between 6.0 and 6.7 µg/dL, with a range of 2–17 µg/dL. There were no statistically significant differences between groups. The five children who lived within 500 m of the lead smelter had a mean blood lead concentration of 9.2 µg/dL, with a range of 5–13 µg/dL, which was significantly higher than the mean blood lead concentration among 485 children in the rest of the country. In a study carried out in Sweden, 1395 blood samples were obtained from children living in an urban or rural area or near a smelter during the period 1978–88. The mean blood lead concentration for all locations together decreased from 6.4 µg/dL (range, 1.8–25 µg/dL) in 1978 to 4.2 µg/dL (range, 1.4–12.9 µg/dL) in 1984, to 3.3 µg/dL (range, 1.5–7.1 µg/dL) in 1988. The decrease was statistically significant for all three areas studied (Skerfving *et al.*, 1986; Schütz *et al.*, 1989).

In Finland, the mean blood lead concentration for the children in two day-care centres in Helsinki was 4.8 µg/dL in 1983 (range, 2.1–8.3 µg/dL), 3.0 µg/dL in 1988 (range, 2.1–4.1 µg/dL), and 2.6 µg/dL in 1996 (range, 1.7–3.7 µg/dL) (Pönkä *et al.*, 1993; Pönkä, 1998).

In 1993, almost 30% of 431 children in a lead-mining community in the Upper Silesian industrial zone of Poland had blood lead concentrations > 10 µg/dL (Zejda *et al.*, 1995). In Belovo, Russian Federation, lead releases from a metallurgy enterprise decreased between 1983 and 1996 from 120 to 9 tonnes per year, due to almost complete cessation of activity. In 1983, mean blood lead concentrations in newborn children and their mothers living in the area were 23.4 and 25 µg/dL, respectively; in 1996, mean blood lead concentrations in 91 children (age, 7–8 years) had decreased to 9.9 µg/dL (range, 0.5–39 µg/dL), with 46% of values still exceeding 10 µg/dL (Revich *et al.*, 1998).

In a community near a smelter in Bulgaria, blood lead concentrations in 109 children varied from 8–63 μg/dL. The higher concentrations in these children were correlated with the consumption of home-grown products. Lower blood lead concentrations were observed in children whose food came from a distant market (Fischer *et al.*, 2003).

The mean blood lead concentration in children in the USA has dropped dramatically since the late 1970s (Brody *et al.*, 1994; Pirkle *et al.*, 1994, 1998; CDC, 1997b, 2003a,b). Results of the NHANES studies in children aged 1–5 years are shown in Table 58.

The NHANES II and NHANES III, Phase I, results showed that from 1976 to 1991, high blood lead concentrations correlated with low income, low educational attainment and residence in the north-eastern region of the USA (Pirkle *et al.*, 1994). Data from Phase II of NHANES III (October 1991 to September 1994) indicated that blood lead concentrations in children aged 1–5 years continued to decrease and were more likely to be elevated among those who were poor, non-Hispanic black, living in large metropolitan areas or living in older housing (with potential exposure to lead from lead-based paint); approximately 4.4% of the children aged 1–5 years had blood lead concentrations ≥ 10 μg/dL (CDC, 1997b). In addition, 1.3% of children aged 1–5 years had blood lead concentrations ≥ 15 μg/dL and 0.4% had concentrations ≥ 20 μg/dL. The downward trends continued in 1999–2000 (CDC, 2003a). For all periods of this study, mean lead concentrations were consistently lower among the older age groups, i.e. age 1–5 years, 2.2 μg/dL; 6–11 years, 1.5 μg/dL; 12–19 years, 1.1 μg/dL in the period 1999–2000 (CDC, 2003a).

A study assessing the source of lead exposure during early childhood in the USA showed that lead-contaminated floor dust was a major source of lead exposure during early childhood, whereas window sills became an increasingly important source as children stood upright (Lanphear *et al.*, 2002).

One of the most serious episodes of general population exposure to lead reported in Latin America occurred in Brazil (Table 62). For 24 years, a lead smelter processing 30 000 tonnes/year operated in the vicinity of Santo Amaro da Purificação (30 000 inhabitants) in the state of Bahia. No proper air pollution control system was used. Smelter dross (solid wastes) was distributed free of charge to the neighbouring population and spread over gardens, backyards, schools and streets, and chimney filters from the smelter were used in homes as carpets, bed spreads and rags. Four cross-sectional studies in children under 9 years of age were conducted in 1980 (Carvalho *et al.*, 1985a), 1985 (Silvany-Neto *et al.*, 1989), 1992 (Silvany-Neto *et al.*, 1996) and 1998 (Carvalho *et al.*, 2003). Blood lead concentrations were among the highest reported in the world. Most children involved in the last study were born after the smelter closed down in December 1993. Five years later, lead concentrations in blood averaged 17.1 ± 7.3 μg/dL, ranging from 2.0 to 36.2 μg/dL. Blood lead concentrations were approximately 5 μg/dL higher in children with pica, with visible presence of dross in home premises, with previous history of lead intoxication in the family and with malnutrition (Carvalho *et al.*, 2003).

In Antofagasta, Chile, a study was conducted with 432 children under 7 years of age living around a minerals storage site, 54 living near the port and 75 in non-exposed areas

(Table 63). Average concentrations of lead in blood of exposed and unexposed children were 8.7 µg/dL and 4.2 µg/dL, respectively. Forty-seven per cent of exposed children, but no unexposed children, had blood lead concentrations > 10 µg/dL. The habit of pica, the number of cigarettes smoked daily at home, the level of education of the mother and having a mother working outside the home were variables that partly explained the variation in blood lead concentrations in the exposed area (Sepúlveda *et al.*, 2000).

In view of airborne lead pollution across the border from a lead smelter in El Paso, TX, USA, an epidemiological study on lead was conducted in 1974 in Juárez City, Chihuahua, Mexico, among 752 children aged 1–9 years. The average blood lead concentration was 29.27 ± 7.30 µg/dL in children living within 8 miles of the lead source. Concentrations decreased with greater distances from the smelter (Ordóñez *et al.*, 2003; see Table 24 and Section 1.4.1(*b*)).

Lead-glazing of ceramics has for many years been a source of exposure of the population of La Victoria, Ecuador, where around 70 kilns operate within an area of 250 km². One hundred and sixty-six children aged 4 months to 15 years living in the area and many of them helping their parents in glazing activities had blood lead concentrations ranging from 6.2 to 119.1 µg/dL (mean, 40.0 µg/dL) compared with an average of 6.6 µg/dL in a reference population of 56 children aged 1–15 years living 500 km away in the province of Zamora. Lead isotope ratios of the soil and blood samples were highly similar and clustered for both study areas, indicating that lead in soil resulting from contamination by the glazing activities is probably one of the main routes of exposure to lead in these children (Counter *et al.*, 2000).

Blood lead concentrations among children in several Asian countries (Table 64) were basically similar to those in adults (Table 60), and were generally between 5 and 15 µg/dL (geometric mean). It should be noted, however, that finger-prick or capillary blood samples were employed in some studies (see Section 1.5 for quality assurance). Blood lead concentrations in children in Mongolia (Burmaa *et al.*, 2002) were substantially lower than in all the other studies listed in Table 64.

In a study carried out at 15 sites in India, the highest (69 µg/dL) and second highest (21 µg/dL) geometric mean blood lead concentrations were observed in children who lived near a scrap-yard and near a lead smelter, respectively. Values for children in the remaining sites were in a range of 9–14 µg/dL (Tripathi *et al.*, 2001). Wu, Y. *et al.* (2002) observed significantly higher blood lead concentrations in children who lived in an area polluted by lead from a battery-recycling plant compared with a control group. Similarly, Zheng *et al.* (2002) described elevated blood lead concentrations (up to 94 µg/dL) in children living in an area with heavy lead pollution. Tantanasrikul *et al.* (2002) found high blood lead concentrations in children in a Thai village area downstream from a lead refinery plant. Wang *et al.* (1998) reported that 22 of 36 children in a kindergarten near a battery recycling factory in Taiwan, China, had blood lead concentrations in excess of 15 µg/dL in comparison with none of 35 children in a kindergarten in a non-exposed area.

In a study of 566 children aged 6–10 years residing in 13 locations in Mumbai, India, a correlation coefficient of 0.88 was observed between air lead and blood lead concentrations. It was also found that a 1-μg/m^3 increase in lead concentration in air resulted in a 3.56-μg/dL increase in blood lead concentration in children (Raghunath *et al.,* 1999).

In another study among children in India, the differences in the mean blood lead concentrations were statistically significant ($p < 0.001$) between the urban, semi-urban and rural populations. The age-related differences in blood lead concentrations were also significant for urban, semi-urban and rural children (Kumar & Kesaree, 1999).

In a study comparing children with and without pica in Delhi, India, only six out of 82 children with no symptoms of pica had a mean blood lead concentration ≥ 30 μg/dL (30–39 μg/dL). Among 88 children with pica, 26 had high blood lead concentrations (30–92 μg/dL) (Gogte *et al.*, 1991).

Among 400 children aged 36–60 months from the city centre, two suburbs, a rural community or an island situated in the harbour at Karachi, Pakistan, about 80% had blood lead concentrations > 10 μg/dL, with an overall mean of 15.6 μg/dL. Housing near a main intersection in the city centre, application of surma (a lead-containing cosmetic) to children's eyes, father's exposure to lead at the workplace, father's illiteracy, child's hand-to-mouth activity and eating from street vendors were among variables found likely to be associated with elevated lead concentrations in blood (Rahbar *et al.*, 2002).

The phase-out of leaded gasoline in Indonesia began in Jakarta on 1 July 2001. In a study conducted before the beginning of the phase-out activities, 35% of children aged 6–12 years in Jakarta had blood lead concentrations ≥ 10 μg/dL and 2.4% had concentrations ≥ 20 μg/dL. Lead concentrations in the blood of children who lived near a highway or major intersection were significantly higher than those in children who lived near a street with little or no traffic. The source of household water was also a significant predictor of blood lead concentrations ≥ 10 μg/dL, after adjustment for age and sex (Albalak *et al.,* 2003).

Hashim *et al.* (2000) measured blood lead concentrations in urban and rural primary-school children in Malaysia; the percentage of children with blood lead ≥ 10 μg/dL was 6.36% overall, and was highest for Kuala Lumpur (11.73%). Urban schoolchildren were found to have higher blood lead concentrations than their rural and semi-urban counterparts, even after controlling for age, sex, parents' education and income levels.

1.4.3 *Occupational exposure*

Potentially high levels of lead may occur in the following industries or workplaces: lead smelting and refining industries, battery manufacturing plants, steel welding or cutting operations, construction, painting and printing industries, firing ranges, vehicle radiator-repair shops and other industries requiring flame soldering of lead solder, and gasoline stations and garages.

Workers in many occupations and job activities within or outside these industries have the potential for relatively high exposures to lead with varying degrees of frequency (Fu & Boffetta, 1995; ATSDR, 1999; NIOSH, 2001). These exposures and workers are (the asterisks indicate occupations for which there is at least one epidemiological study of lead exposure and cancer, as summarized in Section 2 of this volume): *on-going exposure* — battery-production workers*, battery-recycling workers*, foundry workers, lead chemical workers*, lead smelter and refinery workers*, leaded-glass workers*, pigment workers*, vehicle radiator-repair workers and traffic controllers; *moderate frequency of exposure* — firing-range instructors, house renovators, lead miners*, newspaper printers*, plastics workers*, rubber workers, jewellery workers, ceramics workers and steel welders and cutters; *low frequency of exposure* — automobile-repair workers, cable-production workers, construction workers, demolition workers, firing-range participants, flame-solder workers, plumbers and pipefitters, pottery-glaze producers, ship-repair workers and stained-glass producers.

Epidemiological studies have also reported exposure to organic lead compounds, at a chemical plant in Texas, USA, and at an organic lead manufacturing company in New Jersey, USA. However, there are a number of activities that present a potential for high lead exposure but for which no epidemiological data are available.

The most common route of occupational exposure to lead is through inhalation of lead fumes or lead dusts from ambient air, leading to absorption of lead through the respiratory system. Lead may also be ingested and absorbed in the gastrointestinal tract. Organic lead is absorbed through the skin (Bress & Bidanset, 1991).

The lead concentration in air can be measured as a means of monitoring occupational exposure in work areas. However, occupational exposure is more often inferred from measurement of blood lead concentrations in individual workers.

Workers occupationally exposed to lead may carry lead home on their body, clothing and tools. Thus, children of workers exposed to lead can also be at increased risk of exposure. For example, blood lead concentrations of children in households of occupationally-exposed workers were found to be almost twice those of children in neighbouring homes whose parents were not exposed to lead in their occupation (median ranges, 10–14 and 5–8 μg/dL, respectively) (Grandjean & Bach, 1986). Exposures to lead in workers' families have been identified in association with nearly 30 different industries and occupations; the most commonly reported include lead smelting, battery manufacturing and recycling, radiator repair, electrical components manufacturing, pottery and ceramics and stained-glass making (NIOSH, 1995).

The results of surveys of occupational exposure to lead in a large variety of industries in New Zealand, expressed as air lead concentrations and/or blood lead concentrations for the period 1988–89, are presented in Table 65 (Grant *et al.*, 1992).

Lead concentrations in workplace air and in the blood of exposed workers for specific job categories are presented in Tables 66–73. Whereas lead concentrations in air were reported only in a limited number of studies, blood lead concentrations are available for most studies and the exposure intensity is evaluated in terms of blood lead for the groups of exposed workers. Examples of extreme exposures reported in the literature include mean occupational air lead concentrations as high as 1200 μg/m^3 for welding structural steel, 4470 μg/m^3 for primary smelting and 5400 μg/m^3 within a storage-battery plant (WHO, 1977).

Table 65. Occupational exposure to lead in men in New Zealand, 1988–89

Occupation in order of decreasing mean blood lead concentration	No. of workers	Blood lead (µg/dL)		
		Mean	SD	Range
Radiator repairer	51	78.7	47.6	11–155
Smelter/furnaceman	57	78.7	51.8	14–148
Muffler repairer	33	70.4	33.1	31–109
Scrap metal worker	69	66.2	60.0	14–145
Foundryman general	58	64.2	49.7	23–128
Metal moulder	24	64.2	66.2	14–181
Container repairer	13	60.0	26.9	40–61
Engine reconditioner	33	53.8	33.1	23–154
Panel beater	22	55.9	47.6	23–115
Metal machinist	35	55.9	43.5	18–111
Printer	4	55.9	33.1	28–69
Gas cutter/welder	17	43.5	49.7	6–90
Spray painter	42	43.5	29.0	17–80
Plastic worker	55	43.5	35.2	9–124
Metal polisher	29	43.5	55.9	10–119
Paint removal worker	8	41.4	22.8	19–54
Painter/decorator	208	41.4	51.8	5–181
Leadlight worker	11	39.3	29.0	14–64
Metal extruder	16	35.2	31.1	18–77
Garage mechanic	47	35.2	43.5	9–82
Miscellaneous lead product worker	65	31.1	35.2	5–113
Pottery/ceramics worker	3	29.0	24.8	9–46
Workers exposed to exhaust fumes	6	26.9	26.9	14–47
Plumber	10	26.9	20.7	12–46
Cable jointer	174	26.9	26.9	5–91
Car assembler	25	26.9	31.1	5–76
Electroplater	17	22.8	18.6	9–46
Boat builder	30	20.7	18.6	7–47
Bright solderer	9	20.7	20.7	11–49
Petrol pump attendant	10	20.7	14.5	5–33

Adapted from Grant *et al.* (1992)
SD, standard deviation

A NIOSH Health Hazard Evaluation (HHE) is a study of a workplace in the USA conducted to learn whether workers are exposed to hazardous materials or harmful conditions. The HHE is not necessarily representative of an industry or general work practices, since the inspections and measurements are typically done in response to a request by an employee, an officer of a labour union that represents employees, or any management official on behalf of the employer. Table 74 presents data from a series of HHE reports where blood and air concentrations of lead have been measured.

Table 66. Lead concentrations in blood of occupationally exposed subjects: lead–acid battery factories

Country or area	Year(s) of survey	Job/task	Study popu-lation	No. of subjects	Age (years)	Job history (years)	Smoking status	Blood lead (µg/dL)		Lead in air (µg/m³)		Reference
								AM[a]	Range/SD	AM[a]	Range/SD	
Brazil	[1984]	Battery repair[b]	M	5	15–66	≤ 1	NR	35.0[c]		NR		Carvalho *et al.* (1985b)
				11		1–3	NR	37.3[c]				
				23		≥ 4	NR	47.7[c]				
				6	15–18			36.7[c]				
				33	19–66			44.0[c]				
Bulgaria	1992–96	Lead–acid battery	M	103	39.1	9.7	Included	56.2		NR		Vaglenov *et al.* (2001)
China	1950–83	Lead–acid battery										Wang (1984)
		Charging	NR	30	NR	NR	NR	26.2[d]	NR	500		
		Plate moulding	NR	34	NR	NR	NR	25.6[d]	NR	60		
		Printing	NR	30	NR	NR	NR	22.8[d]	NR	5		
China (Province of Taiwan)	NR	Lead–acid battery	M	118	37.0	> 6 months	80%	67.0	± 26	190		Lai *et al.* (1997)
			W	101	36.3	> 6 months	2%	45.0	± 18.7			
	NR	Lead–acid battery	M	120	18–67	0.2–35	38% smokers	67.7	± 28.2	≥ 0.1 in 46% of samples		Wang *et al.* (2002b)
			W	109	18–71	0.2–17		48.6	± 17.0			
	1989–98	Lead–acid battery	17 M 13 W	30	38.3	13.1	NR	20–60[d,e]		NR		Hsiao *et al.* (2001)
	1991	Lead–acid battery	M + W	284	NR	NR	Included	34.7	± 15.0	NR		Chuang *et al.* (1999)
	1997		M + W	392	NR	NR	Included	23.9	± 12.4	NR		
Finland	NR	Lead–acid battery	M + W	91	40.6	12.2	NR	30		NR		Erkkilä *et al.* (1992)
Irak	1996	Lead–acid battery										Mehdi *et al.* (2000)
		Charging	M	11	NR	> 4	40% smokers	36.4	± 11.40	NR		
		Repair	M	8	NR	> 4		58.0	± 13.35	NR		
		Casting	M	18	NR	> 4		71.7	± 24.80	NR		

Table 66 (contd)

Country or area	Year(s) of survey	Job/task	Study population	No. of subjects	Age (years)	Job history (years)	Smoking status	Blood lead (µg/dL)		Lead in air (µg/m³)		Reference
								AM[a]	Range/SD	AM[a]	Range/SD	
Israel	1975	Administration	NR	3	41.3	13.3	Most smokers	28.6	20–34	14.5	11.9–17.0	Richter *et al.* (1979)
		Maintenance	NR	3	41.3	5.5		44.0	43–46	23	–	
		Assembly	NR	6	47.0	9.8		55.0	41–73	49.3	48–50.7	
		Miscellaneous	NR	17	35.2	4.3		59.5	43–87	84.5	71–98	
		Grid smelting and casting	NR	10	43.9	13.1		58.4	43–73	190	118–299	
		Plate drying and formation	NR	15	31.9	4.6		75.2	48–105	399	266–475	
		Oven smelting	NR	3	36.3	6.5		76.3	64–90	885	–	
		Pasting/drying/ oxide formation	NR	4	33.5	6.4		90.7	79–108	1187	1060–1315	
Japan	NR	Lead battery, mostly	M	214	NR	≥ 2	NR	48.9[c]	17.0–101.0	NR		Fukui *et al.* (1999)
			W	44	NR	≥ 2	NR	49.1[c]	28.0–75.0	NR		
Philippines	1990	Lead–acid battery	M	199	33.8	10.7	NR	64.5[b]	23–121	NR		Makino *et al.* (1994)
Republic of Korea	NR	Lead–acid battery	NR	66	40	≥ 3 months	NR	45.7	± 15.7	NR		Kim *et al.* (1995a)
		Casting and pasting		5	39			40.6	± 8.8	83	40–154	
		Plate forming, finishing		17	44			49.2	± 17.4	170	12–468	
		Assembling		22	39			47.2	± 11.6	145	15–411	
		Others		22	39			42.6	± 18.7	NR		
	NR	Lead–acid battery	14 M, 78 W	92	40.1	8.6	NR	27.6		19[c]		Hwang *et al.* (2000)
		Cast-on-strap		37				29.6		32[c]		
		Plate processing		3				36.8		29[c]		
		Battery cell setting		19				22.6		13[c]		
		Finish processing		21				22.4		9[c]		
		Supervisor		12				44.5		27[c]		
	1998	Lead–acid battery	M	156	36.3	8.8	68% smokers	32.0	± 13.0	NR		Hwang *et al.* (2001)
			W	56	47.0	6.2	Nonsmokers	19.8	± 9.2	NR		

Table 66 (contd)

Country or area	Year(s) of survey	Job/task	Study population	No. of subjects	Age (years)	Job history (years)	Smoking status	Blood lead (µg/dL)		Lead in air (µg/m³)		Reference
								AM[a]	Range/SD	AM[a]	Range/SD	
Singapore	NR	Lead–acid battery	M									Chia *et al.* (1991)
			Chinese	11	39.1	10.8	Included	23.6	12.4	35	± 31	
			Malay	25	31.7	7.5	Included	34.3	10.5	51	± 39	
	NR	Lead–acid battery	M	50	38.3	10	NR	32.5	19.1–50.9	88.6	± 176.3	Ho *et al.* (1998)
	1987–89	Lead–acid battery	NR	61	NR	NR	NR	28.4	12.9	NR		Chia *et al.* (1993)
South Africa	NR	Lead–acid battery	M	382	41.2	11.6	52% smokers	53.5	23–110	145	10–5480	Ehrlich *et al.* (1998)
Turkey	NR	Lead–acid battery	M	71	32.7	NR	73% smokers	34.5	13.4–71.8	NR		Süzen *et al.* (2003)
USA	1947–72	Lead–acid battery	M	1083	NR	> 1	NR	62.7		NR		Wong & Harris (2000)

NR, not reported; M, men; W, women

[a] Arithmetic mean, unless stated otherwise

[b] Nineteen different establishments recycling batteries; 76.9% of the workers operating in areas < 30 m² and involved in fusion of lead

[c] Geometric mean

[d] Median value

[e] Values read from graph

Table 67. Lead concentrations in blood of occupationally exposed subjects: mining/primary smelter

Country	Year of survey	Job/task	Study popu-lation	No. of subjects	Age years mean (range)	Years of employ-ment	Smoking status	Blood lead (µg/dL)		Lead in air (µg/m³)		Reference
								AM[a]	Range/ SD	AM[a]	Range	
Canada	1994	Primary smelter	M + W	368	NR	NR	NR	22–25	NR	NR		Fleming *et al.* (1998)
Italy	1977–78	Primary smelter	M	1388	NR	> 1	NR	NR		47.6	1–1650	Cocco *et al.* (1997)
Japan	NR	Copper smelter	M		42.9 (21–60)		Included					Karita *et al.* (2000)
		Blending		13			–	8.9	± 5.5	7	5–8	
		Smelting		51			–	13.5	± 7.2	29	6–67	
		Converter		28			–	15.7	± 7.3	41	17–78	
		Anode		31			–	25.7	± 6.1	313	165–436	
							Current	26.3	14–39			
							Former	21.0	19–23			
							Never	25.9	15–34			
Kazakhstan	1998	Smelter and mining	NR	38	NR	NR	NR	34	13–> 65	NR		Kaul *et al.* (2000)
Sweden	1987	Primary smelter	Active	70	37.4	14.3	NR	32[b]	5.0–47.4	NR		Gerhardsson *et al.* (1993)
			Retired	30	67.9	32.6	NR	9.9[b]	3.3–20.9			
Sweden	1950–87	Primary smelter	M	3979	NR	NR	NR	62.[illegible]–33.1[c]		NR		Lundström *et al.* (1997)
		Other metal workers						55.9–16.6[c]				
		Other personnel						53.8–12.4[c]				
United Kingdom	1970–79	Cadmium plant	M	123	NR	> 1	NR	28		50% > 2000 in whole plant		Ades & Kazantzis (1988)
		Furnace area	M	426	NR	> 1	NR	59				
		Sinter area	M	343	NR	> 1	NR	56				
USA	1976	Primary smelter	M	173	NR	9.9	NR	56.3		3100		Steenland *et al.* (1992)

NR, not reported; M, men; W, women
[a] Arithmetic mean, unless stated otherwise
[b] Median value
[c] Decrease over the study period

Table 68. Lead concentrations in blood of occupationally exposed subjects: secondary smelter

Country or area	Year(s) of survey	Job/task	Study population	No. of subjects	Age years mean (range)	Job history (years)	Smoking status	Blood lead (µg/dL)		Lead in air (µg/m³) AM[a]	Reference
								AM[a]	Range/SD		
China (Province of Taiwan)	NR	Battery recycling									Wang *et al.* (1998)
		Furnace	NR	19	37	11 months	NR	87	14	NR	
		Fragmentation	NR	10	35	15 months	NR	69	16	NR	
		Office, guards	NR	5	52	31 months	NR	38	4	NR	
Ghana	NR	Battery recycling	23 M, 2 W	25	(18–60)	≥ 5	NR	108	60–270	NR	Ankrah *et al.* (1996)
Japan	NR	Secondary lead smelter	19 M, 3 W	22	47 (22–63)	5	NR	43	8–78	NR	Tomokuni *et al.* (1992)
Philippines	NR	Secondary lead smelter (battery recycling)	M	107	32.1	6.6	NR	80.8[b]	19–153	NR	Makino *et al.* (1994)
			W	6	27.8	4.0	NR	44.7[b]	35–61	NR	
Republic of Korea	1996	Secondary lead smelter	83 M, 5 W	88	NR	> 1 month	NR	52.4	17.7	324	Kim *et al.* (2002)
		A	M + W	12				47.4	18.8	310	
		B	M + W	17				47.2	20.7	194	
		C	M + W	18				49.7	13.1	464	
		D	M + W	25				55.4	19.7	316	
		E	M + W	16				60.0	12.1	290	
Sweden	1969–85	Secondary smelter	M	664	28 at entry	2.8[b]	NR	62.1–33.1[c]		NR	Gerhardsson *et al.* (1995a)
USA	1947–72	Smelters (primary, second, recycling)	M	254	NR	> 1	NR	79.7		NR	Wong & Harris (2000)

NR, not reported; M, men; W, women; A–E, five different lead smelters
[a] Arithmetic mean, unlewss stated otherwise
[b] Median value
[c] Decrease over the study period

Table 69. Lead concentrations in blood of occupationally exposed subjects leaded glass

Country or area	Years of survey	Job/task	Study population	No. of subjects	Age (years)	Job history (years)	Smoking status	Blood lead (µg/dL)		Lead in air (mg/m³)		Reference
								AM[a]	Range	AM[a]	Range	
China	NR	Lead-coloured glass	Women	36	21–35	2–17	Never	55.6	25.8–79.3	NR	0.4–1.2	Murata *et al.* (1995)
Japan	1989–90	Lead-coloured glass	NR	5	29–55	2–17	NR					Hirata *et al.* (1995)
		high exposure		(15)[b]				67.1	38–102	1050	741–1658	
		low exposure		(60)[b]				52.3	38–69	286	22–1331	
	NR	Lead glass processing and lead pigment production	Men	160	36	1–28	NR	55.1	18.1–87.9	NR		Oishi *et al.* (1996a)
			Women	138	28	1–28	NR	54.7	21.5–99.4	NR		

NR, not reported
[a] Arithmetic mean
[b] Number of samples collected during 15 months

Table 70. Lead concentrations in blood of occupationally exposed subjects: welders and solders

Country or area	Year of survey	Job/task	Study population	No. of subjects	Age (years)	Job history (years)	Smoking status	Blood lead (µg/dL)		Lead in air µg/m^3)		Reference
								AM[a]	Range/SD	AM[a]	Range	
Welding												
Jordan	NR	Radiator welding	M	22	27.7	1–40	NR	32.8[b]		NR		Hunaiti *et al.* (1995)
Malaysia	NR	Shipyard welding	M	51	> 18	1–17	Included[c]	12	4–31	NR		Mokhtar *et al.* (2002)
Mexico	NR	Radiator repair	NR	73 29 30	33.2	NR	Included Smoker Nonsmoker	35.5 40.4 32.3	6.7–79.4 13.9–79.4 14.6–56.9	19.1	0–99	Dykeman *et al.* (2002)
Philippines	1999	Radiator mechanic	M + W	16	40.2	16.2	NR	20.0	± 10.6	NR		Suplido & Ong (2000)
	NR	Welding mechanic	M	29	NR	NR	Nonsmoker	9.1	5.0–17.0	NR		Suwansaksri *et al.* (2002)
Thailand	NR	Mechanic	NR	40	NR	NR	Never	11.2	3.9–17.0	0.1–0.5		Suwansaksri & Wiwanitkit (2001)
USA	1992	Radiator repair	M	63	39	11	39% current	29[d]	6.6–94	NR		Dalton *et al.* (1997)
	NR	Radiator repair	NR	56	39.5	NR	52% current	37.1	16–73	NR		Goldman *et al.* (1987)
	1990	Radiator repair	NR	7	NR	NR	NR	NR	17–35	PBZ: 209	< 20–810 TWA: < 10–> 40	Tharr (1993)
	1986	Radiator repair	NR	53	37.1	14.3	60% current	31.7	5–58	Area: 40 PBZ: 113	0–281 0–590	Lussenhop *et al.* (1989)
Soldering												
Philippines	NR	Electronic industry	M W	21 193	25.4 21.9	1.8 1.8	NR NR	14.9[b] 9.9[b]	7–45 3–47	NR NR		Makino *et al.* (1994)
Singapore	1987	Electronics industry	NR	118	NR	NR	NR	16.1	± 8.5	110	10–1240	Chia *et al.* (1993)

NR, not reported; M, men; W, women; PBZ, personal breathing zone; TWA, time-weighted average
[a] Arithmetic mean, unless specified otherwise
[b] Geometric mean
[c] Stratification by smoking did not reveal a significant difference between values.
[d] Median value

Table 71. Lead concentrations in blood of occupationally exposed subjects: professional drivers and traffic policemen

Country or area	Year(s) of survey	Job/task	Study population	No. of subjects	Age (years)	Job history (years)	Smoking status	Blood lead (µg/dL)		Lead in air (µg/m³)		Reference
								AM[a]	Range/ SD	AM[a]	Range	
China	1998	Taxi and bus drivers	M	164	NR	NR	75% smokers	10.8[b]	± 1.26	NR		Zhou *et al.* (2001)
Egypt (Alexandria)	NR	Traffic controllers	M	45	20–60	Max., 40	NR	68.3	37–97	NR		Ahmed *et al.* (1987)
Egypt	NR	Traffic policemen	M	126	48.7	9–36	NR	29.2	7.5	NR		Kamal *et al.* (1991)
India	NR	Traffic constables	M	88	41.7	2.7	30%	11.2	0.5–40.2	NR		Potula & Hu (1996a,b)
		Bus drivers	M	22	43.6	5.6	77%	12.1	0.5–35.7	NR		
Indonesia	1983	Policemen	M	24	NR	NR	NR	31	± 18	NR	0.7–6.0	Suzuki (1990)
		Drivers	NR	22	NR	NR	NR	25	± 17	NR	0.7–6.0	
Jordan	NR	Bus drivers, gasoline station workers	NR	47	NR	NR	NR	7.6		NR		Hunaiti *et al.* (1995)
Pakistan	1994–95	Traffic exposed	M	212	19–59	> 1	Included	52.2		NR		Khan *et al.* (1995)
		Traffic police		36				53.4				
		Transportation staff		150				51.1				
		Shopkeepers		36				52.1				

NR, not reported; M, men
[a] Arithmetic mean, unless stated otherwise
[b] Geometric mean

Table 72. Air and blood lead concentrations measured at indoor and outdoor firing ranges

Country	Year(s) of study	Settings/task	No. of subjects and sex	Age (years)	Job history (years)	Blood lead (μg/dL)		Lead in air (μg/m³)		Reference
						AM[a]	Range	AM[a]	Range	
China (Province of Taiwan)	NR	Employees in indoor range	10	NR	4–21	37.2	22.4–59.6	GA, 134; PBZ, 413	NR	Chau *et al.* (1995)
New Zealand	1990–91	Indoor small-bore rifle range	52 M + W	17–68	Recreational shooters	End of season, 55.0; start of season, 33.3		PBZ, 120 GA, 140–210		George *et al.* (1993)
Sweden	NR	Indoor range Powder gun Air gun	 22 M + W 21 M + W	 42.4 46.8	 10.2 13.7	 13.8[b] 8.4[b]	 6.9–22.8 2.0–22.2	 660 4.6	 112–2238 1.8–7.2	Svensson *et al.* (1992)
	1994	On- and off-duty police officers	75 M 3 W	43 32	NR > 9 years	5.0 3.7	1.0–18.2	NR		Löfstedt *et al.* (1999)
United Kingdom	NR	Indoor range for police officers	7	NR	NR	30–59		30–160		Smith (1976)
	NR	Soldiers	35	21.9	4.2	19.25	9.6–30.1	TWA: 190		Brown (1983)
USA	1985	Indoor range Full-time employee Part-time employee	 2 2	NR	NR	 59–77 17–49		Showroom, 2.7 Firing line, 13.6 Midway to target, 57.4; Target, 90.5		Novotny *et al.* (1987)
	1987	Covered outdoor range	15	NR	NR	5.6 (pre-exposure) 10.7 (day 2) 14.9 (day 5) 8.7 (day 69)		GA, 68.4 PBZ, 128.5	3.8–298.6 34.7–314.3	Tripathi *et al.* (1989)

Table 72 (contd)

Country	Year(s) of study	Settings/task	No. of subjects and sex	Age (years)	Job history (years)	Blood lead (µg/dL)		Lead in air (µg/m³)		Reference
						AM[a]	Range	AM[a]	Range	
USA (contd)	1987	Indoor range with training 3 Feb.–28 April	17 M + W	24–40	Trainees					Valway *et al.* (1989)
	Jan.-Feb.					6.45	< 5–23.1	1483–1860	304–2688	
	March (early)					51.4	31.2–73.3	2906–3226	994–5589	
	March (late)					44.5	27.1–62.3	1231	553–2567[c]	
	May					39.3	23.1–51.2			
		Lead bullet						1410		
		Nylon-coated						78.3		
		Copper jacketed						43.1		
	1987	Covered outdoor range using copper-jacketed bullets	6	NR	NR	Before shooting, 6.0 ± 1.7 After shooting, 6.5 ± 1.5		GA, 9.53 PBZ, 5.88	5.50–14.56 0.42–7.66	Tripathi *et al.* (1990)
	1987–88	Uncovered outdoor range		NR	NR					Goldberg *et al.* (1991)
	June 1987		7			28–66		–		
	July 1987					–		460–510 (3-h TWA)		
	Dec. 1987		7			25–70		–		
	April 1988		5			–		100–170 (3-h TWA)		
	June 1988					28–38		–		
	1987	Covered outdoor range		NR	Instructors					Tripathi *et al.* (1991)
		Non-jacketed bullets	2			14.2–24.2[d]	10–27	67.1–211.1	36.7–431.5	
		Jacketed bullets	2				13.1–22.1		5.4–8.7	
	1991–93	University rifle range		College students	Recreational shooters					Prince & Horstman (1993)
		Old ventilation system				11.8–16.4	5–21	176	24–239	
		New ventilation system				13.2–13.6	8–23	129	67–211	

GA, general area; NR, not reported; PBZ, personal breathing zone; TWA, time-weighted average
[a] Arithmetic mean, unless stated otherwise
[b] Median value
[c] New ventilation system installed
[d] Range of means of three sampling dates

Table 73. Lead concentrations in blood of occupationally exposed subjects: miscellaneous

Country	Year(s) of survey	Job/task	Sex	No. of subjects	Age (years) mean and/or range	Years of employ-ment	Smoking status	Blood lead (µg/dL)		Lead in air (µg/m³)		Reference
								AM[a]	Range/SD	AM[a]	Range	
Mechanics/garage												
Denmark	1976	Automobile mechanics	M	138	16–68	NR	NR	40.0–44.8	50–125	3.19	0.2–9.2	Clausen & Rastogi (1977)
Ghana	NR	Automobile mechanics	M	25	17–46	2–29	NR	27.8	0–60	NR		Ankrah *et al.* (1996)
	NR	Gasoline retailers	M + W	40	20–46	0.1–17	NR	8.6	0–20	NR		Ankrah *et al.* (1996)
India	NR	Automobile mechanics	M	22	20–45	NR	NR	NR	24.3–62.4	NR		Kumar & Krishnaswamy (1995b)
	NR	Workers in petrol storage bunkers	NR	22	10–15	> 1	NR	39.3	± 3.7	NR		National Institute of Nutrition (1995–96)
Jordan	NR	Mechanics	M	62	NR	NR	NR	8.1[b]		NR		Hunaiti *et al.* (1995)
Thailand	NR	Repair mechanics	M	23	NR	NR	Non-smokers	8.4	3.9–14.5	NR		Suwansaksri *et al.* (2002)
United Arab Emirates	1999	Heavy industry, garage and painting	M	100	34.8	8.3	NR	77.5		NR		Bener *et al.* (2001)
Others												
Finland	1973–82	Lead-exposed industry workers	M	18 329	33.8 at entry	0–46	NR	29.0–14.5[b,c]		NR		Anttila *et al.* (1995)
			W	2412	37.5 at entry	0–46	NR	20.7–6.2[b,c]				
India	NR	Silver jewellery makers	M	9	25–65	5–40	NR	120.8	40.0–210.0	NR		Behari *et al.* (1983)
	1981	Papier-mâché workers	M + W	30	10–70	NR	NR	69.1	23–122	NR		Kaul & Kaul (1986)
	NR	Silver jewellery workers	M	7	25–70	12–50	NR	113.4	71.0–208.1	NR		Kachru *et al.* (1989)
	NR	Printing press	M	23	20–50	15–30	NR	41.9	± 7.0	NR		Kumar & Krishnaswamy (1995a)
	NR	Papier-mâché workers	M	70	17–40	3–26	NR	68.1	18.2–272.7	NR		Wahid *et al.* (1997)
India	NR	Printing press	M + W	25	18–35	3–5	NR	88	± 30	NR		Agarwal *et al.* (2002)
						6–9		59	± 22			
						9–15		36	± 11			
Italy	NR	Electrician	M	1	20	6	NR	66		NR		Franco *et al.* (1994)

Table 73 (contd)

Country	Year(s) of survey	Job/task	Sex	No. of subjects	Age (years) mean and/or range	Years of employ-ment	Smoking status	Blood lead (µg/dL)		Lead in air (µg/m³)		Reference
								AM[a]	Range/SD	AM[a]	Range	
Japan	NR	Ceramic painting	M	58	54.7	1–53	Refrain	16.5[b]	3.5–69.5	NR		Ishida *et al.* (1996)
			W	70	52.2	3–47	for 12 h	11.1[b]	2.1–31.5	NR		
	NR	Pigment (lead stearate) production	M	49	48.0 (27–63)	14.5 (2–34)	NR	18.0	7–36	NR		Yokoyama *et al.* (1997)
	NR	Crystal toy production	W	123	27.3 (17–44)	7.2 (0.8–25)	NR	55.4	22.5–99.4	920	390–1910	Nomiyama *et al.* (2002)
	NR	Cloisonné production	NR		NR	NR	NR			NR		Arai *et al.* (1994)
		Glazing		49				47.8	11.3–111			
		Silver-plating		16				11.3	3.2–19.5			
Jordan	NR	Metal casting	M	26	NR	NR	NR	41.6[b]		NR		Hunaiti *et al.* (1995)
		Car painting	M	85	NR	NR	NR	10.7[b]		NR		
Malaysia	NR	Shipyard	M		> 18	< 1–17	Included			NR		Mokhtar *et al.* (2002)
		Painting		15				16	8–38			
		Fabrication		19				12	3–28			
Nigeria (SW)	NR	Lead-exposed industry workers	NR	86	24.8	NR	Included	56.3	26–97 40% > 60	NR		Adeniyi & Anetor (1999)
Pakistan	1994–95	Tannery	M	46	19–59	> 1	Included	60.6	± 3.8	NR		Khan *et al.* (1995)
Philippines	NR	Refrigerator production	M	59	25.7	4.7	NR	21.5[b]	8–38	NR		Makino *et al.* (1994)
			W	6	21.8	2.1	NR	17.5[b]	14–22	NR		
Republic of Korea	1999	Various (24 facilities)	M + W	723	39.4	6.3	61% of smokers	31.7	5.4–85.7	NR		Todd *et al.* (2001a)[d]
	1997–99	Various (26 facilities)	639 M, 164 W	803	40.4	8.2	57% of smokers	32.0	± 15	NR		Schwartz *et al.* (2001)[d]
Singapore	1989	Plastics	NR	104	NR	NR	NR	26.0	± 15.8	NR		Chia *et al.* (1993)
		Metal products	NR	70	NR	NR	NR	32.5	± 13.1	NR		
		Solder production	NR	22	NR	NR	NR	25.0	± 9.1	NR		
		Paint production	NR	88	NR	NR	NR	14.3	± 6.8	NR		
		Telecommunication	NR	218	NR	NR	NR	15.4	± 5.7	NR		
		Ship building	NR	92	NR	NR	NR	17.9	± 6.7	NR		
	NR	PVC compounding	M	61	38.3	ca. 10	NR	23.9	6.7–75.8	35.7	ND–277	Ho *et al.* (1998)

Table 73 (contd)

Country	Year(s) of survey	Job/task	Sex	No. of subjects	Age (years) mean and/or range	Years of employ-ment	Smoking status	Blood lead (µg/dL)		Lead in air (µg/m³)		Reference
								AM[a]	Range/SD	AM[a]	Range	
United Kingdom	NR	Painters and decorators	M	3	22–51	NR	NR	[85.5]	84.2–87.1	NR		Gordon *et al.* (2002)
Uruguay	[1993]	Lead–acid battery and lead scrap smelter[e]	M	31	NR	9.5	12	49.7	24.4–87.0	NR	3–1300	Pereira *et al.* (1996)
USA	1984	Electronics industry	M + W	151	> 11	NR	NR	8.0	1–22	NR	61–7000	Kaye *et al.* (1987)
	1994	Custodial activities	NR	13	40	8.5	NR	5.4	2.8–10	0.1–3.9	ND–36	Tharr (1997)
	1994–96	Labourers	M	60	38	15.5	NR	11.2	1.2–50	NR		Reynolds *et al.* (1999)
		Painters	M	83	39	16.4	NR	7.0	1.5–26.3	NR		

NR, not reported; M, men; W, women; ND, not detectable
[a] Arithmetic mean, unless stated otherwise
[b] Geometric mean
[c] Decrease over the 10-year study period
[d] [The participants in the study by Todd *et al.* (2001a) most likely are included in the study by Schwartz *et al.* (2001).]
[e] Two storage battery plants ($n = 16$, $n = 8$); lead scrap smelter ($n = 6$); one self–employed storage battery reconditioner

Table 74. NIOSH Health Hazard Evaluation reports with air and/or blood lead concentration data, 1978–2003

Industry	Year(s) of study	Blood lead (µg/dL)			Air lead (µg/m³)				Reference
		No. of workers tested	AM[a]	Range	No. of samples taken	Type of sampling	AM[a]	Range	
Bridge, tunnel and elevated highway construction: deleading	1980								Landrigan *et al.* (1980)
Grit blasting		13	33	25–47	4	PBZ	305	10–1090	
Scraping and priming		19	61	30–96	3	PBZ	391	24–1017	
Bridge, tunnel and elevated highway construction: repainting	1990–91								Sussell *et al.* (1992a)
Inside containment					8	PBZ	[13 671]	3620–29 400	
Inside containment, inside hood					6	PBZ	[78]	9–194	
Outside containment					16	PBZ		5–6720[b]	
						GA		ND–8170	
Heavy abrasive blasting	Spring 1991	23		5–61					
Moderate abrasive blasting	Summer 1991	12		13–43					
Bridge, tunnel and elevated highway construction: renovation	1993	22	7.2	2.2–16.5					Ewers *et al.* (1995)
Blaster/painter					24	PBZ	250	3–1800	
Apprentice					11	PBZ	110	1–680	
Recycling equipment operator					2	PBZ	140	100–180	
Commercial testing laboratories	1986	10		> 17–192					Gunter *et al.* (1986)
Lakewood, CO					8	PBZ + GA	321	90–800	
Sparks, NV					14	PBZ + GA	114	4–490	
Copper foundries	1991	10	21	10–39	7	PBZ	NA	ND–172	Clark *et al.* (1992)
Electric services	1991	43	20	< 5–43	18	PBZ	[9.4]	1.2–55	Venable *et al.* (1993)
Electric services	1995	NR	NR		43	PBZ	NA	ND–181	Mattorano (1996)
Electronic components	1993	NR	NR		3	PBZ	NA	ND–36	Blade & Bresler (1994)
Electronic components	1993	7	19	9–27			NR		Guo *et al.* (1994)
Fabricated metal products	1987	3	31	25–43	4	PBZ	[803]	7.3–1900	Lee (1987)
Fabricated plate work	1991	9	32	10–51			NR		Hales *et al.* (1991)

Table 74 (contd)

Industry	Year(s) of study	Blood lead (µg/dL)			Air lead (µg/m³)				Reference
		No. of workers tested	AM[a]	Range	No. of samples taken	Type of sampling	AM[a]	Range	
Fabricated plate work	1991	17	34	11–77					McCammon *et al.* (1991)
Lead burners					3	PBZ	[254]	215–307	
Tinning					3	PBZ-LT	[354]	282–390	
Grinding					4	PBZ-LT	[32]	0–46	
General contractors, industrial buildings and warehouses	1989	16	[10]	3–21					Stephenson & Burt (1992)
Oxyacetylene cutting					6	PBZ	522	160–1300	
Other renovation tasks					9	PBZ	NA	ND–2	
General contractors, single family houses: lead paint abatement	1989–91	95		ND–27	1402	PBZ	3.1[c]	< 0.4–916	Sussell *et al.* (1992b)
					1233	GA	2.0[c]	< 0.4–1296	
General contractors, single family houses	1993	53	5.2[c]	NR–17.5	13	PBZ	3.2[c]	0.05–12	Sussell *et al.* (1997)
					37	GA	0.6[c]	0.1–25	
					77	Task-based PBZ	0.2–9.1[c]	0.03–120	
General contractors, single family houses	1998	NR	NR						Sussell & Piacitelli (1999)
Manual paint scraping					5	PBZ-ST	NA	< 1–250	
Power paint removal					6	PBZ-ST	[5054]	54–27 000	
General contractors, single family houses	1996–98	40	16	1–65	20	PBZ	29[c]	1.5–1100	Sussell *et al.* (2000)
					152	Task-based PBZ	1.3–150	0.17–2000	
General contractors, single family houses	1999	NR	NR		128	PBZ	22[c]	ND–660	Sussell & Piacitelli (2001)
					130	GA	1.5[c]	ND–37	
General contractors, single family houses	1999	NR	NR		15	PBZ	100[c]	39–526	Sussell *et al.* (2002)
					5	GA	[2.2]	0.29–6.1	
					79	Task-based PBZ	71[c]	1.4–2240	
Glass products, stained glass art studio	1986	3	[19]	7–33	7	PBZ + GA	80	10–260	Gunter & Thoburn (1986a)
Glass products, made from purchased glass	1991	18	12	< 10–24	4	PBZ	18	7–35	Lee (1991)
Glass products, made from purchased glass	1993	2	2	1.8–2.1	17	PBZ	NA	ND–80	Donovan (1994)
					13	GA	NA	ND–0.7	
Gold ores (fire assay)	1987	NR	NR		4	PBZ	76	36–117	Daniels (1988)
					5	GA	48	14–100	

Table 74 (contd)

Industry	Year(s) of study	Blood lead (µg/dL)			Air lead (µg/m^3)				Reference
		No. of workers tested	AM[a]	Range	No. of samples taken	Type of sampling	AM[a]	Range	
Gold ores (fire assay)	1989								Daniels & Hales (1989)
Assay laboratory personnel		6	42	23–65	1	PBZ	850[d]		
Non-assay laboratory personnel		5	18	7–36	6	GA	NA	ND–110	
Gold ores (fire assay)	1989	6	42	23–65	1	PBZ	170		Daniels *et al.* (1989)
					4	GA	NA	ND–170	
Gold ores (fire assay)	1989	6	37	13–55	3	PBZ	[112]	15–200	Lee *et al.* (1990a)
					5	GA	[26]	6–61	
Gold ores, assay laboratory	1989	2	< 40		1	PBZ		10[d]	Hales & Gunter (1990)
					3	GA		10–30[d]	
Grey iron foundries	1985	NR	NR		4	PBZ	NA	ND–70	Gunter (1985)
					3	GA	53	30–70	
Heavy construction	1991	6							Sussell *et al.* (1992c)
Before blasting			34 before job	15–44	6	PBZ	ND–35		
During blasting, outside containment			28 during job	6–43	5	PBZ	ND–47		
					4	GA	620–3000		
During blasting, inside containment, inside helmet						PBZ		16–25	
Industrial inorganic chemicals	1980–81	79	35	NR–69	75	PBZ	13–79	0–359	Landrigan *et al.* (1982)
Industrial valves	1989	25	15	< 20–33	2	PBZ	[91]	87–94	Kinnes & Hammel (1990)
					4	GA	[69.5]	32–120	
Inorganic pigments	1981	228	8–32						Slovin & Albrecht (1982)
Bagging zinc oxide					11		[33]	9–96	
Mixing zinc oxide					5		[34]	16–68	
Mixing barium ores					7		[9]	ND–15	
Mixing of inert clays					4		[2]	ND–8	
Motor vehicle parts and accessories	1981	65	23	11–52	25	PBZ	37	7–113	Zey & Cone (1982)
Motor vehicle parts and accessories	1983	14	31 ± 12		7	PBZ	[49]	25–104	Ruhe & Thoburn (1984)
Motor vehicle parts and accessories	1986	5	< 29–60		4	PBZ	[172]	40–380	Gunter & Thoburn (1986b)
					4	GA	[68]	20–190	

Table 74 (contd)

Industry	Year(s) of study	Blood lead (µg/dL)			Air lead (µg/m^3)				Reference
		No. of workers tested	AM[a]	Range	No. of samples taken	Type of sampling	AM[a]	Range	
Motor vehicle parts and accessories	1988	8	[29]	8–44	10	PBZ + GA	160	10–290	Gunter & Hammel (1989)
Motor vehicle parts and accessories	1987–88	28	[9]	< 5–43		NR	NR		Driscoll & Elliott (1990)
Motor vehicle parts and accessories	1989	2	[34]	30–37	2	PBZ	[70]	60–80	Gunter & Hales (1990a)
Motor vehicle parts and accessories	1989	7	32	17–64					Gunter & Hales (1990b)
Radiator mechanics		5	38	23–64	4	PBZ	[28]	10–50	
Delivery employees		2	17.5	17–18	2	GA	[55]	20–90	
Motor vehicle parts and accessories	1989								Gunter & Hales (1990c)
Radiator mechanics		4	[30]	13–41	4	PBZ	[98]	30–220	
Delivery employees		2	[18]	14–21					
Motor vehicle parts and accessories: mechanics and delivery employees	1989	4	[21]	11–33	3 1	PBZ GA	[43] 90	20–60	Gunter & Hales (1990d)
Nitrogenous fertilizers	1991	13		4–13	9 7	PBZ GA		ND–7 ND–12	Decker & Galson (1991)
Non-ferrous foundries (castings)	1988	18	[34]	4–67	6	PBZ	[294]	38–520	Montopoli *et al.* (1989)
Police protection (indoor firing range)	1982	NR	NR		5 6	PBZ GA	[1130][d] [1120][d]	940–1300[d] 750–1520[d]	Bicknell (1982)
Police protection (indoor firing range)	1987–88	NR	NR		4	PBZ 8-h TWA	142–2073	102–3361 13–194[d]	Reh & Klein (1990)
Police protection (indoor firing range)	1991	NR	NR		5	PBZ 8-h TWA	14	7–23 < 3[d]	McManus (1991)
Police protection (indoor firing range)	1991	NR	NR						Echt *et al.* (1992)
Student					26	PBZ	26–32[d]	1–116[d]	
Range officer					14	PBZ	16–18[d]	0.15–53[d]	
General area					13	GA		0.15–2450	
Police protection (indoor firing range)	1991	NR	NR		10		5.4[d]	1–16[d]	Lee & McCammon (1992)

Table 74 (contd)

Industry	Year(s) of study	Blood lead (µg/dL)			Air lead (µg/m³)				Reference
		No. of workers tested	AM[a]	Range	No. of samples taken	Type of sampling	AM[a]	Range	
Police protection (outdoor firing range)	1991	NR	NR		16	PBZ	ND–8[d]	NR	Rinehart & Almaguer (1992)
Police protection (indoor firing range)	1992	NR	NR		3 13	PBZ GA	6[d] NA	5–7[d] ND–845	Cook *et al.* (1993)
Police protection (in- and outdoor firing ranges)	1989–91								Barsan & Miller (1996)
Instructor		7–14	8–15	< 4–27	NR	PBZ	12.4	ND–52	
Technician		5	10–16	6–28	12	PBZ	0.6	ND–2.7	
Gunsmith		5–11	11–12	< 4–24	18	PBZ	0.6	ND–4.5	
Custodian		6	< 4		3	PBZ	NA	ND–220	
Police protection (indoor firing range)	1997–98	NR	NR						Harney & Barsan (1999)
1997 (during shooting)					9	PBZ + GA	144[d]	4–190[d]	
1998 (during shooting)					20 8	PBZ + GA[e] PBZ + GA[f]	230[d] 433[d]	ND–640[d] 100–960[d]	
Pressed and blown glass and glassware	1984	12	20	2–36	4 2	PBZ GA	52 75	30–60 70–80	Gunter & Thoburn (1985)
Pressed and blown glass and glassware	1986	9	13	4–33	16	PBZ + GA	NA	ND–80	Gunter (1987)
Pressed and blown glass and glassware	1997	NR	NR		7	GA	[17]	1.6–51	Hall *et al.* (1998)
Primary smelting and refining of copper	1984	49	11	0–24	15	PBZ + GA	NA	< 3–60	Gunter & Seligman (1984)
Secondary smelting and refining of non-ferrous metals	1989	12	29	5–63	5 2	PBZ GA	NA NA	< 2–40 < 2–50	Gunter & Daniels (1990)
Primary and secondary smelting and refining of non-ferrous metals	1981	3	32	26–37	6 9	PBZ GA	123 NA	5–295 ND–1334	Apol (1981)
Refuse systems	1990–91	NR	NR		6 4	PBZ GA	NA NA	ND–30[d] ND–30[d]	Mouradian & Kinnes (1991)
Scrap and waste materials	1987	6		4–33	10	PBZ + GA	NA	ND–2.3	Hills & Savery (1988)
Scrap and waste materials	1991	15	66	9–86		NR			Gittleman *et al.* (1991)
Scrap and waste materials	1993	16	20	4–40		NR			Malkin (1993)

Table 74 (contd)

Industry	Year(s) of study	Blood lead (µg/dL)			Air lead (µg/m³)				Reference
		No. of workers tested	AM[a]	Range	No. of samples taken	Type of sampling	AM[a]	Range	
Ship breaking, ship repair, dismantling ships	1998	NR	NR						McGlothlin *et al.* (1999)
Inside a ship					4	PBZ	[355]	253–435	
Process area					5	PBZ	[189]	41–399	
Inside barge tank					5	PBZ	[198]	79–356	
Under a barge					4	PBZ	NA	< 0.6–2.5	
Shipbuilding and repairing	1985	10	38	25–53	7	PBZ	257	108–500	Landrigan & Straub (1985)
Shipbuilding and repairing	1994	NR	NR		14	PBZ-ST	[133]	3–900	Sylvain (1996)
Shipbuilding and repairing	1997	67	4.4	0–18	347	PBZ	32	0–1071	Kiefer *et al.* (1998)
Special trade contractors: cleaning of lead-based paint	1992	NR	NR		36	PBZ-ST	66	5–360	Sussell *et al.* (1993)
					5	PBZ	30	6–73	
					18	GA-ST	44	4–180	
Steel works, blast furnaces (including coke ovens)	1984	26	33		27	PBZ	40	< 3–190	Gunter & Thoburn (1984)
Steel works, blast furnaces (including coke ovens)	1980–82	79	8–15	1–33	42	NR	NR	NR–79	Hollett & Moody (1984)
Steel works, blast furnaces (including coke ovens)	1989	22	18		20	PBZ	12	< 3–31	Lee *et al.* (1990b)
Steel works, blast furnaces (including coke ovens)	1990	NR	NR		12	[PBZ]	[16]	1.3–44.2	Tubbs *et al.* (1992)
Storage batteries	1983–84	317	10–39	3–58	675	PBZ	30	1–1600	Singal *et al.* (1985)
Storage batteries	1987								Matte & Burr (1989a)
Location 1		27	31–47	NR–64	26	PBZ	[652]	40–5300	
					2	GA	[7]	4–10	
Location 2		12	65[c]	NR–89	10	PBZ	[860]	50–3400	
Location 3		6	28–> 60		3	PBZ	[100]	30–190	
					3	GA	[57]	10–100	
Storage batteries	1987	23	64[c]	28–86	7	PBZ	21[c]	NR–66	Matte & Burr (1989b)
Storage batteries	1991	43	41	12–66	12	PBZ	[276]	9–846	Clark *et al.* (1991)
					2	GA	[59]	10–107	

Table 74 (contd)

Industry	Year(s) of study	Blood lead (µg/dL)			Air lead (µg/m³)				Reference
		No. of workers tested	AM[a]	Range	No. of samples taken	Type of sampling	AM[a]	Range	
Storage batteries	1994–95	111		30–43					Esswein *et al.* (1996)
Pasting operation					19	PBZ	291	68–495	
					4	GA		1–165	
First assembly					12	PBZ	108	15–418	
					5	GA		13–39	
Pouching					7	PBZ	50	31–77	
					8	GA		11–51	
Grid casting					3	PBZ		12–43	
					6	GA		16–141	
Tanks, fabricated plate work	1991	22	23	4–38	22	PBZ	[352]	23–1970	McCammon *et al.* (1992)
Valves and pipe fittings	1981	2	< 30		2	PBZ	[45]	10–80	Ruhe (1982a)
Valves and pipe fittings	1981	2	< 30		2	PBZ	[839]	321–1356	Ruhe (1982b)

AM, arithmetic mean; PBZ, personal breathing zone; NA, not applicable; ND, not detected; NIOSH, National Institute for Occupational Safety and Health (USA); NR, not reported; GA, general area; ST, short-term; TWA, time-weighted average; LT, long-term; [....] calculated by the Working Group

[a] Unless otherwise stated

[b] Highest value probably a contaminated sample; next highest values at 202 µg/m³

[c] Geometric mean

[d] 8-h TWA value calculated from a short-term sample, assuming no other lead exposure during the day than during sampling

[e] Measured with 37-mm cassette

[f] Measured with Institute of Occupational Medicine (IOM) sampler

(*a*) *Lead–acid battery workers*

Blood lead concentrations have been studied most extensively in workers in lead storage-battery factories (Table 66). Occupational exposure to lead may occur during the production of lead–acid batteries, when grids are manufactured either by melting lead blocks and pouring molten lead into molds or by feeding rolled sheets of lead through punch presses. In addition, a lead oxide paste is applied into grid spaces. Average lead concentrations in blood were generally in the range 20–45 μg/dL. Particularly high concentrations (> 65 μg/dL) were detected in workers engaged in grid casting in a study in Iraq (Mehdi *et al.*, 2000), in workers at several workstations in a study from Israel (Richter *et al.*, 1979) and in a study in Taiwan, China (Wang *et al.*, 2002b).

(*b*) *Workers in mining and primary smelting*

The most commonly mined lead ore is *galena* (87% lead by weight), followed by *anglesite* (68%) and *cerussite* (78%). Workers in lead smelter and refinery operations such as sintering, roasting, smelting and drossing are exposed to lead sulfide, sulfates and oxides. Miners of copper and zinc also are exposed to lead.

Relatively high blood lead concentrations (> 60 μg/dL) have been recorded in such workers, in particular in two studies in Nigeria (Adeniyi & Anetor, 1999) and in Uruguay (Pereira *et al.*, 1996) (Table 67).

(*c*) *Workers in secondary smelting*

Battery-recycling workers in secondary smelters are exposed to lead as they convert used batteries and other leaded materials to lead of varying purity. From Table 68, it appears that the mean blood lead concentrations reported for workers in secondary lead smelters were higher than for workers in other occupations (see Tables 66–73). Of the different job categories within secondary smelting, the highest mean blood lead concentrations (87 μg/dL) were observed in workers in charge of furnace operation (Wang *et al.*, 1998). In some individual workers, blood lead concentrations in excess of 150 μg/dL were measured (Makino *et al.* 1994).

(*d*) *Workers in leaded-glass manufacturing*

Leaded glassware is made by combining lead oxide compounds with molten quartz. This process results in lead fumes and dusts, and glass-blowing is an additional activity that involves potential contact with lead. Production of leaded glass has been associated with high lead exposure, with mean blood lead concentrations in excess of 50 μg/dL in all studies (Table 69).

(*e*) *Workers in welding/soldering*

Typical solders contain 60% lead and the high temperatures involved in flame solder work volatilize some of this lead. Workers repairing vehicle radiators are exposed to lead dusts during radiator cleaning in addition to lead fumes during flame soldering (Tharr, 1993).

Surveys on welding work in radiator-repair workers (Table 70) generally showed mean blood lead concentrations in the range of 10–35 μg/dL. A study of 56 mechanics working in radiator shops in the Boston area, USA, reported that 80% had blood lead concentrations greater than 30 μg/dL and 16 had concentrations > 50 μg/dL (Goldman *et al.*, 1987). Relatively high blood lead concentrations (up to 47 μg/dL) were also reported among women engaged in soldering in an electronics plant (Makino *et al.*, 1994).

Welders are exposed to lead in the welding fumes generated by gas metal arc welding of carbon steel. However, in one study, lead concentrations in the welding fumes were found to range from 1.0 to 17.6 μg/m^3, well below the established permissible exposure limit for the workplace (Larson *et al.*, 1989).

(*f*) *Professional drivers and traffic controllers*

Professional drivers (e.g. taxi and bus drivers) and traffic policemen are exposed to lead in ambient air from vehicle exhausts (Table 71). The blood lead concentrations reported are distributed over a wide range, from 10 μg/dL (Zhou *et al.*, 2001) to > 60 μg/dL (Ahmed *et al.*, 1987), probably as a result of variations in traffic intensity and use of leaded gasoline.

(*g*) *Firing-range instructors*

Lead exposure associated with the discharge of firearms at indoor firing ranges began to be monitored in the early 1970s. Over the last 20 years, numerous exposure assessments have been performed at both indoor and outdoor firing ranges (Table 72). Several sources of airborne lead have been identified: fragmentation of bullets during firing; the explosive vaporization of the primer, which can contain both lead styphnate and lead peroxide; and inadequate ventilation of the range (Landrigan *et al.*, 1975b; Fischbein *et al.*, 1979; Muskett & Caswell, 1980; Dams *et al.*, 1988). Instructors are generally exposed to the highest concentrations of airborne lead and tend to have the highest blood lead concentrations due to their regular duties, which include supervising the range, cleaning and test-firing weapons, and preparing training ammunition from commercially purchased components. A positive correlation was reported between exposure of firearms instructors to elemental lead at covered outdoor firing ranges and increased blood lead concentrations (Tripathi *et al.*, 1991). Concentrations of airborne lead can be significantly reduced (97–99%) by using a lead-free primer and bullets jacketed with nylon, brass or copper (Valway *et al.*, 1989; Robbins *et al.*, 1990; Tripathi *et al.*, 1990, 1991; Goldberg *et al.*, 1991; Löfstedt *et al.*, 1999; Bonanno *et al.*, 2002).

(*h*) *Other occupational exposures*

Several studies have found elevated blood lead concentrations in other occupational settings, such as in employees working in automobile garages. Mean blood lead concentrations in children working in petrol storage bunkers in India for more than one year were almost double (39.3 ± 3.7 μg/dL) those of age-matched unexposed children (23.1 ± 0.5 μg/dL) (National Institute of Nutrition, 1995–1996).

Silver jewellery workers are exposed to high concentrations of lead and may have blood lead concentrations > 200 μg/dL (Behari *et al.*, 1983; Kachru *et al.*, 1989).

People working in arts and crafts may be exposed to lead in paints, ceramic glazes and lead solder used in sculpture and stained glass (Hart, 1987; Fischbein *et al.*, 1992).

Newspaper printing has been associated with lead exposure (Agarwal *et al.*, 2002). In one study, more than 3/4 of the monocasters showed some clinical symptoms of lead poisoning (Kumar & Krishnaswamy, 1995a). Where computerized printing techniques have replaced the traditional printing techniques, however, lead exposure is no longer a significant concern in this profession.

1.5 Analysis

Analysis of lead and lead compounds in various matrices has been reviewed (Fitch, 1998).

1.5.1 *Environmental samples*

Although lead occurs in the environment in the form of a range of inorganic or organic compounds, it is always measured and expressed as elemental lead. Determination of lead in environmental samples requires sample collection and sample preparation, often by wet or dry ashing or acid digestion to solubilize lead in aqueous solution before analysis. Care must be taken during sampling and sample preparation to avoid contamination or loss of lead (WHO, 1995).

The techniques most commonly used for the analysis of particulate lead and inorganic lead compounds in air, water, dust, sediments, soil and foodstuffs include flame atomic absorption spectrometry (AAS), graphite furnace–atomic absorption spectrometry (GF–AAS), inductively coupled plasma–mass spectrometry (ICP–MS), inductively coupled plasma–atomic emission spectrometry (ICP–AES), anode-stripping voltametry (ASV) and X-ray fluorescence (XRF).

Organic lead species such as tetramethyl lead and tetraethyl lead can be trapped cryogenically or by liquid or solid sorbents. Gas chromatography (GC) coupled with GF–AAS or photoionization detection (PID) can be used to differentiate between organic lead species (Birch *et al.*, 1980; De Jonghe *et al.*, 1981; Chakraborti *et al.*, 1984; NIOSH, 1994a; ATDSR, 1999).

Selected methods used for the analysis of lead in various matrices are presented in Table 75.

Table 75. Selected methods for analysis of lead in various matrices

Matrix	Method[a]	Detection limit	Method number	Reference[b]
Air	Flame AAS	2.6 µg/sample	Method 7082	NIOSH (1994b)
	GF–AAS	0.02 µg/sample	Method 7105	NIOSH (1994a)
	ICP–AES	0.062 µg/sample	Method 7300	NIOSH (2003a)
	ASV	0.09 µg/sample	Method 7701	NIOSH (2003b)
	XRF	6 µg/sample	Method 7702	NIOSH (1998)
	AAS or AES	0.01 µg/mL (qual.) 0.05 µg/mL (anal.)	Method ID-121	OSHA (2002a)
	ICP–AES	2.1 µg/sample (qual.)	Method ID-125G	OSHA (2002b)
	ICP–AES	0.071 µg/mL (qual.) 0.237 µg/mL (quant.)	Method ID-206	OSHA (2002c)
	XRF	22 µg/sample	Method OSS-1	OSHA (2003)
Air (TEL)[c]	GC–PID	0.1 µg/sample	Method 2533	NIOSH (1994c)
Air (TML)[d]	GC–PID	0.4 µg/sample	Method 2534	NIOSH (1994d)
Water	ICP–AES	42 µg/L	Method D1976	ASTM (2002)
	ICP–MS	0.08 µg/L	Method D5673	ASTM (2003a)
	XRF	1 µg/L	Method D6502	ASTM (2003b)
	AAS	100 µg/L	Method 239.1	US EPA (1978)
Ambient water	ICP–MS	0.0081 µg/L	Method 1640	US EPA (1997a)
	GF–AAS	0.036 µg/L	Method 1637	US EPA (1996c)
	ICP–MS	0.015 µg/L	Method 1638	US EPA (1996d)
Marine water	GF–AAS	2.4 µg/L	Method 200.12	US EPA (1997b)
	ICP–MS	0.074 µg/L	Method 200.10	US EPA (1997c)
Soil, wastes and groundwater	AAS	100 µg/L	Method 7420	US EPA (1986b)
	GF–AAS	1 µg/L	Method 7421	US EPA (1986c)
Marine sediment and soils	GF–AAS	0.2 µg/g	Method 140.0	NOAA (1998a)
	ICP–MS	0.15 µg/g	Method 172.0	NOAA (1998b)
	XRF	0.2 µg/g	Method 160.0	NOAA (1998c)
Aqueous and solid matrices	ICP–AES	28 µg/L	Method 6010C	US EPA (2000)
Food	GF–AAS	0.1 mg/kg	Method 999.10	AOAC (2000a)
	AAS	NR	Method 972.25	AOAC (2000b)
Evaporated milk and fruit juice	ASV	5 ng/sample	Method 979.17	AOAC (2000c)
Sugars and syrups	GF–AAS	3.3 µg/kg	Method 997.15	AOAC (2000d)
Edible oils and fats	GF–AAS	18 µg/kg	Method 994.02	AOAC (1994)

Table 75 (contd)

Matrix	Method[a]	Detection limit	Method number	Reference[b]
Ceramic foodware	AAS GF–AAS	NR NR	Method 4-1 Method 4-2	US FDA (2000a) US FDA (2000b)
Paint, soil, dust, air	ICP–AES AAS GF–AAS	Variable, NR Variable, NR Variable, NR	Method E1613	ASTM (1999)

NR, not reported

[a] AAS, atomic absorption spectrometry; ASV, anode-stripping voltametry; GD–PD, gas chromatography–photoionisation detector; GF–AAS, graphite furnace atomic absorption spectrometry; ICP–AES, inductively-coupled plasma atomic emission spectrometry; ICP–MS, inductively-coupled plasma mass spectrometry; XRF, X-ray fluorescence

[b] NIOSH, National Institute for Occupational Safety and Health; OSHA, Occupational Safety and Health Administration; ASTM, American Society for Testing and Materials; AOAC, Association of Official Analytical Chemists; US EPA, US Environmental Protection Agency; NOAA, National Oceanic and Atmospheric Administration; US FDA, US Food and Drug Administration

[c] TEL, tetraethyl lead

[d] TML, tetramethyl lead

Use of lead isotope ratios in source attribution and apportionment

Stable lead isotopes have been used to identify the source(s) of lead in environmental and biological samples (source attribution and apportionment). Lead isotopes vary over geological time because they are the end-product of radioactive decay of uranium and thorium. Thus, lead deposits of different geological age have different lead isotope ratios; e.g. the major Broken Hill lead–zinc–silver mine deposit in Australia formed approximately 1700–1800 million years ago has an isotope ratio expressed as the $^{206}Pb/^{204}Pb$ ratio of 16.0. In contrast, geologically younger deposits formed approximately 400–500 million years ago, found on the same continent and in various places around the world, have a $^{206}Pb/^{204}Pb$ ratio of about 18.0 (Gulson, 1986, 1996a).

Techniques have been developed to measure lead isotope ratios in environmental and biological samples. Lead is extracted from samples by acid digestion and separated from potentially interfering cations (iron, zinc) by anion-exchange chromatography. Lead isotopes are measured as ratios (e.g. $^{208}Pb/^{206}Pb$, $^{207}Pb/^{206}Pb$, $^{206}Pb/^{204}Pb$) by solid source thermal ionization–mass spectrometry or ICP–MS (Franklin *et al.*, 1997; Eades *et al.*, 2002).

Lead in the environment and in humans (and animals) is often a mixture of lead originally derived from different mines, and it is possible to estimate the relative contribution of the different sources. Where there are two major sources, the estimation is straightforward. For example, if the lead present in a blood sample with a $^{206}Pb/^{204}Pb$ ratio of 17.5 comes from two major sources, the skeleton (ratio of 17.0) and diet (ratio of 18.0), there is an equal contribution to blood from both sources. For three or more sources, the attribution becomes more complex and requires application of specialized computational procedures (Franklin *et al.*, 1997).

1.5.2 *Biological indicators of lead contamination in soil and water*

Lead affects many physiological parameters in plants (Singh *et al.*, 1997). Plants and some fungi synthesize cysteine-rich low-molecular-weight peptides called phytochelatins (class III metallothioneins) in response to heavy metal stress (Grill *et al.*, 1985). Phytochelatins have the general structure $(\gamma\text{-Glu-Cys})_n$-Gly ($n = 2$–11); the majority of legumes (of the order Fabales), on the other hand, synthesize homophytochelatins in which the carboxy-terminal glycine is replaced by β-alanine (Grill *et al.*, 1986). For example, when exposed to lead, roots of *Vicia faba* synthesize phytochelatins, *Phaseolus vulgaris* synthesizes homophytochelatins, and both phytochelatins and homophytochelatins are induced in *Pisum sativum* (Piechalak *et al.*, 2002). These peptides are involved in accumulation, detoxification and metabolism of metal ions including lead (Grill *et al.*, 1985; Mehra & Tripathi, 2000). Phytochelatins detoxify metal by thiolate coordination (Grill *et al.*, 1987). They are synthesized enzymatically from glutathione or its precursor by the enzyme γ-glutamyl cysteine dipeptidyl transpeptidase, also called phytochelatin synthase; the enzyme is present constitutively in cells and is activated by heavy metal ions (Grill *et al.*, 1989). Thus, phytochelatins are synthesized enzymatically in response to exposure to many metals including lead (Grill *et al.*, 1987; Scarano & Morelli, 2002).

Phytochelatins can be detected by high-performance liquid chromatography (HPLC) (Grill *et al.*, 1991) and thus have the potential to be used as plant biomarkers of heavy metal contamination of soil and water. There are ample laboratory and field data indicating that phytochelatins are biological indicators of exposure to metals, including lead (Ahner *et al.*, 1994; Pawlik-Skowronska, 2001; Pawlik-Skowronska *et al.*, 2002).

1.5.3 *Biological samples*

Lead distribution between blood, soft tissue and hard tissue is complex (see Section 4.1 for details). The time required for equilibration of lead between tissues is dependent upon the type of tissue and varies from hours to decades. In addition, equilibration between tissues is subject to a variety of physiological states that affect bone metabolism. Hence, exposure to lead can be estimated by the analysis of various human tissues, either directly for lead or indirectly for biomarkers of exposure to lead. The tissues include blood, plasma, urine, saliva, bone, teeth, nails and hair. The following section summarizes the methods used for the direct determination of lead in tissues and the indirect determination of exposure to lead using biomarkers. Methods that measure distribution of lead throughout the body are discussed in Section 4.1.

(*a*) *Analysis in hard tissues*

(i) *Bone*

Exposure to lead over time results in the progressive accumulation of lead, predominantly (> 95% of total lead burden) in bones (Barry, 1975). Hence, the analysis of lead in bones is a suitable approach to determine exposure to lead during the lifetime of an individual. Using GF–AAS to measure lead concentrations in bone tissue from individuals from prehistoric and modern times, it has been estimated that the body burden of lead in humans in the late 20th century is more than twice that of the late Roman times (Drasch, 1982). Since GF–AAS analysis cannot be performed on human bone *in vivo*, various XRF methods have come into use as a direct measure of lead in bone (Todd & Chettle, 1994). XRF is based on the property of lead to emit X-rays when it is exposed to photons of an appropriate energy; the fluorescence from lead accumulated in bone provides a low-risk, non-invasive measure of total lead content. In the 1990s, XRF analysis was limited to research institutions and was deemed unlikely to become a useful screening tool for exposure to lead (Todd & Chettle, 1994). Intrinsic variability in the instruments used, variability of lead deposition between the two main compartments of bone (cortical versus trabecular), patients' bone density and the use of a minimal detectable limit all increase the complexity of data analysis in epidemiological studies (Hu *et al.*, 1995; Kim *et al.*, 1995b). Efforts continue to improve understanding of the variables that affect the XRF signal (Hoppin *et al.*, 2000; Todd *et al.*, 2000a, 2001b) and to use XRF for meaningful epidemiological analysis (Hoppin *et al.*, 1997; Roy *et al.*, 1997; Markowitz & Shen, 2001). XRF has been used successfully to study the factors involved in the mobilization of lead from bone (Schwartz *et al.*, 1999; Oliveira *et al.*, 2002). With the understanding that bone lead is probably the best overall indication of lifetime exposure to lead (Börjesson *et al.*, 1997; Hu, H. *et al.*, 1998), it is reasonable to consider application of XRF to the analysis of the contribution of exposure to lead to the development of cancer.

(ii) *Teeth*

The dentin of shed deciduous teeth (also known as baby teeth) is a suitable source for analysis of prior and current lead exposure in children during their teeth-shedding years (Gulson, 1996a; Kim *et al.*, 1996a) but this method suffers from the limited availability of samples. It has been estimated that deciduous tooth lead (measured in ppm or μg/g) correlates with about half the value of blood lead (measured in μg/dL), but that this correlation does not hold for the permanent, adult teeth (Rabinowitz, 1995). The studies to determine lead concentrations in teeth each include a specific method for digestion of the tooth, followed by analysis of lead by ASV, ICP–MS or AAS.

(iii) *Hair and nails*

Available data on analysis of lead in hair can be divided into three groups. The first group of studies describe hair analysis as a general toxicological screen for heavy metals. In this case, the primary concerns are sample preparation, i.e. washing, with the intent to remove surface contamination. A recent study of six commercial laboratories advertising multimineral hair analysis showed high variability between laboratories, thus giving cause for concern about the validity of these results (Seidel *et al.*, 2001). The second use of hair lead analysis has been for patients suspected of having chronic, mild or subacute lead poisoning (Kopito *et al.*, 1967). The third documented use is in epidemiologial studies (Tuthill, 1996). However, an analysis of the distribution of heavy metals in tissues of 150 corpses concluded that hair was not an appropriate tissue for monitoring exposure to lead (Drasch *et al.*, 1997). In general, the available data do not support the use of hair as a resource for analysis of exposure to lead.

The use of nails seems attractive as a non-invasive approach to determining exposure to lead. However, lead concentrations in nails is not a reliable indicator of exposure to lead (Gulson, 1996b).

(*b*) *Analysis in soft tissues and body fluids*

(i) *Blood*

The benchmark for analysis of lead exposure is the determination of blood lead concentrations by AAS. Using this method, lead is typically reported in μg/dL, which can be converted to concentration in μM (μmol/L) by dividing the value reported in μg/dL by 20.7.

Analytical methods have changed over time because health-based standards and guidelines have changed. For example, the intervention level set by CDC in the USA has dropped from 60 μg/dL to 35 μg/dL in 1975, to 25 μg/dL in 1985, and to 10 μg/dL in 1991 (CDC, 1991).

Analytical methods used to determine lead concentrations in whole blood detect both the lead associated with proteins in the erythrocytes and that in the plasma (Everson & Patterson, 1980; Cake *et al.*, 1996; Manton *et al.*, 2001). The relationship between lead in whole blood, in erythrocytes and in plasma is discussed in detail in Section 4.2.1. Lead in blood is in equilibrium between the plasma and the erythrocytes. Since the plasma fraction has a greater bioavailability than the lead pool in the red blood cells and is in equilibrium with extravascular compartments, the lead content of plasma should be considered to be a better estimate of the internal dose than the concentration of the metal in whole blood (Cavalleri & Minoia, 1987; Schütz *et al.*, 1996). To obtain an accurate quantification of low concentrations of lead in plasma, Everson and Patterson (1980) introduced the technique of isotope-dilution mass spectrometry and concluded that prior studies had grossly overestimated the amount of lead in the plasma compartment of blood. ICP–MS was also shown to be sensitive enough for monitoring low concentrations of plasma lead, and plasma samples could be frozen prior to analysis without any alteration in the analytical results (Schütz *et al.*, 1996).

As whole blood became the material of choice for the determination of lead exposure, various atomic absorption techniques were introduced and evaluated for this purpose. By the late 1980s, the popularity of GF–AAS stemmed from its high sensitivity (0.05 μg/dL) and small sample-size requirements (< 50 μL); however, there was considerable variation in the different sample preparation techniques and an optimal method could not be defined (Subramanian, 1989). By 2001, commercial laboratories used predominantly electrothermal atomization atomic absorption spectroscopy, ASV and ICP–MS (Parsons *et al.*, 2001). A comparison of GF–AAS and ICP–MS performed in a Japanese laboratory showed the two methods to be equally sensitive but the latter took only one fifth of the time. ICP–MS results tended to be 10–20% lower than those obtained by atomic absorption analysis (Zhang *et al.*, 1997c).

For screening purposes, the simplest blood lead test is conducted with a capillary blood sample obtained from a finger-prick. Concerns over false positives due to skin surface contamination with environmental lead dust have resulted in the recommendation that a positive capillary blood lead test result be followed by a test on venous blood. Following the recommendation of universal screening of children in the USA (CDC, 1991; American Academy of Pediatrics, 1998), an analysis of the cost effectiveness of strategies for screening of lead poisoning concluded that a screening method based on direct analysis of venous blood was the least expensive (Kemper *et al.*, 1998). Other studies have shown an excellent correlation between the results of capillary blood lead analysis and venous blood lead analysis, thus advocating the former as an appropriate method for screening purposes (Parsons *et al.*, 1997).

Regardless of the method chosen, blood lead analysis is the only diagnostic for lead exposure for which there exists an international standard for quality control (ACGIH, 2001; WHO, 1996; see Section 1.6) and an external quality assurance programme (Schaller *et al.*, 2002).

(ii) *Urine*

Urine is a readily available biological sample for the direct analysis of lead content by AAS. This method has been used successfully to monitor relative levels of exposure in workers with chronic occupational exposure to lead (Vural & Duydu, 1995; Jin *et al.*, 2000). One study argued against the routine use of urine as a surrogate for blood lead analysis because of the poor correlation between the two values on an individual person basis, particularly at blood lead concentrations < 10 μg/dL (Gulson *et al.*, 1998b).

(iii) *Placenta*

During development of biomonitoring methods, non-invasive tissue acquisitions are frequently sought and analysis of lead in placental tissue has been suggested and evaluated as a possible indicator of exposure. However, studies show that placenta is not a suitable tissue for exposure monitoring, because lead is not distributed uniformly throughout the tissue (Lagerkvist *et al.*, 1996a).

(iv) *Sweat and saliva*

Lead concentrations in sweat and saliva have been evaluated and are not recommended for exposure monitoring because of the poor correlation with blood lead concentrations (Lilley *et al.*, 1988; Koh *et al.*, 2003).

1.5.4 *Biomarkers of lead exposure*

(*a*) *Biomarkers related to haeme biosynthesis*

It has long been known that lead interferes with haeme biosynthesis (Chisolm, 1964; Lamola & Yamane, 1974). Aberrations in the haeme biosynthetic pathway form the basis for many of the methods used for biomonitoring of human exposure to lead.

Haeme is the tetrapyrrole cofactor component of haemoglobin responsible for direct binding of oxygen. An early step in the pathway of haeme biosynthesis is the synthesis of the monopyrrole porphobilinogen from δ-aminolevulinic acid (ALA). This reaction is catalysed by the enzyme porphobilinogen synthase (PBGS) also commonly known as δ-aminolevulinate dehydratase (ALAD). Despite the fact that the recommended IUPAC name is PBGS, ALAD is still commonly used in the clinical literature. The inhibition of PBGS by lead manifests itself in a decrease in measurable PBGS activity in blood and an accumulation of the substrate ALA in serum, plasma and urine.

Porphobilinogen continues on the pathway to haeme through the action of additional enzymes to form the immediate haeme precursor protoporphyrin IX, also called free protoporphyrin, erythrocyte protoporphyrin (EP) or, erroneously, zinc protoporphyrin (ZPP). Insertion of iron into protoporphyrin IX is then catalysed by the enzyme ferrochelatase to form haeme. When iron is lacking, ferrochelatase inserts zinc into protoporphyrin IX to form ZPP. There is a tight and not fully understood interrelationship between haeme biosynthesis and iron homeostasis such that exposure to lead is seen to increase ZPP (Labbé *et al.*, 1999). Hence, between 1974 and 1991, measurement of ZPP was the method recommended by CDC in the USA for screening for exposure to lead (CDC, 1975).

One limitation in using these biomarkers is that they can be perturbed by conditions other than exposure to lead. The correlation between these biological parameters and a direct measure of blood lead may include significant scatter (Oishi *et al.*, 1996b) and may not be useful at low blood lead concentrations (Schuhmacher *et al.*, 1997). There are both genetic and environmental factors other than lead that can effect ALA in urine or serum, PBGS activity in blood and ZPP in blood (Moore *et al.*, 1971; Labbé *et al.*, 1999; Kelada *et al.*, 2001).

(i) *PBGS (ALAD) activity in blood*

PBGS activity in blood is the most sensitive biomarker of lead exposure (Toffaletti & Savory, 1976; Schuhmacher *et al.*, 1997). Human PBGS is a zinc metalloenzyme in which the catalytically essential zinc is in an unusually cysteine-rich environment that has a very high affinity for lead relative to the corresponding region in other zinc metalloenzymes. Although the activity of PBGS in blood shows normal biological variation, a comparison of the enzyme activity before and after various treatments that displace the inhibiting lead enables the determination of lead-specific enzyme inhibition (Granick *et al.*, 1973; Chiba, 1976; Sakai *et al.*, 1980). The PBGS assay is either a colorimetric determination of the complex of porphobilinogen with Ehrlich's reagent (Berlin & Schaller, 1974) or a quantification by HPLC of the porphobilinogen formed (Crowne *et al.*, 1981). Despite the sensitivity of PBGS to inhibition by lead, determination of the enzyme activity is not widely used in the clinical setting to determine lead exposure. In part, this is due to the fact that the inhibition of PBGS activity is only observed at low levels of exposure and reaches a plateau above 50–80 µg/dL lead (Toffaletti & Savory, 1976). The PBGS assay also gained a reputation for being complex and irreproducible. This may be due to the fact that the enzyme recovers its activity during the assay procedure, thus producing a variation in specific activity with incubation time (Jaffe *et al.*, 1991, 2001). Because assays used clinically require the analysis of a stopped mixture, a fixed incubation time is used, which may vary between laboratories.

PBGS in erythrocytes has a very high affinity for lead (Simons, 1995) and an individual's allotype for the gene encoding PBGS appears to affect the percentage of lead bound by the protein (Bergdahl *et al.*, 1997). Hence, a variety of epidemiological studies have suggested that an individual's PBGS allotype affects the pharmacodynamics of lead poisoning (Sakai, 2000). PBGS activity in blood can also be affected by the condition of hereditary tyrosinaemia, wherein an aberrant metabolic by-product of tyrosine acts as a PBGS inhibitor (Lindblad *et al.*, 1977) (see Section 4.2).

(ii) *ALA in urine and plasma*

Haeme precursors in urine were among the first biomarkers used for detection of lead intoxication. The synthesis of ALA is the primary regulatory target for haeme biosynthesis: haeme down-regulates ALA synthase expression directly by decreasing the half-life of ALA synthase mRNA (Hamilton *et al.*, 1991). Thus, inhibition of PBGS by lead, which results in a decrease in haeme biosynthesis, will upregulate ALA biosynthesis, and increase ALA concentrations in plasma and urine. An increased concentration of plasma ALA in turn increases the affinity of zinc for PBGS, thus giving some reprieve from the lead-induced inhibition of PBGS (Jaffe *et al.*, 2001). This interrelationship between lead, PBGS and ALA contributes to the complex clinical correlations between lead exposure and accumulation of ALA in urine. ALA concentrations in plasma increase slowly below blood lead concentrations of 40 µg/dL and rapidly above this concentration. Significant correlations are found in both the slow and rapid phases (Sakai, 2000). Plasma ALA (expressed in µg/L) is generally found to be about five times the value measured in urine (expressed in mg/g creatinine) (Oishi *et al.*, 1996b).

Analysis of ALA in biological fluids is generally performed either by colorimetry after chemical transformation of ALA into an Ehrlich's-positive pyrrole (Tomokuni & Ichiba, 1988a) or by fluorometry after HPLC analysis using pre- or post-column derivatization (Tabuchi *et al.*, 1989; Okayama *et al.*, 1990; Oishi *et al.*, 1996b).

(iii) *Zinc protoporphyrin in blood*

In the 1970s, the CDC approved ZPP as the preferred biomarker for the monitoring of lead exposure in the USA. The approved assay used spectrofluorometry, could readily be carried out on-site and was widely adopted for screening childhood lead poisoning. However, ZPP is generally not elevated in individuals with blood lead concentrations below 30 μg/dL (Schuhmacher *et al.*, 1997). With the current cut-off for lead poisoning in young children being 10 μg/dL blood lead (CDC, 1991), ZPP has generally fallen out of favour in the USA.

Although ZPP is not expected to be elevated in individuals casually exposed to low concentrations of lead, it continues to be a valuable tool for monitoring occupational exposure (Lee, 1999; Sakai, 2000) and bioresponse to lead (Lauwerys *et al.*, 1995). Also, elevation of ZPP is a diagnostic commonly used to detect iron deficiency (Labbé *et al.*, 1999).

(*b*) *Biomarkers related to pyrimidine nucleotide metabolism*

Although it has received far less attention than PBGS, the enzyme pyrimidine 5′-nucleotidase (P5′N), also known as uridine monophosphate hydrolase-1, is extremely sensitive to inhibition by lead (Paglia & Valentine, 1975). As with other biomarkers, both genetic and environmental factors can affect P5′N activity (Rees *et al.*, 2003). By analogy to the clinical manifestations of hereditary deficiencies in P5′N, the majority of the haematological features of lead poisoning can be explained by inhibition of P5′N (Rees *et al.*, 2003). Although not yet widely used, recent studies suggest that P5′N activity in blood is an excellent biomarker for exposure to lead, although less sensitive than PBGS (Kim *et al.*, 1995a). The three-dimensional structure of human P5′N is not yet known, but the documented sequence contains a cysteine-rich cluster (Amici *et al.*, 2000), which may be the site of lead binding.

P5′N catalyses the hydrolysis of pyrimidine nucleoside 5′-monophosphate to pyrimidine nucleoside and monophosphate (inorganic phosphate). Assays for P5′N activity fall into two categories. Colorimetric assays are based on the determination of inorganic phosphate. These tests require pre-assay sample dialysis and/or lengthy assay times and are not used for monitoring purposes (Sakai, 2000). Assays based on determining pyrimidine nucleosides have been introduced, using either a radiolabelled nucleoside (Torrance *et al.*, 1985) or HPLC analysis of the liberated pyrimidine nucleoside (Sakai & Ushio, 1986). A significant correlation was reported between log P5′N and blood lead concentrations over the range of 3–80 μg/dL (Sakai, 2000). Measurements of concentrations of pyrimidine nucleosides in blood have been suggested as alternative biomarkers for exposure to lead (Sakai, 2000).

(*c*) *Other biomarkers*

Nicotinamide adenine dinucleotide synthetase activity in blood has been suggested as a biomarker for exposure to lead, but this method has received little attention apart from the work of Sakai (2000). Recent investigations into the biological chemistry of lead suggest that lead can bind to a variety of proteins that normally bind zinc and/or calcium, most notably transcription factors. These observations may lead to the future development of alternative biomarkers for measurement of exposure to lead (Godwin, 2001).

1.6 Regulations and guidelines

Regulations and guidelines for lead concentrations in blood in non-occupationally exposed populations, ambient air and drinking-water have been defined in many countries and are given in Table 76.

Regulations and guidelines for occupational exposure to lead and lead compounds from several countries are presented in Table 77; maximum permissible lead concentrations in blood of occupationally exposed populations for several countries are presented in Table 78.

Many countries have set guidelines for lead in drinking water, gasoline, paint, foods, industrial emissions, and other products such as ceramic-ware and solder (Consumer Product Safety Commission, 1977; US DHUD, 1987; OECD, 1993; US Food and Drug Administration, 1994).

JECFA first evaluated lead in 1972, when a provisional tolerable weekly intake of 50 μg/kg bw was established. The value was reconfirmed by the Committee in 1978. In 1986, a provisional tolerable weekly intake of 25 μg/kg bw was established for infants and children for lead from all sources. This value was extended to the general population in 1993 and was reconfirmed in 1999 (WHO, 2000b; JECFA, 2002).

Analytical methods have changed over time (see Section 1.5) because health-based standards and guidelines have changed. A historical review of the CDC guidelines in the USA shows a progressive downward trend in tiered screening and intervention guidelines for childhood lead poisoning. Maximum permissible blood lead concentrations in the USA dropped from 35 μg/dL in 1975 to 25 μg/dL in 1985 to 10 μg/dL in 1991 (CDC, 1975, 1985, 1991). Efforts to maintain this downward trend (Bernard, 2003) may continue to drive development of increasingly sensitive analytical techniques.

The Commission of European Communities reports the following binding biological limit values [maximum allowed lead levels] and health surveillance measures for lead and its ionic compounds: (1) biological monitoring must include measuring the blood lead concentration using absorption spectrometry or a method giving equivalent results. The binding biological limit is 70 μg lead/dL blood; (2) medical surveillance is carried out when exposure occurs to a concentration of lead in air that is greater than 0.075 mg/m^3, calculated as a time-weighted average over 40 h per week, or when a blood lead concentration greater than 40 μg/dL is measured in individual workers; (3) practical guidelines for biological monitoring must include recommendations of biomarkers (e.g. ALA, ZPP, ALAD) and biological monitoring strategies (European Commission, 1998).

The American Conference of Governmental Industrial Hygienists (ACGIH) recommends a biological exposure index (BEI) for lead in blood of 30 μg/dL. Women of childbearing age whose blood lead exceeds 10 μg/dL are at risk of delivering a child with a blood lead concentration above the current CDC guideline of 10 μg/dL (ACGIH Worldwide, 2003). The ACGIH considers analysis of lead in blood by GF–AAS, ASV or ICP–MS to be sufficiently sensitive for concentrations below the recommended BEI (ACGIH, 2001).

Table 76. International standards and guidelines for lead concentrations in blood, air and drinking-water

Country	Blood (µg/dL)	Air (µg/m^3)	Drinking-water (µg/L)
Australia	10 (GP)	0.5 (federal) 1.5 (states)	10–50 (OECD)
Austria			50
Belgium		2.0	
Brazil			10
Canada	10 (GP)	1.0–2.5 (BC) 2.0 (QC) 5.0 (MB, NF, ON)	10
Czech Republic		0.5	50
Denmark		0.4	50
European Union	40[a]	1.0; 40[a]	50
Finland		0.5	10
France		2.0	50
Germany	15 (GP) 10 (C+W)	2.0	40
India			100
Ireland		2.0	50
Israel		0.5	50
Italy		2.0	50
Japan			10
Mexico			50
Namibia		1.5	50
Netherlands		0.5	50
New Zealand		1.0	50 (OECD)
Norway			20
Republic of Korea		1.5	50
Russian Federation		0.3	
Serbia and Montenegro		100–200	50
South Africa		4.0	50–100
Spain		2.0	50
Sweden			10 (OECD)
Switzerland	10–15 (F) 10 (C)	1.0	50 (OECD)
United Kingdom		2.0	50
USA	10 (GP)	1.5	15 (OECD)[a]
WHO	20 (GP)		10

From OECD (1993); International Lead and Zinc Study Group (2000); Ministry of Health, Brazil (2004); IOMC (1998)

BC, British Columbia; C, children; F, fetus; GP, general population; MB, Manitoba; NF, Newfoundland; ON, Ontario; QC, Quebec; W, women of childbearing age

[a] Action level

Table 77. Regulations and guidelines for occupational exposure to lead and lead compounds

Country/Agency	Exposure limit (mg/m^3)	Interpretation[a]
Lead		
Argentina	0.15	TWA
Australia	0.15 (dust and fume)	TWA
Austria	0.10 (men); 0.02 (women)	TWA
Belgium	0.15	TWA
Canada	0.15	
Alberta	0.05 (dust and fume)	TWA
Ontario	0.05 (excluding tetraethyllead)	TWA
Quebec	0.15	TWA
China	0.3 (fume)	Ceiling
	0.05 (dust)	Ceiling
Czech Republic	0.05	TWA
Denmark	0.10	TWA
European Union	0.15	TWA
	0.10 (dust and fumes < 10 μm)	TWA
Finland	0.10	TWA
France	0.15	TWA
Germany	0.1 (excluding lead arsenate and	TWA (MAK)
	8 lead chromate)	STEL (MAK)
India	0.15–0.20	TWA
Ireland	0.15 (excluding tetraethyl lead)	TWA
Israel	0.10 (men); 0.05 (women of fertile age)	TWA
Italy	0.15	TWA
Japan	0.10 (excluding alkyls)	TWA
Malaysia	0.05	TWA
Mexico	0.15 (dust and fume)	TWA
Morocco	0.20	TWA
Namibia	0.15	TWA
Netherlands	0.15 (dust and fume)	TWA
New Zealand	0.1 (dust and fume)	TWA
Norway	0.05	TWA
Peru	0.20	TWA
Poland	0.05	TWA
Republic of Korea	0.05	TWA
Serbia and Montenegro	0.05	TWA
South Africa	0.15	TWA
Spain	0.15	TWA
Sweden	0.10 (total)	TWA
	0.05 (respirable)	TWA
Thailand	0.20	TWA
United Kingdom	0.15	Ceiling (OES)
	0.15	TWA
USA		
ACGIH	0.05	TWA (TLV)
NIOSH	< 0.1	TWA (REL)
OSHA	0.05	TWA (PEL)

Table 77 (contd)

Country/Agency	Exposure limit (mg/m^3)	Interpretation[a]
Lead acetate		
Norway	0.05 (dust and fume)	TWA
Lead hydrogen arsenate ($PbHAsO_4$)		
Canada		
Alberta (as As)	0.15	TWA
	0.45	STEL
China, Hong Kong SAR (as $PbHAsO_4$)	1.5	TWA
Mexico (as Pb)	0.15	TWA
	0.45	STEL
USA (as As)		
NIOSH	0.002	Ceiling (REL)
OSHA	0.01	TWA (PEL)
Lead arsenate (as $Pb_3(AsO_4)_2$)		
Australia	0.15	TWA
Belgium	0.15	TWA
Canada		
Quebec	0.15	TWA
China	0.05 (dust)	TWA
New Zealand	0.15	TWA
USA		
ACGIH	0.15	TWA (TLV)
NIOSH (as As)	0.002	Ceiling (REL)
OSHA (as As)	0.01	TWA (PEL)
Lead chromate (as Cr)		
Australia	0.05	TWA
Belgium	0.012	TWA
Canada		
Alberta	0.05	TWA
	0.15	STEL
Ontario	0.012	TWA
Quebec	0.012	TWA
China	0.012	TWA
China, Hong Kong SAR	0.012	TWA
Finland	0.05	TWA
Germany	0.1 (dusts and aerosols)	TWA (TRK)
	0.05 (NOS[b])	TWA (TRK)
Malaysia	0.012	TWA
Netherlands	0.025	STEL
New Zealand	0.05	TWA
Norway	0.02	TWA
Spain	0.012	TWA

Table 77 (contd)

Country/Agency	Exposure limit (mg/m^3)	Interpretation[a]
USA		
ACGIH	0.012	TWA (TLV)
OSHA	0.001	TWA (REL)
Lead chromate (as Pb)		
Belgium	0.05	TWA
Canada		
British Columbia	0.012	TWA
China, Hong Kong SAR	0.05	TWA
Malaysia	0.05	TWA
Spain	0.05	TWA
USA		
ACGIH	0.05	TWA (TLV)
Lead (II) oxide		
Finland	0.1	TWA
Lead phosphate (as Pb)		
Norway	0.05	TWA
USA		
ACGIH	0.05	TWA (TLV)
OSHA	0.05	TWA (PEL)
Lead sulfide		
China	5	Ceiling
Tetraethyl lead (as Pb)		
Australia	0.1 (sk[c])	TWA
Belgium	0.1 (sk)	TWA
Canada		
Alberta	0.1 (sk)	TWA
	0.3 (sk)	STEL
British Columbia	0.075 (sk)	TWA
Quebec	0.05 (sk)	TWA
China	0.02 (sk)	TWA
	0.06 (sk)	STEL
China, Hong Kong SAR	0.1 (sk)	TWA
Finland	0.075 (sk)	TWA
	0.23 (sk)	STEL
Germany	0.05 (sk)	TWA (MAK)
	0.1 (sk)	STEL (MAK)
Ireland	0.1 (sk)	TWA
Japan	0.075 (sk)	TWA
Malaysia	0.1 (sk)	TWA
Mexico	0.1 (sk)	TWA
	0.3 (sk)	STEL
Netherlands	0.05 (sk)	TWA
New Zealand	0.1 (sk)	TWA

Table 77 (contd)

Country/Agency	Exposure limit (mg/m^3)	Interpretation[a]
Norway	0.01 (sk)	TWA
Poland	0.05 (sk)	TWA
	0.1 (sk)	STEL
Spain	0.1 (sk)	TWA
Sweden	0.05 (sk)	TWA
	0.2 (sk)	STEL
USA		
ACGIH	0.1 (sk)	TWA (TLV)
NIOSH	0.075 (sk)	TWA (REL)
OSHA	0.075 (sk)	TWA (PEL)
Tetramethyl lead (as Pb)		
Australia	0.15 (sk)	TWA
Belgium	0.15 (sk)	TWA
Canada		
Alberta	0.15 (sk)	TWA
	0.5 (sk)	STEL
Quebec	0.05 (sk)	TWA
China, Hong Kong SAR	0.15 (sk)	TWA
Finland	0.075 (sk)	TWA
	0.23 (sk)	STEL
Germany	0.05 (sk)	TWA (MAK)
	0.1 (sk)	STEL (MAK)
Ireland	0.15 (sk)	TWA
Malaysia	0.15	TWA
Mexico	0.15 (sk)	TWA
	0.5 (sk)	STEL
Netherlands	0.05 (sk)	TWA
New Zealand	0.15 (sk)	TWA
Norway	0.01 (sk)	TWA
Spain	0.15 (sk)	TWA
Sweden	0.05 (sk)	TWA
	0.2 (sk)	STEL
USA		
ACGIH	0.15 (sk)	TWA (TLV)
NIOSH	0.075 (sk)	TWA (REL)
OSHA	0.075 (sk)	TWA (PEL)

From ACGIH Worldwide (2003); European Commission (1998); International Lead and Zinc Study Group (2000)

ACGIH, American Conference of Governmental Industrial Hygienists; NIOSH, National Institute for Occupational Safety and Health; OSHA, Occupational Safety and Health Administration

[a] TWA, time-weighted average; STEL, short-term exposure limit; MAK, maximum allowable concentration; OES, occupational exposure standard; TLV, threshold limit value; REL, recommended exposure limit; PEL, permissible exposure limit; TRK, technical exposure limit

[b] NOS, not otherwise specified

[c] sk, skin notation

Note: For the most current information on these regulations and guidelines, the reader is referred to the relevant regulatory authority.

Table 78. Regulations and guidelines for maximum lead concentrations in blood in occupational settings

Country	MLL[a] (μg/dL)	Country	MLL[a] (μg/dL)
Australia	50 (men, and women not capable of reproduction); 20 (women of reproductive capacity)	Japan	60
Austria	45–70	Luxembourg	70
Belgium	80	Morocco	60
Canada	50–80	Namibia	80
Czech Republic	50	Netherlands	70
Denmark	50–70	Norway	2 μmol/L [41.4 μg/dL] (men)
Finland	50	Peru	60 (men)
France	70–80	South Africa	80 (men); 40 (women)
Germany	70 (men); 30 (women under 45 years)	Spain	70
Greece	70–80	Sweden	50 (men and women over 50 years); 30 (women under 50 years)
Ireland	70	Thailand	80
Israel	60 (men); 30 (women of reproductive age)	United Kingdom	60 (men); 50 (adolescents under 18 years); 30 (women of reproductive capacity)
Italy	70	USA	50

From International Lead and Zinc Study Group (2000)
[a] MLL, maximum lead level

2. Studies of Cancer in Humans

2.1 Studies among specific occupational groups

A summary of the epidemiological findings reviewed in this section is presented in Tables 79 (cohort studies) and 80 (population-based case–control studies).

2.1.1 *Battery manufacturing workers*

Fanning (1988) obtained the cause-specific distribution of 867 deaths (in-service deaths and pensioner deaths) occurring in male workers in the United Kingdom who were considered to have been exposed to high or moderate levels of lead whilst engaged in lead battery manufacturing. This distribution was compared with that of 1206 male decedants who had been employed either by other companies that participated in the same pension scheme, or in the lead battery factory but with little potential for exposure to lead. The deaths occurred during the period 1926–85 and the study incorporated data reported previously by Dingwall-Fordyce and Lane (1963) and Malcolm and Barnett (1982). After adjusting for age by 10-year-age groups, there were no significantly elevated proportional mortality odds ratios for cancer risk in relation to lead-exposed employment. A slightly elevated risk was suggested for cancer of the stomach.

There has been an extended study of lead battery and lead smelter workers in the USA (Cooper & Gaffey 1975; Cooper, 1976; Kang *et al.*, 1980; Cooper, 1981; Cooper *et al.*, 1985; Cooper, 1988; Wong & Harris, 2000). The original cohort (Cooper & Gaffey, 1975) included 4680 battery workers from 10 plants; the most recent update (Wong & Harris, 2000) relates to a reduced cohort of 4518 battery workers. All subjects manufacturing lead batteries were employed for at least 1 year during the period 1947–70, and the most recent follow-up has been analysed for the period 1947–95. There were 195 battery workers (4.3%) who were untraced on the closing date of the study. Exposure data were limited but blood lead and urinary lead measurements were taken, mainly after 1960. For lead battery workers with three or more blood lead measurements, the mean blood concentration was 63 μg/dL and, for those with 10 or more urinary lead measurements, the mean urine concentration was 130 μg/dL. Standardized mortality ratios (SMRs) were calculated after comparison with the mortality rates for the male population in the USA, and were adjusted for age and calendar period. For all cancers, the overall SMR was 104.7 (624 observed; 95% CI, 96.6–113.2). There was a significantly elevated SMR for stomach cancer (152.8; 45 observed; 95% CI, 111.5–204.5) and non-significantly elevated SMR for lung cancer (113.9; 210 observed; 95% CI, 99.0–130.4). [The Working Group noted that it is possible that ethnicity, dietary habits, prevalence of *Helicobacter pylori* infection, or socioeconomic status played a role in the excess of stomach cancer.] Findings were also reported for a nested case–control study of stomach cancer, using 30 cases and 120 age-matched controls from a single large battery factory. [The authors noted a large percentage of Italian- and Irish-born members of the study population (23% of the controls in the case–control study). Being Italian- or Irish-born was associated with a twofold excess risk for stomach cancer in this population. The Working Group considered that confounding by place of birth (which is not available for the whole cohort) would probably account for only a proportion of the 1.5-fold excess reported for this whole population.] The nested case–control study did not show any significantly increased odds ratios or trends for any of the three exposure indices that were investigated (duration of employment at the plant, duration of employment in intermediate or high exposure areas of the plant, [crudely] weighted cumulative exposure). [The Working Group noted that the analysis by duration of employment needs to be interpreted with caution, especially among workforces that were subject to active surveillance and potential removal from work.]

Table 79. Cohort studies on cancer risk among occupational groups exposed to lead or lead compounds

Reference, location	Cohort description	Assessment or indices of exposure to lead	Cancer site	Exposure categories	No of cases or deaths	Relative risks	95% CI	Comments
Battery factory workers								
Fanning (1988) United Kingdom	Proportional mortality study; 2073 men; frequency-matched by 10-year age group; 1926–85	Low (1206 men) and high (867 men) exposure groups; defined by job–exposure matrix				**PMOR**		Limited to deaths in service and in pensioners
			All sites		195	0.95		
			Stomach		31	1.34		
			Lung		76	0.93		
Wong & Harris (2000) USA	4518 men employed for > 1 year during 1947–70; follow-up 1947–95; vital status, 95.7%; cause of death, 99.5% (death certificates)	No exposure data; bio-monitoring 1947–72: urinary lead (2275 men), blood lead (1863 men); mean blood lead, 63 µg/dL (n = 1083); mean urinary lead, 130 µg/dL (n = 1550)				**SMR**		Expected deaths based on male mortality rates in the USA
			All sites		624	104.7	96.6–113.2	
			Lung		210	113.9	99.0–130.4	
			Stomach		45	152.8	111.5–204.5	
			Large intestine		59	103.9	79.1–134.0	
			Rectum		14	84.7	46.3–142.1	
			Central nervous system		10	75.0	35.9–137–9	
			Kidney		7	50.2	20.2–103.4	
Lead smelter workers								
Wong & Harris (2000) USA	2300 men employed in 6 smelters for > 1 year during 1947–70; follow-up, 1947–95; vital status, 93%; cause of death, 99.5% (death certificates)	No exposure data; bio-monitoring 1947–72: urinary lead (2275 men), blood lead (1863 men); mean blood lead, 80 µg/dL (n = 254); mean urinary lead, 173 µg/dL (n = 1550)				**SMR**		Expected deaths based on male mortality rates in the USA
			All sites		273	101.8	90.1–114.6	
			Lung		107	121.5	99.5–146.8	
			Stomach		15	133.4	74.6–220.0	
			Large intestine		22	89.0	55.8–134.7	
			Rectum		8	123.0	53.1–242.4	
			Central nervous system		5	74.5	24.2–173.9	
			Kidney		6	92.3	33.9–201.0	
McMichael & Johnson (1982) Australia	241 male smelter workers employed 1–30 years, diagnosed with lead poisoning 1928–59, followed through 1977; 140 deaths identified through death registration records	Lead poisoning; mean urinary lead, 173 µg/L	All sites	Lead-poisoned workers versus other workers	9	**SPMR** 0.59		Reference group: 695 deceased smelter workers without lead poisoning

Table 79 (contd)

Reference, location	Cohort description	Assessment or indices of exposure to lead	Cancer site	Exposure categories	No of cases or deaths	Relative risks	95% CI	Comments
Steenland *et al.* (1992) USA	1990 male smelter workers employed > 1 year, at least 1 day at the smelter 1940–65; subcohort with heavier exposure ($n = 1436$); vital status ≤ 31 December 1979 (95.5%); cause of death, 96.3%	Mean blood lead, 56 µg/dL ($n = 173$); mean air lead, 3.1 mg/m³ ($n = 203$); mean air arsenic, 14 µg/m³ ($n = 89$)				**SMR**		Further follow–up of the cohort from Selevan *et al.* (1985) National standard population No information on smoking
			All sites	Total cohort	192	98	84–112	
			Stomach		15	136	75–224	
			Lung		72	118	92–148	
			Colorectal		9	48	22–90	
			Kidney		9	193	88–367	
			All sites	Subcohort with high lead exposure	137	98	81–115	
			Stomach		10	128	61–234	
			Lung		49	111	82–147	
			Colorectal		8	59	25–116	
			Kidney		8	239	103–471	
Gerhardsson *et al.* (1986) Sweden	Retrospective cohort study; 3832 men followed up 1950–81; subcohort of 437 workers employed ≥ 3 years in high-exposure jobs, 1950–74; based on median value of the cumulative blood lead concentration, subcohort further divided into high ($n = 218$) and low ($n = 219$) mean blood lead (high > 478.5 µg × yr/dL > low) and high ($n = 288$) and low ($n = 149$) peak blood lead (high > 70 µg × yr/dL > low)					**SMR**		National and regional standards specified for cause, sex, age and calendar period Potential exposure to arsenic, chromium and nickel; cohort update in Lundström *et al.* (1997)
			All sites	Cohort	270	[114]	[100–128]	
				Subcohort	23	[87]	[55–131]	
				High mean blood lead	15	[100]	[56–165]	
				High peak blood lead	16	[89]	[51–145]	
			Lung	Cohort	90	[218]	[176–269]	
				Subcohort	8	[160]	[69–315]	
				High mean blood lead	5	[172]	[56–402]	
				High peak blood lead	4	[118]	[32–301]	
			Stomach	Cohort	46	[143]	[105–191]	
				Subcohort	3	[94]	[19–274]	
				High mean blood lead	2	[111]	[13–401]	
				High peak blood lead	3	[136]	[28–399]	

Table 79 (contd)

Reference, location	Cohort description	Assessment or indices of exposure to lead	Cancer site	Exposure categories	No of cases or deaths	Relative risks	95% CI	Comments
Lundström *et al.* (1997) Sweden	3979 workers employed > 1 year 1928–79; sub-cohort of 1992 workers from the lead department and other lead-exposed departments; mortality, 1955–87; vital status, 1955–87; vital status, 88.5%; incidence, 1958–87	Blood lead level 1950–69 (AES) and 1967–87 (AAS); mean blood lead in 1950, 62 μg/dL; mean blood lead in 1987, 33 μg/dL		Total cohort	(*n* = 3979)	**SMR**		Follow-up of the cohort reported in Gerhardsson *et al.* (1986) Regional standard specified for cause, sex, age and calendar period Multifactorial exposure pattern and lack of smoking data
			All sites		126	120	100–150	
			Lung		39	280	200–380	
				Highest exposed subgroup	(*n* = 1026)			
			All sites		55	120	90–150	
			Lung		19	280	180–450	
		≥ 15 year latency period		Total cohort	(*n* = 2353)	**SIR**		
			All sites		172	110	90–120	
			Lung		42	290	210–400	
			Central nervous system		6	110	40–230	
			Gastrointestinal		31	80	50–110	
			Kidney		7	90	40–190	
				Highest exposed subgroup	(*n* = 650)			
			All sites		83	110	90–140	
			Lung		23	340	220–520	
			Central nervous system		4	160	40–420	
			Gastrointestinal		15	80	50–130	
			Kidney		3	90	20–250	
		Lead-only workers or lead department and other lead-exposed departments; ≥ 15 year latency period		Total cohort	(*n* = 1005)	**SIR**		
			All sites		44	90	60–120	
			Lung		14	310	170–520	
			Central nervous system		2	110	10–380	
			Gastrointestinal		6	50	20–110	
			Kidney		0	0	0–150	

Table 79 (contd)

Reference, location	Cohort description	Assessment or indices of exposure to lead	Cancer site	Exposure categories	No of cases or deaths	Relative risks	95% CI	Comments
Lundström *et al.* (1997) (contd)				Highest exposed subgroup	(*n* = 163)			
			All sites		19	120	80–200	
			Lung		7	510	200–1050	
			Central nervous system		1	190	10–1050	
			Gastrointestinal		2	50	10–190	
			Kidney		0	0	0–500	
Englyst *et al.* (2001) Sweden	3979 workers in primary copper and lead smelter; follow-up 1958–87; subcohort (1): 710 workers employed in lead department and other departments during work history; subcohort (2): 383 workers from subcohort (1) only employed in lead department	Estimate based on cumulative blood lead index		Subcohort (1)		**SIR**		Workers also exposed to arsenic. County population reference. Same cohort as Lundström *et al.* (1997)
			All sites		47	100	70–130	
			Lung		10	240	120–450	
			Kidney		2	90	10–320	
			Central nervous system		1	60	2–360	
				Subcohort (2)				
			All sites		18	120	70–190	
			Lung		5	360	120–830	
			Kidney		1	130	3–720	
			Central nervous system		0	0	0–650	
Gerhardsson *et al.* (1995) Sweden	664 male secondary lead smelter workers employed > 3 months 1942–87; incidence 1969–89	Blood lead sampling starting 1969				**SIR**		Regional standard population: county rates specified for cause, sex, age and calendar year
			All sites		40	127	91–174	
			Stomach		3	188	39–550	
			Kidney		1	80	2–448	
			Central nervous system		1	75	2–420	
			Respiratory tract		6	132	49–288	
Cocco *et al.* (1996) Italy	1345 male lead and zinc smelting plant workers followed 1973–91; subcohort of 1222 with known G6PD[a] phenotype	Mean blood lead 1988–92 and mean environmental lead in 1991		Total cohort		**SMR**		Regional reference (Sardinia) Possible healthy worker effect; smoking not addressed
			Lung		2	[57]	[7–206]	
			Stomach		2	[333]	[40–1204]	
						Standardized mortality rates × 10^{-4}		
			All sites	Wild-type G6PD	10	25.7	21.4–30.6	
				G6PD-deficient	2	17.9	4.3–30.1	

Table 79 (contd)

Reference, location	Cohort description	Assessment or indices of exposure to lead	Cancer site	Exposure categories	No of cases or deaths	Relative risks	95% CI	Comments
Cocco *et al.* (1997) Italy	1388 male lead smelter workers, employed > 1 year 1932–71; mortality follow-up 1950–92; vital status 97.3%; cause of death 96%	Lead concentration in respirable dust; air arsenic below level of detection (23/24 samples); geometric mean air lead, 48 µg/m³				**SMR**		National reference (1950–92)
			All sites		149	69	58–81	
			Lung		35	62	43–86	
			Stomach		17	49	29–79	
			Brain		4	125	34–319	
			Kidney		5	142	46–333	
			All sites		132	93	78–110	Regional reference (1965–92)
			Lung		31	82	56–116	
			Stomach		14	97	53–162	
			Brain		4	217	57–557	Exposure to other agents, e.g. cadmium; no smoking data
			Kidney		4	175	48–449	
Ades & Kazantzis (1988) United Kingdom	4173 zinc–lead–cadmium smelter workers; employed > 1 year; all staff employed 1 January 1943 + all staff subsequently employed < 1970; born < 1940; 0.7% lost to follow-up; 3.2% emigrated; ≥ 10 years follow-up	Mean blood lead in cadmium plant, 28 µg/dL (3% of cohort); 59 µg/dL in furnace (10% of cohort); 56 µg/dL in sinter (8% of cohort) Years employed	Lung			**SMR**		Regional standard population. Exposure to lead highly correlated with exposure to arsenic.
				Overall	182	125	107–144	
				Duration of employment (years):				
				1–4	43	86	62–116	
				5–9	23	107	68–161	
				10–19	36	122	86–170	
				20–29	44	190	138–256	
				30–39	28	142	94–205	
				≥ 40	8	292	126–575	
	Nested case–control study with 174 lung cancer cases and 2717 controls frequency-matched on age, employment start date, surviving the case. Subjects followed up < 10 years excluded to allow for latency	Job–exposure matrix; ordered exposure categories	Lung			**RR**		Estimated RR associated with 10 years employment at each exposure level; no. of cases working at least 1 year
				Background	57	1.25		
				Low	73	1.28		
				Medium	72	1.36		
				High	27	1.54		

Table 79 (contd)

Reference, location	Cohort description	Assessment or indices of exposure to lead	Cancer site	Exposure categories	No of cases or deaths	Relative risks	95% CI	Comments
Lead chromate pigment production								
Sheffet *et al.* (1982) USA	1946 men (1296 Caucasian and 650 non-Caucasian) employed ≥ 1 month in a pigment plant 1940–69; followed until 1979	Exposure to chemical dust air samples (airborne chromium)		Caucasian				National standard population. Adjusted to include cases with unknown cause of death
			All sites		50	1.03		
			Lung		21	1.6		
			Stomach		5	2.0		
			Large intestine		2	0.5		
			All sites	Non-Caucasian	25	1.01		
			Lung		10	1.6		
			Stomach		3	1.6		
			Large intestine		0	0.0		
Davies *et al.* (1984a) United Kingdom	1152 male pigment workers first employed 1933, 1949, 1947 and followed until 1981; factories A and B exposure to zinc and lead chromate; factory C exposure to lead chromate only	Jobs categorized into exposure grades: high, medium and low	Lung	Date of first employment		**SMR**		High and medium exposure combined. Reference: specially compiled quinquennial national rates. Adjusted for duration of service
				Factory A				
				1932–45	13	222	120–380	
				1946–54	8	223	100–440	
				1955–mid-1963	2	100	10–360	
				mid-1963–67	0	–		
				Factory B				
				1948–60	6	373	140–810	
				1961–67	5	562	180–1310	
				Factory C				
				1946–60	1	48	0–270	
Davies *et al.* (1984b) United Kingdom	57 male pigment workers with non-fatal clinical lead poisoning; followed from date of poisoning or earliest available record, through 31 December 1981	Not estimated	Lung		4	**SMR** 145	[39–370]	Same factories as in Davies *et al.* (1984a) National reference

Table 79 (contd)

Reference, location	Cohort description	Assessment or indices of exposure to lead	Cancer site	Exposure categories	No of cases or deaths	Relative risks	95% CI	Comments
Glass workers								
Cordioli *et al.* (1987) Italy	468 workers in the glass industry employed ≥ 1 year 1953–1967 and followed until 1985; vital status 98.3%	Not estimated				**SMR**		National standard population
			All sites		28	127	[84–184]	
			Lung		13	209	[111–357]	
			Larynx		4	449	[122–1150]	
			Stomach		2	61	[7–220]	
Sankila *et al.* (1990) Finland	Cohort of 3749 (1803 men and 1946 women) employed ≥ 3 months in 2 glass factories, followed 1953–86; subcohort of 235 glass blowers (201 men and 34 women)	Not estimated		Total cohort		**SIR**		National standard population
			Stomach		34	93	64–129	
			Kidney		3	35	7–102	
			Central nervous system		6	60	22–131	
			Lung		69	128	99–162	
			Colon		7	46	19–96	
			Rectum		14	113	62–189	
			Lung	Subcohort of glass blowers	5	85	28–198	
			Stomach		6	231	85–502	
			Skin		3	625	129–1827	
Wingren & Englander (1990) Sweden	625 male art glassworkers employed ≥ 1 month 1964–85	Air measurements of lead				**SMR**		County reference. Smoking status lower than in the general population
			All sites		26	138	[90–202]	
			Lung		6	240	[88–522]	
			Colon		4	250	[68–640]	
Miners								
Cocco *et al.* (1994a) Italy	4740 men employed ≥ 1 year 1932–71 in 2 lead/zinc mines; mortality 1960–88; vital status 99.5%; cause of death 99.4%	Not estimated				**SMR**		Regional reference Exposure to silica and radon Includes 1741 subjects of the study reported by Carta *et al.* (1994).
			All sites		293	94	83–105	
			Lung		86	95	76–117	
			Stomach		27	94	62–137	
			Bladder		17	115	67–184	
			Intestine and rectum		12	64	33–112	
			Peritoneum; retro-peritoneum		6	367	135–798	
			Kidney		7	128	52–264	
			Nervous system		8	117	50–230	

Table 79 (contd)

Reference, location	Cohort description	Assessment or indices of exposure to lead	Cancer site	Exposure categories	No of cases or deaths	Relative risks	95% CI	Comments
Cocco *et al.* (1994b) Italy	483 women employed ≥ 1 year 1932–71 in the same 2 lead/zinc mines as in Cocco *et al.* (1994a); mortality 1951–88; vital status 96.0%	Not estimated	All sites		32	70	48–99	National reference; availability of death records not mentioned
			Lung		6	232	85–505	
			Stomach		2	32	4–115	
Newspaper printers								
Bertazzi & Zocchetti (1980) Italy	700 men employed ≥ 5 years before 1955 in production department of newspaper plant; mortality 1956–75; vital status 96.7%	Not estimated				**SMR**		National reference
			All sites		51	123	[92–162]	Increase in lung cancer risk confined mainly to packers and forwarders possibly exposed to vehicle exhausts
			Lung		13	148	[79–253]	
			Duration of employment (years):					
			≤ 9		2	167	[20–602]	
			10–19		5	106	[34–247]	
			≥ 20		6	207	[76–450]	
			Digestive organs and peritoneum		19	120	[72–188]	
Michaels *et al.* (1991) USA	1261 men members of typographical union, employed 1 January 1961, followed-up 1961–84, vital status 96.9%	Not estimated				**SMR**		Regional standard (New York City rates)
			All sites		123	84	69–100	Lead phased out during 1974–78; before: low-level exposures documented from other printing industry plants (ranging from < 2% to 40% of the occupational standard)
			Lung		37	89	62–122	
			Stomach		5	55	18–128	
			Bladder		8	151	65–297	
			Leukaemia and aleukaemia		5	104	34–244	

Table 79 (contd)

Reference, location	Cohort description	Assessment or indices of exposure to lead	Cancer site	Exposure categories	No of cases or deaths	Relative risks	95% CI	Comments
Organic lead								
Sweeney *et al.* (1986) USA	Retrospective study; 2510 men (2248 Caucasian and 262 non-Caucasian) employed at chemical plant (tetraethyl lead manufacture) > 1 day 1952–77; vital status 99.3%, cause of death 98.7%	Not estimated						National reference.
		Employment 1952–77, all workers combined	Lung		14	112	68–1.75	One brain tumour appeared to be a metastasis according to pathology reports.
			Larynx		2	364	65–1145	
			Brain and central nervous system		4	213	73–487	
			Lymphatic		4	85	36–343	
		Employment 1952–60, Caucasian only	Lung		13	122	73–194	
			Brain		3	186	51–482	
		Employment prior to 1960 and 15 year latency; duration of employment	Respiratory		14	154	[84–258]	
				< 10 years	6	199	[73–432]	
				> 10 years	8	132	[57–260]	
Fayerweather *et al.* (1997) USA	Case–control study in a tetraethyl lead manufacturing site; 735 male cases and 1423 controls matched on age, sex, payroll class; 1956–87; company mortality registries and employment rosters	Employment in tetraethyl lead areas (ever versus never)		Exposed		**OR**		90% CI
			Digestive	Ever	45	1.3	0.9–1.9	Incidence among active workers only
				Cumulative exposure:				Quartiles of cumulative exposure (low, medium, high, very high) defined as no. of years × rank weight of exposure, ranking variables originating from a variety of sources
				High	10	1.3	0.7–2.7	
				Very high	16	2.2	1.2–4.0	
			Rectum	Ever	9	3.7	1.3–10.2	
				Cumulative exposure:				
				High to very high	7	5.1	1.6–16.5	
			Colon	Ever	16	1.3	0.7–2.5	
				Cumulative exposure:				
				High to very high	8	1.7	0.8–4.0	

Table 79 (contd)

Reference, location	Cohort description	Assessment or indices of exposure to lead	Cancer site	Exposure categories	No of cases or deaths	Relative risks	95% CI	Comments
Biomonitoring								
Anttila *et al.* (1995) Finland	20 741 workers (18 329 men, 2412 women) with monitored blood lead; 1973–83; 2318 industrial plants or workplaces	Highest blood lead (µmol/L)		Blood lead (µmol/L)		**SIR**		Men only [test for trend borderline significant]
			Lung, trachea	< 1.0	25	70	50–110	
				1.0–1.9	35	140	100–190	
				2.0–7.8	11	110	60–200	
			Stomach	< 1.0	11	100	50–190	Men only OR for estimated mean lifetime blood lead ≥ 0.8 µmol/L: 1.1 (95% CI, 0.4–3.2), based on 14 cases
				1.0–1.9	11	140	70–250	
				2.0–7.8	1	30	0–180	
			Kidney	< 1.0	4	60	20–150	Men only OR for estimated mean lifetime blood lead ≥ 0.8 µmol/L: 0.5 (95% CI, 0.2–1.7), based on 7 cases
				1.0–1.9	5	100	30–240	
				2.0–7.8	0	0	0–200	
			Nervous system	< 1.0	8	130	60–260	Men only
				1.0–1.9	6	130	50–270	
				2.0–7.8	3	160	30–460	
		Highest blood lead (µmol/L)				**RR**		Internal comparison; Poisson regression
			Lung, trachea	< 1.0	26	1.0	ref	
				1.0–1.9	36	2.0	1.2–3.2	
				2.0–7.8	11	1.5	0.8–3.1	
	Nested case–control study 1973–90; 53 cases and 156 controls matched on sex, year of birth and vital status	Cumulative exposure (µmol × yr/L)	Lung			**OR**		Test of trend NS Includes pleural cancer Adjusted for smoking
				0	16	1.0	ref	
				1–6	6	0.9	0.2–3.6	
				7–17	15	1.2	0.4–3.1	
				18–70	16	1.4	0.6–3.7	

Table 79 (contd)

Reference, location	Cohort description	Assessment or indices of exposure to lead	Cancer site	Exposure categories	No of cases or deaths	Relative risks	95% CI	Comments
Anttila *et al.* (1996) Finland	Same cohort as Anttila *et al.* (1995)	Blood lead (µmol/L)	Nervous system			**SIR**		Entire cohort analysis
				≤ 0.9	12	[90]	[47–158]	
				1.0–1.9	10	[130]	[62–239]	
				2.0–7.8	4	[138]	[38–353]	
	Nested case–control study 1973–90 with 26 cases and 200 controls matched on sex, year of birth and vital status	Highest blood lead (µmol/L)	Nervous system			**OR**		Internal comparison, 200 controls
				0.1–0.7	7	1.0	ref	
				0.8–1.3	9	1.4	0.5–4.1	
				1.4–4.3	10	2.2	0.7–6.6	
				p for trend		0.17		
			Glioma			**OR**		Internal comparison, 125 controls. Adjusted for year of first personal measurement
				0.1–0.7	1	1.0	ref	
				0.8–1.3	8	6.7	0.7–347	
				1.4–4.3	7	11.0	1.0–626	
				p for trend		0.037		
		Cumulative exposure (year × µmol/L)	Glioma			**OR**		49 controls Adjusted for year of first personal measurement
				0	1	1.0	ref	
				1–6	2	2.0	0.1–116	
				7–14	2	6.2	0.1–816	
				15–49	5	12.0	0.9–820	
				p for trend		0.02		
		Lifetime mean lead (µmol/L)	Glioma	0.1–0.7	1	1.0	ref	49 controls Adjusted for gasoline and cadmium exposure
				0.8–1.3	5	3.5	0.4–171	
				1.4–3.4	4	23.0	0.8–2441	
				p for trend		0.041		
		Duration of occupational exposure to lead (years)	Glioma	0	1	1.0	ref	49 controls Adjusted for gasoline and cadmium exposure
				1–9	1	0.9	0–122	
				10–19	3	3.7	0.2–244	
				20–42	5	6.9	0.6–400	
				p for trend		0.029		

AAS, atomic absorption spectroscopy; AES, atomic emission spectroscopy; RR, relative risk; PMOR, proportional mortality odds ratio; SMR, standardized mortality ratio; SPMR, standardized proportional mortality ratio; SIR, standardized incidence ratio; OR, odds ratio; NS, not significant; [....] calculated by the Working Group

[a] G6PD, glucose-6-phosphate dehydrogenase

Table 80. Population-based case–control studies on cancer risk in relation to exposure to lead or lead compounds

Reference, location and years of study	Characteristics of cases and controls	Assessment or indices of exposure to lead	Cancer site	No. of cases	Odds ratio	95% CI	Comments
Multiple cancer sites							
Siemiatycki (1991) Canada 1979–85	Men aged 35–70 years, resident in the Montreal metropolitan area; hospital records and population files (multi-site cancer and population controls available); response rates: cancer cases 82%, population controls 72% [others not available]; incident cases histologically confirmed	Expert assessment					90% CI; cancer controls for all exposures and sites, except lead fumes and lung cancer (population controls) No data on central nervous system/brain cancer
		Lead compounds:					
		Any[a]	Lung	326	1.1	0.9–1.4	
		Substantial[b]		42	1.5	1.0–2.2	
		Any	Lung, squamous-cell	146	1.3	1.0–1.6	
		Substantial		18	1.5	0.8–2.6	
		Any	Stomach	126	1.2	1.0–1.6	
		Substantial		17	1.8	1.1–2.8	
		Any	Bladder	155	1.3	1.0–1.6	
		Substantial		17	1.1	0.7–1.8	
		Any	Kidney	88	1.2	1.0–1.6	
		Substantial		6	0.8	0.4–1.7	
		Lead dust:					
		Any	Stomach	5	4.7	1.9–11.7	
		Substantial		3	21.6	3.2–99.9	
		Lead oxides:					
		Any	Lung	22	1.9	1.1–3.4	
		Substantial		8	2.2	0.8–5.7	
		Lead carbonate: any	Lung, adenocarcinoma	7	1.9	0.9–4.0	
		Lead chromate: any	Lung	26	1.6	1.0–2.7	
			Bladder	17	1.8	1.1–3.1	
			Kidney	6	2.1	1.0–4.5	
		Lead fumes: any	Lung, oat-cell	12	1.8	1.0–3.2	
			Lung, squamous-cell	16	1.8	0.9–3.6	
			Stomach	10	1.7	0.9–3.0	
			Pancreas	7	1.9	1.0–3.8	
			Non-Hodgkin lymphoma	13	1.8	1.1–3.0	

Table 80 (contd)

Reference, location and years of study	Characteristics of cases and controls	Assessment or indices of exposure to lead	Cancer site	No. of cases	Odds ratio	95% CI	Comments
Stomach							
Cocco *et al.* (1999b) USA 1984–96	Population-based study; 24 states; 41 957 deaths (20 878 Caucasian men, 14 125 Caucasian women, 4215 African-American men, 2739 African-American women) aged ≥ 25 years at the time of death; 2 controls per case, having died from non-malignant diseases	Occupation and industry titles on death certificates plus job–exposure matrix	Stomach				Matching by geographic region, race, sex and age (5-year)
		High probability of lead exposure:					
		Caucasian men		1503	0.92	0.86–0.99	
		African-American men		453	1.15	1.01–1.32	
		White women		65	1.53	1.10–2.12	
		African-American women		10	1.76	0.74–4.16	
		High intensity of lead exposure:					
		Caucasian men		290	1.10	0.95–1.27	
		African-American men		52	0.81	0.59–1.13	
		Caucasian women		37	1.02	0.68–1.51	
		African-American women		3	1.25	0.30–5.23	
Cocco *et al.* (1998b) USA 1984–92	Same design as in Cocco *et al.* (1999b); 1056 cases (1023 Caucasian men and 33 African-American men) and 5280 controls	Occupation and industry titles on death certificates + job–exposure matrix	Stomach				Gastric cardia cancer. [Intercorrelation with other exposures not described]
		High probability of exposure with intensity:					
		Unexposed		841	1.0		
		Low		77	1.3	1.0–1.8	
		Medium		10	1.1	0.5–2.2	
		High		1	–	–	
Kidney							
Partanen *et al.* (1997) Finland 1977–78	Population-based study; 408 incident cases (male and female) aged ≥ 20 years and 819 controls matched on year of birth, sex, survival status; response rate 69% (cases), 68% (controls)	Summary indicators 1920–68; industrial hygienist	Kidney	4	2.77	0.49–15.6	Lead + inorganic lead compounds; adjusted for smoking, coffee consumption and obesity

Table 80 (contd)

Reference, location and years of study	Characteristics of cases and controls	Assessment or indices of exposure to lead	Cancer site	No. of cases	Odds ratio	95% CI	Comments
Pesch *et al.* (2000) Germany 1991–95	Population-based study; 935 cases (570 men, 365 women); 95% histologically confirmed; 4298 controls (2650 men, 1648 women) matched by region, sex and age; response rates 84–95% (cases), 63–75% (controls)	Two job–exposure matrices (lead and lead compounds) used for jobs held > 1 year	Renal-cell carcinoma				Adjusted for age, study centre and smoking
		Job–exposure matrix 1[c]:					
		Men					
		Substantial		29	1.5	1.0–2.3	
		High		71	1.2	0.9–1.6	
		Medium		84	1.2	1.0–1.6	
		Women					
		Substantial		11	2.6	1.2–5.5	
		High		14	1.0	0.6–1.9	
		Medium		8	0.7	0.4–1.6	
		Job–exposure matrix 2[d]:					
		Men					
		Substantial		30	1.3	0.9–2.0	
		High		81	1.2	0.9–1.6	
		Medium		69	0.9	0.7–1.2	
Brain and nervous system							
Cocco *et al.* (1998a) USA 1984–92	Population-based study; 24 states; 27 060 deaths (Caucasian and African-American men and women) and 108 240 controls who died from non-malignant diseases (aged ≥ 35 years)	Occupation and industry titles on death certificates plus job–exposure matrix: *High intensity and high probability of lead exposure*:	Brain				The group with high intensity (estimated mean blood lead > 1.4 μmol/L) and high probability of exposure comprised typesetters and compositors.
		Caucasian men		14	2.1	1.1–4.0	Adjusted for age, marital status, residence (urban versus rural) and socioeconomic status
		Caucasian women		4	1.4	0.4–4.2	
Cocco *et al.* (1999a) USA 1984–92	Same design as in Cocco *et al* (1998a), 12 980 women	Occupation and industry titles on death certificates plus job–exposure matrix	CNS	366	1.1	1.0–1.2	Reference: no exposure
			Meningioma	9	1.9	1.0–3.9	

Table 80 (contd)

Reference, location and years of study	Characteristics of cases and controls	Assessment or indices of exposure to lead	Cancer site	No. of cases	Odds ratio	95% CI	Comments
Hu, J. *et al.* (1998), Heilongjiang Province, China 1989–95	Hospital-based study; 218 cases histologically confirmed (139 astrocytoma and 79 other brain glioma, male and female) 436 controls with non-neoplastic non-neurological diseases, matched on sex, age, residence (rural/urban); 100% response rates for cases and controls	Self-reported exposure to lead	Glioma	0		[4 controls]	
Hu, J. *et al.* (1999), Heilongjiang Province, China 1989–96	Same design as in Hu, J. *et al.* (1998) 183 cases, 366 controls	Self-reported exposure to lead	Meningioma				Adjusted for income, education, fruit and vegetable consumption (men), further adjusted for smoking (women)
		Men		6	7.20	1.00–51.72	
		Women		10	5.69	1.39–23.39	
Other primary sites							
Risch *et al.* (1988) Canada 1979–82	Population-based study; 835 cases histologically confirmed (male and female) and 792 controls, response rates 67% and 53%, respectively; cases and controls matched by year of birth, sex and area of residence	Partially self-reported exposure to lead compounds, men	Bladder				Adjusted for lifetime cigarette consumption; exposure during full-time job ≥ 6 months
		Ever exposed		61	2.00	1.16–3.54	
		OR for trend per 10 years of duration			1.76	0.91–3.51	
		Exposed ≥ 6 months 8–28 years before diagnosis			1.45	1.09–2.02	

Table 80 (contd)

Reference, location and years of study	Characteristics of cases and controls	Assessment or indices of exposure to lead	Cancer site	No. of cases	Odds ratio	95% CI	Comments
Kauppinen *et al.* (1992) Finland 1976–78 1981	Population-based study; 344 cases histologically confirmed (male and female), 476 stomach cancer controls and 385 coronary infarction controls, matched to cases by age and sex; 71% response rates for both cases and controls	*Job–exposure matrix*:	Liver				
		Low exposure to lead and its compounds		52	0.91	0.65–1.29	Men and women combined
		Expert assessment:					
		Any exposure to lead and its compounds		6	1.14	0.44–2.98	Adjusted for alcohol consumption; no cases with heavy exposure; moderate exposure, OR 2.28 (95% CI, 0.68–7.67; 5 cases)

CNS, central nervous system; OR, odds ratio
[a] Any, any exposure
[b] Substantial exposure
[c] Job–exposure matrix 1: British
[d] Job–exposure matrix 2: German

2.1.2 *Lead smelter workers*

The extended study of lead battery and lead smelter workers in the USA (Cooper & Gaffey, 1975; Cooper, 1976; Kang *et al.*, 1980; Cooper, 1981; Cooper *et al.*, 1985; Cooper, 1988; Wong & Harris, 2000) originally included 2352 lead smelter workers from six plants (Cooper & Gaffey, 1975); the most recent update (Wong & Harris, 2000) relates to a reduced cohort of 2300 smelter workers. All lead smelter workers were employed for at least 1 year during the period 1947–70, and the most recent follow-up has been analysed for the period 1947–95. There were 161 lead smelter workers (7.0%) who were untraced on the closing date of the study. Lead exposure data were limited, but blood lead and urinary lead measurements were taken, mainly after 1960. For smelter workers with three or more blood lead measurements, the mean blood concentration was 80 μg/dL and, for those with 10 or more urinary lead measurements, the mean urine concentration was 173 μg/dL. Other exposures may have included cadmium, arsenic and sulfur dioxide. SMRs were calculated after comparison with the mortality rates for the male population in the USA, and were adjusted for age and calendar period. For all cancers, the overall SMR was 101.8 (273 observed; 95% CI, 90.1–114.6). There were non-significantly elevated SMRs for stomach cancer (133.4; 15 observed; 95% CI, 74.6–220.0) and lung cancer (121.5; 107 observed; 95% CI, 99.5–146.8). SMRs were also shown for the lead battery workers and smelter workers combined in relation to three categories of duration of employment (< 10 years, 10–19 years, ≥ 20 years). Positive trends were not found for cancer of the stomach or cancer of the lung. Corresponding findings were not shown separately for smelter and battery workers.

Rencher *et al.* (1977) studied the mortality at a large copper smelter in western USA during the period 1959–69. Death certificates were used to determine the causes of death. The death pattern was compared with regional (state) death rates. [The Working Group did not report the results because the methods of analysis rendered the study uninterpretable and person–time was not defined.]

In a study at a lead smelter in Australia (McMichael & Johnson, 1982), 241 male workers diagnosed with lead poisoning during the period 1928–59 were identified. The list was cross-checked against death registration records in South Australia for the period 1930–77, thereby identifying 140 deaths. Age-standardized proportional mortality rates (SPMR) were calculated after comparison with the mortality pattern in 695 other workers in non-office production jobs at the same smelter, and with the male population in Australia. The SPMR for all cancer mortality was 0.59, based on nine cancer deaths. [The Working Group noted that the low SPMR for cancer may be explained by a very high SPMR for chronic nephritis.]

Selevan *et al.* (1985) studied mortality in a cohort of 1987 men employed between 1940 and 1965 at a primary lead smelter in the USA. Other exposures included zinc, cadmium, arsenic, sulfur dioxide and, in some departments, airborne free silica. In an extended follow-up study of this cohort (Steenland *et al.*, 1992), 1990 male hourly-paid smelter workers were identified. They had worked in a lead-exposed department for at least 1 year, with at least 1 day of employment at the smelter between 1940 and 1965. The vital status of the cohort was determined via the Social Security Administration and the National Death Index. The population of the USA was used as a reference group. For all cancers, the overall SMR was 98 (192 observed; 95% CI, 84–112). There were non-significantly elevated SMRs for stomach cancer and lung cancer. In the subcohort (1436 subjects) with heavier exposure to lead (departments with mean airborne lead concentrations in 1975 that exceeded 0.2 mg/m^3), the SMRs were similar. Eight of the nine kidney cancer deaths occurred in the subcohort with heavier exposure to lead (SMR, 239; 95% CI, 103–471). Analyses by duration of exposure failed to show any significant positive trends with site-specific cancer risks. Detailed data about individual lead exposures were lacking as well as information about potential confounders such as concomitant exposure to cadmium, arsenic and other exposures at the primary smelter. However, some data were available. In 1975, the mean airborne arsenic concentration was 14 µg/m^3, whereas the mean airborne lead concentration was 3.1 mg/m^3. These means were based on 89 and 203 personal 8-h samples, respectively. [This level of arsenic exposure is approximately an order of magnitude lower than that seen in most of the historical cohort studies of arsenic-exposed workers that have shown lung cancer excesses (Steenland *et al.*, 1996). No lung cancer excess was seen in workers with similar average exposure levels (between 7 and 13 µg/m^3) in copper smelters studied by Enterline *et al.* (1987). Similarly, little or no lung cancer excess was seen among workers with this level of exposure in another copper smelter in the USA studied by Lubin *et al.* (2000).] Data on smoking were lacking.

In a study in Sweden (Gerhardsson *et al.*, 1986), 3832 male workers first employed before 1967 at a primary copper smelter in northern Sweden were followed from 1950 to 1981. A subcohort of 437 workers employed for more than 3 years in jobs with high lead exposure had a mean blood lead concentration of 58 µg/dL in 1950, which had decreased to 34 µg/dL in 1974. Workers were also potentially exposed to carcinogenic substances such as arsenic, chromium and nickel. A significant excess of lung cancer and stomach cancer mortality was observed in the whole cohort but was not sustained in the high-exposure subcohort.

In a follow-up study at the same smelter (Lundström *et al.*, 1997), the total cohort was extended to comprise 3979 workers who had been employed for at least 1 year during the period 1928–79 and who had been monitored for blood lead concentrations since 1950. A subcohort of 1992 workers was defined by excluding workers ever employed in the roaster departments, machine shop and any other departments with appreciable exposures to arsenic and nickel. This subcohort comprised workers from the lead department and other lead-exposed departments. Airborne concentrations of arsenic ranged from 0.35 to 1.5 mg/m^3 at the roasters during the late 1940s and decreased to 0.1–0.5 mg/m^3 during the 1950s; those of sulfur dioxide ranged from 70 to 560 mg/m^3 during the 1940s and decreased to 5–10 mg/m^3 during the 1960s. [This subcohort is described in the paper as one of 'lead-only workers', but these workers would have been exposed to some degree to arsenic and nickel.] Expected mortality in 1955–87 and cancer incidence in 1958–87 were calculated relative to county rates, specified for cause, sex, 5-year age groups and calendar year. Information on mortality was obtained from the Cause-of-Death Register at Statistics Sweden. The death certificates were coded according to the 8th revision of the International Classification of Diseases (ICD-8). Information on the incidence of malignant tumours was gathered from record linkage with the National Swedish Tumour Registry, established in 1958. The most highly-exposed subgroup was selected on the basis of a cumulative blood lead dose, which was calculated by summing the annual mean blood lead values for each worker during the period of employment (≥ 207 μg×yr/dL). For the total cohort (*n* = 3979), the overall SMR for all cancers was 120 (126 observed; 95% CI, 100–150). There was a significantly elevated SMR for lung cancer (280; 39 observed; 95% CI, 200–380). The SMR for lung cancer in the most highly-exposed subgroup (*n* = 1026) was 280 (19 observed; 95% CI, 180–450). For cancer incidence in the total cohort (with a 15-year minimum latency period), the overall standardized incidence ratio (SIR) for all cancers was 110 (172 observed; 95% CI, 90–120). There was a significantly elevated SIR for lung cancer (42 observed; SIR, 290; 95% CI, 210–400). The SIR for lung cancer in the most highly-exposed subgroup was 340 (23 observed; 95% CI, 220–520). The risk estimates for lung cancer were further elevated in the subgroup of 'lead-only workers' with the highest exposure (7 observed; SIR, 510; 95% CI, 200–1050). No significantly elevated SIRs were observed for other malignancies. [The multifactorial exposure pattern and the lack of smoking data make it difficult to separate the effects of lead from the effects of other agents, in particular arsenic, in the working environment.]

This cohort from Sweden (described above) was further analysed by Englyst *et al.* (2001) forming two subcohorts from the original cohort of 3979 male smelter workers (Lundström *et al.*, 1997). Subcohort 1 consisted of 710 workers who had been employed in the lead department. Subcohort 2 was nested within subcohort 1 and the subcohort of the 1992 workers defined by Lundström *et al.* (1997) and consisted of 383 workers who had been employed in the lead department at any time but never in the arsenic plant, nickel plant, the roaster department or the machine shop. SIRs for 1958–87 were calculated relative to county rates. The lung cancer incidence was raised in both lead subcohorts. Incidence for all cancers was close to expectation. A detailed study of company records revealed that nine of the 10 lung cancer cases in subcohort 1 and four of the five lung cancers in subcohort 2 had also had some considerable exposure to arsenic. [The Working Group noted that such information on exposure to arsenic was not available for the rest of the cohort.]

Gerhardsson *et al.* (1995) studied the mortality and cancer incidence among workers exposed to lead at a secondary lead smelter in southern Sweden. There was no known concomitant exposure to arsenic, hexavalent chromium, nickel or cadmium. Annual mean blood lead values declined during the follow-up period, from 62 μg/dL in 1969 to 33 μg/dL in 1985. The cohort consisted of 664 male lead smelter workers who had been employed for at least 3 months from 1942 to 1987. The causes of death in 1969–89 were obtained from Statistics Sweden. Death certificates were coded according to ICD-8.

Yearly cancer incidence from 1969 to 1989 was obtained from the National Swedish Tumour Registry, with calendar year-, sex- and 5-year age group-specific incidences for the county population. For all cancers, the overall SIR was 127 (40 observed; 95% CI, 91–174). There were non-significantly elevated SIRs for stomach cancer and cancers of the respiratory tract. [The Working Group noted that the results must be interpreted with caution due to small numbers and lack of data on smoking.]

In a study of 1345 male smelter workers at a lead and zinc smelting plant in south-western Sardinia, Italy, mortality was followed from 1973 to 1991 (Cocco *et al.*, 1996). Death certificates were provided for all deceased subjects by the local health units. SMRs were calculated after comparison with death rates in the general male population in Sardinia. No significant excess of mortality was noted for any single cancer site. There were two deaths from stomach cancer and lung cancer mortality was lower than that expected. The overall SMR was not presented. [The study interpretation is hampered by limited numbers of expected deaths, lack of detailed information about individual exposures to lead, zinc and other substances at the smelter, as well as a lack of data on smoking.]

Cocco *et al.* (1997) also studied 1388 lead workers from another lead smelter in Italy. An industrial hygiene survey carried out in 1977–78 reported concentrations of cadmium in respirable dust below the limit of detection (1 μg/m^3) in 9/39 samples and below 10 μg/m^3 in 28/39 samples. In addition, concentrations of arsenic were reported to be below the limit of detection (1 μg/m^3) in 23/24 samples; the remaining reading was 3 μg/m^3 in the agglomeration area. Concentrations of lead in respirable dust had a wide range of values (1–1650 μg/m^3) with a geometric mean for all work areas of 48 μg/m^3. Vital status of the workers was followed from 1950 to 1992. Fifty-five per cent of the cohort members had died by the end of follow-up. Death certificates were available for 96% of the deceased men. The underlying causes of death were coded according to the 9th revision of the International Classification of Diseases (ICD-9). SMRs were calculated for specific causes of death after comparison with national and regional reference rates. On the basis of national rates, mortality for all cancers, stomach cancer and lung cancer were lower than expected. On the basis of regional rates for a more limited period of follow-up (1965–92), mortality rates for all cancers, stomach cancer and lung cancer were close to those expected.

Lung cancer mortality was investigated in a cohort study of men employed at a zinc–cadmium smelter in the United Kingdom (Ades & Kazantzis, 1988). The study comprised all hourly-paid male workers employed at the smelter on 1 January 1943 and those who subsequently started work before 1970. All subjects were born before 1940 and worked for at least 1 year before 1970. Average arsenic concentrations assessed by static samplers between 1981 and 1983 ranged from 1 to 3 μg/m^3 in the sinter and from 4 to 7 μg/m^3 in the furnace. Airborne cadmium exposure before 1970 was assessed to be 200 μg/m^3 in the sintering plants and 80 μg/m^3 in the cadmium plant. By 1977, these concentrations had decreased to 15 μg/m^3 in both departments. Biological monitoring results showed mean blood lead concentrations of 28 μg/dL in the cadmium plant workers, 59 μg/dL in the furnace workers (10% of the cohort) and 56 μg/dL in the sinter workers

(8% of the cohort). In total, 4173 men were followed up for more than 10 years. SMRs were calculated using regional comparisons. The SMR for lung cancer was 125 (182 observed; 95% CI, 107–144). The lung cancer mortality was positively related to duration of employment. On the basis of a matched case–control study nested in this cohort, the cumulative arsenic and lead exposure (both estimated crudely in terms of 'level–decades'), but not cumulative cadmium exposure, were positively related to lung cancer mortality. [It was not possible, however, to elucidate the independent relationships for arsenic, lead or other concomitant exposures at the smelter.]

2.1.3 *Lead chromate pigment production*

Workers producing lead chromate pigments have been the subject of two cohort studies focused on possible lung carcinogenicity resulting from exposure to hexavalent chromium, which was classified as Group 1 human carcinogen by IARC (IARC, 1990). [It is not possible to separate the effects of chromium on the lung from those of lead in these studies, limiting their usefulness in the evaluation of the carcinogenicity of lead.]

Sheffet *et al.* (1982) studied mortality among 1296 white and 650 non-white men in a pigment plant producing lead and zinc chromates in the USA who were employed for at least 1 month between 1940 and 1969, and followed through 31 March 1979. Moderate exposure was defined as work in jobs with an average exposure of 0.5–2 mg/m^3 airborne chromium, while high exposure was defined as > 2 mg/m^3 airborne chromium; 76% of the cohort had high or moderate exposure. A statistically significant relative risk of 1.6 (95% CI, 1.1–2.2; 31 deaths) for lung cancer was found among male employees, increasing to a significant 1.9 for those exposed for at least 2 years to moderate or high exposure. Stomach cancer had a SMR of 2.0 (95% CI, 0.9–3.6; 8 deaths). SMRs varied depending on whether or not those decedents with cause of death unknown (15%) were excluded from the observed count of lung cancers or added in proportion corresponding to the distribution of observed deaths with known causes. [SMRs for other cancers were calculated, but numbers were small and there were no significant findings.]

Davies *et al.* (1984a) studied 1152 men at three pigment plants in the United Kingdom; two of the plants produced zinc and lead chromates, the third only lead chromate. Workers had at least 1 year of employment between the beginning of complete plant records (1933, 1949 and 1947 for the three plants) and 1967 (with the exception of a few late entrants 1968–74), and were followed up until 1981. Exposure was categorized into high, medium and low grades: jobs in dry departments and full-time stove drying with heavy exposure to chromate-containing dust (high); slight or occasional exposure to chromate, including jobs in management, laboratory, shops, maintenance, etc. (low); and other jobs, e.g. wet departments, men going all over the factories (medium). There was a statistically significant excess of lung cancer mortality at the two factories producing zinc and lead chromate, but no excess was observed at the plant producing only lead chromate, despite small numbers. The authors speculated that zinc chromate was responsible for the lung cancer excess at the first two plants. No quantitative data on exposure were given, although it was mentioned that lead concentrations were high enough to result in frequent lead poisoning until the 1950s.

Davies *et al.* (1984b) studied 57 men with documented lead poisoning who were part of the larger cohort of workers at three pigment plants (Davies *et al.*, 1984a; see above). There were four cases of lung cancer (SMR, 145; 95% CI, 39–370). [Due to small numbers, this study is essentially non-informative regarding cancer risk among these highly-exposed workers.]

2.1.4 *Workers in glass production*

Glass work involves smelting and foundry work, and glass blowing, grinding and polishing with potentially high exposures to lead but also to a variety of other metals (arsenic, cadmium, chromium, antimony, copper), as well as some exposure to silica and, to a lesser extent, possible exposure to asbestos used in insulation. An earlier Working Group (IARC, 1994) concluded that the manufacture of art glass, glass containers and pressed ware entails exposures that *are probably carcinogenic to humans (Group 2A)* and that occupational exposures in flat-glass and special glass manufacture *are not classifiable as to their carcinogenicity to humans (Group 3)*.

Numerous linkage studies on occupation and cancer have been conducted. Some gave positive results for glass workers and lung cancer (Milne *et al*, 1983; Lynge *et al.*, 1986; Levin *et al.*, 1988) or brain cancer (Mallin *et al.*, 1989).

(*a*) *Cohort studies*

Cordioli *et al.* (1987) studied 468 male workers with at least 1 year of employment in a glass factory in Italy between 1953 and 1967 and followed them for mortality until 1985. A SMR for lung cancer of 209 [95% CI, 111–357] was observed, based on 13 lung cancer deaths. An excess of laryngeal cancer was also observed (SMR, 449 [95% CI, 122–1150]), based on four cases.

Sankila *et al.* (1990) studied 3749 workers (1803 men, 1946 women) employed for at least 3 months in two glass factories in Finland and followed them for cancer incidence from 1953–86. An excess of lung cancer was found (SIR, 128; 95% CI, 99–162; 69 cases, 62 men and seven women). The authors noted that a similar excess of lung cancer was found when comparing industrial workers in general with the general population in Finland, suggesting confounding by smoking as a possible explanation of the observed excess. An excess of stomach cancer (SIR, 231; 95% CI, 85–502; six cases) and skin cancer (SIR, 625; 95% CI, 129–1827; three cases) was found in the subcohort of glass blowers ($n = 235$), but no excess of lung cancer was observed in this group.

Wingren and Englander (1990) studied 625 male glass workers employed in Sweden for at least 1 month between 1964 and 1985, for cancer incidence and mortality. Slag from blow pipes contained lead, manganese and nickel. Mortality was emphasized in the results because the follow-up period covered by incidence was shorter, and the incidence results tended to parallel the mortality results. Both national and county (local) standards were used, with county rates being considerably lower for lung cancer. Lung cancer was found in excess using national rates (SMR, 144; 95% CI, 52–311) as well as country rates (SMR, 240; 95% CI, [88–522]), based on small numbers (six lung cancer deaths). Colon cancer (SMR, 250; 95% CI, [68–640]; four deaths) was also elevated, based on county rates. Smoking status was known for 60 workers employed in the 1960s, showing a lower proportion of smokers than in the general population.

(*b*) *Case–control studies*

There have been three case–control studies of glass workers in Sweden, conducted by the same authors, based on death certificates and with some overlapping data (Wingren & Axelson, 1985; 1987; 1993). Initially, three rural parishes in which glass works were common were studied from 1950 to 1982. The initial investigation was expanded to 11 parishes, which included most of the glass works in Sweden, again studying the period 1950–82. To assess past and present exposure, a questionnaire regarding use of different metals was sent to 13 existing glass works of which seven replied. Cancer was not more common in the parishes than in the whole of Sweden in cohort analyses, but in case–control analyses (controls were non-cardiovascular, non-cancer deaths) based on occupation on the death certificate [no information was given on how many were missing], glass workers had elevated odds ratios. There was an excess of lung cancer (odds ratio, 1.7; 90% CI, 1.1–2.5; 21 exposed cases), stomach cancer (odds ratio, 1.5; 90% CI, 1.1–2.0; 44 exposed cases) and colon cancer (odds ratio, 1.6; 90% CI, 1.04–2.5; 18 exposed cases). More detailed data on jobs were available for about half of those who died, and analyses by specific job title suggested that the excess of stomach and colon cancer appeared most strongly among glass-blowers, while the excess of lung cancer was about the same among glass blowers and glass workers without specified job title. However, all glass workers used several metals, which were often used in combination, and it was difficult to identify particular metals as being responsible for particular cancer excesses. Measurement of lead in several worksites showed high air concentrations, with a mean of 61 μg/m^3 in one foundry for heavy crystal glass.

2.1.5 *Studies in miners*

Carta *et al.* (1994) followed mortality among active male employees in two lead and zinc mines in Sardinia, Italy. The study was performed particularly to test the relationships between silica and radon exposures and lung cancer risk. Later, Cocco *et al.* (1994a,b) enlarged the study to include male (n = 4740) and female (n = 483) workers in the mines with at least 1 year of employment between 1932 and 1971. Follow-up of the male cohort was from January 1960 to the end of November 1988, and eligible subjects were men who were still employed on 1 January 1960 or who had worked for a minimum of 12 months during 1960–71. In the study among female workers, follow-up was from 1951 to 1988, and eligible subjects were women who were alive at the onset of follow-up. Vital status was known for 99.5% of the male and 96% of the female cohort members, and death certificates were available for all deceased members. In both mines, the ores mainly consisted of *blende* and *galena* (zinc and lead sulphides). The concentrations of in-air respirable dust averaged 2.5 and 2.6 mg/m^3 in 1962–70 and 1.6 and 1.8 mg/m^3 from 1971 onwards in the two mines, respectively. Dust concentrations at surface workplaces were less than 1 mg/m^3 in the 1970s. Expected rates were derived from the regional rates in the study among men and from the national rates in the study among women. Among men, the overall SMR was 104 (1205 observed; 95% CI, 98–110). The SMR for deaths from all cancers was 94 (293 observed; 95% CI, 83–105) and 95 (86 observed; 95% CI, 76–117) for lung cancer. Except for cancers of the peritoneum and retroperitoneum (SMR, 367; six deaths observed; 95% CI, 135–798), none of the cancer sites studied had a significantly increased SMR. In the study among women, 163 deaths occurred in total (SMR, 78; 95% CI, 67–91); the SMR for lung cancer was 232 (95% CI, 85–505; six deaths observed). Information on lifetime smoking habits were available for 1741 male employees included in a cross-sectional survey in 1973 (Carta *et al.*, 1994). About 65% were current smokers. Further details on exposures to lead were not available.

2.1.6 *Newspaper printers*

Two studies among newspaper printers are described here; these studies aimed at describing explicitly long-term exposures to lead in cohorts not exposed to other known carcinogens (such as other metals, benzene, organic solvents). Other studies of printing workers potentially exposed to lead have not been reviewed in this monograph.

Bertazzi and Zocchetti (1980) studied mortality among workers in a newspaper plant in Milan, Italy. Male workers employed in the production department as of 31 December 1955 and having at least 5 years of employment were considered eligible (n = 700). Mortality follow-up covered the years 1956–75. Follow-up and tracing was successful for 96.7% of the eligible workers. Persons not traced were assumed to be alive at the end of the follow-up period. The expected numbers were calculated using the national rates. For 10 deaths, no specific cause was mentioned on the death certificate. The overall SMR was 108 (199 deaths observed; 95% CI, 94–124). The SMR for any cancer was 123 (51 deaths observed; 95% CI, 92–162), that for lung cancer was slightly elevated (SMR, 148; 13 deaths observed; 95% CI, 79–253) and that for cancers of the digestive organs and peritoneum was 120 (19 observed; 95% CI, 72–188). There were two deaths from brain cancer (expected number not given). SMRs for lung cancer were 167 (two deaths observed), 106 (five deaths observed) and 207 (six deaths observed) in the groups for whom length of employment was 5–9, 10–19 and 20 or more years, respectively. Risk for lung cancer was highest among packers and forwarders (SMR, 250; six deaths; 95% CI, 92–544), who were possibly exposed to vehicle exhausts. Among compositors and stereotypers, who were thought to be the group most probably exposed to moderate concentrations of lead, no excess mortality was found but the study size was small (for lung cancer, there was one death observed and two expected). [The Working Group noted that no data were available on exposure to lead for this cohort.]

Michaels *et al.* (1991) followed mortality among 1261 newspaper printers in New York, USA. The cohort was composed of male members of a typographical union employed at two newspaper printing plants on 1 January 1961. The cohort consisted primarily of compositors and make-up workers, and exposure to lead was assumed to be similar in both groups. No measurements were reported from these two plants, but the authors described measurements of airborne lead at other printing plants in the USA in 1942 as varying from < 1 μg/m^3 to 20 μg/m^3, i.e. below the occupational standard of 50 μg/m^3. According to a survey in 11 plants in the USA in the 1970s, airborne lead concentrations were generally < 10 μg/m^3, most of them < 1 μg/m^3. Of the 1309 male members potentially eligible for the study, 48 (3.7%) were not traced and were excluded. Vital status was known for 1222 subjects (96.9% of the traced). Those with unknown vital status were assumed to be alive at the end of follow-up. Follow-up through death certificates was carried out until December 1984. New York City mortality rates were used as the reference. The overall SMR was 74 (498 deaths observed; 95% CI, 68–81); the SMR for any cancer was 84 (123 deaths observed; 95% CI, 69–100) and that for lung cancer was 89 (37 observed; 95% CI, 69–100). There were no clear increases in SMRs for any of the primary cancer sites studied. [The Working Group noted that the hot lead process was phased out of newspaper printing during the period 1974–78.]

2.1.7 *Exposure to organic lead*

Organo-lead compounds such as tetraethyl and tetramethyl lead have been used historically as components in gasoline. Gasoline engine exhaust has been previously evaluated as *possibly carcinogenic to humans* (Group 2B) (IARC, 1989). Studies on gasoline are not further reviewed here as there are mixed exposures and the effects of lead cannot be characterized separately. A cohort study and a nested case–control study of workers employed in the manufacture of tetraethyl lead are described below.

Sweeney *et al.* (1986) investigated the mortality of 2510 men employed at a chemical plant in east Texas, USA. Tetraethyl lead was produced during the study period from 1952 to 1977, together with ethylene dichloride and chloroethane. Vinyl chloride monomer was also manufactured from 1960 to 1975. Other chemicals (ethylene dibromide, ethylene, inorganic lead, dyes) were used in the manufacturing processes of tetraethyl lead. Male employees who had worked at least 1 day at the factory between 1952 and 1977 were eligible from company records and workers' union files. More than 50% of the total workforce had been employed at the plant for at least 5 years. Vital status was ascertained for 99.3% of the cohort members. Expected numbers were calculated from the national rates by ethnicity, age groups and 5-year calendar periods. Mortality from all causes of death was lower than expected (SMR, 74; 156 observed; 95% CI, 64–84). The SMR for malignant neoplasms was 103 (38 deaths observed; 95% CI, 77–135). The SMR for lung cancer was 112 (14 observed; 95% CI, 68–175). There was a slight excess of laryngeal cancers (SMR, 364; two deaths observed; 95% CI, 65–1145) and of brain and central nervous system tumours (SMR, 213; four deaths observed; 95% CI, 73–487). Among white men employed between 1952 and 1960, when the manufacture of tetraethyl lead was the principal process, the SMR for lung cancer was 122, based on 13 deaths (95% CI, 73–194) and the SMR for brain tumours was 186 (three deaths observed; 95% CI, 51–482). When deaths among male workers employed before 1960 were restricted to those deaths occurring 15 or more years after first employment, the SMR for respiratory cancers was 154 (14 observed; 95% CI, 84–258); for length of employment < 10 years, the SMR was 199 (six observed; 95% CI, 73–432); and for employment > 10 years, the SMR was 132 (eight observed; 95% CI, 57–260). [There were no further details on mortality by employment at departments using tetraethyl lead or with other chemical exposures.]

Fayerweather *et al.* (1997) reported a case–control study among employees who worked at a tetraethyl lead manufacturing company in New Jersey, USA. The plant began producing tetraethyl lead in 1923 and production was closed in 1991; thereafter, the tetraethyl lead plant was involved in lead remediation. The study subjects, 735 male cases of cancer other than non-melanoma of the skin, and 1423 controls matched by year of birth, sex, and most recent payroll class, were drawn from the cancer and mortality registries of the company and from employment rosters. Neoplasms that occurred during 1956–87 were included. The cancer registry mainly covered active workers; workers who left the company were missing from the registry (but those who left the active workforce and were put on the company's disability rolls were included in the registry). The mortality registry covered all active and pensioned employees since 1957. Information on ever having worked in the tetraethyl lead area, years of employment in tetraethyl lead manufacture, rank (degree) of exposure to tetraethyl lead and cumulative exposure to tetraethyl lead were estimated using employment information from the personnel records, industrial hygiene data and records of biological measurements available at the factory. Tetraethyl lead exposure ranks were based on job titles. Employees manufacturing tetraethyl lead could have been exposed both to organic and inorganic lead compounds, but it was not possible to distinguish between these in the exposure assessment because of insufficient data. Exposure (ever/never) to other known or suspected carcinogens (such as aromatic amines, nitriles, benzene, asbestos, radioactive materials) was also assessed. Smoking histories were available from reports of periodical pulmonary function tests for 38% of the cases and 51% of the controls. Cases and controls for whom there was no available information on employment from personnel records were excluded. Odds ratios for cancer of the digestive tract were elevated for the group who had ever worked in the tetraethyl lead manufacturing area compared with the group who had never worked in that area (odds ratio, 1.3; 45 cases observed; 90% CI, 0.9–1.9); the risk was increased for high (odds ratio, 1.3; 90% CI, 0.7–2.7) and very high (odds ratio, 2.2; 90% CI, 1.2–4.0) estimated cumulative exposure. Further latency analyses, adjustments for smoking, and exposure to aromatic amines, radioactive materials and asbestos did not markedly change the results. Risk for rectal cancer was increased (odds ratio, 3.7; nine cases observed; 90% CI, 1.3–10.2), and was associated with high cumulative exposure to tetraethyl lead. The odds ratio for colon cancer was 1.3 (16 observed; 90% CI, 0.7–2.5) and was moderately elevated for the highest cumulative exposure category. [Not all workers exposed to organic lead were followed-up, e.g. workers who had terminated their employment without pension eligibility. Losses in tracing and follow-up were not described in this study. Quantitative information on the exposure categories was not available. Detailed results on other primary cancer sites were not reported.]

2.1.8 *Workers biologically monitored for blood lead concentrations*

Anttila and co-workers (Anttila, 1994; Anttila *et al.*, 1995, 1996) studied mortality and cancer incidence among a worker population biologically monitored for occupational exposure to lead. The biological monitoring programme was undertaken by the Institute of Occupational Health in Finland in order to evaluate the uptake of lead, with the aim particularly to prevent lead poisoning. The database included 63 700 blood lead measurements performed during 1973–83 on workers in approximately 2318 industrial plants or workplaces from all over Finland. Personal identity was traced for 97.0% of the measurements (those for whom the identity could not be traced were excluded). The study population included 20 741 employees, 18 329 men and 2412 women. In the cohort analyses, follow-up was done through cause-of-death records, and records from the nationwide cancer registry from 1973 to 1988. In addition to the cohort follow-up, a nested case–control study was performed, extending the incidence follow-up to 1990. The case–control study included 10 common primary cancer sites and controls were selected from monitored workers not registered for cancer. Controls were matched with the cases by sex, year of birth, age and vital status. In the case–control study, information on occupational histories and on smoking and alcohol consumption were requested from the study subjects or their next-of-kin using a postal questionnaire. Lifetime exposures to lead, and eight other groups of occupational carcinogens, were estimated by an industrial hygienist; the assessment was blinded as to the case–control status. Assessment of lifetime exposures to lead was based on a combination of average individual blood lead values and exposure profiles within lead-exposed worker groups/industries.

Yearly median concentrations of blood lead decreased from 1.4 μmol/L in 1973 to 0.7 μmol/L in 1982 among men and from 1.0 μmol/L to 0.3 μmol/L among women. The blood lead concentrations exceeded 1.0 μmol/L (the administrative reference value of 'occupationally unexposed' during that time) in 9100 (42%) of the employees. Workers monitored most regularly for blood lead concentrations were from the lead battery industry (about 1300 employees from five plants), lead smelting and metal scrap business (692 employees from 36 plants), metal foundries (419 employees from 30 plants), railroad equipment machine shops (434 employees from 14 plants) and manufacture of some industrial chemicals (100 employees from seven plants). Lead-exposed employees monitored less frequently were those working, for example, in automobile repair shops and related industries (1290 employees from 292 workplaces), the graphics industry (1238 employees from 166 plants), the manufacture of glass, pottery, PVC plastics and paints (1220 employees from 68 plants), shipyards (1113 employees from 23 plants) and miscellaneous metal and engineering (2844 employees from 335 plants) (Anttila, 1994).

Altogether 1082 deaths (1007 men and 75 women; SMR, 84; 95% CI, 79–89) and 469 incident cancer cases (SIR, 99; 95% CI, 90–108) were observed in the cohort follow-up. Three exposure categories, based on the highest personal blood lead concentration, were used: low, < 1.0 μmol/L; intermediate, 1.0–1.9 μmol/L; and high, 2.0–7.8 μmol/L. [Compared with many other occupational cohorts, there were rather low levels of exposure to lead in this cohort and small numbers of highly-exposed employees; there were only a few cancer cases among women.] In the low exposure group, the SIR for any cancer was 80 (95% CI, 70–100; $p < 0.05$); the SIRs were 120 (95% CI, 100–140) and 100 (95% CI, 70–140) in the intermediate and high exposure categories, respectively. The SIRs for lung cancer were, respectively, 70 (95% CI, 50–110), 140 (95% CI, 100–190) and 110 (95% CI, 60–200) for the three groups. [The Working Group noted that the reference population has a deficit in all cancers and lung cancer incidence, which affects internal comparisons.] In the internal comparison, there was a twofold risk for lung cancer (relative risk, 2.0; 95% CI, 1.2–3.2) for the intermediate and a 1.5-fold risk (relative risk, 1.5; 95% CI, 0.8–3.1) in the high exposure groups, compared with the low exposure group [no *p*-value for trend available]. Additional analyses were done by cumulative exposure for which the *p*-value for trend was not statistically significant (Anttila *et al.*, 1995).

In the nested case–control study on lung cancer, there were initially 121 male cases and 363 controls. The final population was restricted to 53 cases and 156 controls for whom complete occupational histories were obtained. The nested case–control analyses gave results similar to those of the cohort analyses. There was a positive trend, although not statistically significant, of odds ratios increasing with increasing cumulative exposure to lead, with odds ratios for lung cancer being 0.9, 1.2 and 1.4 for three groups of estimated lifetime cumulative exposure to lead of 1–6, 7–17 and 18–70 μmol/L × year as compared with the unexposed, adjusted for smoking and vital status. Compared with non-adjusted results, the odds ratio for lung cancer increased slightly in the highest exposure group and remained unaltered in the intermediate category when adjusted for smoking and vital status, suggesting that smoking was not a confounder in the internal comparison. In this study (Anttila *et al.*, 1995), a significant fourfold difference was reported between the risk for lung cancer for raised blood lead alone and raised blood lead with estimated co-exposure to exhaust. [The Working Group noted that information on exposure to engine exhaust was of limited quality and the results were difficult to interpret.] There were no clear increases in risk for stomach or kidney cancer associated with lead exposure.

In a further study on brain and nervous system cancers in the same cohort (Anttila *et al.*, 1996), the observed/expected numbers of brain and other nervous system cancers were 12/13.3, 10/7.7 and 4/2.9 over three categories of blood lead (< 1.0, 1.0–1.9, 2.0–7.8 μmol/L). Internal analyses using Poisson regression showed 1.6-fold (95% CI, 0.7–3.8) and 1.8-fold (95% CI, 0.6–5.8) risks for the intermediate and high blood lead categories in comparison with the low. Histology-specific risk estimates could be computed only in the case–control design. There was a statistically significant increase in the risk for gliomas in the high blood lead category (*p*-value for trend = 0.037; 16 gliomas in total), whereas there were no associations between exposure to lead and cancers with other or unknown histology (10 cases; p-value for trend = 1.00). Among those subjects for whom lifetime exposures could be assessed (including 10 of the glioma cases), the risk was associated with the estimated level and duration of lifetime occupational exposure to lead as well as with the cumulative exposure (p-values for trend = 0.041, 0.029 and 0.020, respectively).

2.1.9 *Register linkage studies*

McLaughlin *et al.* (1987) studied the occurrence of meningioma in men using the Cancer–Environmental Registry of Sweden, which linked cancer incidence from 1961–79 with 1960 census information on employment. Analyses included all intracranial and intraspinal meningiomas (n = 1092), 98% of which were coded as histologically benign. Among glassmakers, a regionally-adjusted fivefold risk was observed (6 cases; SIR, 5.2; $p < 0.01$).

Navas-Acién *et al.* (2002; discussed in a letter to the editor by Costa, 2003) investigated occupational risks for gliomas and meningiomas in Sweden. The study was based on a linkage of census records with cancer registry files, and exposures were estimated based on the occupational and industrial titles in the 1970 census. A job–exposure matrix was used that classified probability (no/possible/probable) of exposure, based on estimated proportions of exposed workers. Possible exposure meant that between 10 and 66% of the subjects were exposed at a level > 10% of the threshold limit value. Probable exposure meant that more than 66% of the subjects were exposed. The job–exposure matrix was aimed to be representative for the labour force in Sweden. There were 3363 gliomas and 1166 meningiomas in men, and 1561 gliomas and 1273 meningiomas in women in the follow-up from 1971 to 1989, including those aged 25–64 years at the beginning of follow-up. Risk for glioma in men with possible exposure to lead was not increased (10 cases; relative risk, 1.08; 95% CI, 0.58–2.01; adjusted for age, period, geographical category, town size and other chemical exposures); there were no cases with probable exposure to lead. Risk for meningioma was elevated (seven cases; relative risk, 2.36; 95% CI, 1.12–4.96) for possible exposure to lead; no cases had probable exposure. There were fewer than four cases exposed to lead in the female study population, and the risk estimates were not reported. [The Working Group noted that it is difficult to be confident about the exposure classification.]

Wesseling *et al.* (2002) carried out a study on brain and nervous system cancer risk among women in Finland, based on linkage of census and cancer registry data. Occupation titles were drawn from the 1970 census, and follow-up was performed from 1971 to 1995 among a cohort of 413 887 women with blue-collar occupations. There were 693 cases of brain and nervous system cancers, 43% of which were meningiomas, 29% gliomas and 28% of other types. In a Poisson regression model with multiple agents, adjusted for year of birth, period of diagnosis, and turnover rate, exposure to lead was not statistically significantly elevated: the SIR for low exposure (blood lead < 0.3 μmol/L) was 1.24 (95% CI, 0.95–1.62) and the SIR for medium/high exposure (blood lead > 0.3 μmol/L) was 1.27 (95% CI, 0.81–2.01).

2.1.10 *Population-based case–control studies*

(*a*) *Multiple cancer sites*

A population-based case–control study of cancer associated with occupational exposure among male residents of Montreal, Canada, aged 35–70 years, included histologically-confirmed cases of several types of cancer newly diagnosed between 1979 and 1989 in 19 hospitals (Siemiatycki, 1991). Interviews were carried out with 3730 cancer patients (response rate, 82%) and 533 age-stratified controls from the general population (response rate, 72%). The main cancer sites included were oesophagus, stomach, colon, rectum, pancreas, lung, prostate, bladder, kidney, skin melanoma and non-Hodgkin lymphoma. For each cancer site analysed, two controls were available: a population control and a control selected among cases of cancer at other sites. The interview was designed to obtain lifetime job histories and information on potential confounders. Each job was reviewed by a team of chemists and industrial hygienists who translated the jobs into occupational exposures using a checklist of 293 substances found in the workplace. For exposure to lead compounds or various other forms of lead, no excess risk of cancer was seen for most of the primary sites examined. For substantial exposure to lead compounds, there was a statistically significant 1.8-fold increase in the risk of stomach cancer and a statistically significant 1.5-fold increase in the risk of lung cancer. Substantial exposure to lead dust was associated with an increased risk of stomach cancer, but there were only three exposed cases. The odds ratio for kidney cancer for any exposure to lead was 1.2 (90% CI, 1.0–1.6; 88 exposed cases) and that for substantial exposure was 0.8 (90% CI, 0.4–1.7; six cases). For other forms of exposure to lead, there were smaller numbers, and there were some excess risks reported only with the category 'any exposure'. [The Working Group noted that this study reported significant associations between estimated exposure to lead compounds and both stomach cancer and (to a lesser extent) lung cancer. However, the study involved multiple comparisons of exposures and cancer sites, as well as some uncertainties in exposure classifications, and so reliance has been placed in this monograph primarily on the results from cohort studies of lead-exposed populations.]

(*b*) *Stomach*

Cocco *et al.* (1999b) reported a population-based case–control study on occupational risk factors for stomach cancer associated with 12 workplace exposures, based on information from a national surveillance programme for occupational diseases at the National Cancer Institute, USA. The main study included 41 957 deaths from stomach cancer during 1984–96. Two controls per case were selected from those who died from non-malignant diseases; controls were matched to cases by geographic region, race, sex and 5-year age group. An investigation of deaths from cancers of the gastric cardia (ICD-9 code 151.1), including 1056 cases during 1984–92 and 5280 controls, was also undertaken (Cocco *et al.*, 1998b). The study classified probability and intensity of exposures to lead with help of a job–exposure matrix composed from occupational and industry titles reported as the 'usual' occupation and industry on the death certificate. Overall, risk for stomach cancer was not increased among Caucasian men with either increasing probability or intensity of exposure to lead. There were some slight increases in the risk among African-American men, Caucasian women and African-American women with high probability of lead exposure. Risk for gastric cardia cancer was slightly elevated with increasing probability or intensity of exposure to lead. There was only one case, however, in the group with high probability and intensity and the risk estimate was not provided. [The reliability of the lead exposure data and intercorrelations with other exposures were not described.]

(*c*) *Kidney*

A population-based case–control study among residents of Finland (Partanen *et al.*, 1991) was conducted in 1977–78 involving 672 incident cases of primary renal adenocarcinoma and 1344 controls matched on age, sex and survival status. A questionnaire including information on job history, smoking and obesity was sent to all participants or to the next-of-kin of deceased participants. Response rates for cases and controls were 69% and 68%, respectively. After exclusion of non-eligible subjects, 408 cases and 819 controls remained in the study. Summary indicators of occupation were calculated for the period 1920–68 to allow for a 10-year latency and occupational histories were scored by an industrial hygienist. The annual exposure to lead and inorganic lead compounds was categorized as background (< 0.001 mg/m^3), low (0.001–0.05 mg/m^3), high (> 0.05 mg/m^3) and 'not known'. Four cases of kidney cancer (all men) had been exposed to lead and inorganic lead compounds. After adjusting for smoking, coffee consumption and obesity, an odds ratio of 2.77 (95% CI, 0.49–15.6) was observed in subjects with at least 5 years of high- or low-level exposure before 1968, or less than 5 years of exposure but at least 1 year of high-level exposure during 1920–68, versus background exposure. When the white-collar and farming occupations were excluded, the odds ratio was 5.6 (95% CI, 0.6–54.8).

A population-based case–control study on renal-cell cancer from 1991 to 1995 (Pesch *et al.*, 2000) enrolled 935 cases from five regions in Germany and 4298 population controls, matched to the cases by region, sex and age. Information on occupational history and other risk factors was collected in face-to-face interviews. The response rates were 84–95% and 63–75% for cases and controls, respectively. Information on occupational risk factors was based on two job–exposure matrices (British and German) and used on every job task held for at least 1 year. For each job title and job task the exposure matrix provided an expert rating in terms of the probability and the intensity of exposure to an agent. Slight increases were suggested in the renal-cell cancer risk for estimated exposures to lead, with some dose–response patterns. [Descriptions of tasks with estimated exposures were not provided. Inter-correlations or confounding from other occupational exposures were not tested. It was not possible to check whether differential response rates between cases and controls affected the results.]

(*d*) *Brain and nervous system*

A population-based case–control study using information from a national surveillance programme for occupational diseases at the National Cancer Institute, USA, classified probability and intensity of exposures to lead with help of a job–exposure matrix composed from occupational and industry titles (Cocco *et al.*, 1998a). No information on the duration of exposure was available. Cases were 27 060 Caucasian and African-American subjects (14 655 men and 12 405 women) who died during the period 1984–92 from cancer of the brain at age 35 years or older. Four controls per case were selected from among subjects who died from non-malignant diseases. When all levels of exposure to lead were combined, brain cancer risk did not increase with increasing probability of exposure. When all probabilities of exposure were combined, there was no overall increase in the risk by exposure level, except among the African-American population (for most of whom low probability of exposure was coded, however, if the estimated level was medium or high). The risk estimate for brain cancer with high probability and level of exposure to lead was 2.1 (95% CI, 1.1–4.0; 14 cases observed) among Caucasian men and 1.4 (95% CI, 0.4–4.2; four cases observed) among Caucasian women. Among Caucasian men, the category with high probability and level of exposure appeared to be only one occupational group, i.e. typesetters and compositors. In a later study on central nervous system tumours in women in the USA, Cocco *et al.* (1999a) reported a slightly increased risk for meningiomas (odds ratio, 1.9; 95% CI, 1.0–3.9; nine cases observed) for any versus no exposure to lead.

Hu, J. *et al.* (1998) performed a hospital-based case–control study on risk factors for glioma in the province of Heilongjiang, China. Altogether 218 consecutive incident cases of primary glioma diagnosed between 1989 and 1995 were identified from six hospitals, and two controls were recruited per case from patients with non-neoplastic, non-neural disease. The reported response rates were 100% for both cases and controls. Based on self-reported exposure (request to describe chemical or other occupational exposures using a pre-specified list of agents), there was no increase in the risk related to lead exposure (no cases and four controls). The study was extended to December 1996 with 183 cases of meningioma and 366 controls (Hu *et al.*, 1999). This study suggested an increased risk for meningioma with exposure to lead. [Only self-reported exposure was available. Occupations or exposure levels among lead-exposed respondents were not detailed.]

(*e*) *Other primary sites*

Risch *et al.* (1988) conducted a population-based case–control study of bladder cancer during 1979–82 in Canada. Cases aged 35–79 years diagnosed through the tumour registry or hospital files were eligible (n = 1251) and population controls were used (n = 1483). Information on occupational history and jobs held in some pre-selected industries, together with self-reported exposure to fumes, dusts, smoke or chemicals, were collected for 835 (67%) eligible cases and 792 (53%) controls through face-to-face interviews. Information on family, medical and residential histories, use of tobacco, socioeconomic factors and diet was also collected. Among men who had worked full-time for at least 6 months, exposure to lead compounds was associated with risk for bladder cancer (twofold risk among ever exposed, adjusted for smoking) and there was a trend with duration of exposure/employment as estimated per 10 years. [Exposure to lead was not reported among women. Exposures were partially self-reported. It was not clearly stated if the information on work tasks was used in defining exposure status in the assessment. It was not possible to check whether the differential response rate affected the results.]

Kauppinen *et al.* (1992) conducted a population-based case–control study on primary liver cancer and occupational exposures in Finland. Cases were drawn from 1976–78 and 1981 from the files of the nationwide cancer registry (cases from 1979–80 had been used in another study by the same group); two reference groups were formed from patients with stomach cancer in 1977 and persons who had died from coronary infarction. There were 344 liver cancer cases, 476 controls with stomach cancer and 385 controls with coronary infarction. Controls were matched to cases by age and sex. Information on work history was collected, with the aid of a postal questionnaire, from the closest next-of-kin traced for the study subjects. Response rates were 71% for both cases and controls. Exposure assessment was made using a job–exposure matrix and by a team of occupational hygienists. In the analyses using the job–exposure matrix, no association between the risk for liver cancer and exposure to lead and lead compounds was seen (odds ratio, 0.91; 95% CI, 0.65–1.29 for a combined group of low level or probability of exposure). Based on the hygienists' assessments, the odds ratio for any exposure to lead was also close to unity (1.14; 95% CI, 0.44–2.98 after adjustment for alcohol consumption). No cases and four controls had had heavy exposure to lead (they were all typesetters with more than 10 years of employment) and five cases had had moderate exposure (odds ratio, 2.28; 95% CI, 0.68–7.67). Moderate exposure was defined as a duration of at least 10 years with low-level exposure or a duration of less than 10 years with high-level exposure; the group included workers in plumbing, welding and crystal glass manufacture. [Comparison between stomach cancer and infarction controls as to their exposures to lead was not available.]

2.1.11 *Meta-analyses*

Fu and Boffetta (1995) reviewed reports of 16 cohort studies and 13 case–control studies (nested and population-based) relating to lead exposure and cancer risk. Meta-analyses were performed for all cancers (12 studies), stomach cancer (10 studies), lung cancer (15 studies), kidney cancer (five studies) and bladder cancer (five studies). [The Working Group noted that most of the studies included in the meta-analyses of Fu and Boffetta (1995) and Steenland and Boffetta (2000) (see below) have been considered in this monograph. Neither meta-analysis included exposures to organo-lead or in the mining industry, both of which are discussed in detail in this volume. The meta-analysis of Fu and Boffetta (1995) included two studies of oil mist exposure in the printing industry (Goldstein *et al.*, 1970; Pasternack & Ehrlich, 1972), which have not been discussed here. These two studies lacked specific lead exposure data, did not adjust for smoking nor for other occupational exposures and did not have appropriate reference groups.] Fu and Boffetta (1995) included only the most recent publications if several reports were available for the same study population. Fixed-effect models were used; random-effect models were also applied when there was significant heterogeneity in a set of relative risks. The meta-analysis was limited to overall study findings (SMRs from cohort studies, and odds ratios from case–control studies); quantitative data or analyses in relation to categories of cumulative exposure were not considered. The meta-analyses (fixed-effect models) provided significantly elevated summary relative risks for all cancers (relative risk, 1.11; 95% CI, 1.05–1.17), stomach cancer (relative risk, 1.33; 95% CI, 1.18–1.49), lung cancer (relative risk, 1.29; 95% CI, 1.10–1.50) and bladder cancer (relative risk, 1.41; 95% CI, 1.16–1.71). A non-significantly elevated risk was shown for kidney cancer (relative risk, 1.19; 95% CI, 0.96–1.48). Significant heterogeneity in the set of study-specific relative risks was only shown for lung cancer ($p < 0.001$) but a highly significant summary relative risk was also obtained for this cancer from a random-effect model (odds ratio, 1.29; 95% CI, 1.10–1.50). When meta-analysis was restricted to studies conducted in industries involving higher lead exposures (battery and smelter industries), significantly elevated summary relative risks were shown for all cancers (five studies: relative risk, 1.08; 95% CI, 1.02–1.15), stomach cancer (four studies: relative risk, 1.50; 95% CI, 1.23–1.83) and lung cancer (random-effect model applied to three studies: relative risk, 1.42; 95% CI, 1.05–1.92). A non-significantly increased relative risk was shown for kidney cancer (three studies: relative risk, 1.26; 95% CI, 0.70–2.26). [Most of the studies included in this meta-analysis were of occupational groups with exposure to carcinogens such as chromium and arsenic as well as lead. Most of the studies were cohort studies entailing comparison with the general population without adjustment for potential confounding from smoking or diet. Many of the cohort studies did not report data for all of the cancers of interest and there is considerable scope for publication bias for the meta-analyses of kidney and bladder cancer; however, this is not an issue for the lung cancer findings.]

In their review of lead and cancer in humans, Steenland and Boffetta (2000) included a meta-analysis of eight cohort studies of highly exposed workers. Four studies analysed cancer mortality (of which one study used a nested case–control design); the remaining four studies analysed cancer incidence (cancer registrations). The results of meta-analyses for all cancers (n = 1911) and cancers of the lung (n = 675), stomach (n = 181), kidney (n = 40) and brain (n = 69) were presented. The investigators first determined whether there was significant heterogeneity in each set of cause-specific relative risks (estimated by overall site-specific SMRs, summary relative risks or odds ratios obtained from internal comparison). There was an absence of such heterogeneity for all cancers, and cancers of the stomach, kidney and brain. Therefore, fixed-effect models were used for these groupings of cancer sites to combine relative risks across the studies. A significantly elevated relative risk was shown for cancer of the stomach (relative risk, 1.34; 95% CI, 1.14–1.57) but not for kidney cancer (relative risk, 1.01; 95% CI, 0.72–1.42), brain cancer (relative risk, 1.06; 95% CI, 0.80–1.40) or all cancers (relative risk, 1.04; 95% CI, 1.00–1.09). There was significant heterogeneity in the set of relative risks for lung cancer and the investigators applied a random-effect model, leading to an overall relative risk of 1.30 (95% CI, 1.15–1.46). A previous study (Englyst *et al.*, 1999) had shown that there was significant arsenic exposure in the outlier study (Lundström *et al.*, 1997), and exclusion of this study led to a much lower summary relative risk for lung cancer (1.14;

95% CI, 1.04–1.25). [This meta-analysis is limited to overall summary findings; quantitative data or possible dose–response effects within the eight studies were not available for meta-analysis. It was not possible to adjust for potential confounders such as smoking and occupational exposure to arsenic and other chemicals.]

2.2 Studies based on general population (environmental) exposures

Studies in the general population involve exposures to lead in the environment which are usually much lower than lead exposures in occupational studies, sometimes by as much as an order of magnitude. Exposure effects at low doses can differ from those at high doses with regard to the type of cancer. Furthermore, low-dose effects may involve biological mechanisms different from those involved in high-dose effects, even for the same cancer site. Nevertheless, when considering the same cancer site, in general, one should expect that higher doses should cause more disease than lower doses.

Five ecological studies deal with exposure to lead and cancer. Correlations between levels of trace metals in water supplies and cancer mortality in the USA were investigated by Berg and Burbank (1972). Lung cancer mortality rates for Caucasian men and women in the former 'Tri-State mining district' of the USA (Cherokee County, KS; Jasper County, MO and Ottawa County, OK) were investigated by Neuberger and Hollowell (1982). Correlations between lead concentrations (and other aspects of air pollution) and lung cancer incidence rates (standardized for age, sex and race) were investigated in 1973–76 by Vena (1983) for 125 census tracts in New York State, USA. Correlations between blood lead concentrations and age were investigated by Hussain *et al.* (1990) for cancer patients and other residents of the Lahore district in India. Relationships between mineral and trace elements in drinking-water and gastric cancer mortality in 34 municipalities in the Aomori Prefecture of Japan were investigated by Nakaji *et al.* (2001). [The Working Group judged these studies to be uninformative due to the poor classification of exposure and the considerable scope for confounding.]

2.2.1 *Cohort studies*

McDonald and Potter (1996) conducted a mortality study in a cohort of 454 paediatric patients resident in Massachusetts, USA, and diagnosed with lead poisoning at Boston Children's Hospital between 1923 and 1966. Diagnosis of lead poisoning was based on the presence of at least two of the following clinical criteria: (1) history of lead exposure or of lead poisoning in a sibling; (2) radiographic lead lines in the bones; (3) gastrointestinal, haematological and/or neurological symptoms of lead poisoning. Cohort members were traced until 1991 to ascertain mortality; 153 (33.7%) were lost to follow-up. Numbers of observed deaths were compared with those expected, based on population statistics in the USA. Eighty-six deaths were observed (observed/expected, 1.74; 95% CI, 1.40–2.15), 10 of which were due to cancer (observed/expected, 1.14; 95% CI, 0.55–2.10). Seventeen deaths were directly attributed to lead poisoning. Mortality from cardiovascular disease was elevated (observed/expected, 2.09; 95% CI, 1.29–3.19). [The study is limited by the high percentage of cohort members lost to follow-up.]

2.2.2 *Cohort studies of the general population based on blood lead concentrations*

The National Health and Nutrition Examination Survey (NHANES II) conducted two studies between 1976 and 1980 on the same population in the USA, based on a national probability sample of the civilian non-institutionalized population, aged 6 months to 74 years at baseline (n = 27 801) (Jemal *et al.*, 2002; Lustberg & Silbergeld, 2002) (see also Section 1.6). Data were obtained from standardized questionnaires, physical examinations and laboratory tests. Single blood lead measurements were made for all children below 7 years of age and for a random subsample of half of the subjects aged 7 years or more. Mortality was investigated for the period 1976–92 via internal comparisons of rates for those with high blood lead concentrations versus those with low blood lead concentrations [a single blood lead estimation may misrepresent long-term exposure].

Jemal *et al.* (2002) restricted their analyses to 3592 Caucasian subjects (1702 men, 1890 women) aged 30 years or more at baseline. The study had a complex sample design with multistage stratified cluster sampling and sample weighting of study participants. Cox proportional hazard regression models were used to estimate dose–response relationships between blood lead and mortality from all cancers (203 deaths), as well as some specific cancers. Log-transformed blood lead was both categorized into quartiles and treated as a continuous variable in a cubic regression spline. Median blood lead concentrations for the quartiles were 7.3, 10.6, 13.8 and 19.7 μg/dL. In analyses that adjusted for baseline values of age (continuous variable), poverty, annual alcohol and tobacco use, region and year of examination, there were no significant trends between blood lead concentrations (quartile analyses) and risk for cancer mortality in men and women combined (p = 0.16), men (p = 0.57) or women (p = 0.22). None of the examined site-specific cancer risks showed a significant association with blood lead at baseline. For lung cancer (71 deaths), the rate ratio comparing subjects with blood lead concentrations above the median versus below the median, adjusted for smoking and age, was 1.5 (95% CI, 0.7–2.9). Based on five stomach cancer deaths, the relative risk for those with blood lead concentrations above the median versus those below the median was 2.4 (95% CI, 0.3–19.1). [The Working Group noted the strong reported correlation between smoking and baseline blood lead concentration and that adjustment for smoking did not consider duration of smoking, which may have led to some residual confounding.]

NHANES II was used by another research group to analyse associations between blood lead concentrations at baseline and subsequent mortality (Lustberg & Silbergeld, 2002). This report made use of data for non-Caucasian as well as Caucasian subjects. A total of 4292 male and female participants aged 30–74 years with baseline blood lead concentrations were considered; follow-up identified 929 deaths (240 cancer deaths) before the end of 1992. In order to exclude those with high blood lead concentrations due to possible occupational exposure, the authors did not consider subjects who had blood lead concentrations ≥ 30 μg/dL. [The Working Group noted that elimination of those with highest exposure may weaken dose–response analyses.] In analyses that adjusted for baseline values of age, sex, race, education, income, smoking, body mass index, exercise and location (urban, rural, suburban), there was a positive trend with blood lead concentration for all causes of death (referent < 10 μg/dL; 10–19 μg/dL: relative risk, 1.17; 95% CI, 0.90–1.52; 20–29 μg/dL: relative risk, 1.46; 95% CI, 1.14–1.86), for diseases of the circulatory system (referent < 10 μg/dL; 10–19 μg/dL: relative risk, 1.10; 95% CI, 0.85–1.43; 20–29 μg/dL: relative risk, 1.39; 95% CI, 1.01–1.91) and for all cancers (referent < 10 μg/dL; 10–19 μg/dL: relative risk, 1.46; 95% CI, 0.87–2.48; 20–29 μg/dL: relative risk, 1.68; 95% CI, 1.02–2.78). The only specific cancer for which results were given was lung cancer, for which rate ratios were 1.70 (95% CI, 0.60–4.81) and 2.20 (95% CI, 0.80–6.06), for the middle and high exposure groups, respectively. [The Working Group noted that residual confounding by smoking may have resulted from failure to consider duration in the adjustment for smoking. Data for all cancers show large decreases in rate ratios after control for smoking, suggesting that better control over smoking might lead to further decreases, especially for lung cancer. The Working Group also noted that the generalized increase in all deaths, all cancers and all circulatory diseases with increasing blood lead concentration suggests possible residual confounding by socioeconomic status.]

2.2.3 *Case–control studies*

The possible relationship between laryngeal cancer and subclinical lead intoxication (assessed both by blood lead concentrations and ALAD activity in the blood) has been investigated (Kandiloros *et al.*, 1997). A total of 58 patients underwent surgery for cancer of the larynx over a period of 8 months at a hospital in Athens, Greece. After excluding patients with a history of lead intoxication, professional exposure to lead, previous renal or haematological diseases, or with other health problems, a total of 26 patients (24 men, two women) aged 42–75 years were included in the study. All patients had histologically-confirmed squamous-cell laryngeal carcinoma; none of the patients had received chemotherapy. Fifty-three patients with no history of cancer, suffering from other diseases, mainly otitis media, comprised the control group. There was no significant difference in the mean blood lead concentration between the two groups (patients: mean, 8.5 μg/dL; controls: mean, 7.9 μg/dL). However, ALAD activity was significantly lower ($0.001 < p < 0.01$) in the cases (patients: mean, 50.9 U/L; controls: mean, 59.8 U/L). [The Working Group noted that the exclusion of lead-exposed cases may have biased the results and that the ALAD concentration could have been affected by the case–control status.]

The possible relationships between cancer of the gallbladder and biliary concentrations of heavy metals have been investigated (Shukla *et al.*, 1998). Cases comprised 38 patients (11 men, 27 women) with histologically-diagnosed cancer of the gallbladder admitted to the surgical unit of the University Hospital, Varanesi, India, from January 1995 to March 1996. Controls comprised 58 patients with gallstones (14 men, 44 women). The mean age of the cases was 53.5 years and that of the controls was 48.3 years. Bile was taken by needle aspiration from the gallbladder of all patients at the time of surgery for estimation of cadmium, chromium and lead concentrations. Statistical comparisons were made using Student's *t*-test. Highly significant differences between cases and controls ($p < 0.001$) were observed for the mean values of all the metals under study (cadmium: cases, 0.19 mg/L; controls, 0.09 mg/L; chromium: cases, 1.26 mg/L; controls, 0.55 mg/L; lead: cases, 58.4 mg/L; controls, 3.99 mg/L). There was no overlap in the observed ranges of biliary lead concentrations (cases, 35–76 mg/L; controls, 0–19 mg/L). [The Working Group noted that age and sex differences in the two groups (cases were on average 5 years older than controls and included a higher percentage of men) were not taken into account, but judged this to be an unlikely explanation of the study findings. The results could indicate that lead exposure is an important risk factor for cancer of the gallbladder, but no attempt was made to determine whether the cases had been more exposed to lead than had the controls. Alternatively, the lead concentration findings may reflect a consequence of gallbladder cancer or gallstones.]

At a hospital clinic in Lucknow, India, blood lead, zinc and copper concentrations in 17 patients undergoing surgery for cancer of the prostate, 41 patients undergoing surgery for benign hyperplasia of the prostate and 20 controls (men without any symptoms of bladder flow obstruction) were investigated (Siddiqui *et al.*, 2002). Patients (mean age: cancer cases, 71.0 years; benign disease, 70.0 years) were older than controls (mean age, 53.1 years) [no information was supplied on how controls were selected]. Mean blood lead concentrations were significantly higher ($p < 0.05$) in patients with prostate diseases (cancer cases, 28.2 μg/dL; benign hyperplasia, 23.4 μg/dL) than in controls (10.2 μg/dL). Blood concentrations of zinc and copper were significantly lower ($p < 0.05$) both in prostate cancer cases and cases of benign hyperplasia than in controls. [The comparisons were unadjusted for age.] None of the subjects reported any previous occupational or accidental exposure to lead. [The Working Group noted that the disease status may have affected the blood lead concentrations.]

2.3 Studies on parental exposure and childhood cancer

2.3.1 *Cohort studies*

Wulff *et al.* (1996) conducted a cancer incidence study among a cohort of 30 644 children born between 1961 and 1990 in the municipality of Skellefteå, Sweden, to determine whether children born to women living near the Rönnskär smelter during pregnancy ($n = 4400$) had an increased incidence of cancer compared with children born to women living at a distance from the smelter ($n = 26\ 244$). The Rönnskär smelter is a significant source of environmental pollutants, including lead, arsenic, copper, cadmium and sulfur dioxide. People living in two parishes within a 20-km radius of the smelter (St. Örjan and Bureå) were considered to be the exposed group, based on environmental sampling data. People in all other parishes within the municipality were considered to be unexposed.

Through linkage to the Swedish Cancer Registry, cancer diagnoses were obtained and compared with expected numbers based on national incidence rates in Sweden. Thirteen cases of childhood cancer (four leukaemia, three brain, one kidney, one eye and four other cancers) were identified among children born in the exposed area, versus 6.7 expected (SIR, 195; 95% CI, 88–300). Among children born to women living in the unexposed area, the observed number of cancer cases ($n = 42$) was similar to that expected ($n = 41.8$). [The focus on incidence of disease, the large size of the population and the linkage to national data sets are strengths of this study, but the lack of individual exposure data or blood lead concentrations are weaknesses. The presence of multiple contaminants makes etiological assignment difficult.]

In a study in Norway, Kristensen and Andersen (1992) used multistep register linkage to measure cancer incidence in a cohort of children who were the offspring of men who were members of the Oslo printers' unions. A file of these workers' children was established through linkage with the Central Population Register. Children born between 1950 and 1987 (n = 12 440) were traced for cancer incidence during the years 1965–87 in the Cancer Registry of Norway (193 406 person–years). Thirty-three incident cases of cancer were found. To account for the fact that the use of lead in the Oslo printing industry ended in the mid-1970s, an examination of cancer incidence was undertaken in the subcohort of 3221 children born before 1975. In this group, none developed cancer before age 15 (32 532 person–years) compared with 3.7 expected (upper limit of the 95% CI, 100). [The Working Group noted that exposure was uncertain.]

2.3.2 *Case–control studies*

(*a*) *Wilms' tumour*

In a case–control study of Wilms' tumour incidence (Kantor *et al.*, 1979), 149 children born in Connecticut, USA, aged 0–19 years (80 males, 69 females) with Wilms' tumour recorded in the Connecticut Tumor Registry during the period 1935–73 were compared with 149 matched controls selected from Connecticut birth certificates and matched by sex, race and year of birth. The occupation of the father at the time of the child's birth was determined from the birth certificate and used as an indicator of potential sources of exposure to carcinogens. An association was found between paternal occupations related to lead (driver, motor-vehicle mechanic, service-station attendant, welder, solderer, metallurgist and scrap metal worker) in the children with Wilms' tumour compared with the controls. Fathers of 22 cases and of six controls had been employed in lead-related occupations (odds ratio, 3.7; 95% CI, 1.5–11.1). Fathers of five cases and of one control had been employed in jobs with potential exposure to lead (odds ratio, 5.75). [The Working Group noted that no confidence interval was given and that exposure was uncertain.]

In a case–control study conducted by Wilkins and Sinks (1984a,b), an occupation–exposure linkage system was used to examine the possible association between paternal occupation and Wilms' tumour incidence. The study was undertaken in Ohio, USA, and was based on 62 cases with histologically-confirmed tumours, registered through the Columbus

Children's Hospital Tumor Registry between 1950 and 1981. Cases from certain counties in Ohio were excluded from analysis because they fell outside a particular catchment area. Two controls per case were selected from birth certificate files in Ohio and matched on year of birth, sex and race. Job-related exposure of the father was inferred from the occupational and industry notation on the birth certificates, using a job–exposure matrix developed by Hoar *et al.* (1980). The first part of the study was designed to test the hypothesis that paternal exposure to lead is a risk factor for Wilms' tumour in offspring. There was no statistical difference in the frequency of occupational exposure to lead (odds ratio, 1.1; 95% CI, 0.6–2.0), lead alkyls (odds ratio, 1.3; 95% CI, 0.5–3.3) or lead salts (odds ratio, 0.7; 95% CI, 0.1–4.1) between fathers of children with Wilms' tumour and fathers of controls. Occupations associated with exposure to lead were examined by calculating odds ratios, all of which were greater than unity but not statistically significant. For exposure to lead, the odds ratio was 1.25 (95% CI, 0.56–2.70).

Olshan *et al.* (1990) undertook a case–control study in the USA to examine the possible relationship between Wilms' tumour and paternal occupational exposure. Cases consisted of 200 children with Wilms' tumour diagnosed by histopathological examination, who were registered at selected National Wilms' Tumour Study institutions between 1 June 1984 and 31 May 1986. The National Wilms' Tumour Study registers an estimated 84% of all cases of Wilms' tumour diagnosed in the USA. Disease-free controls ($n = 233$) of the same age (± 2 years) and geographic area were matched to each case using a random-digit dialling procedure. To ascertain history of occupational exposure, the parents of cases and controls completed a self-administered questionnaire that provided information on all jobs held for more than 6 months since 18 years of age. Questionnaires were completed by the parents of 234 cases (61% of eligible cases), but only 200 (52% of eligible) were successfully matched with a control. Questionnaires were completed by parents of 233 controls (52% of eligible). Paternal exposures were assessed for three separate time periods in the period between birth and diagnosis: preconception, during pregnancy and postnatal. Exposure was determined by juxtaposition of each occupational exposure history with a job–exposure matrix developed by NIOSH. Specific analyses linking exposure to lead with the incidence of Wilms' tumour gave odds ratios of 1.07 (37 exposed cases/33 exposed controls; 95% CI, 0.58–1.98) for preconception exposure; 1.14 (24/24; 95% CI, 0.56–2.36) for exposure during pregnancy; and 1.31 (21/22; 95% CI, 0.61–2.77) for postnatal exposure.

(*b*) *Other cancer sites*

Buckley *et al.* (1989) conducted a case–control study to examine the incidence of acute non-lymphocytic leukaemia in relation to parental occupational exposures in children in the USA and Canada under 18 years of age. Of 262 eligible cases, mothers of 204 children (78%) were interviewed successfully. Controls were obtained through random-digit dialling and matched on date of birth (± 2 years for children aged more than 4 years and ± 12 months for children aged 1–3 years) and race. Information on occupational exposure was sought through interview with the mother, and exposures were ascertained either by direct reporting of chemical name or inference from job title. The fathers of five cases and five controls had been exposed to lead between 1 and 1000 days (odds ratio, 1.0; 95% CI, 0.3–3.5); the fathers of six cases and of none of the controls had had exposure to lead for more than 1000 days (p for trend = 0.03). [The Working Group noted that the positive trend with increasing duration is based on a small number of cases and on retrospective ascertainment of exposure without any blood lead data.]

A case–control study conducted during 1976–87 in the USA included all residents of New York State, excluding New York City, diagnosed with neuroblastoma (Kerr *et al.*, 2000). A total of 216 cases aged < 15 years and born to Caucasian mothers was ascertained from the NY State Cancer Registry. Controls were sampled from the NY State Department of Health live birth certificate registry and matched on ethnicity of the mother and age. Telephone interviews were conducted with the mothers during 1992–93 with a completion rate of 85% (final number of cases = 183). Interviews gathered information on gestation, drug use and medical history during pregnancy, parents' lifestyle, occupation, and socio-demographic attributes. Using self-reported occupational exposure and a list of industries and occupations with potential for exposure, exposure certainty indexes were coded for each of 25 physical and chemical agents as: category 1, reported exposure and potential for exposure; category 2, no report of exposure but potential for exposure; category 3, report of exposure but no potential for exposure; category 4 (no reported exposure and no potential for exposure) was used as reference. Odds ratios of 4.7 (95% CI, 1.3–18.2) for self-reported maternal exposure to lead (nine cases, four controls) and 2.4 (95% CI, 1.2–4.8) for self-reported paternal exposure (21 cases, 18 controls) were observed. Odds ratios for categories 1, 2 and 3 for maternal exposure were 3.5 (95% CI, 0.7–22.6), 0.8 (95% CI, 0.4–1.8) and 8.3 (95% CI, 0.8–412.1), respectively, and for paternal exposure, 2.2 (95% CI, 0.9–5.4), 1.0 (95% CI, 0.7–1.6) and 3.3 (95% CI, 1.0–11.5), respectively.

3. Studies of Cancer in Experimental Animals

3.1 Lead acetate

3.1.1 *Mouse*

(*a*) *Oral administration*

In a study by Waszynski (1977), a total of 137 male and female F1(RIII × C57Bl) mice, 6–8 weeks of age, were divided into four groups and fed diets containing lead acetate (analytical grade) (daily intake, 6 mg/mouse), sulfathiazole (daily intake, 0.3 mg/mouse), lead acetate plus sulfathiazole, or unaltered diet (control) for 18 months and were observed for an additional 7 months. Some animals died during the observation period. Histological analysis revealed that none of the treatments produced renal tumours. [The Working Group noted that the group sizes were not specified.]

Blakley (1987) exposed groups of 42–46 female albino Swiss mice, 8 weeks of age, to lead acetate [purity unspecified] in drinking-water at concentrations of 0 (control), 50 or 1000 μg/mL for up to 280 days. This mouse strain has a high spontaneous incidence of lymphocytic leukaemia. Mice that died during exposure or were killed at the end of the study were examined grossly for evidence of lymphocytic leukaemia of thymic origin (enlarged thymus). Survival was significantly reduced ($p = 0.007$, Lee-Desu survival statistic) in the lead-treated mice, suggesting that lead enhanced death due to leukaemia. [The Working Group noted the absence of histological analysis of the tumours.]

(*b*) *Pre- and perinatal administration*

In a study by Waalkes *et al.* (1995), groups of 10–15 primigravid C57Bl/6NCr mice, previously bred with C3H/HeNCr males to produce B6C3F$_1$ offspring, were given *ad libitum* drinking-water containing lead acetate [purity unspecified] at doses that provided lead concentrations of 0 (control), 500, 750 and 1000 ppm, from gestation day 12 through to birth and until 4 weeks postpartum when offspring were weaned. Exposure to lead acetate did not alter litter size. The offspring were placed into same-sex groups of 23–25 based on maternal exposure level to lead acetate. They were given water without added lead and with or without 500 ppm sodium barbital as a renal tumour promoter and observed for a total of 112 weeks postpartum. Exposure to lead acetate did not alter body weight of the offspring nor the survival of any group during the observation period. A complete necropsy was performed on each animal. In male offspring, histological examination of the kidneys revealed that exposure to lead acetate was associated with a dose-related increase ($p = 0.0006$, Cochran-Armitage test for trend) in the incidence of proliferative lesions (including atypical tubular-cell hyperplasia) and a significant increase in the incidence of renal adenomas ($p < 0.05$, two-tailed Fisher's exact test) and occasional renal carcinomas. In female offspring, exposure to lead acetate was associated with a significant dose-related increase ($p = 0.017$; Cochran-Armitage test for trend) in the incidence of renal proliferative lesions, including hyperplasia, adenoma and carcinoma. Proliferative lesions were exclusively of renal tubular cell origin. Sodium barbital did not increase the incidence of renal proliferative lesions in any group. The authors noted that the transplacental/translactational lead acetate-induced tumours arose in the absence of extensive chronic nephropathy typically seen in lead carcinogenesis in rodents chronically exposed as adults. Exposure to lead acetate was not associated with tumours at extra-renal sites in any of the experimental groups (Waalkes *et al.*, 1995).

(*c*) *Administration with known carcinogens or modifiers of carcinogenesis*

Bull *et al.* (1986) tested various chemicals with potential to initiate tumours, including lead acetate (purity, > 99%), in groups of 30 female SENCAR mice, 6–8 weeks of age. The mice received a single oral dose of 600 mg/kg bw [presumably by gastric intubation; vehicle either emulphor, saline or water] or a single dermal application of 600 mg/kg bw to the shaved back [vehicle either acetone or ethanol]. Two weeks later, mice received dermal applications of 1.0 μg of the skin tumour promoter, 12-*O*-tetradecanoyl phorbol-13-acetate (TPA), in 0.2 mL acetone three times per week for up to 52 weeks. Skin tumours were assessed histologically; other tumours were not reported. Oral and topical applications of lead acetate did not affect the incidence of skin tumours. [The Working Group noted that the study was limited by the use of a single dose and the inadequate reporting of experimental details.]

Blakley (1987) also studied the effects of oral administration of lead acetate on the incidence of urethane-induced lung adenoma in female Swiss mice. Groups of 19–25 mice, 3 weeks of age, were exposed to lead acetate [purity unspecified] in the drinking-water at concentrations of 0 (control), 50, 200 or 1000 μg/mL for 15 weeks. A single intra-peritoneal injection of 1.5 mg/kg bw urethane was administered 3 weeks after the start of lead treatment. The lead acetate and urethane treatments did not alter water consumption or body weight gain. The animals were killed at the end of the lead exposure period (15 weeks). Lungs were inflated, fixed and inspected visually for the number and size of adenomas. Treatment with lead acetate did not alter average lung tumour size or multi-plicity (tumours/animal). [The Working Group noted that the absence of a group treated with lead acetate alone limited the utility of this study.]

3.1.2 *Rat*

(*a*) *Oral administration*

Boyland *et al.* (1962) fed a group of 20 male Wistar rats, 10 weeks of age, a diet containing 1% lead acetate [purity unspecified] for 1 year and observed them for up to 629 days. Histological evaluation of rats that died revealed the first renal tumour after 331 days. Subsequently, 14 more rats died with renal tumours. Among the total of 15 renal tumours, 14 were carcinomas. [The Working Group noted the absence of a control group but the remarkable incidence of renal carcinomas in lead acetate-exposed animals.]

In a lifetime study testing metals for nutritional essentiality, groups of 50 male and 50 female Long Evans rats [age unspecified] were exposed to 5 ppm lead as lead acetate [purity not specified] in drinking-water from weaning to natural death and compared with control animals given water without added lead. Lead acetate significantly increased mortality in both sexes ($p < 0.05$, Student's *t*-test). Not all animals underwent necropsy and only grossly visible tumours were evaluated microscopically [tumour location not specified]. The authors indicated no significant differences in total tumour incidence between control and lead acetate-treated rats (Chi-squared test) (Schroeder *et al.*, 1965; Kanisawa & Schroeder, 1969). [The Working Group noted the low dose used, the limited pathological evaluation, that animals would have been deficient in other metals, and that the data were inconsistent between the two reports.]

Zawirska and Medras (1968) gave groups of 94 male and 32 female Wistar rats [age not specified] a diet supplemented with lead acetate [purity unspecified] to achieve a dose of lead of 3 mg/rat per day for 2 months followed by a dose of 4 mg/rat per day for 16 months. The groups were compared with 19 male and 13 female control rats fed unaltered diets. After 18 months, 40 of the lead acetate-treated rats [sex unspecified] were killed while the rest were allowed to live to a natural death. Weight loss was evident in the lead acetate-treated rats [actual body weight data not given; survival data not given]. Extensive histological examination was performed on all animals. The authors stated that no tumours were observed in control rats except for one adenoma and one carcinoma of the mammary gland. This included an absence of spontaneous tumours of the kidney and endocrine organs in control animals. The 94 lead acetate-treated male rats had 58 renal tumours (43 adenomas, 15 carcinomas), 23 adrenal gland tumours (22 adenomas, one carcinoma), 23 interstitial-cell tumours of the testes, 22 prostatic tumours (21 adenomas, one carcinoma), 10 lung tumours (eight adenomas, two carcinomas), four pituitary adenomas, three liver tumours, three brain gliomas, three thyroid adenomas, two spermatic duct carcinomas, one leukaemia and one sarcoma [given a tumour incidence of 0/19 in control males, incidences of renal, adrenal, testes and prostatic tumours were significantly increased in lead acetate-treated male rats ($p < 0.05$, two-tailed Fisher's exact test)]. The 32 lead acetate-treated female rats had 14 renal tumours (12 adenomas, two carcinomas), nine adrenal gland adenomas, five lung tumours (four adenomas, one carcinoma), three mammary gland tumours, two liver tumours, two thyroid tumours, one pituitary adenoma, one oesophageal carcinoma, one leukaemia and two sarcomas [given a tumour incidence of 0/13 in control females, incidences of renal and adrenal tumours were significantly increased in lead-treated female rats ($p < 0.05$, two-tailed Fisher's exact test)]. [The Working Group noted that the spontaneous incidence of gliomas in rats is a very rare event.]

In further studies (Zawirska & Medras, 1972; Zawirska, 1981), groups of 47 male and 47 female Wistar rats, 31 weeks of age, were fed lead acetate [purity unspecified] in the diet to achieve a dose of lead of 3 mg per day [based on 20 g food/rat given to 10 rats/cage] for periods ranging between 60 and 504 days and were observed for times ranging from 60 days to the point of natural death (maximum 572 days). Control animals [stated variously as 31 males and 31 females or 47 males and 47 females] were fed unaltered diet and were observed for up to 800 days [survival was imprecisely defined]. All rats were examined histologically. No tumours were reported in the control group. In the 94 lead acetate-treated rats, examination revealed 102 tumours including 12 rats with kidney adenomas, 15 with lung adenomas, 17 with pituitary adenomas, 10 with brain gliomas, 11 with thyroid adenomas, five with parathyroid adenomas, 11 with prostate adenomas, eight with mammary adenomas and 13 with adrenal cortical adenomas [all incidences were significantly increased, except parathyroid adenoma incidence, versus 0/62 control animals ($p < 0.05$, two-tailed Fisher's exact test)]. The authors stated that renal tumour incidence appeared to be related to length of treatment with lead acetate. [The Working Group noted some inconsistencies between the two reports. The Working Group also noted that the spontaneous incidence of kidney adenomas and brain gliomas is a very rare event.]

Azar *et al.* (1973) fed groups of 50 male and 50 female rats [strain and age unspecified] diets containing concentrations of lead acetate [purity unspecified] to give 10, 50, 100 or 500 ppm lead for 2 years. A control group of 100 males and 100 females remained untreated.

In a second study, started shortly after the first, groups of 20 male and 20 female rats were fed 0, 1000 and 2000 ppm lead [presumably as lead acetate] for 2 years. Weight gain was depressed in animals receiving 1000 and 2000 ppm lead. Data on survival rates at 2 years indicated increased mortality in males fed 500 and 2000 ppm lead [test not specified]. Complete necropsy with histological examination was carried out on all animals. No pathological lesions were reported in rats fed up to 100 ppm lead. No renal tumours occurred in either male or female control rats. In male rats treated with lead, the incidence of renal tumours was 5/50, 10/20 and 16/20 in groups fed 500 ppm, 1000 ppm and 2000 ppm, respectively [all three incidences were statistically significant, two-tailed Fisher's exact test; a χ^2 test for trend proved significant ($p < 0.001$)]. In female rats treated with lead, the incidence of renal tumours was 0/50, 0/20 and 7/20 in the groups fed 500 ppm, 1000 ppm and 2000 ppm, respectively [the incidence in the last group was significantly increased; two-tail Fisher's exact test]. Most renal tumours were adenomas derived from the tubular epithelium. The doses of lead acetate used resulted in the following blood lead concentrations: no treatment, 12.7 μg/dL; 10 ppm lead acetate, 11.0 μg/dL; 50 ppm, 18.5 μg/dL; 100 ppm, 35.2 μg/dL; 500 ppm, 77.8 μg/dL.

Waszynski (1977) fed groups of 15–20 male and 19–26 female [individual group size not specified] Wistar rats, aged 2–2.5 months, diets containing either lead acetate (analytical grade) alone, sulfathiazole alone, lead plus sulfathiazole or unaltered diet (control) for 18 months and observed them for an additional 7 months. Diets were prepared to give a dose of 3 mg/rat per day lead acetate and 54 mg/rat per day sulfathiazole. Some animals died during the observation period. Histological examination of the 42 male and female rats that survived until the end of the observation period showed that lead acetate treatment alone induced 14 renal tumours including five carcinomas in males and one carcinoma in a female. In 43 male and female rats that survived until the end of the observation period, lead plus sulfathiazole treatment induced 17 renal tumours including one renal carcinoma in a female. Controls and rats fed sulfathiazole alone did not develop renal tumours. [The Working Group noted some deficiencies in reporting. The Working Group also noted that the spontaneous occurrence of renal carcinomas in rats is a very rare event.]

Nogueira (1987) fed groups of 10–12 male Wistar rats, 6 weeks of age, diets containing 0 (control), 0.5 or 1.0% lead acetate [purity unspecified] for up to 24 weeks. Survival and body weight were unaltered by lead acetate treatment. At necropsy, kidneys were assessed histologically in a median transverse section and tumours were categorized as basophilic or chromophobic, and the incidence was reported separately. Renal tumours were not reported in the 10 control rats [the Working Group noted the absence of other data on tumours in controls]. Renal tumours did not occur in the 12 rats fed 0.5% lead acetate, but of the 10 rats fed 1.0% lead acetate, two developed basophilic tumours and seven developed chromophobic tumours [it is unclear if any rats had both types of tumours].

In a study by Fears *et al.* (1989) on carcinogenic mixtures, groups of 24 male and 24 female Fischer 344 rats [age unspecified] were fed 500, 2000 or 8000 ppm lead as lead acetate [purity unspecified] in the diet for up to 725 days. Control groups of 213 male and 214 female rats received unaltered diet. Other groups of male and female rats received lead together with various other carcinogens (*N*-butyl-*N*-(4-hydroxybutyl)nitrosamine [NBBN], aflatoxin B_1 or thiouracil) in the diet to evaluate carcinogenic synergy. Survival of lead-treated rats did not differ from that of controls. All animals underwent complete necropsy. Tissues were examined histologically, and only malignant tumours were tabulated [pathological type not specified]. No malignant renal tumours were found in the 213 male and 214 female control rats. In male rats treated with lead acetate alone, the incidence of malignant renal tumours was 0/24, 11/24 [statistically significant, two-tailed Fisher's exact test, $p < 0.05$], and 19/24 [statistically significant; two-tailed Fisher's exact test, $p < 0.05$; χ^2 test for trend, $p < 0.0001$] in animals that received 500 ppm, 2000 ppm and 8000 ppm lead, respectively. In female rats treated with lead acetate alone, the incidence of malignant renal tumours was 0/24, 1/24, and 4/24 [statistically significant, two-tailed Fisher's exact test] in animals that received 500 ppm, 2000 ppm and 8000 ppm lead, respectively. No carcinogenic interactions were observed between lead and NBBN, aflatoxin B_1 or thiouracil.

(*b*) *Subcutaneous administration*

In a study undertaken by Teraki and Uchiumi (1990) to analyse the metal content in metal-induced injection-site tumours, a group of 13 male Fischer 344/NSle rats, 5 weeks of age, received subcutaneous dorsal injections of 60 mg/kg bw lead acetate [purity unspecified] in distilled water weekly for 5 weeks. Another group of 13 rats was injected with saline and served as controls. Rats were observed for 80 weeks following the start of the injections [survival data not given]. [Although not explicitly stated, histological analysis appears to have been performed.] Of the rats injected with lead acetate and available for review, 42% [probably five rats with tumours/12 rats injected] developed injection-site sarcomas [No data were given for the incidence of injection-site tumours in controls and the Working Group noted the incomplete reporting of experimental details.]

(*c*) *Administration of lead with known carcinogens or modifiers of carcinogenesis*

Hinton *et al.* (1979) fed groups of 150 male Fischer 344 rats, weighing 125–175 g [age unspecified], unaltered diet (control) or diets containing 1% lead as lead acetate [purity unspecified], 0.04% *N*-(4′-fluoro-4-biphenyl) acetamide (FBPA) or 1% lead acetate plus FBPA. Ten to 20 rats from each group were killed after 3, 7 and 14 days and 4, 8, 16, 24, 36 and 52 weeks of exposure [survival unspecified] and a gross examination of the kidneys and livers for the appearance of tumours was made. This revealed one mass in the kidney of a rat fed lead acetate alone for 52 weeks. Lead acetate treatment also appeared to increase FBPA-induced gross renal tumour multiplicity [not statistically evaluated]. Upon histological examination, these lesions were confirmed as renal adenocarcinomas. [The Working Group noted that the experimental design and reporting was insufficient to evaluate the role of lead acetate on FBPA-induced carcinogenesis.]

Tanner and Lipsky (1984) fed groups of male Fischer 344 rats [initial group size of 50 but substantially reduced due to lead-induced mortality], weighing 125–175 g, diets containing either 10 000 ppm lead as lead acetate [purity unspecified], 400 ppm FBPA, FBPA plus lead, or unaltered diet (control). Five to 10 animals per group were killed after 16, 24, 36 and 52 weeks of feeding and kidneys were examined microscopically. No details were given on survival. The number of control animals killed at each time point was 5–10 [exact number unspecified]. No renal lesions were seen in the controls at any time. The incidence of renal hyperplasia, adenoma and adenocarcinoma was reported irrespective of concurrent lesions in the same animal. Of the 26 rats fed FBPA alone, 19 had hyperplasia, eight had adenomas and eight had carcinomas. Of the 29 rats fed lead alone, 21 had hyperplasia, two had adenomas and one had an adenocarcinoma. Of the 27 rats fed FBPA and lead, 27 had hyperplasia, 18 had adenomas and 10 had carcinomas. Statistical evaluation was not carried out. [The Working Group noted the incomplete reporting and the high early mortality of the treated rats.]

Koller *et al.* (1985) gave groups of 7–16 male weanling Sprague-Dawley rats 0, 26 or 2600 ppm lead as lead acetate [purity unspecified] in drinking-water continuously for a total of 76 weeks. Twenty-eight weeks after start of lead acetate exposure, each group was simultaneously exposed to diets containing sodium nitrite (6.36 g/kg diet) and ethyl urea (2.0 g/kg diet) for 20 weeks and thereafter to unaltered diet until the end of the study (76 weeks). A control group received unaltered water and feed, and a group received 2600 ppm lead acetate alone for 76 weeks. Of the lead-exposed animals, 3/36 were lost to observation due to early death. All rats were subjected to histological examination. Renal tumours occurred with the following incidence (tumour bearing rats/number of rats examined): control, 0/7; ethyl urea and sodium nitrite only, 0/8; 26 ppm lead acetate plus ethyl urea and sodium nitrite, 0/7; 2600 ppm lead acetate plus ethyl urea and sodium nitrite, 6/10 [statistically significant versus controls, two-tailed Fisher's exact test]; 2600 ppm lead acetate only, 13/16 [statistically significant versus controls, two-tailed Fisher's exact test]. All kidney tumours were classified as renal tubule carcinomas with the exception of a clear cell adenoma in the group of rats treated with 2600 ppm lead plus ethyl urea and sodium nitrite.

Nogueira (1987) fed groups of 10–12 male Wistar rats, 6 weeks of age, diets containing 0 (control), 0.5 or 1.0% lead acetate [purity unspecified] for up to 24 weeks. Separate groups were given 0.01 or 0.025% *N*-nitrosodiethylamine (NDEA) in water at a dose of 5 mg/kg per day [presumably 5 mg of solution/kg per day by intubation] with or without 0.5 or 1.0% lead acetate. Lead acetate did not appear to affect NDEA-induced carcinogenesis.

In a study of the effects of calcium and lead on blood pressure, Bogden *et al.* (1991) fed groups of 4–8 male weanling Wistar rats diets containing either 0.2% or 4.0% calcium. The animals were given drinking-water containing 0, 1 or 100 μg/mL lead as lead acetate [purity unspecified]. After 31 weeks, rats were killed and one kidney from each rat was prepared for histological examination. Proliferative lesions of the kidney were observed only in rats fed the 4.0% calcium diet and given 100 μg/mL lead in drinking-water; among five rats there were three with transition cell hyperplasia and two with invasive carcinoma. [The Working Group noted the small group sizes.]

3.1.3 *Dog*

Azar *et al.* (1973) fed groups of four male and four female beagle dogs [age unspecified] diets containing 0 (control), 10, 50, 100 and 500 ppm lead acetate [purity unspecified] for 2 years, at which time the experiment was terminated. These doses of lead did not affect weight gain or mortality. A complete necropsy with histological examination was carried out on all animals. There were no pathological effects of dietary lead in any organ system in the females. Two male dogs fed 500 ppm lead showed a slight degree of cytomegaly in the proximal convoluted tubule of the kidneys. No tumours of any type were reported. [The Working Group noted the small group sizes and the short duration of treatment.]

3.1.4 *Monkey*

A case of a rhesus macaque (*Macaca mulatta*) that developed chronic myelocytic leukaemia after having been exposed to lead acetate has been reported by Krugner-Higby *et al.* (2001). The malignancy occurred in a female monkey that had received daily oral exposures to lead for a total of 2 years in order to achieve a target blood lead concentration of 35 μg/dL. Beginning at day 8 postpartum and continuing for the next 6 months, lead was given to the monkey mixed in a commercial milk formula [dose unspecified]. After weaning at 6 months, lead was administered in a fruit-flavoured diet for an additional 18 months [dose unspecified]. Regular blood samples were drawn to test for blood lead concentrations. The mean concentration of lead in blood over the lifetime of the leukaemic macaque was 37.6 μg/dL. The first symptoms of haematopoietic abnormality developed when the monkey was 25 months of age and, after an attempt at chemotherapeutic intervention, the animal was sacrificed 4 months later. The author noted that this was the first report of chronic myelocytic leukaemia in this species and that it is a rare malignancy in non-human primates. The animal was seronegative for several retroviruses that have been associated with lymphoid neoplasia in non-human primates.

3.2 Lead subacetate

3.2.1 *Mouse*

(*a*) *Oral administration*

Van Esch and Kroes (1969) fed groups of 25 male and 25 female Swiss mice, 5 weeks of age, diets containing either 0 (control), 0.1% or 1.0% lead subacetate [purity unspecified] for up to 2 years. The higher dose caused an early decrease in survival. Although the dose was reduced to 0.5% at 92 days of treatment for male mice and 114 days for female mice, few animals survived beyond 1 year. Survival was similar in controls and mice fed 0.1% lead subacetate. In the latter group, histological examination showed renal tumours in six males (two adenomas, four carcinomas) and one female (adenoma) while none occurred in controls. One carcinoma occurred in a female fed 1.0/0.5% lead subacetate. [The Working Group noted that the number of mice subjected to pathological analysis was not specified].

Stoner *et al.* (1986) gave groups of 16 male and 16 female strain A/J mice, 6–8 weeks of age, three oral doses of lead subacetate [purity unspecified] per week for up to 24 weeks (total dose, 190 mg/kg bw) and compared them with untreated controls. Of the lead-treated mice, 81% of the females and 100% of the males survived to the end of the study. At the end of the experiment, lungs were removed, fixed, and gross lesions representing lung tumours were counted. A few lesions were subjected to histological examination to confirm typical histopathology of pulmonary adenoma. Lead subacetate-treated mice did not show a significant lung tumour response.

(*b*) *Intraperitoneal administration*

In an earlier study, Stoner *et al.* (1976) gave groups of 20 male and female strain A/Strong mice, 6–8 weeks of age, intraperitoneal injections of lead subacetate (> 97% pure) dissolved in tricaprylin, three times per week for 5 weeks (total doses, 30, 75 or 150 mg/kg bw) and observed them for up to 30 weeks after the first injection. The high dose was considered to be a maximum tolerated dose. Of the lead-treated mice, 60–75% survived to the end of the study compared with 90% of the controls. At the end of the experiment, lungs were removed, fixed, and gross lesions representing lung adenomas were counted. A few lesions were subjected to histological examination and confirmed the typical histopathology of pulmonary adenoma. Lung tumour multiplicity (average number of tumours/mouse) was increased approximately threefold in mice given the highest dose of lead subacetate compared with controls given vehicle alone (1.47 ± 0.38 versus 0.50 ± 0.12; $p < 0.05$, Student's *t*-test) (Stoner *et al.*, 1976; Shimkin *et al.*, 1977).

Poirier *et al.* (1984) gave groups of 30 (equal numbers of male and female) strain A/Strong mice, 6–8 weeks of age, intraperitoneal injections of lead subacetate (reagent grade) dissolved in tricaprylin (0.04 mmol/kg per injection) three times per week (total of 20 injections; total dose, 0.8 mmol/kg) and observed them for up to 30 weeks after the first injection. This dose schedule was said to constitute a maximum tolerated dose of lead in this strain of mouse. To define potential antagonism, separate groups received intraperitoneal injections of calcium acetate or magnesium acetate at 1:1, 3:1 and 10:1 molar ratios with lead subacetate. Calcium or magnesium were admixed with the lead prior to injection and given with the same dosage schedule as lead subacetate. Survival of mice to the end of the study was 70–87% in controls, 67% in mice treated with lead alone and 53–77% in mice treated with combined calcium and lead. Survival ranged from 43–60% in mice given magnesium at 3:1 or 10:1 molar ratios with lead. When magnesium was given as an equimolar mixture with lead, only 1/30 mice survived, preventing further analysis of this group. At the end of the experiment, surviving animals were killed, lungs were removed and fixed, and gross lesions representing lung adenomas were counted. A few lesions were subjected to histological examination and confirmed the typical histopathology of pulmonary adenoma. Lead alone caused a significant increase ($p < 0.05$, Student's *t*-test) in lung tumour multiplicity compared with controls (0.86 ± 0.20 versus

0.32 ± 0.12). At all doses used, calcium significantly reduced lead-induced increases in lung tumour multiplicity ($p < 0.05$). In the study with magnesium, lead alone caused a significant increase in lung tumour multiplicity ($p < 0.05$) compared with mice given the vehicle while magnesium given at molar ratios of 3:1 or 10:1 with lead significantly reduced lead-induced increases in lung tumour multiplicity ($p < 0.05$).

Stoner *et al.* (1986) gave groups of 16 male and 16 female strain A/J mice, 6–8 weeks of age, intraperitoneal injections of lead subacetate [purity unspecified] dissolved in water three times per week for up to 24 weeks (total doses, 38, 95 or 190 mg/kg bw) and compared them with water-treated controls. Of the lead-treated mice, 81–100% survived except in the group of males that received the high dose, of which only 3/16 (19%) survived to the end of the study. At the end of the experiment, surviving animals were killed, lungs were removed and fixed, and gross lesions representing lung tumours were counted. A few lesions were subjected to histological examination and confirmed the typical histopathology of pulmonary adenoma. Lung tumour multiplicity was significantly increased in the males at the low dose (38 mg/kg bw; 0.5 ± 0.18) and at the high dose (190 mg/kg bw; 0.67 ± 0.33), compared with controls (0.07 ± 0.07) ($p < 0.05$; Wilcoxon nonparametric rank test). The four other lead-treated groups did not show a significant lung tumour response. [The Working Group noted the mortality in the high dose-treated male group.]

(*c*) *Administration of lead with known carcinogens or modifiers of carcinogenesis*

Sakai *et al.* (1990) gave groups of 14–18 of male ddy mice [age unspecified], weighing 22–24 g, weekly intraperitoneal injections of 10 mg/kg bw lead subacetate [purity, > 99.99%] suspended in 50% glycerine solution for 18 weeks with or without either two or three intraperitoneal injections of 10 mg/kg bw *N*-nitrosodimethylamine (NDMA) in saline per week. Controls received injections of vehicles alone (saline and 50% glycerine solution). The treatments did not affect survival [test unspecified]. Lung tumours were evaluated histologically [stage was not specified, but included adenomas and adenocarcinomas]. Control mice and mice given lead alone did not develop lung tumours. Although lead did not alter NDMA-induced lung tumour incidence, lung tumour multiplicity was significantly increased in groups given lead compared with those that received NDMA alone. Animals given two injections of NDMA per week developed an average of 0.33 tumours/lung compared with 0.78 tumours/lung in mice also receiving lead ($p < 0.05$, Student's *t*-test) [descriptive statistics not given]. Mice injected three times a week with NDMA developed an average of 3.4 tumours/lung compared with 5.7 tumours/lung in mice also receiving lead subacetate ($p < 0.05$, Student's *t*-test) [standard errors not given].

3.2.2 *Rat*

(*a*) *Oral administration*

Van Esch *et al.* (1962) fed groups of 11–16 male and 11–16 female Wistar rats [age incompletely specified] diets containing 0.1% lead subacetate [purity unspecified] or unaltered diet (control) for 29 months or 1.0% lead subacetate or unaltered diet (control) for 24 months. Both concentrations of lead reduced body weight ($p < 0.005$, Wilcoxon's test) and 1.0% dietary lead subacetate reduced survival [test unspecified]. The incidence of renal tumours in rats fed 0.1% lead subacetate was 5/16 in males and 6/16 in females compared with 0/14 in control males and 0/15 in control females [incidences in both males and females were significantly elevated, Fisher's exact test]. The incidence of renal tumours in rats fed 1.0% lead subacetate was 6/13 in males and 7/11 in females compared with 0/13 in control males and 0/13 in control females [incidences in both males and females were significantly elevated, Fisher's exact test; χ^2 test for trend for both male and female, and $p < 0.006$ and $p < 0.0004$ respectively]. Three carcinomas occurred in rats fed 0.1% lead subacetate and six occurred in rats fed 1.0% lead subacetate; the remainder were adenomas. In the group fed 1.0% lead subacetate, one animal had a carcinoma with multiple metastases.

Mao and Molnar (1967) fed a group of 40 male Wistar rats (weighing ~200 g) [age unspecified] a diet containing 1% lead subacetate [purity unspecified] and a group of 20 rats an unaltered diet. Rats were killed or died from 238 to 690 days (controls) or from 213 to 677 days (lead-treated) [average survival unspecified]. Necropsies were performed on all animals and kidneys were examined histologically. Evaluation [presumably of the kidney only] revealed a single renal sarcoma among the 20 control rats while 31/40 lead-treated rats developed renal tumours [significantly different from controls, Fisher's exact test], including adenomas and carcinomas. One lead-treated rat with a renal tumour showed a pulmonary metastasis.

In a study by Oyasu *et al.* (1970) in which the effects of 2-acetylaminofluorene (2-AAF) in combination with lead subactate was studied, two groups of male CD Sprague-Dawley rats, 5–8 weeks of age, were fed diets containing 1.0 % lead subacetate [purity unspecified] or 1.0% lead subacetate and 1.6% indole and were observed for 12–17 months. Average survival in these groups was 53–69 weeks. A pool of various control groups (age range, 58–67 weeks) was used, including a mixed group of 130 male and female CD Sprague-Dawley ex-breeders over 60 weeks of age, a mixed group of 155 male and female CD Sprague-Dawley rats fed unaltered diets, 23 Wistar rats [sex unspecified] fed 3.2% indole in the diet and 17 CD Sprague-Dawley rats [sex unspecified] fed unaltered diets but whose cerebrum was damaged by focal freezing. Necropsy and histological examination was performed on all animals. The authors pooled the groups of rats fed lead subacetate alone with those fed lead acetate plus indole for statistical analysis. The reported incidence (tumour bearing rats/rats examined) of cerebral gliomas was: 1/325 (0.3%) in control rats; and 5/58 (8.6%) ($p < 0.05$, test unspecified) in rats fed either lead subacetate alone or lead subacetate plus indole. Two of 17 rats fed lead subacetate alone developed gliomas and 3/41 rats fed lead subacetate + indole developed gliomas. [The Working Group considered there were only 285 untreated controls, in which one glioma occurred.] The incidence of renal cortical tumours [pathological stage undefined] was: 13/17 (76%) in rats fed lead subacetate alone and 25/41 (61%) in rats fed lead subacetate plus indole. The incidence of renal tumours in controls was not reported. [The Working Group noted the unusual design of analysis and incomplete reporting of this investigation.]

In a study of the histopathology of chemically-induced renal tumours carried out by Ito *et al.* (1971), a group of 10 male Wistar rats, 6–8 weeks of age, was fed 1.5% lead subacetate [purity unspecified] in the diet for 48 weeks and renal tumours were assessed histologically. All 10 rats developed either renal adenomas (60%) or renal carcinomas (40%). [The Working Group noted the absence of a control group.]

In another study by Ito (1973) focusing on the histopathology of tumours of the urinary system of rats, groups of 11–13 male Wistar rats, 6–8 weeks of age, some of which were also subjected to unilateral nephrectomy, were fed 1.5% lead subacetate [purity unspecified] in the diet for 23 weeks (intact or nephrectomized) or 48 weeks (intact). Tumours of the urinary system were assessed histologically. In the 13 intact rats fed the lead subacetate-containing diet for 23 weeks, no renal tumours were observed while 2/11 lead subacetate-treated unilaterally-nephrectomized rats developed renal tumours. After 48 weeks of exposure, renal tumours developed in 9/11 lead subacetate-treated intact rats. Lead subacetate-induced tumours were either renal-cell adenomas (64%) or carcinomas (36%). [The Working Group noted the absence of control groups.]

In a study performed by Kasprzak *et al.* (1985) of the effects of dietary calcium on the carcinogenicity of lead subacetate in the kidney, groups of 28–30 male Sprague-Dawley rats were fed 1% lead subacetate (AR grade) admixed with 0, 0.3, 1, 3 or 6% calcium acetate in the diet and observed for 79 weeks. Controls received unaltered basal diet and a separate group was fed 3% calcium acetate alone. All additions to the basal diet caused significant suppression of weight gain ranging from 7 to 46% ($p < 0.05$, Student's *t*-test). No significant differences in survival were observed (two-tailed Fisher's exact test). At the time of the detection of the first renal tumour (58 weeks), surviving rats were killed, tissues were examined microscopically and renal tumour incidence was determined. Renal tumours did not occur in control rats or rats fed calcium alone. In rats fed lead subacetate alone, 13/29 (45%) developed renal tumours [statistically significant; Fisher's exact test, $p < 0.05$] including 11 adenomas and two adenocarcinomas. Addition of 0.3, 1, 3 or 6% calcium (calcium reduced renal lead content by up to 72%) to the diet significantly increased ($p = 0.035$–0.014, two-tailed Fisher's exact test) the incidence of renal tumours in lead-treated rats to 62–79%. The number of rats with bilateral renal tumours was also significantly increased ($p < 0.05$, two-tailed Fisher's exact test) in comparison with rats treated with lead subacetate alone.

(*b*) *Administration of lead with known carcinogens or modifiers of carcinogenesis*

The effects of lead subacetate in combination with 2-AAF, indole or boiled linseed oil containing 'lead drier' [lead drier is a compound made of lead, cobalt and manganese naphthenates that was added to improve the drying qualities of oil-based paints made with boiled linseed oil] on renal carcinogenesis were studied by Hass *et al.* (1967) in male CD rats, 6–8 weeks of age. For up to 74 weeks the animals were fed diets supplemented with two or more of the following components: 0.06% 2-AAF, 1.6% indole, 1.0% lead subacetate [specified as 'chemically pure'] and 10.0 g/100 mL [presumably mL of diet] commercial boiled linseed oil containing 'lead drier'. Some animals in each group were killed at 52 weeks. The concentrations of naphthenates in the linseed oil were given as 0.20% lead, 0.35% manganese and 0.30% cobalt. In total, 64 rats received 2-AAF plus indole, 24 rats received lead subacetate plus indole, 50 rats received lead subacetate, indole and linseed oil, and 74 rats received lead subacetate, 2-AAF, indole and linseed oil. A few rats died during exposure [precise survival and body weight data not given]. Complete autopsies were done and tissues from all tumours were examined microscopically. None of the animals fed diets containing 2-AAF and indole developed renal tumours. All of the groups fed diets containing lead subacetate developed renal cortical tumours. Of the 24 rats fed lead subacetate plus indole, 22 had 'cystomas' [presumably cystic adenomas], 19 had adenomas [presumably solid adenomas] and 11 (46%) had adenocarcinomas. Of the 50 rats fed lead acetate, indole and linseed oil, 30 had cystomas, 20 had adenomas and 14 (28%) had adenocarcinomas. Of the 74 rats fed lead subacetate, indole, linseed oil and 2-AAF, 37 had cystomas, 29 had adenomas and 25 (34%) had adenocarcinomas. [The Working Group noted the absence of a control group or a group receiving lead subacetate alone].

Oyasu *et al.* (1970) fed three groups of male CD Sprague-Dawley rats, 5–8 weeks of age, diets containing 1.0 % lead subacetate [purity unspecified], or 1.0% lead subacetate and 1.6% indole, or 1.0% lead subacetate, 1.6% indole (added to prolong the lifespan of 2-AAF-treated rats) and 2-AAF. The animals were observed for 12–17 months. Average survival was 53–69 weeks. Histological examination was performed on all animals that died or were killed at the end of the experiment. For statistical analysis the authors pooled the groups of rats fed lead subacetate alone with those fed lead acetate plus indole. The reported incidence (tumour bearing rats/rats examined) of cerebral gliomas was 5/58 (8.6%) in rats fed either lead subacetate alone or lead subacetate plus indole (2/17 rats fed lead subacetate alone developed gliomas and 3/41 rats fed lead subacetate + indole developed gliomas), and 6/72 (8.3%) in rats fed lead subacetate, indole and 2-AAF. The incidence of renal cortical tumours [pathological stage undefined] was 13/17 (76%) in rats fed lead subacetate alone; 25/41 (61%) in rats fed lead subacetate plus indole, and 36/72 (50%) in rats fed lead subacetate, indole and 2-AAF. [The Working Group noted the unusual design of analysis and incomplete reporting of this investigation.]

Hiasa *et al.* (1983) studied the development of renal tumours in groups of 17–24 male Wistar rats, 6 weeks of age, fed diets containing 500 or 1000 ppm *N*-ethyl-*N*-hydroxyethylnitrosamine (EHEN) for 2 weeks followed by 1000 ppm lead subacetate (purity, 99.5%) for 20 weeks with an additional observation period of 10 weeks (total duration, 32 weeks). Two groups were fed EHEN alone (1000 ppm) and lead subacetate alone, respectively. Controls received unaltered diets for 32 weeks. Rats that died before the end of the study were excluded from evaluation; these included two rats given EHEN alone and four rats given EHEN plus lead subacetate. All groups fed lead subacetate and the group fed 1000 ppm EHEN alone showed significant reduction ($p < 0.05$, test unspecified) of final body weight (maximum, 14%). Histological examination revealed the following renal tumour incidence (tumour-bearing rats/rats examined): 500 ppm EHEN, 0/24; 1000 ppm EHEN, 9/18 ($p < 0.05$ versus control, χ^2 test); 500 ppm EHEN plus lead subacetate, 10/22 ($p < 0.05$ versus 500 ppm EHEN alone); 1000 ppm EHEN plus lead subacetate, 17/17 ($p < 0.05$ versus 1000 ppm EHEN alone); lead subacetate alone, 0/24; control 0/24. No adenocarcinomas occurred in rats fed EHEN alone, one renal adenocarcinoma occurred in a rat fed EHEN 500 ppm plus lead subacetate and 10 adenocarcinomas in rats fed 1000 ppm EHEN and lead subacetate. [The Working Group noted the short duration of the study for the assessment of lead-induced tumours.]

The effects of various nephrotoxic chemicals, including lead subacetate, in promoting EHEN-induced renal carcinogenesis were studied by Shirai *et al.* (1984) in groups of 23–25 male Fischer 344 rats [age unspecified; weighing ~130 g] that were given 0.1% EHEN in the drinking-water for 1 week followed by 0.1% lead subacetate [purity unspecified] in the diet for 35 weeks. A separate group received lead subacetate alone from week 2 to week 36. All rats were subjected to unilateral nephrectomy during the third week of the experiment. All rats were killed after 36 weeks and five transverse kidney sections from each animal were taken for histological evaluation. Lead subacetate alone did not induce renal tumours. EHEN alone induced renal-cell tumours [size and histology unspecified] in 5/23 rats (22%); exposure to lead subacetate after EHEN increased the incidence of renal-cell tumours to 13/25 ($p < 0.05$ versus EHEN alone, test unspecified). [The Working Group noted that no untreated control group was included and noted the short duration of the study for the assessment of lead subacetate-induced tumours.]

Groups of 15 male Wistar rats, 6 weeks of age, were fed diets containing 1000 ppm EHEN for 2 weeks. Unilateral nephrectomies were then performed on all rats and they were provided with unaltered diets or diets containing 1000 ppm lead subacetate [purity unspecified] for up to 18 additional weeks. Five animals from each group were killed at weeks 8, 12 and 20 of the experiment. In rats given EHEN alone, 2/15 had simple renal hyperplasia (hyperplasia with a tubular pattern), 0/15 had renal 'adenomatous hyperplasia' (hyperplasia with loss of tubular pattern) and 0/15 had renal tumours. In rats given EHEN plus lead subacetate, 11/15 had simple hyperplasia, 8/15 had adenomatous hyperplasia and 1/15 had a renal-cell tumour. Incidence and multiplicity (lesions/rat) of simple hyperplasia was increased in the rats fed EHEN plus lead and killed at week 20 versus rats fed EHEN alone ($p < 0.05$, tests unspecified) (Hiasa *et al.*, 1991; Nishii 1993). [The Working Group noted that no untreated control group was included and noted the short duration of the study for the assessment of lead subacetate-induced tumours.]

3.2.3 *Hamster*

Van Esch and Kroes (1969) fed groups of 22 male and 23–24 female Syrian golden hamsters, 3–4 weeks of age, either 0 (control), 0.1 or 0.5% lead subacetate [purity unspecified] in the diet for up to 2 years. The higher dose in females and both doses in males appeared to reduce survival, mostly during the first year [not statistically evaluated]. At the end of the experiment all animals were killed and underwent histological examination. No renal tumours or hyperplasia occurred in any group, although pleomorphic cells with hypertrophic nuclei were commonly observed in the kidneys of lead-treated hamsters.

3.2.4 *Rabbit*

Hass *et al.* (1967) fed a total of 85 male rabbits (primarily New Zealand albino with a few German Checker and Belgian Hare), 3 months of age, diets containing 0.5–1.0% lead subacetate (specified as chemically pure) for 3–78 weeks. Twenty-one animals received lead alone while the others were given various other compounds (linseed oil containing lead drier, 2-AAF, cholesterol, chloroform, carbon tetrachloride and vitamin D) in the diet or by injection. Precise survival and body weight data were not given. None of the lead-treated rabbits developed renal tumours, although chronic lead nephropathy was common. [The Working Group noted the absence of a control group, the use of a variety of strains of rabbits and the incomplete reporting of the study.]

3.3 Lead carbonate

3.3.1 *Rat*

Oral administration

Fairhall and Miller (1941) fed male albino rats, 70–90 g, [strain and age unspecified] diets that contained 0.1% lead arsenate (49 rats) (see section 3.10 for assessment of the lead arsenate experiment) or an equivalent amount of lead as lead carbonate (55 rats) for up to 2 years. A control group of 24 rats of similar age and weight was fed the same diet without the test substances. At the end of the first year, approximately half of the surviving rats in each group were killed, and tissues were taken for histological examination. The remaining rats in each group were maintained on the same treatments and were killed at the end of the second year; their tissues were examined similarly. Histological examinations performed at 1 and 2 years showed moderate to marked kidney changes (enlargement of cells in the convoluted tubules, intranuclear inclusions and accumulation of brown pigment in cells of the convoluted, proximal and distal tubules), but no tumours in the rats fed lead carbonate. No pathological changes of note were observed in other tissues and organs in the lead carbonate-treated rats compared with controls. No tumours were observed at any site in any of the groups. [The Working Group noted the incomplete reporting of the study.]

3.4 Lead nitrate

3.4.1 *Mouse*

Administration of lead with known carcinogens or modifiers of carcinogenesis

Litvinov *et al.* (1984) gave groups of 50 female CBA × C57/BL6 mice [age unspecified] 10 mg/L NDMA or 0.3 mg/L lead nitrate or both compounds together in drinking-water for either 26 or 39 weeks. None of the mice receiving lead nitrate alone for 39 weeks developed tumours. Treatment with lead nitrate did not appear to impact NDMA-induced renal tumours. [The Working Group noted the short duration of the study for assessment of lead-induced tumours.]

3.4.2 *Rat*

(*a*) *Oral administration*

Schroeder *et al.* (1970) gave groups of male Long-Evans rats [age and initial number unspecified] 25 ppm lead nitrate (25 mg/L lead) in the drinking-water from weaning until death. An epidemic of pneumonia of 3 weeks duration killed 22 lead-treated rats and 19 controls. Sufficient rats survived in each group (52 lead-treated rats and 52 controls) to continue the experiment. After corrections for the early mortality, the survival of lead-treated rats was lower ($p < 0.05$) than that of the controls. Grossly visible tumours [type and location unspecified] were found in 7/43 lead-treated rats at necropsy; the tumour incidence (10/50) in controls was not significantly different. [The Working Group noted the low dose of lead nitrate that was used and the incomplete reporting of this experiment.]

(*b*) *Administration of lead with known carcinogens or modifiers of carcinogenesis*

Litvinov *et al.* (1982) gave groups of 50 albino outbred male rats, weighing 150–200 g, NDMA in the drinking-water (effective dose, 0.5 mg/kg bw per day) alone or in the presence of lead nitrate (0.5 mg/L drinking-water). A group of 50 control rats were given drinking-water only; no group treated with lead nitrate alone was available. The experiment lasted 19 months. A complete necropsy was performed on all animals and tissues were examined histologically. No renal or liver tumours occurred in control animals. Renal tumours occurred in 8/42 rats treated with NDMA alone and in 19/41 rats treated with NDMA and lead nitrate. Liver tumours occurred in 15/42 rats receiving NDMA alone compared with 5/41 rats receiving NDMA and lead nitrate combined. The authors concluded that lead nitrate increased the incidence of kidney tumours and decreased the incidence of liver tumours.

3.5 Lead powder

3.5.1 *Rat*

(*a*) *Oral administration*

Furst *et al.* (1976) gave groups of 25 male and 25 female young Fischer 344 rats [age unspecified] weighing ≤ 119 g, lead powder (99.9% pure; 10 mg lead; particle size unspecified) in corn oil by stomach tube twice a month for 12 months and observed them for 24 months. Groups of 20 male and 20 female control rats were given 0.5 mL corn oil by stomach tube according to the same schedule. A complete necropsy was performed on all of the animals that were killed and included histological examination of suspicious tissues. Survival data were not reported. One lymphoma and four leukaemias were found at necropsy in 47 lead powder-treated rats; this did not differ significantly from the incidence of three lymphomas found at necropsy of 29 controls. No other neoplasms were reported in the lead powder-treated or control rats.

(*b*) *Intramuscular administration*

In a similar experiment, Furst *et al.* (1976) gave groups of 25 male and 25 female young Fischer 344 rats [age unspecified], weighing ≤ 111 g, monthly intramuscular injections of 10 mg lead powder (99.9% pure; particle size unspecified) in trioctanoin for 9 months and then monthly injections of 5 mg lead powder for 3 months and observed the animals until the end of the experiment (24 months). Equal numbers of rats were given the trioctanoin vehicle alone and served as controls. A complete necropsy was performed on all animals that were killed and included histological examination of suspicious tissues. Fibrosarcomas developed at the injection site in one of the lead powder-treated rats and in one of the control rats. The incidences of lymphoma were 6/50 in the lead powder-treated rats and 3/50 in the trioctanoin-treated controls. The authors noted the following tumours in the lead powder-treated rats that were not seen in the controls: a metastasis of an osteogenic sarcoma in the lungs without primary site identification, a mesothelioma of the urogenital tract and two tumours of the pancreas (a fibrolipoma and a villous adenoma). Statistical analyses were not reported, but the authors concluded that 'lead powder did not seem to produce any appreciable number of tumours'.

(*c*) *Intrarenal administration*

Jasmin and Riopelle (1976) gave a group of 20 young female Sprague-Dawley rats, weighing 120–140 g, injections of 5 mg lead powder [purity and particle size not specified] suspended in 50 μL glycerine into the cortical sections of both poles of the right kidney (total dose, 10 mg lead powder/rat). A negative control group of 16 rats received similar intrarenal injections of 50 μL glycerine alone and a positive control group of 16 rats received intrarenal injections of 5 mg nickel subsulfide powder (total dose, 10 mg/rat) in 50 μL glycerine. The experiment lasted 12 months, during which time the animals were examined at regular intervals for development of erythrocytosis and renal tumours. All of the kidneys were removed at necropsy for histological examination. No erythrocytosis or renal tumours developed in the lead powder-treated rats or in the negative controls, whereas marked erythrocytosis ($p < 0.05$ versus controls) developed in all of the 16 positive control rats, and renal carcinomas were found in 7/16 of these near the nickel subsulfide injection sites [p-value not reported].

3.6 Lead oxide

3.6.1 *Rat*

Inhalation exposure

Monchaux *et al.* (1997) exposed a group of 50 male Sprague-Dawley rats, 12 weeks of age, to lead oxide particles [purity unspecified] (mean particle size, 0.69 μm; mass median aerodynamic diameter (MMAD), 5.1 μm) in a whole-body chamber. The mean airborne concentration of lead oxide measured within the chamber was 5.3 ± 1.7 mg/m^3, and rats were exposed for 6 h per day on 5 days per week for 1 year. The authors estimated that this exposure was approximately equivalent to the dose of oral lead acetate that would give rise to a 10% incidence of kidney cancers in rats, according to the experiments of Azar *et al.* (1973). A group of 785 untreated rats served as the control. In addition to the rats treated with lead oxide alone, a group of 63 rats was initially exposed to 0.6 Gy fission neutrons by placing the animals at a distance of 4 m from a Silene experimental reactor core (time unspecified); another group of 50 rats was exposed to fission neutrons and 2 months later to lead oxide by inhalation. A fifth group of 25 rats was exposed to lead oxide by inhalation and then received six intramuscular injections of 25 mg/kg bw 5–6 benzoflavone (βNF) [schedule unspecified] for lung tumour promotion starting 1 month after lead exposure ended. All animals were kept until moribund [precise survival time unspecified] except those exposed to lead oxide and βNF, which were killed 100 days after the last injection of βNF. A complete necropsy was performed on each animal. Lungs were fixed by intratracheal instillation of fixative. Lead oxide exposure did not reduce survival compared with controls. No lung tumours occurred. One renal tumour occurred among the group of animals receiving lead oxide alone. The addition of βNF did not alter lead oxide-induced tumours. Lead oxide did not alter cancer rates induced by neutron exposure.

3.6.2 *Hamster*

Intratracheal administration

Kobayashi and Okamoto (1974) gave groups of 15 male and 15 female Syrian golden hamsters, 6 weeks of age, intratracheal instillations weekly for 10 weeks of either 1 mg lead oxide powder (99.8% purity; particle diameter < 20 μm), or a mixture of 1 mg benzo[*a*]pyrene and lead oxide, or 1 mg benzo[*a*]pyrene alone. Each treatment sample was suspended in 0.2 mL isotonic saline plus 0.5% carboxymethylcellulose solution. One group received vehicle alone. All suspensions were ultrasonicated and homogenized, so that the final size of most of the particles (95%) within the mixture was < 10 μm. Fifteen males and 15 females were kept as untreated controls. The hamsters were killed when moribund or at 60 weeks after the initial intratracheal instillation. The hamsters treated with lead oxide alone, benzo[*a*]pyrene alone or the combination showed lower survival rates than those that received the vehicle alone or untreated controls. At necropsy, in addition to examination of any visible tumour foci, the five pulmonary lobes of each hamster were sectioned for histological examination. Atypical epithelial proliferations, adenomas (11 in males and females) and an adenocarcinoma (in a female) were observed in the lungs of hamsters given benzo[*a*]pyrene mixed with lead oxide. The neoplastic changes originated mostly in the bronchiolo-alveolar area. No neoplastic changes were found in the other groups. Lead oxide alone induced hyperplastic and squamous metaplastic foci of the alveolar area, while benzo[*a*]pyrene alone affected the lung only slightly. Although statistical confirmation was not provided, the authors concluded that lead oxide showed a cocarcinogenic effect with benzo[*a*]pyrene in the bronchiolo-alveolar area of hamster lungs. [The Working Group noted that lead could have acted as a carrier for benzo[*a*]-pyrene as in other particle studies, but this does not exclude other lead-related mechanisms of carcinogenesis.]

3.7 Lead naphthenate

3.7.1 *Mouse*

Skin application

Baldwin *et al.* (1964) painted a 20% solution of lead naphthenate [purity unspecified] in benzene on shaved dorsal skin of a group of 59 adult male Schofield albino mice. The total dose of 6 mL was administered over 12 months as weekly or twice-weekly applications [dosing schedule unclear]. Kidney damage [no further details reported] was observed in treated animals and, after 648 days, less than 50% of the mice had survived. Of the 59 treated animals, two developed skin papillomas, one developed renal carcinoma and four showed tubular adenomas of the kidney. [The Working Group noted that no vehicle-control group was included and that a known carcinogen was used as the vehicle.]

3.8 Lead chromate

Chromium[VI] was previously evaluated as *carcinogenic to humans* (Group 1) in the Monograph on Chromium and Chromium Compounds (IARC, 1990).

3.8.1 *Mouse*

Intramuscular administration

Furst *et al.* (1976) gave a group of 25 female weanling NIH-Swiss mice intramuscular injections of 3 mg/mouse lead chromate (98% pure) in trioctanoin (tricaprylin; total dose,

12 mg/mouse) monthly for 4 months. The authors noted that a higher dose (8 mg/mouse) of lead chromate was not tolerated. Two control groups of mice were included; one received the vehicle alone and the other served as uninjected controls. Necropsies were performed at termination of the study at around 25 months, and showed that 2/17 mice in the lead chromate-treated group had developed lymphoma and 3/17 had alveologenic carcinomas [further details not reported]. Necropsies of 22/25 mice in the vehicle-control group revealed two animals with lymphocytic leukaemia and one with an alveologenic carcinoma. In the uninjected controls, necropsies of 15/25 mice showed one lymphoma, five lymphocytic leukaemias and one alveologenic carcinoma. [The Working Group noted the incomplete reporting of the study.]

3.8.2 *Rat*

(*a*) *Subcutaneous injection*

Groups of 40 male and 40 female Sprague-Dawley rats, 13 weeks of age, were given a single subcutaneous injection of 30 mg/rat lead chromate (chromium yellow) or basic lead chromate (chromium orange) [purity unspecified] suspended in saline. Within 150 weeks, 26/40 animals injected with lead chromate and 27/40 injected with basic lead chromate had developed sarcomas (rhabdomyosarcomas and fibrosarcomas). No sarcomas developed in 60 control animals (Maltoni, 1976; Maltoni *et al.*, 1982).

(*b*) *Intramuscular administration*

Hueper (1961) gave a group of 33 rats [strain, age and sex unspecified] intramuscular implantations of lead chromate [amount and purity unspecified] in sheep fat. One tumour was reported at the implantation site [no further details stated]. None of the rats in two vehicle-control groups developed tumours. [The Working Group noted the incomplete reporting of the study.]

Furst *et al.* (1976) gave groups of 25 male and 25 female weanling Fischer 344 rats intramuscular injections of 8 mg lead chromate (98% pure) in trioctanoin (tricaprylin) once a month for 9 months. At the termination of the study at around 25 months, two lymphomas, 11 injection-site fibrosarcomas, 10 injection-site rhabdomyosarcomas and one osteogenic sarcoma had developed in 24 lead-chromate-treated female rats. Among 23 lead chromate-treated male rats, three injection-site fibrosarcomas, seven rhabdomyosarcomas and three renal carcinomas had developed. In the vehicle-control group, necropsy revealed two lymphomas among 16 females and one lymphocytic leukaemia and one injection-site fibrosarcoma among 12 males. [The Working Group noted the development of tumours of the kidney distant to the site of administration in male rats.]

(*c*) *Intrapleural administration*

Hueper (1961) also gave a group of 33 rats [strain, age and sex unspecified] intrapleural implantations of lead chromate [amount and purity unspecified] in sheep fat. Three tumours were reported at the implantation site [no further details stated]. None of the rats in two vehicle-control groups developed tumours. [The Working Group noted the incomplete reporting of the study.]

(*d*) *Intrabronchial administration*

In a study to investigate the potential carcinogenicity of a range of chromium-containing materials, groups of 50 male and 50 female Porton-Wistar rats, 8–10 weeks of age, received intrabronchial implantations of stainless-steel mesh pellets (5 × 1 mm) loaded with about 2 mg of a series of seven commercial types of lead chromate test materials (lead chromate (99.8% pure), primrose chrome yellow, Supra LD chrome yellow, molybdate chrome orange, light chrome yellow, medium chrome yellow and silica-encapsulated medium chrome yellow). The lead chromates contained between 60–64% lead with the exception of the silica-encapsulated medium chrome yellow (40% lead). Groups of 50 male and 50 female rats receiving pellets loaded with cholesterol alone acted as negative controls and similar groups receiving pellets loaded with 2 mg calcium chromate (96.7% purity) suspended in 50:50 cholesterol acted as positive controls. Animals were maintained for 24 months at which time surviving animals were killed and full necropsies were performed. All lungs and any suspected lesions were examined histologically. Survival was 95.7% at 400 days and overall, 53.9% at 700 days. No bronchial carcinomas (0/100) were seen in the cholesterol-alone control group whilst 25/100 bronchial carcinomas (24 squamous-cell carcinomas and one adenocarcinoma) were found in the calcium chromate positive control group. Among the seven lead chromates tested, one squamous-cell tumour of the lung was found in one male in each of the four groups which received lead chromate (99.8% pure), primrose chrome yellow, Supra LD chrome yellow or medium chrome yellow, respectively (in each of the four groups, incidence was 1/100, males and females combined; $p = 0.37$; χ^2 test) (Levy & Venitt, 1986; Levy *et al.*, 1986).

3.8.3 *Guinea-pig*

Intratracheal administration

Steffee and Baetjer (1965) gave a group of 13 guinea-pigs [strain and sex unspecified], 3 months of age, 0.3-mL intratracheal instillations of 1% lead chromate [purity and particle size unspecified] in saline at 3-monthly intervals for 18 months with no further exposure until death or termination of the experiment. After an experimental period of 40–50 months, none of the lead chromate-exposed animals and none of the vehicle-control animals (18 guinea-pigs) had developed pulmonary tumours. [The Working Group noted the small numbers of animals and the insufficient experimental details provided.]

3.8.4 *Rabbit*

Intratracheal administration

Steffee and Baetjer (1965) gave a group of seven rabbits [strain and sex unspecified], 4 months of age, 1-mL intratracheal instillations of 1% lead chromate [purity and particle size unspecified] in saline at 3-monthly intervals for 9–15 months with no further exposure until death or termination of the experiment. After an experimental period of 40–50 months, none of the lead chromate-exposed animals and none of the vehicle-control animals (five rabbits) had developed pulmonary tumours. [The Working Group noted the small numbers of animals and the insufficient experimental details provided.]

3.9 Lead phosphate

3.9.1 *Rat*

(*a*) *Subcutaneous injection*

Zollinger (1953) gave groups of 10 albino randomly-bred rats [strain, age and sex unspecified] weekly subcutaneous injections of 20 mg lead phosphate [purity unspecified] as a 2% suspension in 1 mL [vehicle unspecified] for up to 16 months (total doses, 40–760 mg/rat). No kidney epithelial tumours were reported for the 40 rats in an untreated control group. Among treated rats, many animals died during the experiment and the incidence of renal tumours (adenomas, cystadenomas, papillomas and cortical carcinomas) was 19/29 for rats surviving ≥ 10 months from the start of treatment. Each of the 19 had received a total dose of 120–680 mg lead phosphate. Histological analysis revealed that 21/112 treated rats had renal tumours (the earliest developing 4 months after the start of treatment), and in 11, the renal tumours were bilateral. The author reported that tumour incidence increased with time. [The Working Group noted the renal tumour response with a water-insoluble lead compound.]

Tönz (1957) gave groups of 36, 33, 14 and 29 albino rats [strain, age and sex unspecified] subcutaneous injections of 20 mg lead phosphate [purity unspecified] suspended in pectin weekly for up to 9.5 months and observed them for a total experimental period of up to 16.5 months after the start of the injections. Total doses were: 340 mg over 4 months; 440 mg over 4–9.5 months; 250 mg over a total experimental period of 10 months or less; and 360 mg from a total experimental period of 10 to 16.5 months; for the above four groups, respectively. Kidney weight increased in all animals given lead phosphate. All 36 rats that received a total dose of 340 mg and all 33 rats that received a total dose of 440 mg lead phosphate died during or shortly after the treatment. The incidences of renal adenomas and carcinomas were 19/29 and 3/29 respectively in the group that received an average total dose of 360 mg lead phosphate. Spontaneous epithelial kidney tumours were not observed in more than 2000 historical control animals in the author's laboratory. [The Working Group noted that no concurrent control group was included but noted the renal tumour response with a water-insoluble lead compound.]

Baló *et al.* (1965) gave a group of 80 albino rats [age and sex unspecified] subcutaneous injections of lead phosphate [purity and vehicle unspecified] at weekly or fortnightly intervals for 18 months. Rats surviving to the end of treatment had received a total dose of 1.3 g lead phosphate. Renal adenomas developed in 29 lead phosphate-treated rats and in none of 20 control animals. [The Working Group noted the renal tumour response with a water-insoluble lead compound.]

(*b*) *Subcutaneous and intraperitoneal administration combined*

Roe *et al.* (1965) gave three groups of 24 male Chester Beatty Wistar rats [age unspecified] combined subcutaneous and intraperitoneal injections of a technical grade of lead phosphate in distilled water at repeated intervals for 34 weeks (total doses, 29, 145 and 450 mg lead phosphate for the three groups, respectively). No carcinoma developed in the 23 rats that survived to 200 days in the lowest-dose group. Twenty-one animals in the highest-dose group died before 200 days and two of the three remaining animals developed renal adenomas. In the mid-dose group, 14/23 rats surviving to 200 days developed renal tumours (13 adenomas, seven adenocarcinomas and one undifferentiated malignant renal tumour) [statistically significant, Fisher's exact test; $p < 0.05$]. Two of the 24 control rats developed renal tumours (one undifferentiated malignant tumour and one transitional-cell carcinoma in the renal pelvis).

3.10 Lead arsenate

Arsenic compounds were previously evaluated as *carcinogenic to humans* (Group 1) in Supplement 7 of the *IARC Monographs* (IARC, 1987) and in the Monograph on Arsenic in Drinking-Water (IARC, 2004b).

3.10.1 *Rat*

(*a*) *Oral administration*

Fairhall and Miller (1941) fed a group of 49 white male rats [strain unspecified], weighing 70–90 g, a diet containing 10 mg/animal lead arsenate [purity unspecified] daily for 2 years (total approximate dose, 7.2 g). Of the animals that were given lead arsenate 45% had died after 1 year and 61% at 2 years [cause of death unspecified]. No tumours were reported from necropsies of the experimental animals nor from the 24 animals in the control group. [The Working Group noted the high early mortality.]

Kroes *et al.* (1974) fed groups of 40 or 29 male and 40 or 19 female weanling Wistar rats a diet containing 463 or 1850 ppm, respectively, of technical-grade lead arsenate (60% lead; 20.9% arsenic) for up to 120 weeks. At necropsies of 17 surviving males that had received the higher dose, one bile duct adenocarcinoma, one renal cortical adenoma and one lymphangioma were observed. No tumours were seen at necropsies of 11 surviving females that received the higher dose. In 38 males in the low-dose group, one renal hamartoma and two pituitary adenomas were observed. Among 40 females in the low-dose group, eight developed pituitary adenomas. In the control groups, necropsy of 39 males revealed one nephroblastoma, one pituitary adenoma, one lymphatic leukaemia and one lymphoblastosarcoma, and among 59 females, one thoracic sarcoma and 13 pituitary adenomas were observed. The authors stated that no definite conclusions could be drawn from the study.

(*b*) *Administration of lead with known carcinogens or modifiers*

Kroes *et al.* (1974) also fed two groups of 40 male and 40 female weanling SPF-derived Wistar rats a diet containing 463 ppm technical-grade lead arsenate (60% lead; 20.9% arsenic) and 0.3 mL water by intubation (five times/week for the duration of the study) for up to 120 weeks. One of the groups also received 5 μg/rat NDEA in water by intubation five times/week for the duration of the study. Control groups comprised 50 male and 60 female rats receiving 0.3 mL water by intubation and 50 male and 60 female rats receiving 5 μg/day NDEA as well as 0.3 mL water by intubation (five times/week for the duration of the study). Necropsies were performed on all the animals at the end of the study. In the group that received lead arsenate plus NDEA, one heart endothelial sarcoma and one pituitary adenoma were seen among 34 male rats; in the corresponding 40 females, seven pituitary adenomas were observed. In the water-only control group, one nephroblastoma, one pituitary adenoma, one lymphatic leukaemia and one lymphoblastosarcoma were observed among 39 males. In the corresponding group of 59 females, one thoracic sarcoma and 13 pituitary adenomas were observed. In the water plus NDEA control groups, one splenic lymphosarcoma, three pituitary adenomas, one lymphosarcoma and one lymphatic leukaemia were observed among 40 males. In the corresponding female group of 58 rats, one renal hamartoma, 14 pituitary adenomas and one lymphosarcoma were observed. [The Working Group noted the absence of an effect of lead arsenate on NDEA-induced tumours.]

3.11 Tetraethyl lead

3.11.1 *Mouse*

Subcutaneous administration

Epstein and Mantel (1968) gave groups of 109, 79 and 69 male and female randomly bred neonatal (0–21 days old) Swiss mice subcutaneous injections of total doses of 0.6, 1.2 and 2.0 mg/mouse, respectively, of tetraethyl lead [purity unspecified] in tricaprylin into the nape of the neck. The low-dose group received 0.1 mg on days 1 and 7 and 0.2 mg on days 14 and 21; the mid-dose group received 0.2 mg on days 1 and 7 and 0.4 mg on days 14 and 21; and the high-dose group received a single injection of 2 mg on day 1. All 69 mice injected with 2 mg, 92% of the 79 mice injected with 1.2 mg and 20% of the 109 mice injected with 0.6 mg tetraethyl lead died prior to weaning. At 36 weeks, the incidence of lymphomas in the mice that survived treatment with 0.6 mg tetraethyl lead (low dose) was 1/26 males and 5/41 females. The incidence of lymphomas in vehicle-control animals was 1/39 males and 0/48 females. Thus the incidence of lymphomas in treated female mice was significantly elevated ($p < 0.05$, χ^2 test) compared with female control mice but not in treated male mice compared with male control mice. [The Working Group felt that this study was limited by high mortality and the lack of concordance in tumour response between lead-treated male and female mice.]

4. Other Data Relevant to an Evaluation of Carcinogenicity and its Mechanisms

4.1 Absorption, distribution, metabolism and excretion

4.1.1 *Inorganic lead compounds*

(*a*) *Humans*

(i) *Absorption*

Absorption of lead is influenced by the route of exposure, the physicochemical characteristics of the lead and the exposure medium, and the age and physiological status of the exposed individual (e.g. fasting, concentration of nutritional elements such as calcium, and iron status). Inorganic lead can be absorbed by inhalation of fine particles, by ingestion and, to a much lesser extent, transdermally.

Inhalation exposure

Smaller lead particles (< 1 µm) have been shown to have greater deposition and absorption rates in the lungs than larger particles (Hodgkins *et al.*, 1991; ATSDR, 1999). In adult men, approximately 30–50% of lead in inhaled air is deposited in the respiratory tract, depending on the size of the particles and the ventilation rate of the individual. The proportion of lead deposited is independent of the absolute lead burden in the air. The half-life for retention of lead in the lungs is about 15 h (Chamberlain *et al.*, 1978; Morrow *et al.*, 1980). Once deposited in the lower respiratory tract, particulate lead is almost completely absorbed, and different chemical forms of inorganic lead seem to be absorbed equally (Morrow *et al.*, 1980; US EPA, 1986).

In two separate experiments, male adult volunteers were exposed to aerosols of lead oxide (prepared by bubbling propane through a solution of tetraethyl lead in dodecane and burning of resulting vapour) containing 3.2 µg/m^3 lead (15 subjects) or 10.9 µg/m^3 lead (18 subjects) in a room for 23 h/day for up to 18 weeks (Griffin *et al.,* 1975a). Six unexposed controls were included in each experiment. For those volunteers who remained until the end of the study, blood lead concentrations increased for about 12 weeks and then remained at ~37 µg/dL and ~27 µg/dL for the groups with higher and lower exposure, respectively. The concentration in the blood of controls was ~15 µg/dL. Lead content in blood declined after cessation of exposure, returning to near pre-exposure concentrations after 5 or 2 months for higher and lower exposure, respectively. Chamberlain *et al.* (1978)

suggested that some residual unburnt tetraethyl lead vapour may have been present in these experiments.

Twelve volunteers exposed to 150 μg/m^3 lead as lead oxide for 7.5 h per day on 5 days per week for 16–112 weeks exhibited elevated concentrations of lead in blood and urine, with one subject achieving a blood lead concentration of 53 μg/100 g (Kehoe, 1987). An average respiratory intake of 14 μg lead per day was reported for five male volunteers while exposed to an ambient concentration of 0.4–2.1 μg/m^3 airborne lead (Rabinowitz *et al.*, 1977).

Oral exposure

Most data on gastrointestinal absorption of lead are available for adults; there have been very few studies in children. Absorption of lead occurs primarily in the duodenum (reviewed in Mushak, 1991). The mechanisms of absorption have yet to be determined but may involve active transport and/or diffusion through intestinal epithelial cells (transcellular) or between cells (paracellular), and may involve ionized lead (Pb^{2+}) and/or inorganic or organic complexes of lead (Mushak, 1991). The extent and rate of gastrointestinal absorption are influenced by physiological conditions of the exposed individual such as: age, fasting, the presence of nutritional elements including calcium, phosphorus, copper and zinc, iron status, intake of fat and other calories; and physicochemical characteristics of the medium ingested, including particle size, mineral species, solubility and lead species.

Studies in adults

The experimental studies in adults have mainly employed lead chloride and radioactive tracers (^{212}Pb and later ^{203}Pb). Other evidence, often indirect, comes from stable lead isotope methods and epidemiological studies. Representative studies in adults are summarized in Table 81. The experimental studies generally had small numbers of subjects, ranging from one to 23 and the studies with ^{203}Pb were very short-term, due to the short half-life of the tracer (52 h). There was a wide variation in absorption between individuals in most studies; absorption was up to 96% in subjects who ingested lead with alcohol whilst fasting (Graziano *et al.*, 1996) but was generally less than 10% in subjects who received lead with food.

Studies in children

Dietary data for very young infants (< 6 months old) are scarce; results of some studies are listed in Table 82. For example, of the eight children investigated by Alexander *et al.* (1974), only one was aged less than 6 months. In the study by Ziegler *et al.* (1978), only one infant was studied from 14 days of age, two were studied from 72 and 83 days of age, respectively, and the rest were over 118 days (~4 months) old. In a study by Gulson *et al.* (2001a), 15 newborn infants were monitored for at least 6 months postpartum. Infants were breastfed or formula-fed or both and, aged about 91–180 days, usually fed solid foods (baby food called beikost). Daily lead intake ranged from 0.04 to 0.83 μg/kg bw with a geometric mean of 0.23 μg/kg bw and the excretion/intake ratio ranged from 0.7 to 22 with a geometric mean of 2.6. In a stable-isotope study, the mean value of blood

Table 81. Absorption of lead in adults after ingestion

No. and sex of subjects	Percentage ± SD absorption (range)	Exposure conditions	Reference
Radioactive tracer $^{203}PbCl_2$[a] or $^{203}PbAc$[a]			
11 men +	65	Fasting	James *et al.* (1985)
12 women	3.5	Meal with calcium + phosphorus	
	16	3 h after breakfast	
	43	5 h after breakfast	
10 men	21 ± 16 (10–67)	2 h after meal	Blake (1976)
6 men	8 (4–11)	Meal	Chamberlain *et al.* (1978)
	45 ± 17 (24–65)	Fasting	
7 men	21 (10–48)	2 h after meal	Moore *et al.* (1979)
4 women	70 (67–74)	Fasting	Blake & Mann (1983)
	17 (7–26)	Fasting + 175 mg calcium/250 mg phosphorus	
	2 (1–5)	Fasting + 1750 mg calcium/2500 mg phosphorus	
8 men	63 (59–67)	Fasting	Heard & Chamberlain (1982)
6 men	3 (2–5)	In liver and kidney of lamb[b]	
2 men	44 (37–56)	Fasting	Heard *et al.* (1983)
9 men	5.5 (2–14)	In spinach[c]	
8 men	10 (5–15)	Normal meal + 200 mg calcium/ 140 mg phosphorus	
2 men	14 (3–28)	With coffee and tea (and normal meal) (nine tests)	
4 men	19.5 (11–23)	With beer 10 min before light lunch	
9 men	14 ± 3 (8–18)	Tracer given 2 h after meal	Newton *et al.* (1992)
Stable lead isotopes[d]			
9 men	13.8 ± 3.1	'Contaminated' beer, 0.5 L/d for 5 d	Newton *et al.* (1992)
5 men	10 ± 2.7 (6.5–14)	With food: lead nitrate	Rabinowitz *et al.* (1976)
4 men	8.2 ± 2.8 (6–10)	With food: lead nitrate/cysteine	Rabinowitz *et al.* (1980)
4 men	35 ± 13 (30–37)	Fasting: lead nitrate/sulfide/cysteine	
2 men, 4 women	76 (46–96)	Fasting: Sherry in lead crystal decanter	Graziano *et al.* (1996)
1 man	34	Fasting: Wine doped with tracer ^{207}Pb	Gulson *et al.* (1998c)
	2.3	Wine doped with ^{207}Pb consumed with meal	

[a] Volunteers ingested ^{203}Pb as lead chloride or lead acetate in various media, e.g. in water, beverages and meal, with varying amounts of calcium and phosphorus under fasting and non-fasting conditions. Venous blood samples were taken at various times, e.g. 24 and 48 h. Body burden was measured by γ-ray counting, 4–9 days after dosing.

[b] Portions of liver or kidney from lamb injected with ^{203}Pb as lead chloride and butchered after 6 days were cooked and served in meals to volunteers.

[c] The plants of spinach were placed in water containing the ^{203}Pb as lead chloride for 48 h. The tops were then harvested, cooked and eaten with normal meal.

[d] Volunteers ingested non-radioactive enriched lead isotopes ^{204}Pb, ^{206}Pb or ^{207}Pb as lead nitrate, lead cysteine or lead sulfide in various media, e.g. in water, beverages and meal. Lead in samples (blood, urine or faeces) was determined by thermal ionization mass spectrometry.

Table 82. Daily lead intakes in children and absorption of lead after ingestion

Study group	Exposure	Daily intakes (µg/kg bw per day) mean (range)	Mean absorption[a] (%)	Mean retention[b] (%)	Reference
4 boys and 4 girls, aged 3 months to 8 years	11 balance studies in own homes. One child was studied 4 times from 3 months to 1.08 years.	10.6 (5–17)	53	18	Alexander *et al.* (1974)
6 boys and 6 girls, aged 14–746 days	2 separate balance studies 11–18 days apart in metabolic unit; 61 studies with variable lead intakes > 5 µg/kg bw per day	> 5	42	32	Ziegler *et al.* (1978)
9 children in hospital, aged 3–13 weeks; part of group of 29 children aged 3 weeks–14 years	104 balance studies with 29 children	6.5 [1.5–17]	Between –79% and 12% for the 9 subjects, but high inter-subject variability, some in negative balance; –40% for all 29 children		Barltrop & Strehlow (1978)

[a] Absorption denotes total intake minus faecal excretion
[b] Retention denotes total intake minus total excretion

lead coming from diet was 50% (Ryu *et al.*, 1983, 1985). This value was consistent with earlier estimates of uptake of lead in blood in newborn infants when environmental lead concentrations were much higher (Alexander *et al.*, 1974; Ziegler *et al.*, 1978). In contrast, Manton *et al.* (2000) suggested that the absorption in one child aged 4 months was only 1–5%. [The Working Group noted that the percentage absorption observed in this study is at variance with the majority of observations in infants.]

It should be noted that no absorption studies have been conducted in children older than 8 years. However, the changes in stable isotope tracers of blood lead in mothers and their children present similar profiles; both reach equilibrium with a unique exogenous lead isotope profile suggesting that children aged 6–11 years and their mothers may absorb a similar percentage of ingested lead from dietary sources (Gulson *et al.*, 1997a).

Nutritional factors affecting absorption

Mineral content is one factor that may lower the absorption of lead when it is ingested with food. For example, the presence and amount of calcium and phosphorus in a meal depress the absorption of ingested lead. The effect is greater for the two elements together than for either alone, with calcium showing a stronger effect than phosphorus (Blake & Mann, 1983; Heard *et al.*, 1983; James *et al.*, 1985). In children, an inverse relationship has been observed between dietary calcium intake and retention of lead, suggesting that children who are deficient in calcium may absorb more lead than calcium-replete children (Ziegler *et al.*, 1978). Several studies have drawn attention to the potential toxicity of lead in calcium or vitamin supplements (Capar & Gould, 1979; Roberts, 1983; Boulos & von Smolinski, 1988; Bourgoin *et al.*, 1993; Rogan *et al.*, 1999; Scelfo & Flegal, 2000). However, a study using isotope differences between lead in two types of calcium supplements and that in the blood of adults showed that the supplements did not increase blood lead concentration over a 6-month trial (Gulson *et al.*, 2001b).

A higher dietary intake of iron is associated with lower blood lead concentrations among children and iron deficiency may result in higher absorption of lead (Watson *et al.*, 1980; Mahaffey & Annest, 1986; Watson *et al.*, 1986; Marcus & Schwartz, 1987; Hammad *et al.*, 1996; Wright *et al.*, 2003). Evidence for the effect of iron deficiency on lead absorption has been provided also from animal studies (see Section 4.1.1(*b*)).

In a metabolic study of 10 adult subjects who ingested copper, zinc or iron supplements incorporated into a basal diet, higher faecal lead losses and lower blood lead concentrations were observed only with the copper supplements (Kies & Ip, 1991). [This could be an effect on either absorption or retention.]

A positive correlation has been observed between blood lead in children and total and saturated fat and caloric intake (Lucas *et al.*, 1996; Gallichio *et al.*, 2002). No relationship between intake of fat and protein and lead concentrations in bone and blood was found in middle-aged to elderly men in the Normative Aging Study (Cheng *et al.*, 1998).

Ascorbic acid is known to enhance the urinary elimination of lead from blood, liver and kidney in rats (Flora & Tandon, 1986). However, evaluation of the data from the Third National Health and Nutrition Examination Survey showed that there is no significant relationship between ascorbic acid intake in diet and blood lead concentrations in humans (Simon & Hudes, 1999; Houston & Johnson, 2000).

Absorption of lead from soil

In a study to mimic the soil ingestion habits of children, six adult subjects ingested soil (particle size less than 250 μm) from the Bunker Hill (ID, USA) mining site, resulting in a dose of 250 μg lead/70 kg bw. Based on stable lead isotope analysis, the subjects absorbed 26 ± 8% of the lead in the soil when they were in the fasted state and 2.5 ± 1.7% when the same soil lead dose was ingested with a meal (Maddaloni *et al.*, 1998). There are no reported measurements of the absorption of soil-borne lead in infants or children. Evidence for a lower absorption of soil-borne lead compared with dissolved lead is provided from studies in laboratory animals (see Section 4.1.1(*b*)). Experiments with lead-bearing mine waste soil suggested that surface area characteristics determine dissolution rates for particles < 90 μm in diameter, whereas dissolution of 90–250-μm particles appeared to be controlled more by surface morphology (Davis *et al.*, 1994). Similarly, in-vitro experiments showed that the solubility of 30-μm particles of lead sulfide in real gastric fluid [origin not specified] was much greater than that of 100-μm particles (Healy *et al.*, 1982).

Dermal exposure

Little information is available regarding absorption of lead in humans after dermal exposure. Moore *et al.* (1980a) conducted a study in which commercially-available lead acetate solution (6 mmol/L lead acetate) or skin cream (9 mmol/kg lead), labelled with [^{203}Pb]acetate, was applied to the forehead skin of eight male volunteers for 12 h and then washed off. Blood and urine samples were collected. The percentage of absorption was estimated by measuring the ^{203}Pb activity in blood samples, by counting over the subject's calf region using a whole-body monitor, and also by counting 24-h and 48-h urine samples. Absorption through intact skin was 0.18 ± 0.15% of the dose applied; that through scratched skin was 0.26 ± 0.46%. Lead exposure from the use of hair-colouring agents containing lead acetate was reported to be insignificant (Moore *et al.*, 1980a; Cohen & Roe, 1991). However, this assumes that only adults will be in contact with the colouring agents and ignores human behaviour in the home environment (Mielke *et al.*, 1997b). Measurements of lead on hands and surface wipes (including combs, hair dryer, faucet) from subjects using hair-colouring agents showed between 150 and 700 μg lead per hand and more than 100 μg/9.3 dm^2 [~10 μg/dm^2] on the surfaces. At such concentrations, there is a potential for hand-to-mouth and hand-to-surface transfer of lead not only to adults but also to children (Mielke *et al.*, 1997b).

The dermal absorption studies of Florence and colleagues (1988), although limited in subject numbers (nine workers), remain the most comprehensive to date. Following observations that workers in a lead battery factory exhibited high concentrations of lead in sweat, Florence *et al.* (1988) and Lilley *et al.* (1988) showed that finely-powdered lead metal and lead oxide (20 mg; particle size < 0.45 μm) or 60 μL of 0.5 M lead nitrate solution (6 mg lead) placed on the skin of one arm was rapidly absorbed. The absorbed lead appeared in sweat (induced by pilocarpine iontophoresis) on the other arm and in saliva, but was not detectable in blood or urine. The authors found that the rate of lead absorption through the skin increased with increased sweating and, as observed by Moore *et al.* (1980a), suggested that the mechanism was one of rapid diffusion through filled sweat ducts followed by a slower diffusion through the stratum corneum (Lilley *et al.*, 1988). The authors (as also observed by Moore *et al.*, 1980a) noted that the absorbed lead must be transported in the plasma and concentrated quickly into the extracellular pool (sweat and saliva), that its mean residence time in the plasma is very short and that little lead enters the erythrocytes (Lilley *et al.*, 1988). [No quantification of the amount of lead absorbed was undertaken and there were inconsistencies between the concentrations of lead in sweat from the two arms on certain days.]

In later experiments using compounds made with ^{204}Pb tracer and employing the sensitive thermal ionization–mass spectrometry (TIMS) and ICP–MS methods, lead acetate or lead nitrate was applied to the skin of four volunteers and perspiration induced by either pilocarpine iontophoresis or thermally in a sauna (Stauber *et al.*, 1994). The lead compounds were rapidly absorbed through the skin and detected in sweat, blood and urine within 6 h of application. In one subject, 4.4 mg lead (as lead nitrate) was applied to the skin under a patch and perspiration induced by iontophoresis. Of the applied dose, 1.3 mg lead was not recovered from skin washings, indicating that 29% of the applied dose was absorbed into or through the skin. The authors suggested that some of the absorbed lead was still present in the epidermis and had not entered the circulatory system as the other experiments indicated that an equivalent of only 0.2% of the ^{204}Pb applied to the skin was detected in blood. However, no measurable increase of total lead in blood or urine was found in this study. [The Working Group agreed with the authors in their concern about this lack of increase in total lead in blood or urine, since blood lead is the accepted biomarker of exposure.]

(ii) *Distribution*

Lead enters and leaves most soft tissues reasonably freely. The clearance from the blood into both soft tissues and bone dominates lead kinetics during the first few weeks after an exposure, with an apparent half-life of several weeks (Table 83). Once an approximate equilibrium is reached between soft tissues and blood, the concentration of lead in blood is determined almost entirely by the balance among absorption, elimination, and transfer to and from bone. In the absence of continuing exposure, the whole-body half-life represents the loss of lead from bone. Lead enters and leaves bone by physiologically-distinguishable mechanisms (reviewed and summarized in O'Flaherty, 1991a, 1992, 1993), which include rapid exchange between blood plasma and bone at all bone surfaces, incorporation of lead into forming bone and its loss during bone resorption, and very slow diffusion of lead throughout undisturbed bone. Slow diffusion accounts for the gradual build-up of large quantities of bone-seeking elements such as lead in quiescent, largely cortical bone (Marshall & Onkelinx, 1968).

Table 83. Kinetic parameters for lead in blood of non-occupationally exposed adults and young children

Study group and exposure	No. and sex of subjects	Age range (years)	Lead half-life in days ± SD (range)	Comments	Reference
Adults					
Inhalation of lead oxide	24 men 21 men	24–49 24–50	~1 month ~1 month	10.9 μg/m³ lead 3.2 μg/m³ lead	Griffin *et al.* (1975a)
Ingestion of stable ^{204}Pb and ^{207}Pb as nitrate	5 men	25–53	25 ± 3	With meals	Rabinowitz *et al.* (1976)
Ingestion of lead-contaminated beer for 28 days	9 men	23–65	30 ± 4 (19–46)	No standardization of meals	Newton *et al.* (1992)
Ingestion of wine doped with ^{207}Pb tracer	1 man	NR	23	With meals	Gulson *et al.* (1998c)
Exposed to environments with different lead isotopes	7 (of 8) women (immigrants[a])	26–36	59 ± 6 (50–66)	Isotopic changes in blood lead monitored monthly	Gulson *et al.* (1995, 1999)
Children					
Newborn infants of immigrant mothers[a]	9	0–0.5	91 ± 19 (65–131)	Isotopic changes in blood lead monitored every 2 months	Gulson *et al.* (1999)

NR, not reported

[a] The Working Group noted the longer half-lives of lead in blood for the immigrant women and their newborn infants. The timing of sampling for the immigrant women, usually at least 1 month after their arrival in Australia, suggests that the longer half-life observed was a whole-body half-life, reflecting a primary contribution from bone.

Bone formation and bone resorption are generally tightly coupled. During infancy and childhood, the bones grow rapidly and they are continually reshaped. Although the formation rate may greatly exceed the resorption rate, both processes are active throughout bone. When full growth is reached in the late teens, bone formation and resorption rates are equal. Subsequently, resorption of old bone and formation of new bone, which take place throughout the entire bone volume, serve to maintain healthy bone tissue and to restructure the bone in response to changing physical demands. The bulk of this activity takes place in trabecular bone. The coupling of bone formation and bone resorption is a two-edged sword: it is necessary to think of bone as both a sink for lead and a source of endogenous lead, since both processes operate simultaneously. During childhood, when the formation rate is high, so is the resorption rate, so that little bone lead from an early childhood exposure will persist into adulthood. On the other hand, generally whenever resorption is high, so is formation, so that return of lead to blood plasma with resorbing bone will be partially compensated by its redeposition into forming bone. Since trabecular bone generally turns over more rapidly than cortical bone, the lead content of trabecular bone should respond more rapidly than the lead content of cortical bone to changes — either increases or decreases — in lead exposure (O'Flaherty, 1993).

Beginning as early as at age 25–30 years, bone resorption rate rises slightly while bone formation rate does not change, so that slow net bone loss begins in early adulthood (Jowsey *et al.*, 1965; Mazess, 1982). There are also physiological states in which bone resorption and formation become temporarily partially uncoupled. During the first five or more years following menopause in women, the bone resorption rate is temporarily increased without a compensatory increase in bone formation rate, after which bone resorption rate drops back to a level about the same as that observed in older men (and in women before menopause) (Mazess *et al.*, 1987; Nilas & Christiansen, 1988). During pregnancy and lactation, the bone resorption rate is increased in order to supply calcium to the fetus and neonate.

The distribution of lead in various body compartments is considered in greater detail below.

Blood

Lead in blood is found primarily in the red blood cells (> 99%) rather than the plasma (Hursh & Suomela, 1968; Everson & Patterson, 1980; DeSilva, 1981; US EPA, 1986; Bergdahl *et al.*, 1997a). Bergdahl *et al.* (1997b,c, 1998a) showed that the principal lead-binding protein was delta-aminolevulinic acid dehydratase (ALAD), also known as porphobilinogen synthase (PBGS). Human ALAD has two alleles, ALAD-1 and ALAD-2, with three phenotypes (and their percentages in Caucasian populations): ALAD 1-1 (80%), ALAD 1-2 (19%) and ALAD 2-2 (1%) (Battistuzzi *et al.*, 1981; Benkmann *et al.*, 1983). It has been proposed that this polymorphism causes differential sensitivity to lead exposure (see Section 4.2.2).

Half-life of lead in blood

The half-life of lead in human blood has been determined experimentally, primarily in adult men. These studies were carried out on small numbers of subjects, usually fewer than ten, exposed only for up to 124 days. There are very limited data for children. A summary of estimated half-lives from experimental studies is given in Table 83. The mean half-lives of loss of lead from the blood immediately following an exposure are similar across studies and are independent of the route of exposure, although there are large differences between individuals. The mean half-lives for adult men in these studies ranged from 19–30 days. However, in lead workers exposed for periods of up to 10 years, with high blood lead concentrations, the half-life of initial loss from the blood following cessation of exposure is of the order of 20–130 days; the half-life in lead workers was a function of cumulative occupational exposure (O'Flaherty *et al.*, 1982).

When equilibrium is reached between soft tissues and blood, the net rate of loss of lead from the blood decreases. Subsequently, the rate-determining step for whole-body loss is the return of lead from the bone; in environmentally exposed subjects at equilibrium with their environment, 40–70% of lead in blood derives from bone (Manton, 1985; Gulson *et al.*, 1995; Smith *et al.*, 1996). Because of the nature of the mechanisms responsible for return of lead from bone to blood, the overall process is not correctly described by a half-life; however, it is convenient to continue to use half-lives to characterize whole-body loss as expressed by the decline of blood lead concentrations. In adult women of child-bearing age, Gulson *et al.* (1995, 1999) determined a mean whole-body half-life of 59 ± 6 days. Infants born to mothers immigrant to Australia had whole-body half-lives of 65–131 days, considerably longer than the 50–66-day half-lives observed for the adult women (Gulson *et al.*, 1999). Manton *et al.* (2000) observed longer whole-body half-lives of lead during the first 2 years of life in the blood of two groups of children who had been exposed to lead from residential remodelling over varying periods of time. Half-lives of lead in children exposed for unspecified brief periods of time were between 8 and 11 months, while half-lives in those with longer exposures varied from 20 to 38 months.

Whole-body half-lives of lead in blood estimated for workers occupationally exposed to lead are commonly much greater than those shown in Table 83 for non-occupationally exposed individuals, and reflect a much greater loading of the skeleton with lead (O'Flaherty *et al.*, 1982; Hryhorczuk *et al.*, 1985; Schütz *et al.*, 1987; Nilsson *et al.*, 1991; Fleming *et al.*, 1997, 1999). They are comparable to half-lives of lead measured in cortical bone (Christoffersson *et al.*, 1986; Erkkilä *et al.*, 1992).

Serum–whole blood relationships

Several authors have proposed that measurement of lead in serum may better reflect the fraction of lead that is available in the circulation for exchange with target organs such as the central nervous system and kidneys, and with the developing fetus (Manton & Cook, 1984; Schütz *et al.*, 1996; Hernandez-Avila *et al.*, 1998; Hu, H. *et al.*, 1998; O'Flaherty, 1998; O'Flaherty *et al.*, 1998; Smith *et al.*, 1998; Bergdahl *et al.*, 1999). A stronger association was found between the ratio plasma lead/blood lead with bone lead concentrations (measured by X-ray fluorescence) than with whole blood lead concentrations (Cake *et al.*, 1996; Hernandez-Avila *et al.*, 1998). Using urine as a proxy for plasma, Tsaih *et al.* (1999) observed significant associations between bone lead and urinary lead.

The low concentration of lead in plasma, relative to red blood cells, has made it extremely difficult to measure accurately plasma lead concentrations in humans, particularly at blood lead concentrations less than 20 μg/dL (Schütz *et al.*, 1996; Hernandez-Avila *et al.*, 1998). Serum analyses, especially at lower blood lead concentrations, are complicated by erythrocyte contamination (haemolysis), sampling and laboratory contamination, measurement error and misinterpretation of the data (Manton *et al.*, 2001).

Plasma is generally accepted as the source of lead available to distribution and excretion processes. Urinary lead excretion in humans is directly proportional to plasma lead concentration but not to blood lead concentration (O'Flaherty, 1993). Breast milk lead has been considered an indirect measure of plasma lead. A number of studies have shown significant linear relationships between lead in human breast milk and whole blood collected at delivery (cord blood) or post partum (Moore *et al.*, 1982; Ong *et al.*, 1985; Rabinowitz *et al.*, 1985; Namihira *et al.*, 1993; Palminger Hallén *et al.*, 1995a; Gulson *et al.*, 1998a).

Physiologically-based kinetic models in which transfers of lead (other than into bone) are assumed to be proportional to plasma lead concentration have been successful in a variety of different applications (O'Flaherty, 1998, 2000).

The relationship between serum lead and blood lead concentrations is not linear, due at least in part to limited availability of lead binding sites in the erythrocyte (DeSilva, 1981; Marcus, 1985; O'Flaherty, 1993). This binding is highly variable among individuals; it is influenced by extrinsic factors, such as iron nutritional status; and there is some evidence for its inducibility (Raghavan *et al.*, 1980; Marcus & Schwartz, 1987). The saturable binding of lead to erythrocytes has been interpreted as binding to three principal components, the tightest binding of which is to ALAD (Bergdahl *et al.*, 1998a). Thus, the fraction of blood lead in the plasma, the driving compartment for transfer into tissues, increases disproportionally with increasing blood lead concentration (Figures 1 and 2). The disproportionality becomes more pronounced as blood lead concentrations increase above about 40 µg/dL. Below this concentration, the relationship of serum lead concentration to blood lead concentration can be approximated by a straight line (Manton *et al.*, 2001).

Figure 1. The relationship between plasma lead and blood lead

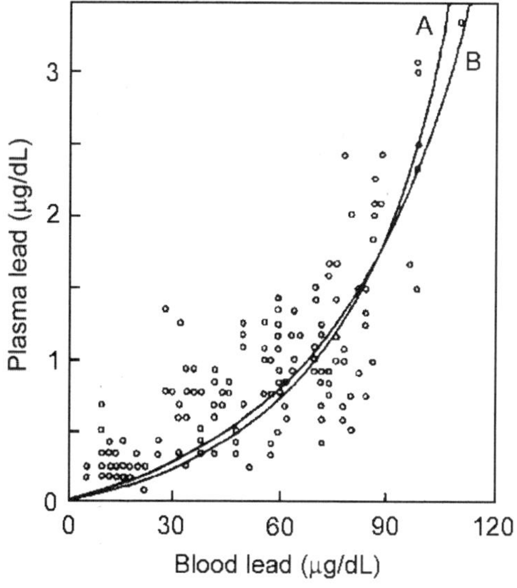

Adapted from O'Flaherty (1993)
Data points are from DeSilva (1981) as shown in Marcus (1985). Curve A is the model simulation. Curve B is Marcus' fit to the data, using a no-intercept model (Marcus' Model 4) consistent with the concept of a maximum erythrocyte binding capacity for lead.

Figure 2. Plot of serum lead concentration *vs* blood lead concentration for 73 subjects

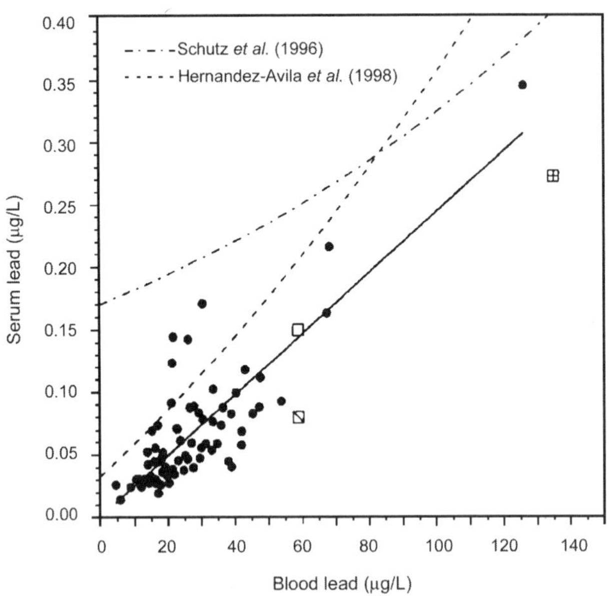

Adapted from Manton *et al.* (2001)
The line fitted to the points has the equation y = 0.00246 + 0.00236x (r = 0.82). Curves for workers obtained by Schütz *et al.* (1996) and Hernandez-Avila *et al.* (1998) are those calculated by Manton *et al.* (2001). The curves of both groups of workers were defined down to blood lead concentrations of 23 µg/dL so that at the lower end of their ranges, the observations for the workers overlap with those of Manton *et al.* (2001). See Manton *et al.* (2001) for further details.

In summary, in more recent investigations within this apparently linear range, there is convergence towards a percentage of serum lead/whole blood lead of < 0.3% (Cake *et al.*, 1996; Bergdahl & Skerfving, 1997; Bergdahl *et al.*, 1997a; Hernandez-Avila *et al.*, 1998; Bergdahl *et al.*, 1999; Manton *et al.*, 2001; Smith *et al.*, 2002; see Table 84). These investigations confirm earlier studies with radioactive ^{203}Pb tracers that showed that 0.2% of the ^{203}Pb was present in plasma at 50–100 h after exposure (Heard & Chamberlain, 1984).

Soft tissues

Lead has been measured in a variety of tissue samples in humans but care needs to be taken when comparing results because of the different reporting of measures for wet, dry and ashed weights.

In a study of lung tissues collected at autopsy from individuals with no known occupational exposure to lead [no details given], an average lead concentration of 0.22 ± 0.11 µg/g tissue was found (Barry, 1975). In 42 non-occupationally exposed subjects, Gross *et al.* (1975) detected 0.36 ± 0.12 µg/g wet weight (ashed, 23.9 ± 10.6 µg/g) in lung tissue. In a

Table 84. Analyses of blood lead concentrations in serum and whole blood samples

Subjects (no.) exposed or not to lead	Analytical method[a]	Blood lead concentration (μg/dL)	% serum/whole blood (mean or range)	Curvilinear relationship	Reference
Women, non-exposed (73)	TIMS	0.6–12.6	0.1–0.4	Linear < 10 μg/dL	Manton *et al.* (2001)
Women and men, non-exposed (26)	ICP-MS	2.3–41.6	0.2–0.7	Yes	Hernandez-Avila *et al.* (1998)
Women, non-exposed (63)	ICP-MS	< 25	0.099–0.48	For samples > 10 μg/dL	Smith *et al.* (2002)
Men, exposed (143)	ICP-MS	10–30 30–90	0.4 (read from the graph) 0.35 (read from the graph)	Yes	Bergdahl *et al.* (1997a); Bergdahl & Skerfving (1997)
Men, exposed (49)	TIMS	16.5–55.2	0.8–2.5	Not stated	Cake *et al.* (1996)
Children (44), exposed (31) Considerably lower exposed: 'Unexposed' (13)	ICP-MS	9.9–92 3.9–12	0.24–2.0 (median, 0.79) 0.23–0.49 (median, 0.36)	Yes (for exposed and unexposed children)	Bergdahl *et al.* (1999)

[a] TIMS, thermal ionization–mass spectrometry; ICP–MS, inductively-coupled plasma mass spectrometry

similar study, Mylius and Ophus (1977) reported an average of 0.56 μg/g dry weight (range, 0.28–1.14 μg/g) in lung tissue from 10 non-occupationally exposed individuals.

Gerhardsson *et al.* (1995b) showed that in 32 deceased smelter workers with known lead exposure history, the major soft tissue organs of lead accumulation were: liver > kidney > lungs > brain. Lyon *et al.* (2002) measured lead in liver tissue of 157 subjects aged < 1 day to 6 years. Lead concentrations ranged from 0.0083 to 0.407 μg/g wet weight. The median fetal liver concentration in 10 subjects was 0.0256 μg/g dry weight (Lyon *et al.*, 2002), comparable with the value in a Canadian study of 21 fetal livers of 0.061 ± 0.023 μg/g dry weight as calculated by Lyon *et al.* (2002) from the reported value, 0.243 ± 0.092 μg/g wet weight (Gélinas *et al.*, 1998). These values are considerably lower than those found in adults before 1994 (0.25–2.30 μg/g; Caroli *et al.*, 1994), in 73 adults in Canada (0.01–1.2 μg/g; Treble & Thompson, 1997) and in children aged 0–10 years for the period 1975–89 (0.08–1.37 μg/g; Patriarca *et al.*, 2000).

Barregård *et al.* (1999) measured lead in the renal cortex from 36 living healthy kidney donors in Sweden and found mean values of 0.18 μg/g dry weight. This was the first study of heavy metals in kidney cortex of living, healthy subjects.

Al-Saleh and Shinwari (2001b) measured concentrations of lead in tumour tissue from 23 patients (17 women, six men) with malignant brain tumours and 21 patients (11 women,

10 men) with benign brain tumours who were undergoing treatment at a Saudi Arabian hospital. Mean lead concentrations were similar in malignant and benign tumours (0.65 ± 1.7 and 0.61 ± 1.7 μg/g, respectively). In a study of a population in the USA, however, the concentration of lead in brain was below the limit of detection of 0.0008 μg/g (Bush *et al.*, 1995). [The Working Group noted the lack of a proper control group and other indices of cumulative lead exposure, and the limited statistical analyses of this study.]

Bone

In human adults, more than 90% of the total body burden of lead is found in the bone, whereas bone lead accounts for ~70% of the body burden in children (Barry, 1975). Lead is not distributed uniformly in bone (Somervaille *et al.*, 1986; Wittmers *et al.*, 1988; Aufderheide & Wittmers, 1992; Hoppin *et al.*, 2000; Todd *et al.*, 2000b, 2001c,d, 2002).

Estimates of the half-life of lead in trabecular bone are partly dependent on the tissue analysed and the 'purity' of the trabecular component [patella, calcaneus, finger bone (phalanx)]; current estimates range from about 12–16 years although earlier estimates ranged from 2–7 years (Christoffersson *et al.*, 1986; Schütz *et al.*, 1987; Gerhardsson *et al.*, 1993; Bergdahl *et al.*, 1998b). Earlier estimates for the half-life of lead in cortical bone were of the order of 13–27 years (Rabinowitz, 1991; Gerhardsson *et al.*, 1993; Bergdahl *et al.*, 1998b).

Studies over the past two decades using X-ray fluorescence methods have shown that trabecular bone — which has a faster turnover rate — (measured at the calcaneus or patella) has higher concentrations of lead/mg bone mineral than cortical bone (measured at the tibia) in the same subjects. The ratio of the concentration of lead in trabecular *vs* cortical bone generally ranges from 1.1 to 2.0; it appears to be independent of duration of exposure, occupation, age, sex, life-stage, pregnancy status, trabecular bone site, or blood lead concentration (Hu *et al.*, 1996b,c; Bergdahl *et al.*, 1998b; Fleming *et al.*, 1998; Hernandez-Avila *et al.*, 1998; Tsaih *et al.*, 1999; Brown *et al.*, 2000; Hu *et al.*, 2001; Elmarsafawy *et al.*, 2002; Korrick *et al.*, 2002; Rothenberg *et al.*, 2002; Hernandez-Avila *et al.*, 2003; Garrido Latorre *et al.*, 2003). A ratio of 3.6 in trabecular/cortical bone lead was measured in active workers exposed to lead in Finland (Erkkilä *et al.*, 1992). The higher ratio is consistent with the more rapid turnover of trabecular bone, which would be expected to be responsive to current exposure. [There may be a possible bias in the studies reported here since the majority of the subjects were from the Normative Aging Study].

Maternal patella bone lead concentrations have been shown to be superior to tibia bone lead concentrations in predicting lower infant birth weight (Gonzalez-Cossio *et al.*, 1997) and reduced growth rate from birth to 1 month of age (Sanín *et al.*, 2001).

In two of three adult males studied after cessation of occupational exposure to lead, lead concentrations in the patella (representative of trabecular bone) decreased more rapidly than those in the tibia (representative of cortical bone), consistent with the estimates of a shorter lead half-life in trabecular bone (Hu *et al.*, 1991).

Fleming *et al* (1997) and, in a follow-up study, Brito *et al* (2001) observed non-linear relationships between cumulative blood lead index (CBLI) and bone lead concentrations in groups of 367 and 519 active lead-smelter workers. By subdividing their study groups by date of hire, the authors showed that the apparent half-life of bone lead increased with length of employment (Brito *et al.*, 2001). They suggested that the increase was attributable to the age-dependence of bone turnover; i.e. that turnover was lower in the older men with longer employment histories. However, since blood lead concentrations in both groups of smelter workers exceeded 60 μg/dL during their earlier employment years (before the mid-1970s) and declined thereafter, the curvilinearity in the bone lead concentration/CBLI relationship could also be explained simply as a reflection of that of the plasma lead/whole blood lead relationship. This curvilinearity would have led to a disproportionate loading of bone with lead relative to blood lead concentrations (but not relative to plasma lead concentrations) during the early employment years when blood lead concentrations were high (Fleming *et al.*, 1997).

Cortical bone lead concentrations gradually increase with age whereas concentrations in trabecular bone (rib, vertebrae) level-off in the fifth decade of life and then may decrease (Gross *et al.*, 1975; Drasch *et al.*, 1987; Wittmers *et al.*, 1988; Kosnett *et al.*, 1994; Hu *et al.*, 1996c).

Analyses of bone and teeth can provide an integrated biomarker of previous lead exposure and can be used in a variety of investigations. For example, K-X ray fluorescence (K-XRF) analysis of bone has shown strong associations between bone lead and hypertension, cognitive functioning (e.g. Korrick *et al.*, 1999; Cheng *et al.*, 2001; Gerr *et al.*, 2002; Rothenberg *et al.*, 2002) and delinquency (Needleman *et al.*, 2002).

(iii) *Metabolism*

Ionic lead in the body is not known to be metabolized or biotransformed. It does form complexes with a variety of proteins and non-protein ligands (US EPA, 1994; ATSDR, 1999).

(iv) *Excretion*

Lead in the faeces includes both lead that has not been absorbed in the gastrointestinal tract and lead excreted in the bile (endogenous faecal excretion). When lead exposure is by ingestion, more than 90% of excreted lead is found in the faeces (Kehoe, 1987; Smith *et al.*, 1994). Biliary clearance is also a major route of excretion of absorbed lead. Excretion of lead does not appear to depend on exposure pathway (ATSDR, 1999), but the ratio of urinary to faecal excretion is variable. Values of from 1:1 to 3:1 have been reported for the ratio of urinary lead clearance to endogenous faecal lead clearance in adult humans after injection, inhalation or ingestion of ^{203}Pb-lead (Chamberlain *et al.*, 1978; Campbell *et al.*, 1984).

Excretion of lead through sweat is a minor process. Concentrations of lead in sweat vary depending on exposure and can be significantly elevated in workers in the lead industry (Stauber & Florence, 1988; Omokhodion & Howard, 1991; Omokhodion & Crockford, 1991a) compared with unexposed subjects (Omokhodion & Howard, 1991; Omokhodion & Crockford, 1991b). In healthy subjects who volunteered to ingest small amounts of lead, the lead concentrations in sweat were less than 10 μg/L and were about 20% of the concentrations found in urine and 6% of those in blood (Rabinowitz *et al.*, 1976; Omokhodion & Crockford, 1991b). [The Working Group noted the possibility of contamination of samples during collection and/or the lack of baseline lead concentrations reported in some of these studies.]

(v) *Mobilization of lead*

Although earlier investigators (Brown & Tompsett, 1945; Ahlgren *et al.*, 1976) had suggested that the skeleton was a potential endogenous source of lead poisoning, the opposing concept of the skeleton as a 'safe' repository for lead persisted until the mid-1980s and early 1990s. Potential mobilization of lead from the skeleton can occur at times of physiological stress associated with enhanced bone remodelling, such as during pregnancy and lactation (Manton, 1985; Silbergeld, 1991; Hertz-Picciotto *et al.*, 2000), menopause (Silbergeld *et al.*, 1988; Silbergeld, 1991), extended bed rest (Markowitz & Weinberger, 1990), hyperparathyroidism (Kessler *et al.*, 1999) and weightlessness. The lead deposited in the bone of adults can serve to maintain blood lead concentrations long after exposure has ended (O'Flaherty *et al.*, 1982; Manton, 1985; Kehoe, 1987; Schütz *et al.*, 1987; Nilsson *et al.*, 1991; Gulson *et al.*, 1995; Inskip *et al.*, 1996; Smith *et al.*, 1996; Fleming *et al.*, 1997).

Pregnancy and lactation

During pregnancy, the mobilization of bone lead increases. The increase in blood lead concentrations during the third trimester has been attributed to increased bone resorption to meet the calcium requirements of the developing fetal skeleton (Manton, 1985; Rothenberg *et al.*, 1994; West *et al.*, 1994; Lagerkvist *et al.*, 1996b; Schuhmacher *et al.*, 1996b; Gulson *et al.*, 1997b; Hertz-Picciotto *et al.*, 2000).

Manton (1985) monitored blood lead of one woman by use of high-precision measurement of stable lead isotopes and attributed the almost doubling of blood lead concentrations during pregnancy to skeletal sources. In subjects who had been exposed in their earlier life to lead from sources different from their current environment, Gulson *et al.* (1995) and Smith *et al.* (1996) — using the same methods — estimated that 40–70% of lead in blood is derived from the skeleton. In Australia, Gulson *et al.* (1997b) monitored two immigrant cohorts longitudinally during and after pregnancy over a 10-year period using the same study design and monitoring protocols. The first cohort (Gulson *et al.*, 1997b, 1998a), comprising 16 pregnant immigrants, six long-term Australian women and six non-pregnant immigrant controls, showed that concentrations of blood lead increased during pregnancy by an average of about 20% compared with the non-pregnant immigrant controls. The increases were attributed to release of lead from the skeleton associated with increased bone remodelling, and were possibly related to the low calcium intake of most of the subjects.

Berglund *et al.* (2000) determined lead in blood and urine in relation to bone turnover in pregnant and lactating women in Stockholm, Sweden. In contrast to many of the studies cited above, no increase in blood lead during pregnancy was detected. The authors suggested that this could be attributed to normal physiological haemodilution (Hytten, 1985), a diet relatively high in calcium and low in lead, transfer of lead to the fetus and a possibly relatively low body burden of lead in younger women in Sweden. However, significant increases in concentrations of blood during pregnancy have been observed in women whose blood lead concentrations were also low (Gulson *et al.*, 1997b, 1998a; Rothenberg *et al.*, 2000). In addition to increases in blood lead during later stages of pregnancy, blood lead concentrations have been observed to decrease in the early stages of pregnancy. The mechanisms for these changes are not understood, although increased mobilization of bone lead during pregnancy may contribute partly to the increase (Lagerkvist *et al.*, 1996b; Schuhmacher *et al.*, 1996b; Gulson *et al.*, 1997b, 1998a). Increased blood volume and haemodilution may contribute to the decrease observed in the first half of pregnancy, whereas increased absorption of lead during pregnancy or decreased elimination may also occur (Rothenberg *et al.*, 1994; Franklin *et al.*, 1997; Gulson *et al.*, 1997b).

Transplacental transfer/breast milk

Transplacental transfer of lead in humans has been demonstrated in a number of studies indicating that the ratio of cord/maternal blood lead concentration at delivery ranges from about 0.6 to 1.0 (Barltrop, 1969; Rabinowitz *et al.*, 1984; McMichael *et al.*, 1986; Goyer, 1990a; Graziano *et al.*, 1990; Al-Saleh *et al.*, 1995; Schuhmacher *et al.*, 1996b; Gulson *et al.*, 1997b). Diffusion has been proposed as the primary mechanism for transplacental lead transport (Goyer, 1990a).

Evidence for maternal-to-fetal transfer of lead in humans can be gained from stable lead isotope measurements. For example, a 0.99 correlation in lead isotopic ratios for maternal and cord blood (Manton, 1985; Gulson *et al.*, 1997b) and similarity of isotopic ratios in maternal blood and in blood and urine of newborn infants provide strong evidence of placental transfer (Gulson *et al.*, 1999; Gulson *et al.*, 2004). The presence of lead in neonatal liver provides further direct evidence that it crosses the human placental barrier (Lyon *et al.*, 2002).

Breast milk can also be a vehicle for maternal excretion of lead. However, given the very low lead concentrations and the analytical difficulties arising from the high fat content of breast milk, lead analyses require careful attention (Gulson *et al.*, 1998a). For breast milk collected serially, the mean lead concentration was found to be 0.73 ± 0.70 μg/L for mothers whose blood lead concentration was less than 5 μg/dL. For the first 60–90 days postpartum, the contribution from breast milk to blood lead in the infants varied from 36–80%. Gulson *et al.* (1998a) evaluated studies published over the last 15 years of lead concentrations in breast milk and suggested that studies in which the ratio of lead concentration in breast milk to lead concentration in maternal whole blood were greater than 0.15 should be viewed with caution because of potential contamination during sampling and/or laboratory analyses. Several studies appear to show a linear relationship between lead in breast milk and maternal whole blood lead. The percentage of lead in breast milk was comparable with that in whole blood in subjects with blood lead concentrations ranging from

2–34 μg/dL. Gulson *et al.* (1998a) suggested that breastfed infants are only at risk if the mother is exposed to high concentrations of lead contaminants either from endogenous sources such as the skeleton or exogenous sources.

Reduction of lead mobilization during pregnancy and lactation

Studies that focused on the reduction of lead mobilization during pregnancy and lactation in humans have usually employed calcium supplementation. Increased intake of calcium has been suggested as a measure to prevent mobilization of extra lead during pregnancy and lactation (Farias *et al.*, 1996; Hernandez-Avila *et al.*, 1996; Gulson *et al.*, 1998d; Hertz-Picciotto *et al.*, 2000; Gulson *et al.*, 2003). Calcium supplementation at the recommended level of approximately 1000 mg/day (NIH, 1994) was found to almost halve the extra lead released during pregnancy but offered no benefit during lactation (Gulson *et al.*, 2004). In contrast, calcium carbonate supplementation of 1200 mg/day elemental calcium during lactation gave a modest reduction of 16% in blood lead concentrations amongst women with relatively high bone lead burdens (Hernandez-Avila *et al.*, 2003). In an earlier report that apparently used the same cohort but with smaller numbers, there did not seem to be any benefit from calcium supplementation during lactation (Téllez-Rojo *et al.*, 2002). Using concentrations of cross-linked N-telopeptides of type I collagen (NTX), a sensitive biomarker of bone resorption, Janakiraman *et al.* (2003) observed that a 1200-mg calcium supplement taken at bedtime during the third trimester of pregnancy reduced maternal bone resorption by an average of 14%.

Menopause

Increases in blood lead in postmenopausal women have been attributed to release of lead from the skeleton associated with increased bone resorption during menopause (Silbergeld *et al.*, 1988; Symanski & Hertz-Picciotto, 1995; Muldoon *et al.*, 1994; Weyermann & Brenner, 1998; Hernandez-Avila *et al.*, 2000). Most of these studies were based on blood lead concentrations. More recent investigations employing bone X-ray fluorescence measurements as well as blood lead concentrations have supported an endogenous contribution of bone lead to blood (Webber *et al.*, 1995; Korrick *et al.*, 2002; Garrido Latorre *et al.*, 2003). Postmenopausal women using hormone replacement therapy may have lower blood lead concentrations and higher bone lead values than non-users (Webber *et al.*, 1995; Garrido Latorre *et al.*, 2003). In contrast, in a cross-sectional study of 264 women (46–74 years old) in Boston, USA, both tibia and patella lead values were significantly and positively associated with blood lead but only among postmenopausal women not using estrogen (Korrick *et al.*, 2002). In a pilot study of immigrant women in Australia, Gulson *et al.* (2002) found a decrease in blood lead concentrations and changing lead isotopic composition in women treated for 6 months with a powerful anti-bone resorptive bisphosphonate drug. Upon cessation of treatment, the blood lead concentrations increased and the isotopic composition changed.

Preferential partitioning of bone lead into plasma

Several authors have proposed that lead released from the skeleton is preferentially partitioned into serum rather than erythrocytes; one explanation being that the lead from endogenous sources was in a different form to that from exogenous sources (Cake *et al.*, 1996; Hernandez-Avila *et al.*, 1998; Tsaih *et al.*, 1999). In a study employing similar methods, Bergdahl and Skerfving (1997) disputed the findings of Cake *et al.* (1996). Chettle *et al.* (1997) also challenged the hypothesis of Cake *et al.* (1996) that the ratio of serum lead to whole blood lead increases with increasing amounts of lead released from bone. Using urine as a proxy for serum, Gulson *et al.* (2000) compared lead isotopic ratios and lead concentrations in 51 matched blood and spot urine samples from 13 subjects, covering the interval from before pregnancy through 180 days postpartum. There was no evidence for preferential partitioning of lead into serum compared with whole blood.

Pharmacokinetic models

Several pharmacokinetic models for lead have been proposed to explain and predict physiological processes, including intercompartmental lead exchange rates, retention of lead in various pools, and relative rates of distribution among the tissue groups. Comprehensive discussions of these models have been published by ATSDR (1999). One of the earliest was a three-compartment model based on stable lead isotope tracer experiments and balance data from five healthy men (Rabinowitz *et al.*, 1976). A physiologically-based pharmacokinetic (PBPK) model developed initially for rats by O'Flaherty (1991a,b,c, 1993, 1995) uses physiologically-based parameters to describe the volume, composition and metabolic activity of blood and tissues that determine the disposition of lead in the human body. The compartments and pathways in the O'Flaherty model are shown in Figure 3 (ATSDR, 1999). Two other models in current use are compartmental pharmacokinetic models; the integrated exposure uptake biokinetic (IEUBK) model for lead in children (Figure 4) (US EPA, 1994) and the Leggett model (Leggett, 1993), which simulate the same general processes as those in the PBPK model, although transfer rate constants and kinetic coefficients may not have precise physiological correlates. All three models have been calibrated, to varying degrees, against empirical physiological data from animals and humans, and blood lead concentrations observed in exposed populations of children and adults. Pharmacokinetic models have been used to estimate the probability distribution of blood lead concentrations in children potentially exposed to lead via multiple exposure pathways at hazardous waste sites. The O'Flaherty and Leggett models have accurately reproduced adult blood lead concentrations, and may be modified to reflect changes in lead associated with pregnancy, ageing, or disease states (Pounds & Leggett, 1998; O'Flaherty, 2000).

Figure 3. Compartments and pathways of lead exchange in the O'Flaherty model

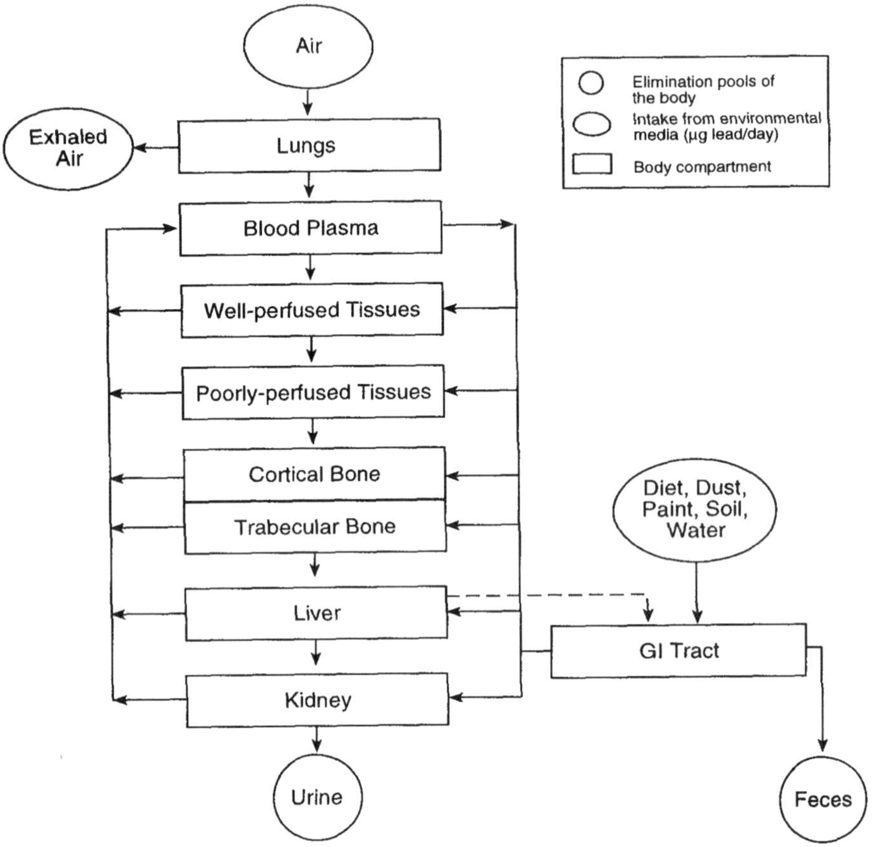

From ATSDR (1999), derived from O'Flaherty, 1991b, 1993, 1995

(*b*) *Animals*

(i) *Absorption*

Ingestion

Absorption of lead from the gastrointestinal tract in experimental animals is age-dependent and is influenced by the amount of food intake.

Prior to weaning, rodents absorbed from 50% to more than 80% of a single oral dose of radiolabelled lead, while older rodents absorbed < 1–15% (Forbes & Reina, 1972; Garber & Wei, 1974; Kostial *et al.*, 1978; Flanagan *et al.*, 1979).

In rats receiving a carrier-free oral dose of 0.02 µCi ^{212}Pb, absorption of lead from the gut declined steadily from 74–89% in animals 16–22 days of age to 15–42% in animals 24–32 days old and to only 16% in 89-day-old animals (Forbes & Reina, 1972). [It was

Figure 4. Structure of the IEUBK model for children

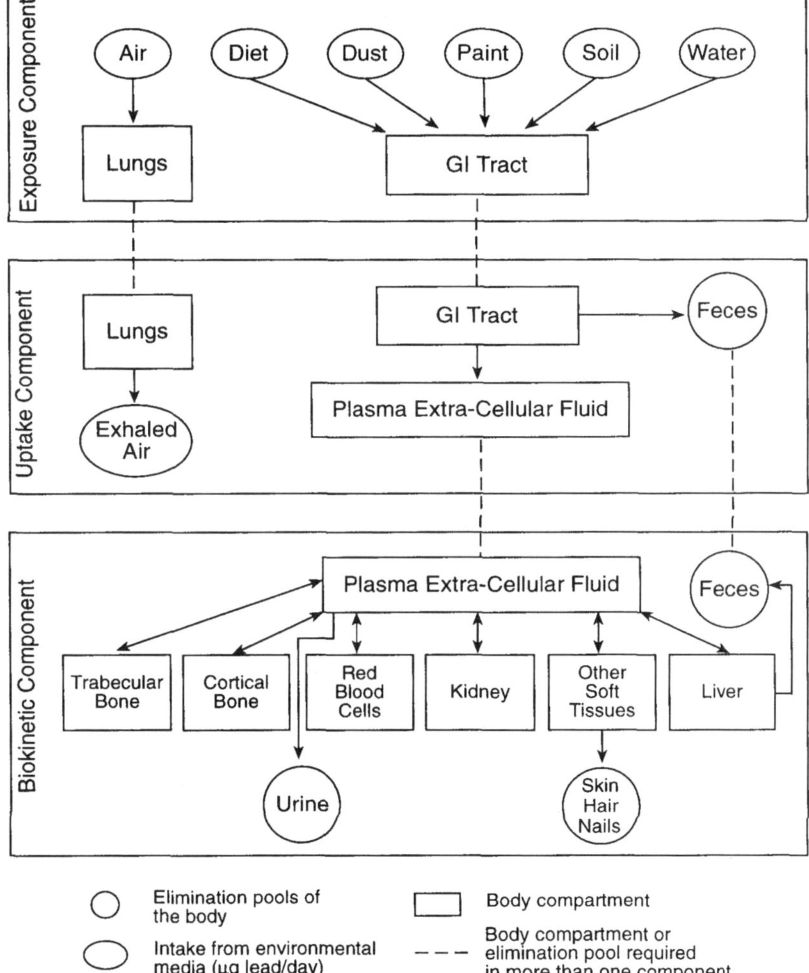

From ATSDR (1999)

unclear whether the study was conducted with fasted animals.] A single oral dose of ^{203}Pb-lead chloride resulted in 52% absorption in 1-week-old suckling rats compared with 0.4% in 6-week-old adults on a standard diet (Kostial *et al.*, 1978). Lead absorption from an intragastric dose of 2 µCi ^{210}Pb-lead acetate was 5.4% and 9.7% in adult C56Bl/6 Jax mice that were given an iron-supplemented diet or an iron-deficient diet, respectively (Flanagan *et al.*, 1979).

The presence of food in the intestine was shown to reduce by more than 80% the absorption of a 10-mg/kg oral dose of lead acetate in Sprague-Dawley rats (Aungst & Fung, 1981). In Swiss-Webster mice, food reduced lead absorption from 14% to 7.5%, when a single tracer dose of ^{210}Pb-lead acetate (3 µg/kg bw) was administered. However, the absorption rate (4–5%) was similar in fasted and non-fasted mice receiving a higher dose of lead (2 mg/kg bw) (Garber & Wei, 1974).

In non-human primates, the absorption of lead ranged from 38–65% in young animals and from ~3–40% in mature animals (Willes *et al.*, 1977; Pounds *et al.*, 1978; O'Flaherty *et al.*, 1996; Cremin *et al.*, 2001).

Fasted young monkeys (*Macaca fascicularis*; 10 days of age) absorbed 64.5% of an oral dose of 10 µg/kg bw ^{210}Pb-lead nitrate, while only 3.2% was absorbed by fasted mature adults (Willes *et al.*, 1977). Similarly, the gastrointestinal absorption of an oral dose of 72.6 µg ^{206}Pb-lead acetate (352 nmol) in 12 mL apple juice was ~65% in fasted infant rhesus monkeys (Cremin *et al.*, 2001). Fasted adult cynomolgus monkeys absorbed 22–44% of a single dose of lead given as ^{210}Pb-lead nitrate, depending on the dose (O'Flaherty *et al.*, 1996). In fed juvenile rhesus monkeys (5–7 months old), lead absorption was 38% versus 26.4% in fed adults following a single gavage dose of 10 mg/kg bw ^{210}Pb-lead acetate (Pounds *et al.*, 1978).

Experiments in mice and rats provide evidence that lead absorption is increased in the later stages of pregnancy and during lactation (Donald *et al.*, 1986; Maldonado-Vega *et al.*, 1996). The gastrointestinal absorption of ^{203}Pb in lactating rats was found to be about 2–3.5 times that in controls (Kostial & Momcilovic, 1972; Momcilovic, 1979).

There is experimental evidence that gastrointestinal absorption of lead is a saturable process. In mice, single administrations of 0.2, 2 or 20 mg/kg ^{210}Pb-lead acetate resulted in similar absorption rates (Garber & Wei, 1974). Duodenal perfusate experiments in mice have shown that lead uptake from the lumen increased in proportion to lead concentration in the perfusate but that the transfer of lead across isolated mouse duodenum to the carcass was saturable (Flanagan *et al.*, 1979).

The extent of absorption decreased from 42% in fasted adult Sprague-Dawley rats administered a single oral dose of 1 mg/kg bw lead (as lead acetate) to 2% when the dose was increased to 100 mg/kg bw. Furthermore, the percentage of the dose recovered from the tissues (brain, liver, kidneys, blood) decreased from 6.9% after 1 mg/kg bw lead to 0.6% after 100 mg/kg bw in adults and from 11.0% to 0.6% in pups (Aungst *et al.*, 1981). A 100-fold increase in a single oral dose from 10 µg to 1 mg ^{203}Pb-lead chloride was accompanied by an increase of only 20-fold in the quantity of lead absorbed in fasted Wistar rats (Conrad & Barton, 1978). Studies by Polák *et al.* (1996) demonstrated a dose-dependent biovailability in rats of both soluble lead and lead in mine waste or in mine waste-contaminated soils. Fractional absorption decreased as lead intake increased, regardless of the source of the lead, but the magnitude of this dose dependence was lead source-dependent. Fractional absorption varied from 4–5% at low exposure rates (1–2 mg/kg bw lead per day) when lead acetate was added to the diet, to 0.24% at a high exposure rate (24 mg/kg bw lead per day) when a test soil of mine waste contaminated with lead was added to the diet (Polák *et al.*, 1996).

The absorption of an intraluminal dose of ^{203}Pb-lead acetate in chicks was impaired by the presence of lead (as lead chloride) in the diet, in a dose-dependent fashion from 43% at a dietary concentration of 0.1% lead to 16 % at a dietary concentration of 0.8% (Fullmer, 1991).

Fractional absorption of ^{210}Pb-lead nitrate decreased from 44% of a single oral dose of 750 μg/kg bw to 22–28% of a dose of 1500 μg/kg bw in fasted adult cynomolgus monkeys (O'Flaherty *et al.*, 1996).

The bioavailability of lead is dependent on its chemical form and its particle size as well as the matrix and the source of environmental lead. Absorption of lead from the gastrointestinal tract of Wistar rats (30-day-old) varied greatly with chemical form; lead carbonate administered in the diet showed a 12-fold greater absorption coefficient than metallic lead. Relative to the absorption of lead acetate taken as 100%, the absorption coefficients of lead salts were: 44% for lead chromate, 62% for lead octoate, 64% for lead naphthenate, 67% for lead sulfide, 121% for lead tallate and 164% for lead carbonate (basic) (Barltrop & Meek, 1975). In studies performed by Dieter *et al.* (1993), rats were fed ≤ 38-μm size particles of lead sulfide, lead oxide, lead acetate and a lead ore concentrate from Skagway, Alaska, USA, mixed into the diet at doses of 0, 10, 30 and 100 ppm for 30 days. Bioavailability was found to be highest for lead acetate, intermediate for lead oxide and lowest for lead sulfide and Alaskan mixed-ore concentrate. Lead concentrations in bone and kidney were about 20- and 10-fold greater, respectively, in rats fed the more soluble compared with the less soluble lead compounds (Dieter *et al.*, 1993). Experimental studies on fed young rats showed that the mean relative bioavailability (compared with lead acetate) of lead in the Butte mining waste soil was 20%, 9% and 8% based on measurements of lead in blood, bone and liver, respectively (Freeman *et al.*, 1992). In further studies by these authors, the absolute bioavailability of ingested lead acetate in feed was estimated to be 15% based on measurements of blood lead concentrations after oral administration. The addition of control soil to the diet with lead acetate resulted in a significant decrease in lead bioavailability. The absolute bioavailability to rats of mining waste lead in soil administered in feed was approximately 3% based on blood lead concentration and less than 1% based on bone and liver lead concentrations (Freeman *et al.*, 1994). The bioavailability of lead sulfide was found to be approximately 10% that of lead acetate (Freeman *et al.*, 1996).

In immature swine, the relative bioavailability (compared with lead acetate) of lead from soil samples from the Smuggler Mountain Superfund Site in Aspen (CO, USA) was shown to range from 57% based on blood lead area-under-the-curve (AUC) to about 80% based on liver lead concentration. The absolute bioavailability was estimated to be from 28% (via blood AUC) to about 40% (via liver uptake) (Casteel *et al.*, 1997).

An inverse relationship was found between the particle size of metallic lead (6–250 μm) administered in the diet and absorption in rats. This relation was more marked in the 6–100-μm range; a fivefold enhancement of absorption was observed when rats were fed with lead particles of mean size 6 μm compared with 197-μm particles. A marked enhancement of absorption (1.5–1.8-fold) was also found on feeding lead chromate and lead octoate when particle size was reduced from 500–1000 μm to less than 50 μm (Barltrop & Meek, 1979).

The bioavailability of lead is influenced by dietary habits. Regular rat chow attenuates the absorption of lead by the strong binding or precipitative action of the chow diet (Freeman *et al.*, 1996). Lead absorption of a single oral dose of ^{203}Pb-lead chloride in adult rats fed several 'human' diets ranged from about 3% to more than 20% above that in controls receiving regular rat chow food. Highest absorption values were observed in animals fed fruit and cow's milk (Kello & Kostial, 1973; Kostial *et al.*, 1978; Kostial & Kello, 1979).

Palminger Hallén and Oskarsson (1995) studied the effects of milk on lead absorption in rat pups. At 2 h after gastric intubation of various liquid diets labelled with ^{203}Pb, the lead bioavailability was 47% from water, 42% from human milk, 40% from infant formula, 31% from cows' milk and 11% from rat milk. After 6 h, the bioavailability of lead was about 50% from water and human milk, 45% from infant formula and cow's milk and 36% from rat milk. Rat pups given lead in human milk had lead concentrations in blood and brain approximately twice as high as those of pups given lead in rat milk.

Other investigators have not found any effect of milk on lead absorption in suckling or adult rodents (Garber & Wei, 1974; Meredith *et al.*, 1977; Henning & Leeper, 1984). Kinetic analysis of pups' blood lead concentration revealed a rate-limited absorption in suckling mice exposed to milk from mothers administered lead, with a slower absorption of lead in the offspring compared with dams. The conflicting evidence on whether milk influences absorption of lead in infant rodents might be resolved, at least in part, by measurements of lead absorption at different time periods after its administration to the animals (Palminger Hallén *et al.*, 1996a).

Nutritional status has been shown to influence lead absorption and/or retention in experimental animals. Vitamin D, calcium and phosphorus have complex and interrelated effects on lead absorption (Fullmer, 1990, 1991, 1997). Diets deficient in calcium and/or phosphate are associated with increased intestinal absorption and/or retention of lead in experimental animals (mice, rats, chicks, monkeys) (Six & Goyer, 1970; Quarterman & Morrison, 1975; Jacobson & Snowdon, 1976; Barton & Conrad, 1981; Mykkänen *et al.*, 1984; Aungst & Fung, 1985; Van Barneveld & Van den Hamer, 1985). Simultaneous reduction of both dietary calcium and phosphate content produced an additive effect on absorption of lead (Quarterman & Morrison, 1975; Barltrop & Khoo, 1976). However, experimental studies in chicks have shown that variations in the extent and duration of lead ingestion and calcium deficiency may result in increases or decreases in lead absorption (Fullmer, 1991). In chicks fed standard diet but administered a single injection into the lumen of the intestine of ^{203}Pb-lead acetate, lead absorption increased from 18.8% in animals with adequate calcium content in the diet to 54.5% in animals fed a severely calcium-deficient diet. In calcium-deficient chicks on a diet containing lead, a biphasic response was observed; intestinal absorption of lead was enhanced by calcium deficiency initially, in a manner similar to the groups not fed lead, but this response was inhibited by prolonged dietary lead intake (Fullmer, 1991).

Calcium supplemention has been shown to reduce lead absorption in several animal species when administered at the same time as lead (Barltrop & Khoo, 1976; Meredith *et al.*, 1977; Barton *et al.*, 1978a; Varnai *et al.*, 2001) but not when administered separately (Quarterman *et al.*, 1978; Aungst & Fung, 1985; Van Barneveld & Van den Hamer, 1985). Calcium supplementation caused a statistically significant dose-related decrease in lead in tissues (liver, kidneys, brain and carcass) of suckling rats exposed to lead orally but had no effect on lead incorporated in tissues after parenteral exposure to lead, suggesting that calcium primarily reduced lead absorption from the gastrointestinal tract (Varnai *et al.*, 2001).

Administration of cholecalciferol (vitamin D3) or 1,25-dihydroxycholecalciferol (1,25-$(OH)_2D$), the active metabolite of vitamin D3, was found to increase gastrointestinal absorption of lead in rats and chicks (Smith *et al.*, 1978; Hart & Smith, 1981; Mykkänen & Wasserman, 1982; Edelstein *et al.*, 1984; Fullmer, 1990). Dietary vitamin D deficiency or depletion resulted in increased intestinal absorption of lead in intact animals, but the manipulation of dietary phosphate and vitamin D3 content had no significant effect upon the absorption of lead from isolated gastrointestinal segments of rats. Hence, this increased absorption was attributed to a decrease of gastrointestinal motility with a prolonged transit time (Barton *et al.*, 1980; Barton & Conrad, 1981). However, the administration of cholecalciferol to rachitic chicks resulted in an increase in the transepithelial transport of ^{203}Pb in the intestine (Mykkänen & Wasserman, 1982). The vitamin D-induced intestinal calcium-binding proteins bind lead with higher affinity than calcium suggesting a co-transport mechanism whereby lead absorption would be increased by calcium deficiency (Fullmer *et al.*, 1985; Fullmer, 1997). However, the effect of 1,25-$(OH)_2D$ appeared to be dependent upon the duration of exposure to lead and the magnitude of lead stores in the body. The efficiency of intestinal ^{203}Pb absorption was significantly diminished by dietary lead in an apparently dose-dependent fashion (Fullmer, 1990).

Iron status also influences the absorption and/or retention of dietary lead in rodents (Six & Goyer, 1972; Ragan, 1977; Barton *et al.*, 1978b; Conrad & Barton, 1978; Robertson & Worwood, 1978; Flanagan *et al.*, 1979; Morrison & Quarterman, 1987; Crowe & Morgan, 1996). Lead absorption was found to be promoted by iron deficiency and inhibited by iron loading (Barton *et al.*, 1978b). Rats fed iron-deficient diets had increased concentrations of lead in kidney and bone (femur) when compared with rats ingesting equivalent quantities of lead (as lead acetate) in drinking-water while being fed an iron-adequate diet (Six & Goyer, 1972). The degree of iron deficiency does not need to be severe to increase lead retention. A sixfold increase in tissue lead was demonstrated in rats when body iron stores were reduced, but before frank iron deficiency developed (Ragan, 1977). ^{203}Pb absorption in fasted rats was found to be increased by a short period of severe iron restriction before any change in haematological parameters became apparent. An extended period of moderate iron restriction, causing a reduction in haemoglobin concentration, resulted in increased iron and lead absorption. When iron dietary concentrations were made adequate to meet essential requirements produced by blood loss or hypoxia, lead absorption was similar to that in controls (Morrison & Quarterman, 1987). The ion lead Pb^{++} is a substrate for the divalent-cation metal transporter 1 (DMT1). This transporter is expressed most significantly in the proximal duodenum in the rat and is upregulated by dietary iron deficiency (Gunshin *et al.*, 1997). In a yeast model, it was demonstrated that DMT1 transports lead and iron with similar affinity and that iron inhibits the transport of lead (Bannon *et al.*, 2002).

Other dietary factors reported to influence absorption of lead in experimental animals are lipids (Barltrop & Meek, 1975; Barltrop & Khoo, 1976; Quarterman *et al.*, 1977; Ku *et al.*, 1978), amino acids and proteins (Conrad & Barton, 1978; Quarterman *et al.*, 1980), citrate and ascorbic acid (Garber & Wei, 1974; Conrad & Barton, 1978; Spickett *et al.*, 1984) and lactose (Bushnell & DeLuca, 1983).

Blood lead concentrations measured in rats after controlled oral exposure to lead as lead acetate are given in Table 85.

Table 85. Blood lead concentrations in rats during chronic oral exposure to lead acetate

Strain of rat	Age at start of exposure	Duration of exposure (days)	Lead acetate added to diet (ppm as lead)	Blood lead concentration (µg/dL ± SD)	Reference
Fischer 344/N	6–7 weeks	30	0	–	Dieter *et al.* (1993)
			10	16 ± 1.7	
			30	31.8 ± 3.8	
			100	84.8 ± 8.9	
Fischer 344	4 weeks	7	0	5.0 ± 0.9	Freeman *et al.* (1996)
			17.6	32.0 ± 6.9	
			42.8	37.6 ± 5.4	
			127	77.1 ± 11.2	
		15	0	2.7 ± 0.3	
			17.6	20.5 ± 1.6	
			42.8	42.4 ± 8.4	
			127	67.6 ± 8.1	
		44	0	1.2 ± 0.1	
			17.6	24.9 ± 1.9	
			42.8	40.5 ± 2.8	
			127	70.6 ± 3.4	
Sprague-Dawley	24 days	31	*In drinking-water*	*Read from graph*	O'Flaherty (1991c)
		60	1000	~100	
			1000	~100	
	22 days	418	*In drinking-water*	*Read from graph*	
			1000	~120	
			2000	~135	

Intratracheal instillation, inhalation

The bioavailability of lead from inhaled particles depends on the particle size and is affected by the particle matrix.

A study by Eaton *et al.* (1984) showed that five weeks after exposure by intratracheal instillation, the vast majority of a lead chromate paint particulate suspension (median particle diameter, 6 μm) remained in the lung of rats (ratio lung lead:bone lead, 540). In contrast, after exposure to lead acetate, little remained in the lung, but significant elevations were found in bone (ratio lung lead:bone lead, 0.5) and kidney. Intratracheal instillation of lead tetraoxide showed an intermediate absorption rate (ratio lung lead:bone lead, 73).

Grobler *et al.* (1988) showed that in rats exposed to aerosols of lead chloride (0.05, 77, 249 and 1546 μg lead/m³) (mass median diameter (MMD), < 5.8 μm; 56% of the total particles at 77 μg/m³, 44% at 249 μg/m³, 37% at 1546 μg/m³) for 28, 50 and 77 days, blood lead concentrations reached relatively stable plateaux, which differed significantly with lead exposure. Stability was reached after 10 days at the highest exposure concentration and after 30 days when rats were exposed to 249 μg/m³. When exposure ceased, blood lead concentrations declined with a half-life of 3–5 days.

In baboons, the rate of absorption of lead into the bloodstream after exposure to coarse (mean particle size, 1.6 μm; MMD, 5.9 μm) airborne particles of lead oxide was faster and the concentration reached was higher than that after exposure to fine (mean particle size, 0.8 μ; MMD, 2 μm) particles (Rendall *et al.*, 1975). This finding contrasts with the greater deposition and absorption rates of fine particles (< 1 μm) reported in humans exposed by inhalation (ATSDR, 1999; see also Section 4.1.1(*a*)(i)).

Blood lead concentrations measured in the studies by Rendall *et al.* (1975) and Grobler *et al.* (1988) are given in Table 86.

Skin absorption

After application of a solution of lead acetate or nitrate (6.4 mg of lead) to the skin of female BALB/c mice, an analysis of the organs, faeces and urine showed that 0.4% of the applied dose was absorbed through the skin and entered the circulatory system. In less than 24 h significant increases in lead concentrations were observed in the skin, muscle, pancreas, spleen, kidney, liver, caecum, bone, heart and brain but not in the blood (Florence *et al.*, 1998).

Sun *et al.* (2002) measured the urinary lead content of rats after application of a patch of linen cloth containing lead compounds (100 mg lead in petrolatum on a 2 × 6-cm cloth), under occlusive conditions, for 12 days. Total amounts of lead in urine increased from 10.8 ng in the controls to 3679.3 ng for lead naphthenate, 146.0 ng for lead stearate, 736.6 ng for lead nitrate, 123.1 ng for lead sulfate, 115.9 ng for lead oxide and 47.8 ng for lead metal powder.

In studies by Bress and Bidanset (1991), in-vivo absorption was measured by applying 300 mg/kg bw tetrabutyl lead, lead nuolate, lead naphthenate, lead acetate or lead oxide to the shaved backs of guinea-pigs for 7 days under occluded wrappings. Tetrabutyl lead was

Table 86. Blood lead concentrations in baboons and rats during and after inhalation exposure

Species	Exposure protocol	Mean blood lead concentration (µg/dL ± SD)	Reference
Baboon (*Papio ursinus*)	Dust clouds of Pb_3O_4; target conc., 2 mg/m^3 lead; mean particle size: group A, 1.6 µm; group B, 0.8 µm; 5 days/week for 4 weeks	At the end of exposure: group A, ~50*; group B, ~18* 6 weeks after end of exposure: group A, 40 ± 19.7; group B, 20 ± 7.7	Rendall *et al.* (1975)
BD IX rats	Aerosol of lead chloride; 4 groups;	During exposure (plateau conc.)	Grobler *et al.* (1988)
	0.05 µg/m^3 lead (controls)	0.5–4	
	77 µg/m^3 lead for 77 days	~15*	
	249 µg/m^3 lead for 28 days	~25*	
	1546 µg/m^3 lead for 50 days	~60*	
	All groups, 22 h/day, 7 days/week		

*Read from the graph

present in blood, brain, liver and kidney in the highest quantities. Lead nuolate was found in greater amounts than lead naphthenate in the liver and kidneys. Lead acetate was poorly absorbed while lead oxide showed no absorption (see also Section 4.1.2(*b*)(i)).

(ii) *Distribution*

Experimental studies have shown that lead is rapidly distributed into soft and mineralizing tissues after acute and chronic exposures. The initial distribution of lead into soft tissues has a half-life of 3.5 days in rats (O'Flaherty, 1991c).

In rodents and non-human primates, 98–99% of the blood lead content is associated with erythrocytes, the remainder being found in the plasma (Morgan *et al.*, 1977; Willes *et al.*, 1977; Keller & Doherty, 1980a; Palminger Hallén & Oskarsson, 1993). As in humans, plasma lead is the source of lead available to distribution and excretion processes. Keller and Doherty (1980a) found that milk lead concentration in lactating mice was linearly related to plasma lead concentration but not to blood lead concentration. Similarly, Oskarsson *et al.* (1992) were able to fit the relationship between lead concentrations in whole blood and milk in cows with an exponential expression, demonstrating its nonlinearity.

A physiologically-based model in which soft-tissue distribution and excretion of lead are assumed to be proportional both to the rate of blood flow to the tissue (which is proportional to plasma flow) and to the concentration of lead in blood plasma has successfully reproduced the time-profile of concentration changes in blood lead after cessation of chronic feeding of lead to rats (O'Flaherty, 1991c). Because of the high dose rates used in these studies (blood lead concentrations in excess of 100 μg/dL) and the disproportionality between plasma lead and blood lead, a model that assumed distribution to be proportional to whole blood lead could not have duplicated the observed blood lead concentration profiles.

After acute exposure by inhalation, lead content expressed as percentage of the dose in rats has been shown to be highest in kidneys, liver and lung, with concentrations increasing in bone as those in soft tissues declined and stabilized (Morgan & Holmes, 1978). After oral exposure, lead concentrations in rats were highest in kidneys (Aungst *et al.*, 1981). After intravenous injection of ^{203}Pb-lead chloride to rats, 20% of the dose was found initially in the kidney; subsequently, long-term deposition of 25–30% occurred in bone (Morgan *et al.*, 1977). At steady state, the pattern of distribution of lead is bone > kidney > liver > brain (Griffin *et al.*, 1975b; Morgan *et al.*, 1977; Conrad & Barton, 1978; Kostial *et al.*, 1978; Aungst *et al.*, 1981; Rader *et al.*, 1981; Mykkänen *et al.*, 1982; Cikrt *et al.*, 1983; Miller *et al.*, 1983; Cory-Slechta *et al.*, 1989; P'An & Kennedy, 1989).

When Sprague-Dawley rats (44–48 days old at the beginning of the study, maturc adult at the end) were given intraperitoneal injections of lead acetate (10 or 20 mg/kg bw) at 1, 2, 4, 8, 12, 16, 20 and 24 weeks, lead accumulated steadily in the bone, kidney and brain and reached high concentrations in bone and kidney, but remained low in brain. The authors suggested that although brain lead values increased, some regulatory mechanisms limited access of lead to the adult brain (P'An & Kennedy, 1989). In a study reported by Crowe and Morgan (1996), rats were exposed to lead acetate from 3 days prior to birth (day 18 of pregnancy) until 15, 21 or 63 days postpartum, via the placenta, and then via the milk. This was achieved by giving a diet containing 0 or 3% lead acetate to pregnant Wistar rats, as well as 0.2% lead acetate in their drinking-water. After weaning, 0.2% lead acetate in the drinking-water became the sole source of dietary lead for the offspring. To study the effect of iron deficiency on lead absorption, low-iron diets were given to mothers from day 18 of pregnancy and were continued with the young offspring rats after weaning. It was found that iron deficiency did not increase lead deposition in the brain and brain lead concentrations were relatively low (< 0.1 μg/g) in all rats. Lead concentrations in the liver were below 2 μg/g, whereas kidneys had almost 20-fold higher concentrations. Compared with other tissues, the blood–brain barrier appeared to restrict lead uptake by the brain independent of the iron status of the animals; the functional blood-brain barrier is present very early in development, possibly before birth (Crowe & Morgan, 1996). In other studies in rats, following intravenous administration, lead has been shown to cross the blood–brain barrier (Bradbury & Deane, 1993).

In rats exposed almost continuously (22 h/day, 7 days/week) to lead oxide particles (MMD, 86% ≤ 0.18 μm) at an average concentration of 21.5 μg/m³ for 12 months, the concentrations of lead in blood, kidney and liver were found to reach a maximum at 3–4 months of exposure and did not increase significantly after that time. The concentration of lead in soft tissues decreased after the exposure, but remained elevated in bone (Griffin *et al.*, 1975b). In a subsequent study in which rats were exposed to lead oxide particles (20 μg/m³) for 15 months, a small increase in tissue lead was found between the sixth and the fifteenth months of exposure, but in the femur the increase during this period was nearly 70% (Russell *et al.*, 1978).

In studies conducted by Maldonado-Vega *et al.* (1996), rats were given 100 ppm [100 μg/mL] lead acetate in distilled water either before and during lactation (during 158 days), or before lactation only (144 days), or during lactation only (14 days). Results were compared with those obtained from non-pregnant lead-exposed matched rats and non-exposed pregnant and non-pregnant control rats. During lactation, lead concentrations in blood, liver and kidney increased while those in bone decreased. The increase in tissue concentrations was shown to result from increased intestinal absorption (exogenous exposure) and bone resorption (endogenous exposure). Significant deposition of lead in bone was observed in rats exposed to lead only during lactation indicating that both processes (deposition and bone resorption) take place in this period (Maldonado-Vega *et al.*, 1996, 2002).

There is experimental evidence of lead mobilization from bones to blood (Grobler *et al.*, 1991). In studies in monkeys, 17–20% of the total blood lead originated from historical bone stores (Inskip *et al.*, 1996; O'Flaherty *et al.*, 1998). Increased lead release from the skeleton occurs during pregnancy and lactation (Buchet *et al.*, 1977; Maldonado-Vega *et al.*, 1996; Franklin *et al.*, 1997; Maldonado-Vega *et al.*, 2002). Maternal-to-fetal transfer of lead appears to be related partly to the mobilization of lead from the maternal skeleton. Evidence for transfer of maternal bone lead to the fetus has been provided by studies with stable lead isotopes in cynomolgus monkeys (*Macaca fascicularis*). The study by Franklin *et al.* (1997) showed that 7–39% of the maternal lead burden that is transferred to the fetus appears to derive from the maternal skeleton (see Section 4.1.1(*a*)(v)).

The mean half-life of lead in bone was found to be 3.0 ± 1.0 years in the rhesus monkey (McNeill *et al.*, 1997). Injection of 25 μCi of an aqueous solution of ^{210}Pb and its daughters into adult rats and analysis of bone tissue over the subsequent 140 days showed a half-life of lead in bone of 64–109 days (Torvik *et al.*, 1974).

Age-related differences in the distribution of lead have been reported in experimental animals. After intraperitoneal injection of ^{203}Pb, marked differences were observed in the kinetics of lead retention and distribution in suckling as compared with adult rats. Compared with older rats, suckling rats showed 2.3-fold higher whole-body retention, higher blood concentrations and an almost 8-fold greater accumulation in the brain. Retention in the kidneys was one third lower in the suckling rats (Momcilovic & Kostial, 1974; Kostial *et al.*, 1978).

Similar findings have also been reported for kidney and bone in neonatal monkeys exposed to a single oral dose of ^{210}Pb lead nitrate. Bone lead concentrations and bone:blood lead ratios were significantly higher in infant monkeys than in adults. Brain:blood lead ratios were significantly greater in 10-day-old infants than in adult monkeys. The liver lead concentration was also higher in neonates and young monkeys than in adults (Willes *et al.*,

1977). Lead concentrations in fetal bone of monkeys have been reported to exceed maternal bone lead concentrations (Franklin *et al.*, 1997).

Ageing has also been shown to alter the pattern of distribution of lead in rats administered lead acetate in drinking-water. In studies reported by Cory-Slechta *et al.* (1989), blood lead concentrations in adult (8-month-old) and old (16-month-old) rats showed different trends over the course of exposure; values in adults declined, while those of old rats tended to increase. Brain lead concentrations and, to a marginally significant extent, liver lead concentrations were higher in old rats than in adult rats, while bone lead concentrations were significantly lower in old rats than in adult rats. The pattern of distribution, namely femur > liver > brain, was similar in all age groups, but age-related increases in lead concentrations in brain and kidney were noted, along with decreases in femoral bone lead content. This shift did not appear to reflect enhanced lead uptake from the gastrointestinal tract but rather a change in bone physiology with age, combined with altered patterns of urinary lead excretion over time (Cory-Slechta, 1990).

The intracellular bioavailability of lead in major target organs such as the kidney and brain appears to be determined largely by formation of complexes with a group of low-molecular-weight proteins. Several distinct high-affinity cytosolic lead-binding proteins (PbBP) have been identified in the rat kidney and brain that appear to act as receptors for lead (Oskarsson *et al.*, 1982; DuVal & Fowler, 1989). The PbBP from rat kidney has been shown to be a specific cleavage product of α_{2u}-globulin, produced most extensively in the livers of male rats and to a much lesser extent in female rats of breeding age. The PbBP was shown to migrate to the nucleus and form complexes with nuclear chromatin (Mistry *et al.*, 1985; 1986; Fowler & DuVal, 1991). The renal PbBP is selectively localized in only certain nephrons and only specific segments of the renal proximal tubule. Short-term, high-dose lead exposure (1% or 7% lead acetate in drinking-water for 7 weeks) resulted in increased excretion of this protein in the urine with a concomitant decrease in renal concentrations of PbBP (Fowler & DuVal, 1991). The brain PbBP appears to be a chemically similar but distinct molecule (DuVal & Fowler, 1989). High-affinity PbBPs have also been identified in the kidney and brain of monkeys (Fowler *et al.*, 1993).

(iii) *Excretion*

Excretion of lead occurs mainly in the faeces and urine (WHO, 1985). Adult mice were found to excrete about 62% of intravenously injected lead within 50 days; cumulative lead concentrations in faeces were 25–50% of the administered dose (Keller & Doherty, 1980b). Adult rats excreted 24.4% and 9.5% of intravenously injected lead in faeces and urine, respectively, within 48 h (Kostial & Momcilovic, 1974). In rats and monkeys exposed by inhalation to lead oxide (21.5 μg/m^3) for 1 year, lead excretion was greater in faeces than in urine, but wide variations between individual animals were noted (Griffin *et al.*, 1975b). Five days after a single intravenous dose of ^{203}Pb in rats, total lead excretion was found to amount to 53%, with similar amounts being excreted in urine and faeces, except on day 2 (ratio faeces:urine, 2) (Morgan *et al.*, 1977). Studies on rats exposed for 30–45 min to an 'urban-like' aerosol of ^{210}Pb-dibenzoylmethane (added to gasoline and burned in a tubular furnace heater at 600 °C) showed that, 6 days after inhalation, less than 1% of the total absorbed dose of lead was retained in lung, 40% had been eliminated in faeces and 15% in urine, 40% was fixed in the skeleton and 4–5% in soft tissue (Boudene *et al.*, 1977).

Studies on dogs after intravenous administration of ^{210}Pb showed that 56–75% of the total dose of lead was excreted in the faeces (Hursh, 1973; Lloyd *et al.*, 1975).

Adult monkeys have been shown to excrete more absorbed lead in faeces than young animals (13% versus 3.45%), while urinary excretion was similar (5.31% versus 3.84%) (Pounds *et al.*, 1978).

Marked species differences in the biliary excretion of lead have been reported (Castellino *et al.*, 1966; Klaassen & Shoeman, 1974; Conrad & Barton, 1978; Cikrt *et al.*, 1983; Gregus & Klaassen, 1986). A relatively high biliary excretion of lead was reported in rats (Klaassen & Shoeman, 1974). About 6.5–8.5% of a dose of ^{210}Pb-lead nitrate or ^{203}Pb-lead chloride administered intravenously to rats was excreted in the bile within 24 h; biliary excretion thus plays an important role in the enterohepatic circulation of lead in rats (Cikrt, 1972; Cikrt & Tichy, 1975). In a further study, biliary excretion of lead was analysed in three groups of rats given drinking-water containing lead acetate (at 100, 250 and 2500 mg lead/L) for 80 days. Biliary excretion of lead in the exposed groups reached 0.08 ± 0.01, 0.20 ± 0.04 and 1.46 ± 0.09 μg/mL, respectively, compared with 0.05 ± 0.04 μg/mL in a control group (Cikrt *et al.*, 1983). Rabbits have been shown to excrete lead in the bile at < 50% and dogs at < 2% of the rates of biliary excretion of lead in rats (Klaassen & Shoeman, 1974).

Studies on the renal handling of lead (^{203}Pb) in dogs showed that plasma lead is filtered and reabsorbed but that there is no evidence of tubular secretion of lead (Vander *et al.*, 1977). Urinary clearance of lead was calculated to be 19% of the estimated glomerular filtration rate in two cynomolgus monkeys (O'Flaherty *et al.*, 1996).

In rodents, lead is transferred across the placenta to fetuses and during lactation to the litter (Kostial & Momcilovic, 1974; McClain & Siekierka, 1975; Hackett *et al.*, 1982a,b; Donald *et al.*, 1986; Maldonado-Vega *et al.*, 1996, 2002). The lactational transfer after current or recent exposure of dams to lead is considerably higher than the placental transfer (Kostial & Momcilovic, 1974; Palminger Hallén *et al.*, 1995b). A high transfer of lead into milk was demonstrated in rodents, as well as a high uptake of lead in the tissues of suckling pups. About 20–33% of an initial maternal dose of lead was transferred to suckling rats or mice (Momcilovic, 1978; Keller & Doherty, 1980a; Palminger Hallén *et al.*, 1996b). In a study by Palminger Hallén & Oskarsson (1993), rat and mouse dams were administered a single intravenous dose of ^{203}Pb on day 14 of lactation in four or five doses ranging from 0.0005 to 2.0 mg/kg bw. The concentration of ^{203}Pb in plasma was linearly correlated with that in milk. The milk:plasma ratios were 119 and 72 in mice and 89 and 35 in rats at 24 and 72 h after administration, respectively. Excretion into milk appeared more efficient in mice than in rats, but rat pups had higher tissue concentrations than mouse pups; this may be due to a higher bioavailability and/or a lower excretion of lead in rat pups (Palminger Hallén & Oskarsson, 1993). Continuous exposure of rats to lead in drinking-water during gestation and lactation resulted, at day 15 of lactation, in milk lead concentrations about 2.5-fold higher than blood lead concentrations. When exposure to lead was terminated at parturition, the milk lead concentrations were similar to those of blood lead at day 15 of lactation, and were only 10% of the milk lead concentrations found after continuous exposure to lead during gestation and lactation. Exposure of offspring to lead via placenta and milk from dams exposed continuously resulted in blood and brain lead concentrations sixfold higher than those in offspring exposed via the placenta only. Exposure of offspring via milk only from dams exposed to lead until parturition resulted in blood lead concentrations that were higher than those in offspring exposed to lead via the placenta only (Palminger Hallén *et al.*, 1995b).

(*c*) *Experimental systems* in vitro

In vitro, intestinal permeability to lead has been shown to be similar in intestines from fasted and fed rats (Aungst & Fung, 1981).

Healy *et al.* (1982) showed that the rate of dissolution of lead sulfide in gastric acid *in vitro* was dependent on particle size, being much greater for particles of 30 μm diameter than for particles of 100 μm diameter.

Studies in kidneys of rats *in vitro* have shown that the kidney PbBP facilitates the nuclear uptake of lead followed by its binding to chromatin (Mistry *et al.*, 1985, 1986; Fowler & DuVal, 1991; Goering, 1993; Fowler, 1998).

Bress and Bidanset (1991) measured the degree of in-vitro penetration of lead acetate and lead oxide, using diffusion tubes in excised guinea-pig skin and human skin from autopsy. The percentage recovery of lead acetate in guinea-pig skin and human skin was 0.03% and 0.05%, respectively. There were no measurable amounts of lead oxide absorbed in either species.

Steady-state kinetic analyses of ^{210}Pb in hepatocytes from rats demonstrated three compartments, more than 85% of the lead being found in the kinetic pool associated with mitochondria (Pounds *et al.*, 1982). In osteoclastic bone cells from mouse calvaria, three similar kinetic pools of intracellular lead containing approximately 10%, 12% and 78% of total cellular lead were identified; as in hepatocytes, the bulk of cellular lead was associated with mitochondria. The half-times for isotopic exchange were 1, 27 and 480 min, respectively (Pounds & Rosen, 1986).

4.1.2 *Organic lead compounds*

The toxicity of organic lead compounds is generally high, but varies widely between animal species and according to the chemical structure of the compound. Most of the information available concerns tetraethyl lead, but the toxicity of tetramethyl lead and some of its metabolites is also well described. Organic lead compounds are toxicokinetically distinct from inorganic lead compounds in terms of absorption and distribution and, owing to their greater lipophilicity, they are rapidly partitioned into soft tissues.

(*a*) *Humans*

(i) *Absorption*

Inhalation exposure

Inhaled tetraethyl and tetramethyl lead vapours behave as gases in the respiratory tract and, as a result, their pattern and extent of deposition and absorption differ from that of inhaled inorganic lead particles (US EPA, 1994; ATSDR, 1999). These differences result in a higher fractional absorption: approximately 60–80% of the deposited tetraethyl and tetramethyl lead was absorbed by the lungs (Heard *et al.*, 1979).

Dermal exposure

Tetraethyl lead is a lipophilic substance that can penetrate intact skin in lethal quantities. The amount absorbed is proportional to the surface area exposed and the concentration. Accidents involving transdermal absorption of tetraethyl lead and tetramethyl lead in humans have been described (Hayakawa, 1972; Gething, 1975). Due to its higher lipophilicity, tetraethyl lead is more readily absorbed than tetramethyl lead.

(ii) *Distribution*

Inhalation of tetraethyl lead results in much higher concentrations of lead in the brain than does inhalation exposure to inorganic lead.

Distribution of organic lead in humans has been observed to be highly variable and measurements are complicated by metabolism of the alkyl lead to inorganic lead. For example, in a man who ingested a chemical mixture containing 59% tetraethyl lead (38% lead w/w), the highest concentrations of triethyl lead and inorganic lead were found in the liver and kidneys followed by the brain, pancreas and heart (Bolanowska *et al.*, 1967). In another report in which a man and a woman accidentally inhaled a solvent containing 31% tetraethyl lead (17.6% lead w/w), concentrations of triethyl lead and inorganic lead were highest in the liver and lower in the kidney, brain, pancreas, muscle and heart (Bolanowska *et al.*, 1967), although the liver/kidney ratio for triethyl lead was 5:1 in the woman compared with that of 1.3:1 in the man. Trialkyl lead metabolites have also been detected in brain tissue of subjects not occupationally exposed to air pollution (Nielsen *et al.*, 1978).

Organic lead compounds are ultimately metabolized to inorganic lead and the latter is stored in the bones (Schwartz *et al.*, 1999, 2000a).

(iii) *Metabolism*

Alkyl lead compounds are actively metabolized in the liver through oxidative dealkylation catalyzed by cytochrome P-450. Relatively few human studies that address the metabolism of alkyl lead compounds were found in the available literature (Bolanowska *et al.*, 1967; Nielsen *et al.*, 1978; ATSDR, 1999).

(iv) *Excretion*

Tetraethyl lead is excreted in the urine as diethyllead and inorganic lead (Turlakiewicz & Chmielnicka, 1985; Vural & Duydu, 1995). Following inhalation exposure, exhalation of tetraalkyl lead compounds is a major pathway of elimination in humans. Heard *et al.* (1979) showed that 48 h after inhalation exposure, 40% and 20% of inhaled tetramethyl and tetraethyl lead doses, respectively, that were initially deposited in the lung, were exhaled, and there was little urinary excretion.

(*b*) *Animals*

(i) *Absorption*

Bress and Bidanset (1991) measured absorption *in vivo* by applying 300 mg/kg tetrabutyl lead, lead nuolate, lead naphthenate, lead acetate or lead oxide to the shaved backs of guinea-pigs for 7 days under occluded wrappings. Tetrabutyl lead was present in tissues in the highest quantities: mean (± SD) total lead concentration reached 7.46 (± 0.68) μg/g in blood, 8.52 (± 0.46) μg/g in kidney, 4.31 (± 0.21) μg/g in liver and 4.02 (± 0.29) μg/g in brain (see also Section 4.1.1(*b*)(i)).

(ii) *Distribution*

Previous monographs (IARC, 1972; 1980) have summarized many studies on the distribution of lead published before 1980. In more recent studies in rabbits (Arai *et al.*, 1998), total lead in the brain 1 day after intravenous injection of triethyl neopentoxy lead consisted of triethyl lead alone; total lead in liver and kidney was about 72–78% triethyl lead, about 14–19% inorganic lead and about 8–9% diethyl lead. Lead in blood was about 34% triethyl lead, about 38% inorganic lead and about 28% diethyl lead. In bile, it was about 2% triethyl lead, about 9% inorganic lead and about 89% diethyl lead. These ratios of lead species in the organs were similar 7 days after injection, but only inorganic lead was detected in blood.

Studies by Morgan and Holmes (1978) using adult rats exposed for 40–60 min by inhalation to an aerosol containing ^{203}Pb-tetraethyl lead added to lead-free petrol showed that less than 2% of the dose was present in the lungs after 1 week. Mean total deposition of lead was calculated to be 30.5%. At least half of the ^{203}Pb deposited in the lungs was absorbed with a half-life of less than 1 h. To investigate whether lead in ingested exhaust particles is absorbed from the gastrointestinal tract, exhaust particles from an engine running on ^{203}Pb tetraethyl-enriched gasoline were collected on millipore filters, which were then fed to rats. Less than 0.5% of the ^{203}Pb lead associated with the particles was found to be absorbed.

(iii) *Metabolism*

Tetraethyl and tetramethyl lead undergo oxidative dealkylation and are metabolized to the highly neurotoxic metabolites triethyl and trimethyl lead, respectively. In rabbit liver, the reaction is catalysed by a cytochrome P-450-dependent monoxygenase system

(Kimmel *et al.,* 1977). Complete oxidation of alkyl lead to inorganic lead also occurs in rat, mouse and rabbit (Bolanowska, 1968; ATSDR, 1999).

(iv) *Excretion*

Previous monographs have summarized many studies on the excretion of lead published before 1980 (IARC, 1972; 1980). Kozarzewska and Chmielnicka (1987) studied the excretion of tetraethyl lead in rabbits. After intragastric or intravenous administration to rabbits of 12 mg/kg bw tetraethyl lead, diethyl lead constituted 70–90% and 50%, respectively, of the total lead excreted in urine during the first seven days, and 70% and 40%, respectively, after 30 days. Maximum diethyl lead excretion occurred on the first three days regardless of the route of the administration. After administration of a 3 mg/kg bw dose, excretion of diethyl lead did not vary so much between the intragastric and the intravenous routes of administration; in this case, during 30 days of observation, diethyl lead constitued about 40% of the total lead excreted in urine. In rabbits exposed for 5 h to tetraethyl lead by inhalation at a concentration of 200 μg/m^3 in air, maximum diethyl lead excretion was recorded on day 2 after exposure and constituted about 20% of total lead excreted in the urine. On day 7, only trace quantities of this metabolite were found.

Arai and Yamamura (1990) showed that in rabbits, after a single intravenous dose of 9.9 mg/kg bw tetramethyl lead (7.7 mg/kg bw lead), the mixture of lead compounds excreted in urine was composed of about 73% dimethyl lead, 19% trimethyl lead, 6% inorganic lead and 2% tetramethyl lead on the day following injection. The excretion on day 7 was entirely composed of trimethyl lead. In rabbits injected with 39.7 mg/kg bw tetramethyl lead (30.8 mg/kg bw lead), total urinary lead excretion was composed of about 67% dimethyl lead, 14% trimethyl lead, 17% inorganic lead and 2% tetramethyl lead on the day following administration and about 8% dimethyl lead, 74% trimethyl lead, 17% inorganic lead and 1% tetramethyl lead on day 7 after dosing. In both groups of rabbits, total lead excretion in faeces during the 7 days after injection was entirely composed of inorganic lead. During the same period, 1–3% of either administered dose of tetramethyl lead was excreted in the urine and 7–19% in the faeces.

Further studies (Arai *et al.*, 1998) showed that about 4% of an intravenous dose of triethyl neopentoxy lead (10 mg/kg bw; 4 mg/kg bw lead) administered to rabbits was excreted in the urine within 7 days and about 68% in the faeces. Urinary excretion of total lead was composed of about 85% diethyl lead, 8% triethyl lead and 7% inorganic lead. The 7-day faecal excretion was composed of about 92% inorganic lead, 4% diethyl lead and 4% triethyl lead. Hence, the major chemical species of lead excreted in the urine was diethyl lead, while the major species excreted in the faeces was inorganic lead.

(*c*) *Experimental systems* in vitro

Bress and Bidanset (1991) measured the degree of in-vitro penetration of tetrabutyl lead, lead naphthenate, lead nuolate, lead acetate and lead oxide, using diffusion tubes in excised guinea-pig skin and human skin from autopsy. The percentage recovery of lead in guinea-pig skin ranged from 1.3% with tetrabutyl lead, demonstrating the highest skin penetration, followed by lead naphthanate (0.45%), lead nuolate (0.25%), lead acetate (0.03%) and lead oxide (< 0.01%). The same rank order of recovery was seen in excised human skin where recovery of tetrabutyl lead was 6.3%.

4.2 Toxic effects

The extensive literature on the toxic properties of lead up until 1998 has been reviewed in the Toxicological Profile for Lead (ATSDR, 1999) and earlier by the National Research Council (NRC, 1993).

4.2.1 *Overt symptoms of lead intoxication*

Mankind has been using lead for over 6000 years and the widespread contamination of the environment with lead is solely the result of anthropogenic activities. In 370 BC, the Greek physician Hippocrates was probably the first to recognize lead as the cause of colic in a man who was a metal worker. In the 1st century AD, Dioscorides, another Greek physician, noted that exposure to lead could cause paralysis and delirium in addition to intestinal problems and swelling (Cilliers & Retief, 2000; Hernberg, 2000). In Roman times winemakers used lead pots or lead-lined kettles to boil the crushed grapes, and added lead acetate to their wine as a sweetener (Aitchinson, 1960). References to paralysis in miners exposed to lead increased in Europe in the 1600s, as did reports of colic in wine-drinkers (Lin-Fu, 1992).

One of the earliest manifestations of lead intoxication in adults is so-called lead-induced colic, which is a syndrome characterized by a combination of abdominal pain, constipation, cramps, nausea, vomiting, anorexia and weight loss. Various pathogenic mechanisms have been proposed for this syndrome: it may result from changes in visceral smooth muscle tone secondary to the action of lead on the visceral autonomic nervous system; from lead-induced alterations in sodium transport in the small-intestinal mucosa; and from lead-induced interstitial pancreatitis. The possible presence of this syndrome should be considered in the differential diagnosis of abdominal pain of obscure etiology, and whenever a disparity is observed between the symptoms and the abdominal findings in a patient with abdominal pain, especially in the presence of a history of occupational exposure to lead (Janin *et al.*, 1985).

Many cases of acute lead intoxication have been described in the literature (for reviews, see Srianujata, 1998; Vig & Hu, 2000; Matte, 2003). Only a few studies are discussed below.

The effects on health of occupational exposure to lead have been investigated in 92 exposed workers in a lead–acid battery factory and 40 non-exposed workers who served as a control group. The two groups were closely similar in age, stature, body weight and socioeconomic status. In the factory, concentrations of lead in air varied between 1.8 and 2.2 mg/m^3. In 46 workers, average concentrations of lead in blood were 48–81 μg/dL, depending on job title. In 12 controls, an average blood lead concentration of 21 μg/dL was measured. A highly significant increase ($p < 0.01$) was also recorded in urinary coproporphyrin and basophilic stippled red blood cells of the exposed group in comparison with the control group. Central nervous system symptoms (insomnia, fatigue, weakness and drowsiness) were reported by 50% of the workers, and other symptoms such as abdominal colic and constipation were noted by 41% of the exposed group (Awad el Karim *et al.*, 1986).

Three cases of acute lead poisoning in adults were reported to be caused by exposure to old leaded paint. Initial concentrations of lead in blood in the three subjects were 84.2, 85.2 and 87.1 μg/dL, respectively, and all complained of abdominal pain, malaise and nausea. The patients received sodium calcium edetate and/or succimer for three weeks, which reduced their blood lead concentrations by 50–75%. Despite removal from the source of exposure, lead concentrations remained elevated in two cases, which may be explained by release of lead from the skeleton (Gordon *et al.*, 2002).

A case of severe lead poisoning in a young woman was reported to be caused by prolonged use of eye make-up ('kohl') made of lead sulfide. Clinically, the patient presented with abdominal cramps, anxiety and irritability, and microcytic sideropenic anaemia. Emergency chelate treatment improved her condition and decreased lead concentrations in blood from their initial value of 490 μg/dL to 49 μg/dL 6 weeks after treatment (Bruyneel *et al.*, 2002).

4.2.2 *Effects on haeme-containing systems*

(*a*) *Humans*

Interaction with enzymes and high-affinity metal-binding proteins is probably the most important mechanism of lead toxicity. This interaction usually consists of reversible binding of lead to sulfhydryl groups or to other protein sites capable of binding divalent cations. In this regard, the most well-known example is the inhibition by lead of δ-aminolevulinic acid dehydratase (ALAD) (also known as porphobilinogen synthase, PBGS), a key enzyme in the pathway of haeme synthesis (Figure 5). This enzyme has a unique zinc binding site (Jaffe *et al.*, 2001) that confers a very high affinity for Pb^{2+} (Simons, 1995).

Over the past 10 years, attention has been paid increasingly to early, subtle (subclinical) effects of lead on haeme systems, the hypothesis being that these form a physiopathogenetic continuum with the clinical or overt effects. The only difference between early and clinical effects of a given type depends on their degree and not on their nature (Goyer, 1990b). The effects on haeme synthesis and haematological effects are dose-dependent (Table 87) and become manifest at blood lead concentrations < 10 μg/dL (ALAD inhibition), at 15–30 μg/dL (inhibition of iron chelation in haeme), and 50–60 μg/dL (reduction of haemoglobin concentrations).

Effects of lead, such as inhibition of ALAD, elevation of aminolevulinic acid (ALA) in urine and increase of free erythrocyte protoporphyrin in blood, have been observed in humans exposed to lead (Lauwerys *et al.*, 1973; Alessio *et al.*, 1976; Tomokuni & Ogata, 1976; Horiguchi *et al.*, 1981; Moore, 1988). These biological indicators correlate more or

Figure 5. Haeme biosynthesis in the cell

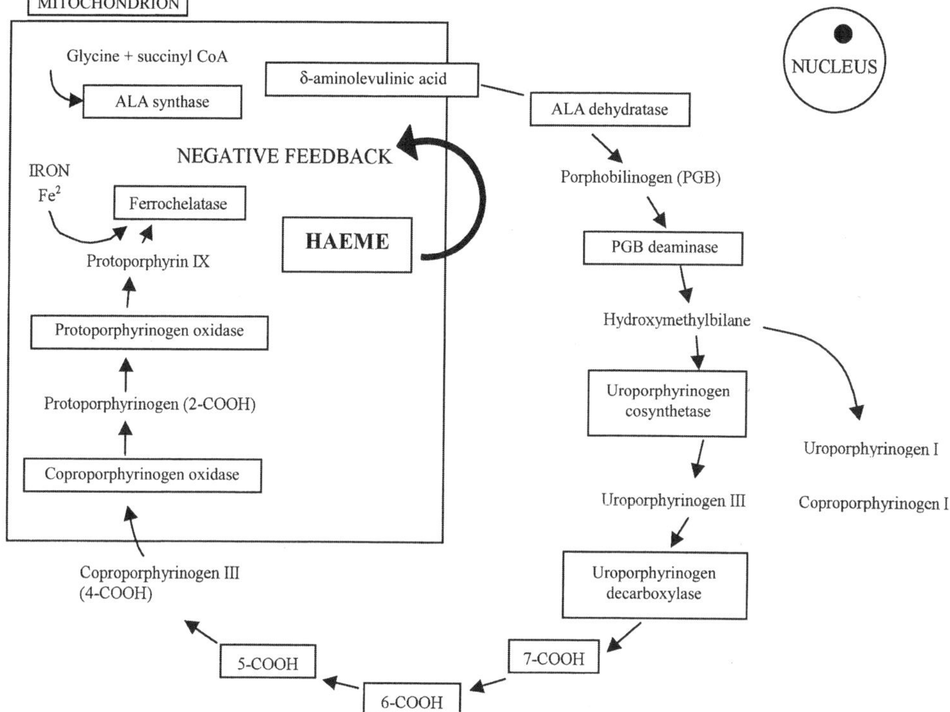

Modified from Moore (1988)
Lead inhibits ALA dehydratase, coproporphyrinogen oxidase and ferrochelatase with consequent increases in the urinary excretion of ALA and coproporphyrin III together with accumulation of protoporphyrin 9 in the erythrocyte. Primary control of the rate-limiting enzyme, 5-aminolaevulinate synthase is vested in the end product of the pathway, haeme through the 'pool' of free haeme in the cell. This pool is depleted in lead poisoning through diminished synthesis of haeme and enhanced catabolism of the haeme by haeme oxygenase. The net result is increased synthesis of ALA synthase and excessive production of pathway intermediates. There is, in addition, some deleterious influence on haemoprotein synthesis because of the lack of haeme substrate for their formation.

less closely with the concentration of lead in peripheral blood (see Section 1.6.2), and are therefore useful in evaluating the effect of lead in individuals exposed occupationally or environmentally to the metal. They have also been used for assessing exposure to lead.

In addition to effects on haeme in erythropoiesis, attention has also been paid to the possible effects of lead on other haeme-containing enzymatic systems, such as P450 cytochromes or systems involved in the metabolism of vitamin D (Silbergeld *et al.* 1988; Goyer, 1990b). Such effects result in a decreased availability of cytochromes for the respiratory chain and the accumulation of toxic metabolites such as ALA.

Table 87. Effects of lead on haeme synthesis in adults and relative concentrations of lead in blood at which they become manifest

Lowest observed effect level (blood lead concentration, µg/dL)	Haeme synthesis and haematological effects
80	Frank anaemia
50	Reduced haemoglobin production
40	Increased urinary ALA and elevated coproporphyrins
25–30	EP elevation in men
15–20	EP elevation in women
< 10	ALAD inhibition

Adapted from US EPA (1986)
ALA, delta-aminolevulinic acid; ALAD, delta-aminolevulinic acid dehydratase; EP, erythrocyte protoporphyrin

(i) *Inhibition of ALAD by lead*

Inhibition of ALAD by lead is discussed in Section 1.6.2. It is responsible in part for increases in ALA in plasma, in blood and in urine. ALA synthase is induced by negative feedback from the depression of haeme synthesis. ALA in plasma and blood should reflect the effects of lead more directly than ALA in urine (Moore *et al.*, 1980b; WHO, 1980; see Section 1.6.2 for analytical methods).

In subjects recently exposed to lead, there is a latency period of about 2 weeks before ALA in urine increases. After cessation of exposure, the excretion of ALA in urine returns to normal relatively quickly; thus this parameter is not suitable for detecting past exposure to lead (Tola *et al.*, 1973; Haeger-Aronsen *et al.*, 1974; Benson *et al.*, 1976).

(ii) *ALAD gene polymorphism*

ALAD is a well-known enzyme that is essential to tetrapyrrole biosynthesis (e.g. haeme, chlorophyll and vitamin B12). In humans, ALAD is a polymorphic enzyme with two common alleles, $ALAD_1$ and $ALAD_2$ (Battistuzzi *et al.*, 1981; Petrucci *et al.*, 1982). The enzyme is polymorphic due to a G-to-C transversion of nucleotide 177 in the coding region, which results in replacement of lysine by asparagine at position 59 in the protein (Wetmur *et al.*, 1991a).

Numerous studies have investigated the role of the ALAD polymorphism in relation to blood lead concentrations. The data indicate that at equivalent exposures, homozygotes or heterozygotes for $ALAD_2$ have significantly higher mean blood lead concentrations, and lower concentrations of ALAP (only at high blood lead concentrations, 40–60 µg/dL) than homozygotes for $ALAD_1$ (Wetmur *et al.*, 1991b; Smith *et al.*, 1995; Sithisarankul *et al.*, 1997; Sakai, 2000). However, no differences in the net accumulation of lead in bone were found (Fleming *et al.*, 1998). Lead (Pb^{2+}) has been shown to bind the ALAD enzyme by displacement of zinc (Zn^{2+}) (Simons, 1995; Bergdahl *et al.*, 1998a). The difference in haeme precursor concentrations in people carrying different ALAD genotypes is thought to be due to a difference in binding affinity of lead for the ALAD isoenzymes (Bergdahl *et al.*, 1997b). However, the model of human ALAD based on homologous crystal structure showed no obvious structural variation that would affect either metal binding to, or catalytic function of, the different ALAD isoenzymes. In in-vitro binding experiments, no differential displacement of Zn^{2+} by lead (Pb^{2+}) was found between the $ALAD_1$ (K59) and $ALAD_2$ (N59) protein variants (Jaffe *et al.*, 2000), but the two allozymes show a small difference in the kinetics of lead displacement by zinc (Jaffe *et al.*, 2001). This implies that differences in susceptibility to lead of subjects carrying different ALAD genotypes may be related to a difference in direct binding of lead to the gene products. However, other indirect mechanisms leading to differences in lead retention in carriers of the different genotypes cannot be ruled out.

(iii) *Other gene polymorphisms*

An additional polymorphism that may modify the toxicity of lead involves the vitamin D receptor (*VDR*) gene. This gene can exist in two alleles (B and b) and experimental data suggest that bone calcium content increases with increasing copy number of the b allele. Because lead can substitute for calcium in many biological systems, and since both lead and calcium are divalent cations, it has been suggested that the toxicity of lead may be modified by polymorphisms in the *VDR* gene which could explain the increased concentrations of lead in dense cortical bone in populations occupationally exposed to lead (Schwartz *et al.*, 2000b). The *VDR* gene is involved in the absorption of calcium through the gut and into calcium-rich tissue such as bone. However, effects of *VDR* polymorphism on a number of parameters of lead toxicity were not observed in a recent study of 798 workers exposed to lead (Weaver *et al.*, 2003).

Schwartz *et al.* (2000b) evaluated the association of tibial lead concentration with polymorphisms in the vitamin D receptor (*VDR*) gene in 504 former organolead manufacturing workers (mean age, 57.4 years). Tibial lead concentrations were measured by X-RF spectrometry in subjects with different *VDR* genotypes, adjusting for confounding variables. All study subjects had low tibial lead concentrations (mean, 14.4 μg/g bone mineral) and there were only small differences by *VDR* genotype. In a multiple linear regression model, the *VDR* genotype modified the relation between tibial lead concentration and age or years since last exposure. Although the influence of the *VDR* genotype on bone mineral density is a matter of debate, the data suggest that variant VDR alleles modify lead concentrations in bone.

Another gene that may influence the absorption of lead is the haemochromatosis gene encoding the HFE protein. Mutations in the *HFE* gene give rise to haemochromatosis in homozygous individuals. Because of the associations between iron and lead transport, it is possible that polymorphisms in the *HFE* gene may also influence the absorption of lead. Patients homozygous for the *HFE* mutation accumulate more lead than those who do not carry two mutated alleles (Barton *et al.*, 1994). The role of these genes in the effects of lead is not fully understood (Onalaja & Claudio, 2000).

(iv) *Lead and coproporphyrins*

Lead may inhibit other enzymes in the metabolic pathway of haemoglobin synthesis. Inhibition of coproporphyrinogen decarboxylase results in accumulation of coproporphyrins and their increased urinary excretion. Urinary coproporphyrin is not, however, a specific indicator of exposure to lead, since it may also result from porphyria cutanea tarda, liver disease, haemolytic anaemia, infectious disease and alcohol consumption. The influence of lead on disorders of porphyrin metabolism, which are more evident in women than in men, have been documented among lead-exposed workers.

No effects are detected on urinary coproporphyrin at blood lead concentrations ≤ 40 μg/dL and, in constantly exposed subjects, blood lead and urinary coproporphyrin correlate well, with a positive linear relation (Williams *et al.*, 1969; US EPA, 1986). Increased excretion of urinary coproporphyrin occurs with a latency of about 2 weeks, when blood lead concentrations are slightly higher than those at which ALAU increases (Tola *et al.*, 1973; Benson *et al.*, 1976). After cessation of exposure, the urinary coproporphyrin concentrations normalize with a few weeks (sometimes within a few days). The validity of urinary coproporphyrin to predict different blood lead concentrations is rather modest, so its use as a screening test is limited. In addition, subjects with severe lead exposure may in some cases show normal concentrations of urinary coproporphyrin (Alessio *et al.*, 1976).

(v) *Lead and free erythroprotoporphyrin*

Lead causes an increase in free protoporphyrin IX in blood, which is measured as zinc protoporphyrin (ZPP). This is possibly due to the interrelationship between iron availability and haeme biosynthesis (Labbé *et al.*, 1999). An increase in ZPP results from the ferrochelatase enzyme inserting Zn^{2+} in place of Fe^{2+} (Bloomer *et al.*, 1983).

ZPP is a normal metabolite that is formed in trace amounts during haeme biosynthesis. During periods of iron insufficiency or impaired iron utilization, zinc becomes an alternative metal substrate for ferrochelatase, leading to increased ZPP formation. Evidence suggests that this zinc-for-iron substitution occurs predominantly within the bone marrow, and the ZPP:haeme ratio in erythrocytes reflects the iron status in the bone marrow. In addition, ZPP may regulate haeme catabolism through competitive inhibition of haeme oxygenase, the rate-limiting enzyme in the haeme degradation pathway that produces bilirubin and carbon monoxide (Labbé *et al.*, 1999).

Roh *et al.* (2000) showed that ZPP concentrations measured by haematofluorometry were consistently higher than those measured by HPLC and spectrofluorometry in non-exposed adults, but were lower in exposed workers. They also found a positive correlation between blood lead and ZPP in workers exposed to high concentrations of lead, but not in non-exposed controls. The increase in ZPP is observed only at exposures resulting in blood lead concentrations > 20 μg/dL and good correlations have been found with blood lead concentrations > 40 μg/dL (Leung *et al.*, 1993; Froom *et al.*, 1998) (see also Section 1.6.2).

The best-fitting correlation between blood lead and ZPP is an exponential curve, with an *r*-value ranging from 0.38 to 0.69. In a group of 97 subjects selected in a stratified sample, in whom the blood lead values ranged from 10–120 μg/dL, there was a very good correlation between blood lead and log ZPP ($r = 0.87$). When the diagnostic validity of the ZPP test was analysed in various groups of workers, a high number of false negatives was observed at various ZPP cut-off values. ZPP cannot be applied in screening of workers with medium or low exposures to lead. In such situations, it is considered advisable to use blood lead as an indicator (Apostoli & Maranelli, 1986).

At blood lead concentrations < 20 μg/dL, ZPP concentrations were not found to be significantly different between the genotypes $ALAD_1$ and $ALAD_2$. Furthermore, ALAD genotypes did not affect the concentrations of haeme precursors at low blood lead concentrations (Alexander *et al.*, 1998; Zhang *et al.*, 1998). At blood lead concentrations of 20–60 μg/dL, ZPP concentrations in $ALAD_1$ homozygotes were significantly higher than those in $ALAD_2$ carriers (Schwartz *et al.*, 1995; Alexander *et al.*, 1998).

(vi) *Lead and pyrimidine 5′-nucleotidase*

Lead may affect haematocrit and haemoglobin concentrations also via the haemolytic effect of pyrimidine nucleotide accumulation due to the inhibition of pyrimidine 5′-nucleotidase (P5N) (Sakai, 2000). Following initial observations on the inhibitory effects of lead on P5N (Paglia *et al.*, 1975; Angle & McIntire, 1978), a number of studies have been carried out mainly to develop adequate analytical methods for measuring P5N activity in the general population and to study its relationship with blood lead concentrations and with other enzymes such as deoxy-P5N and arginase (Cook *et al.*, 1985, 1986; Sakai & Ushio, 1986). It was reported that ALAD is more sensitive to lead than P5N (Tomokuni & Ichiba, 1988b; Ong *et al.*, 1990; Pagliuca *et al.*, 1990; Kim *et al.*, 1995a). It has been suggested that P5N is the 45-kDa protein component in the lysate from erythrocytes of exposed workers that is seen to bind Pb^{2+} (Bergdahl *et al.*, 1998a).

(vii) *Lead and indicators of anaemia*

Anaemia following exposure to lead is caused by the decreased synthesis of both haeme and globin and by a haemolytic mechanism that is due partly to inhibition of P5N (Sakai, 2000). Anaemia induced by lead poisoning is normocytic in children and women and commonly associated with iron deficiency, which may produce a more severe microcytic hypochromic anaemia (Clark *et al.*, 1988). Anaemia may also result in part from the inhibitory action of lead on erythropoietin (Graziano *et al.*, 1991).

A threshold lead-in-blood concentration resulting in a decrease in haemoglobin has been estimated to be 50 μg/dL for occupationally exposed adults (US EPA, 1986).

A cross-sectional epidemiological study was conducted to assess the association between blood lead concentration (11–164 μg/dL) and hematocrit value in 579 children (age, 1–5 years) living near a primary lead smelter. There was a non-linear dose–response relationship between blood lead concentration and hematocrit, which was influenced by age. In one-year-olds, the age group most severely affected, the risk of having an hematocrit < 35% — indicative of anemia — was 2% at a blood lead concentration of 20–39 μg/dL, 18% at 40–59 μg/dL, and 40% at a PbB > 60 μg/dL. The data suggest that lead-induced anemia is an important consequence of lead absorption, even at low exposure levels (Schwartz *et al.*, 1990).

(viii) *Lead and other haeme-containing systems*

Lead inhibits the synthesis of cytochromes, such as cytochrome C, in both animal and human systems (Bull *et al.*, 1983). It also affects other haeme-requiring enzymes, such as cytochrome C oxidase in muscle (Goldberg *et al.*, 1985).

A decrease in haeme will also alter the activity of other haeme-requiring proteins (Figure 6).

(*b*) *Animal studies*

The effects of lead on the haematopoietic system in experimental animals have been studied extensively (see WHO, 1995; ATSDR, 1999).

A decrease in ALAD activity in erythrocytes was observed in rats given lead acetate at 1000 ppm in the drinking-water for 6 days. Blood lead concentrations increased to 44 μg/dL after the first day and remained within 10 μg/dL of that value until the end of the exposure period (Simmonds *et al.*, 1995).

In subchronic exposure studies, decreased haematocrit values and impaired haeme synthesis were reported, the lowest effective dose being dependent on the exposure route and on the chemical form of lead. When administered to rats by gavage, lead acetate caused a decrease in haematocrit values at a dose of 30 mg/kg bw per day given for 19 days (Overmann, 1977). When rats received 1% lead acetate in the diet for 7 weeks, a similar decrease in haematocrit value was seen (Walsh & Ryden, 1984). In contrast, rats that received lead acetate in their drinking-water at 34 mg lead/kg bw per day did not show adverse effects on haematocrit (Fowler *et al.*, 1980).

Urinary excretion of ALA was significantly increased in rats that received lead acetate or lead oxide at 5 mg lead/kg bw per day for 30 days, but no effect was seen with lead sulfide or a lead ore (Dieter *et al.*, 1993). Likewise, ALAD activity in serum was more strongly inhibited by lead acetate than by lead sulfide or lead-contaminated soil (Freeman *et al.*, 1996).

The effect of ingestion of lead on haematological parameters was investigated in male and female Swiss mice. Eight different doses of lead were administered through preparation of different feeds. The amounts of lead in the diet were designed to provide blood lead concentrations below (0.6–< 2.0 μg/dL) and above (> 2.0–13 μg/dL) the normal background. One litter of mice was exposed to each dose by feeding the mother with the lead-containing diet starting 1 day after mating, and mother and offspring continued to receive the feed until the litter was 90 days old. Male and female mice receiving concentrations of dietary lead below normal background displayed enhanced erythrocyte production as measured by higher cell numbers and increased haemoglobin and haematocrit values. However, as the blood lead concentrations approached 10 μg/dL, there was a marked decrease in erythrocyte production. These findings are significant since lead appeared to stimulate erythrocyte production at low concentrations (2.0 μg/dL) while adversely affecting red cell synthesis at higher concentrations (7.0–13 μg/dL) (Iavicoli *et al.*, 2003).

(*c*) *Experimental systems* in vitro

Acute toxic effects of lead (at 0.5, 1.0, 2.5 and 5.0 μM for 24 h) on coproporphyrinogen oxidase activity have been evaluated in an in-vitro model using HepG2 cells, a hepatoma cell line of human origin (Hernández *et al.*, 1998). The cells were treated with 150 μM ALA to induce porphyrins. Cellular protoporphyrin increased in a dose-dependent manner, reaching a maximum at 2.5 μM lead, but no changes in extracellular protoporphyrin were found. Extracellular coproporphyrin concentration was increased two-fold at all concentrations of lead, without changes in cellular content. The coproporphyrinogen oxidase activity was depressed in a dose-dependent manner to 62% of control activity at 5.0 μM lead. The dose-dependent increase in coproporphyrin secretion accompanied by the depression of coproporphyrinogen oxidase activity supports the hypothesis that lead inhibits coproporphyrinogen oxidase.

4.2.3 *Nephrotoxicity*

The renal effects of lead in humans and experimental systems have been reviewed (Goyer, 1989; Nolan & Shaikh, 1992; Goyer, 1993; WHO, 1995; Loghman-Adham, 1997). Acute and chronic effects of lead on the kidney are summarized in Figure 7. Acute exposure to high concentrations of lead results in disruption of proximal tubular architecture with disturbances in proximal tubular function. Histological changes include intranuclear inclusions in proximal tubular cells and mitochondrial swelling. Renal manifestations of acute lead poisoning include glycosuria, aminoaciduria and phosphaturia, collectively presented as the Fanconi syndrome. Chronic exposure to low concentrations of lead is also associated with increased urinary excretion of low-molecular-weight proteins and lysosomal enzymes. Chronic exposure to high concentrations of lead results in irreversible changes in the kidney, including interstitial fibrosis, tubular atrophy, glomerular sclerosis and ultimately chronic renal failure. It has also been implicated in the development of gout and hypertension secondary to nephropathy.

It has become evident that concentrations of lead as low as 10 μg/dL in blood, previously considered to be safe, may also be associated with renal function abnormalities, such as changes in serum creatinine concentration or in creatinine clearance (Staessen *et al.*, 1992; Kim *et al.*, 1996b). Whether such small changes in renal function result in clinically-significant health problems is uncertain.

The renal effects of lead in humans and experimental systems reviewed below are summarized in Table 88.

Figure 6. Multiorgan impact of reduction of haeme body pool by lead

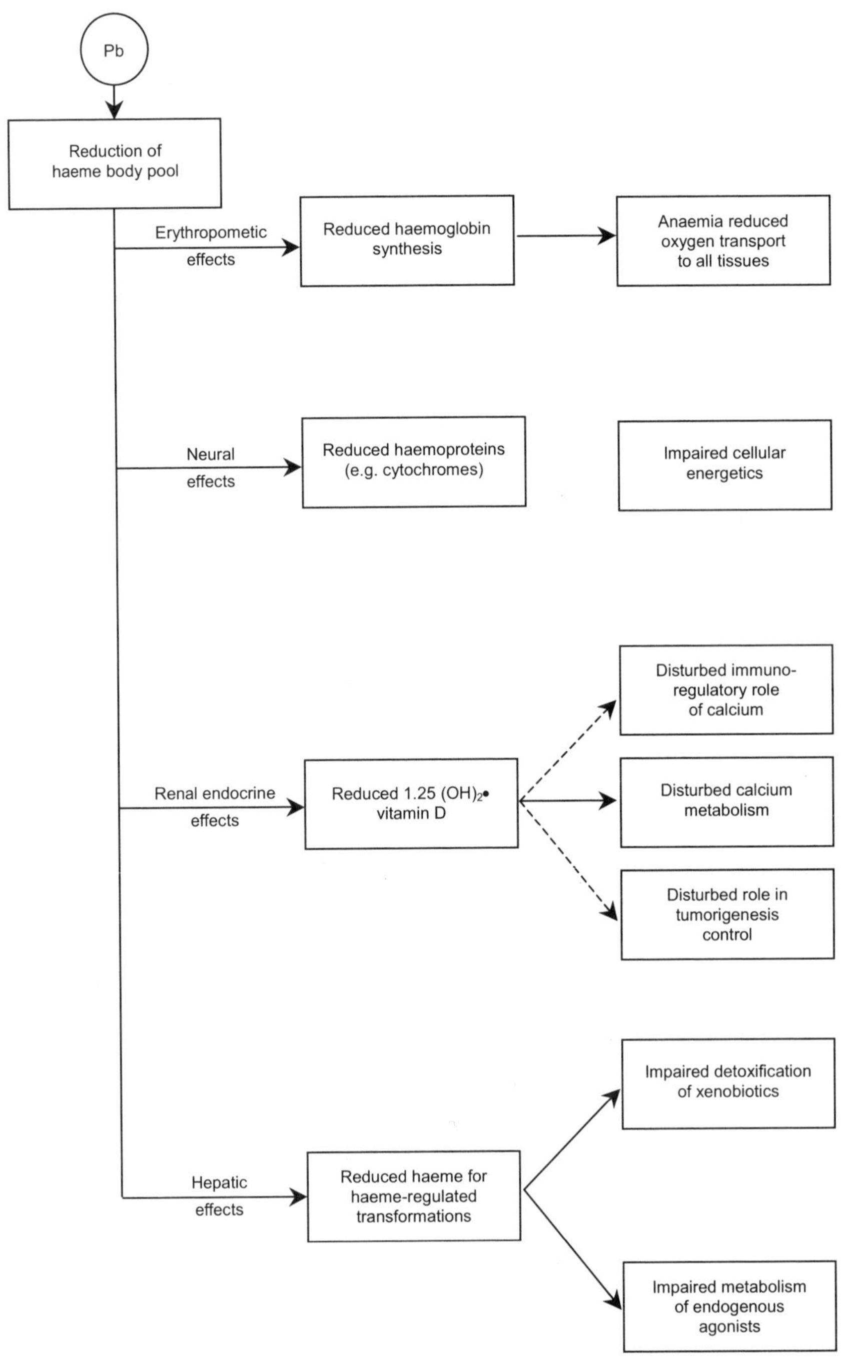

Modified from ATSDR (1999)

Figure 6 (contd)

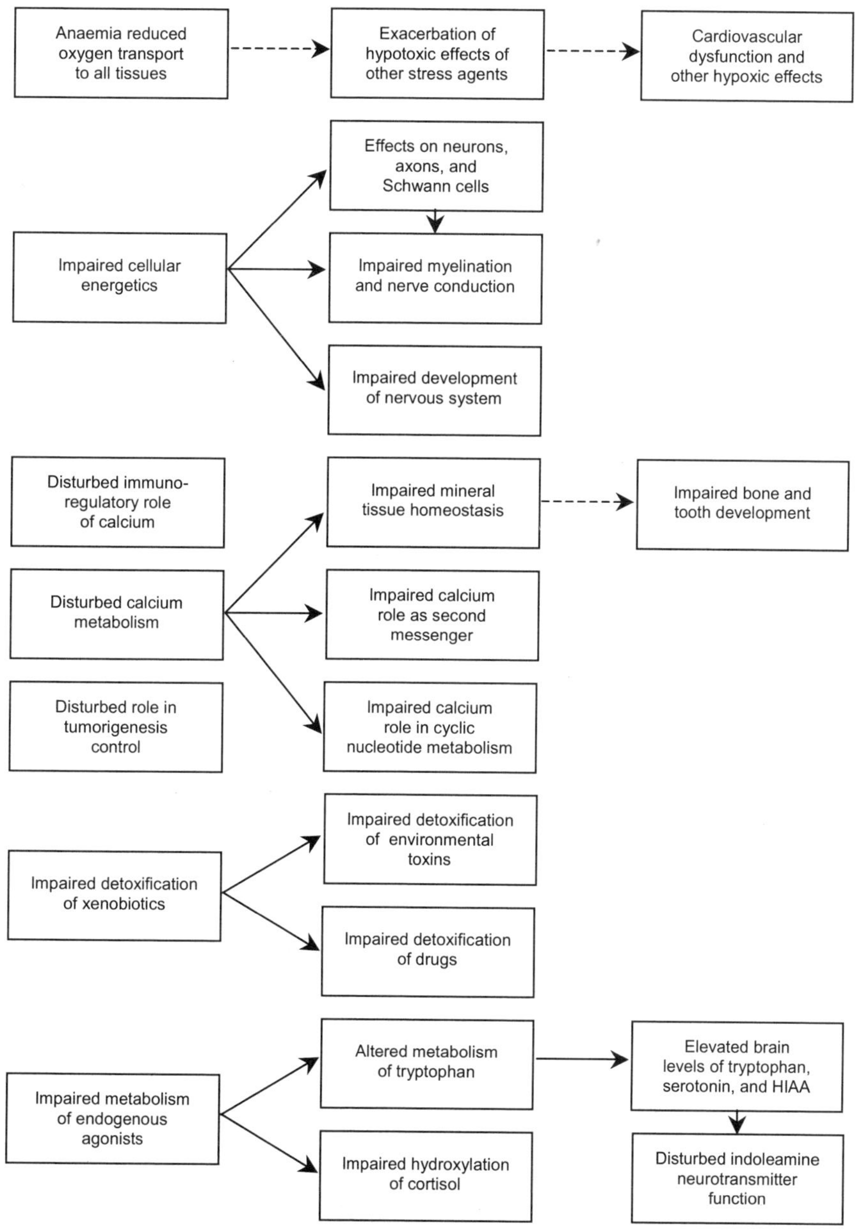

Figure 7. Consequences of excessive lead exposure

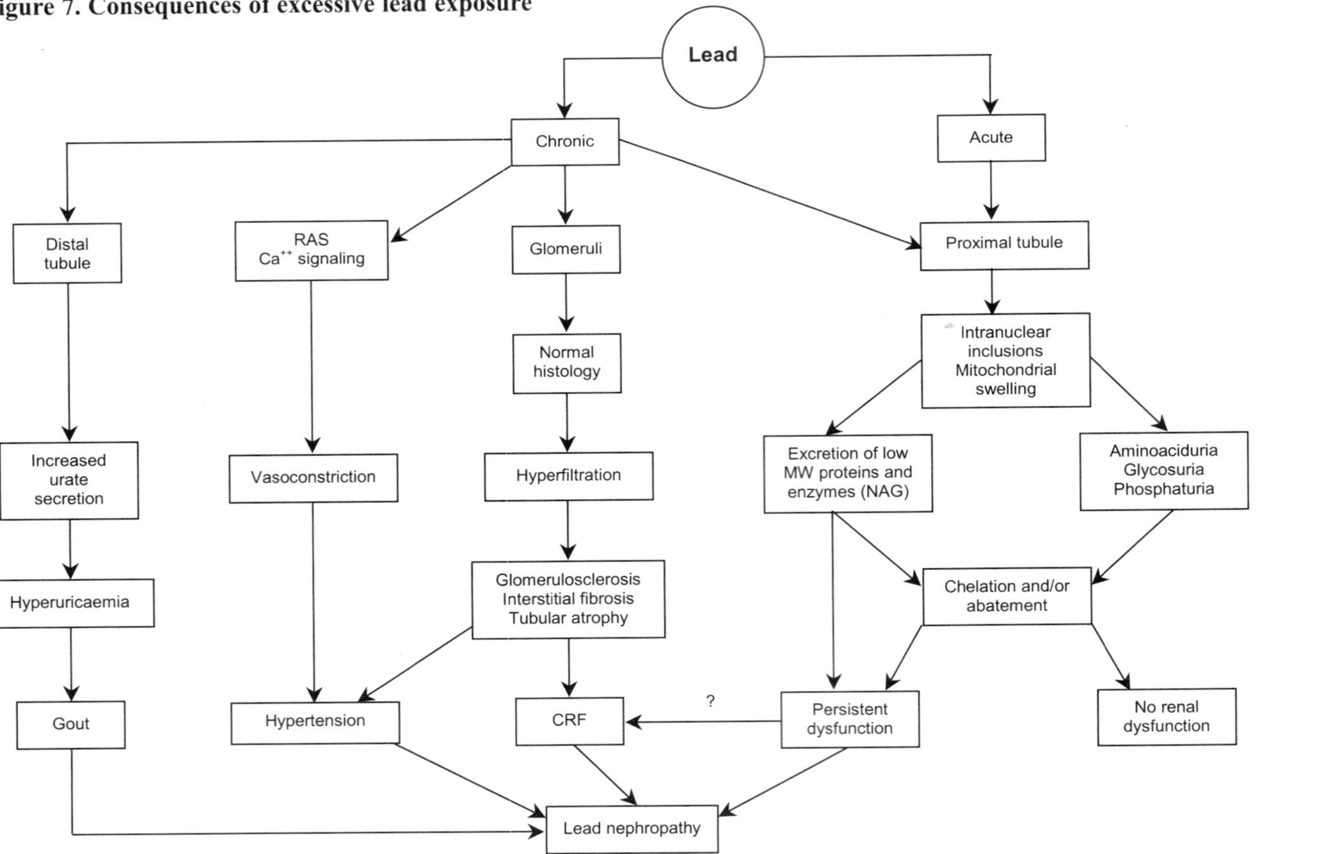

Modified from Loghman-Adham (1997); CRF, chronic renal failure; NAG, *N*-acetyl-β-D-glucosaminidase
Acute lead poisoning results in proximal tubular dysfunction; these changes usually disappear with chelation therapy or removal from lead sources. Chronic lead poisoning can affect glomerular function when blood lead levels exceed 60 µg/dL. After an initial period of hyperfiltration, the glomerular filtration is reduced and nephrosclerosis and chronic renal failure ensue. Prolonged lead exposure also interferes with distal tubular secretion of urate, leading to hyperuricaemia and gout. Finally, chronic lead exposure may cause hypertension, resulting from vasoconstriction due to the action of lead on the renin–angiotensin system (RAS) and on calcium signaling.

Table 88. Summary of published studies of the renal effects of lead

Effects	General population	Occupational exposure	Clinical studies	Animal studies
Acute				
Hypophosphaturia, aminoaciduria, glycosuria (Fanconi syndrome)	–	–	Chisholm (1962)	–
Glomerular filtration rate	–	–	Wedeen *et al.* (1979)	Khalil-Manesh *et al.* (1992a, 1994)
γ-Glutamyl transferase natriuria	–	–	–	Huguet *et al.* (1982)
Tubular change (inclusion bodies, mitochondria)	–	Cramér *et al.* (1974)	Biagini *et al.* (1977)	Moore & Goyer (1974); Goyer & Wilson (1975); Fowler *et al.*, (1980)
Chronic				
S-Creatinine	Staessen *et al.*, (1990); Kim *et al.* (1996)	Ong *et al.* (1987)	–	–
Creatinine clearance	Staessen *et al.* (1992)	Ong *et al.* (1987)	–	–
S-Urea (BUN)	Campbell *et al.* (1977)	Baker *et al.* (1979); Maranelli & Apostoli (1987); Ong *et al.* (1987)	–	–
Hyperuricaemia	Campbell *et al.* (1977)	Maranelli & Apostoli (1987)	–	–
α1-Microglobulin		Chia *et al.* (1995)	–	–
β2-Microglobulin	Staessen *et al.* (1992)	Huang, J.-X. *et al.* (1988)	–	–
N-Acetyl-β,D-glucosaminidase	Verberk *et al.* (1996)	Meyer *et al.* (1984); Ong *et al.* (1987); Verschoor *et al.* (1987)	–	–
Glutathione *S*-transferase	–	–	–	Khalil-Manesh *et al.* (1992a); Moser *et al.* (1995)
Serum proline	–	Cramér *et al.* (1974)	–	–
6-kPGF1α, TXB2, tubular antigen	–	Cárdenas *et al.* (1993)	–	–
Gout	–	Batuman *et al.* (1981); Pollock & Ibels (1988)	–	–
Renal mortality	–	McMichael & Johnson (1982)	–	–

–, no data; BUN, blood urea nitrogen; 6-kPGF1α, 6-ketoprostaglandin F1 alpha; TXB2, thromboxane B2

(*a*) *Humans*

(i) *General population*

In a longitudinal study of 459 men, Kim *et al.* (1996b) reported a positive correlation between blood lead concentration and impairment of renal function measured by serum creatinine concentrations. A weak positive correlation between serum creatinine and blood lead concentrations had also been found by Staessen *et al.* (1990) in a study conducted among civil servants not subject to industrial exposure to heavy metals. Staessen *et al.* (1992) examined a random population sample, including 965 men and 1016 women (geometric mean blood lead concentrations, 11.4 μg/dL and 7.5 μg/dL, respectively), and reported that creatinine clearance was inversely correlated with blood lead concentrations. A positive correlation was found in this study between serum β2-microglobulin and blood lead concentrations in men.

Verberk *et al.* (1996) reported a positive relationship between concentration of lead in blood (mean ± standard deviation, 34.2 ± 22.4 μg/dL) and the activity of *N*-acetyl-β-D-glucosaminidase (NAG) in urine in 151 children (3–6 years old) who resided at different distances from a lead smelter in Romania. There was a 13–14% increase of urinary NAG activity per 10 μg/dL increase in blood lead concentration, which was indicative of renal tubular damage. Campbell *et al.* (1977) found that increased blood lead concentrations were associated with increased serum urea concentrations and hyperuricaemia in 283 people living in houses known or believed to have lead plumbing systems, with lead concentrations in the drinking-water > 0.1 mg/L.

(ii) *Occupational exposure*

Buchet *et al.* (1980) examined 25 male lead-smelter workers (blood lead concentration range, 33.8–61.3 μg/dL; mean (range) duration of exposure, 13.2 (3.1–29.8) years) and 88 male controls (blood lead concentration range, 5.5–34.2 μg/dL), and found no differences in renal function between the groups and no clinical signs of renal impairment. The authors concluded that blood lead concentrations less than 62 μg/dL were not associated with renal toxicity.

Ong *et al.* (1987) examined renal function in 158 male and 51 female lead-exposed workers (age range, 17–68 years) with mean (± SD) blood lead concentrations of 42.1 (± 16.6) and 31.9 (± 14.3) μg/dL, respectively. Serum creatinine, blood urea nitrogen and creatinine clearance were significantly correlated with blood lead concentrations. After adjusting for age of the subjects, the increase in NAG excretion with increasing blood lead concentration was found to be statistically significant ($p < 0.001$).

Meyer *et al.* (1984) found significant increases in median urinary NAG activity in 29 workers exposed to lead, but there was no correlation with blood lead concentrations. In a later study by Verschoor *et al.* (1987), the excretion of NAG was reported to be a consistent and sensitive parameter of early effects on renal tubular function in workers occupationally exposed to low concentrations of lead. No significant differences were found in various indicators of renal function between 148 male workers exposed to lead (blood lead, 2.29 μM (geometric mean); range, 1.63–3.21 μM) [47.4 μg/dL; range, 33.8–66.5 μg/dL] and 125 non-exposed workers (blood lead, 0.40 μM (geometric mean); range, 0.27–0.58 μM) [8.3 μg/dL; range, 5.6–12.0 μg/dL] matched for age, smoking habits, socioeconomic status and duration of employment. There were no differences in protein excretion patterns and no signs of renal impairment. However, regression and matched-pair analyses suggested that renal tubular parameters as measured by NAG excretion might be more strongly influenced by exposure to lead than the glomerular parameters. Changes in renal function parameters may occur at blood lead concentrations below 60 μg/dL.

Chia *et al.* (1995) suggested that time-integrated blood lead indices were the most important descriptors of the variability in urinary α1-microglobulin, urinary β2-microglobulin and urinary retinol binding protein in 128 workers exposed to lead (current blood lead concentration range, 7.6–66.2 μg/dL). Urinary α1-microglobulin was the only marker that was significantly higher in the lead-exposed group than in controls, with a good dose–response and dose–effect relationship with the time-integrated blood lead indices.

No clinical signs of renal impairment were observed among active and retired lead-smelter workers with long-term exposure whose blood lead concentrations were below 70 μg/dL (Gerhardsson *et al.,* 1992; see also Roels *et al.,* 1999)

Elevated concentrations of blood urea nitrogen (≥ 20 mg/dL) were reported in 28 of 160 lead-exposed workers whose blood lead concentrations ranged from 16–280 μg/dL (Baker *et al.*, 1979). Maranelli and Apostoli (1987) reported significantly higher concentrations of blood urea nitrogen and serum uric acid in 60 workers with lead poisoning (mean ± SD of blood lead, 71.9 ± 16.5 μg/dL) compared with 76 control subjects.

Cramér *et al.* (1974) found significantly lower plasma concentrations of proline, valine, tyrosine and phenylalanine, but no excessive aminoaciduria in five men with heavy occupational exposure to lead (blood lead concentration range, 71–138 μg/dL) compared with non-exposed controls. Typical lead-induced intranuclear inclusion bodies were found only in renal biopsies of the workers with short exposure. Mitochondrial changes were found in all subjects.

Cárdenas *et al.* (1993) reported interference of lead (mean blood lead concentration, 48 μg/dL) with the renal synthesis of eicosanoids, resulting in lower urinary excretion of 6-keto-prostaglandin $F_{1\alpha}$ and an enhanced excretion of thromboxane. As this was not associated with any sign of renal dysfunction, it may represent a reversible biochemical effect or contribute to the degradation of renal function after the onset of clinical lead nephropathy. The urinary excretion of some tubular antigens (BBA, BB50 and HF5) was positively associated with duration of exposure to lead.

(iii) *Clinical studies*

Chisholm (1962) examined renal tubular injury in 23 lead-intoxicated children and compared the pattern of aminoaciduria with that seen in 56 patients with other diseases that impair renal function. Acute lead intoxication in children produced disorders of renal tubular function similar to those of Fanconi syndrome. Hypophosphataemia, aminoaciduria and glycosuria were found in 8/23 children, and most frequently in those with severe clinical manifestations. The abnormalities disappeared within 2 months, showing that the effect of lead was reversible.

Biagini *et al.* (1977) studied renal morphology in eight patients with chronic lead poisoning (blood lead concentration range, 90–200 μg/dL). The ultrastructural changes, which mainly involved the proximal tubules, were (1) a degenerative pattern (swollen mitochondria, dilated endoplasmic reticulum and scanty microvilli), (2) signs of metabolic hyperactivity (intranuclear granular inclusions, oddly shaped nuclei) and (3) a regenerative pattern (poorly differentiated cells with few microvilli, shallow infoldings of basal cell membranes). In the glomeruli, the most characteristic finding was a mesangial reaction. In some cases, the basement membrane appeared to be thickened and the visceral epithelial cells were hypertrophic. Interstitial fibrosis was present, as well as a certain degree of arteriolar hyperplasia. These findings appear to confirm chronic lead nephropathy.

Wedeen *et al.* (1979) reported reduced glomerular filtration rates (GFR; < 90 mL/min/1.73 m^2; see McIntosh *et al.*, 1928) in 21 of 57 workers with excessive lead body burdens (urinary lead > 1000 μg/24 h, after edetate disodium calcium lead mobilization test). In seven of eight renal biopsy specimens examined by immunofluorescence microscopy, the finding of glomerular and tubular immunoglobulin deposition raises the possibility that an autoimmune response may contribute to the interstitial nephritis that occurs in occupational lead nephropathy.

Batuman *et al.* (1981) examined 44 male patients with gout by using the ethylenediaminetetracetic acid (EDTA) lead-mobilization test. The amount of mobilizable lead was significantly greater in patients with gout who had renal impairment than in patients with gout who had normal renal function, although lead blood concentrations were not significantly different between the groups (26 ± 3 and 24 ± 3 μg/dL, respectively). Renal function (determined by the serum creatinine concentration) correlated with mobilizable lead in all 44 patients. The data indicate that lead plays a role in gout nephropathy. If lead nephropathy with gout or hypertension is suspected, the diagnosis may be confirmed using an EDTA chelation test (Pollock & Ibels, 1988).

An age-standardized proportional mortality analysis was conducted among 241 lead-smelter workers diagnosed with 'lead poisoning' between 1928 and 1959. Among the 140 deaths in this group, the study showed a substantial excess in the numbers of deaths from chronic renal disease, particularly prior to 1965 (see also Section 2.1.2). A moderate excess was also apparent for other smelter workers, not diagnosed with lead poisoning. In recent years, these excesses of mortality in lead-exposed workers have largely disappeared (McMichael & Johnson, 1982).

(*b*) *Animal studies*

Chronic intoxication with lead is associated with the presence of characteristic intranuclear inclusions in proximal tubular epithelial cells of the kidney. Chemical analysis of these inclusion bodies has indicated the presence of lead as well as of protein, presumably of the non-histone type. The inclusion bodies are eosinophilic and do not appear to contain DNA or RNA. Lead-induced formation of nuclear inclusion bodies has been observed in kidneys of rabbits (Hass *et al.*, 1964), rats (Goyer *et al.*, 1970; Choie & Richter, 1972a,b), monkeys (Allen *et al.*, 1974) and dogs (Stowe *et al.*, 1973).

Moore and Goyer (1974) used differential centrifugation to isolate inclusion bodies from renal tubular cells of rats exposed to lead and studied their biochemical composition. The inclusion bodies contain about 40–50 μg lead/mg protein and may function as an intracellular depot of non-diffusible lead. Further studies indicated that protein-bound lead in renal tubular cells may be partitioned between insoluble and non-diffusible, morphologically-discrete inclusion bodies and a soluble, extractable fraction that is presumably diffusible.

Goyer and Wilson (1975) demonstrated that the nuclear inclusion bodies formed in lead-treated rats could be disrupted and removed from the nuclei by the administration of EDTA and that this removal corresponded to peak urinary excretion of lead. The sharp increase in urinary lead following EDTA therapy is the result, at least in part, of chelation and excretion of sequestered lead bound to nuclear protein and indicates that the formation of inclusion bodies is reversible.

The lowest chronic exposure to lead resulting in a detectable renal effect in rats has been reported to be 5 mg/L in drinking-water, which resulted in a median blood lead concentration of 11 μg/dL (Fowler *et al.*, 1980). At this exposure level, cytomegaly and karyomegaly were found in renal proximal tubular cells. Proximal tubular cells from rats exposed to 50 and 250 ppm lead for 6 or 9 months showed intranuclear inclusion bodies. Inhibition of renal mitochondrial respiration and swollen mitochondria were seen at 9 months of exposure, but these changes were not evident at 6 months.

Huguet *et al.* (1982) reported acute kidney damage following intraperitoneal administration of lead acetate (0, 0.05, 0.15 and 0.30 mmol Pb^{2+}/kg bw) to groups of five male and five female rats. Minimal kidney damage shown by increased urinary γ-glutamyl transferase activity was observed only in males given the highest dose. In all animals and at all doses, natriuria was significantly decreased on the first day (from 4 h after administration). Such changes evoke mild tubular abnormalities but glomerular disturbances may also be involved.

Khalil-Manesh *et al.* (1992a) studied the progression of lead nephropathy in rats given lead acetate at a high dose (5% in drinking water) for 1–12 months. Control animals were pair-fed. In the exposed rats, the glomerular filtration rate (GFR) was significantly higher than in the controls after 3 months of lead exposure, but was lower than the controls after 12 months. Lead inclusion bodies were found in nuclei of proximal convoluted tubules and the pars recta in all lead-treated animals from 1 month onwards. Tubular atrophy and interstitial fibrosis first appeared at 6 months, and increased in severity thereafter. Brush borders of proximal tubules were disrupted at 1 and 3 months, but recovered thereafter. After 3 and 6 months of lead exposure, urinary NAG and glutathione *S*-transferase (GST) concentrations were elevated in the exposed rats compared with controls, but at 9 and 12 months the differences were not all significant. Concentrations of urinary brush border antigens were also increased above controls at 1 and 3 months, but were decreased at 6 and 12 months, correlating with morphological changes in the brush border. The authors concluded that a high dose of lead in rats may initially stimulate both renal cortical hypertrophy and an increase in GFR. Later, the adverse effects of lead on the tubulointerstitium predominate, and the GFR decreases. The urinary marker, NAG, was found to be abnormal in the early stages post-exposure, but age-related changes obscured this abnormality at later stages and urinary GST appeared to be a more consistent marker of injury.

In the same experimental system, administration of the chelator dimercaptosuccinic acid (DMSA) resulted in an improvement in GFR and a decrease in albuminuria, together with a reduction in size and number of nuclear inclusion bodies in proximal tubules (Khalil-Manesh *et al.*, 1992b). Overall, treatment with DMSA improved renal function but had less effect on pathological alterations.

In rats exposed via drinking-water to 5000 mg/L or 100 mg/L lead acetate for 1–12 months, GFR and blood lead concentrations correlated positively during the first 6 months of treatment. GFR and red blood cell membrane Na-K-ATPase correlated negatively at 6 and 12 months in rats given the high dose (Khalil-Manesh *et al.*, 1994).

Moser *et al.* (1995) reported effects of acute and chronic exposure to lead on GST isoforms during kidney development in rats. In the acute exposure experiment, rats of 14 and 50 days of age were given three daily intraperitoneal injections of lead acetate (114 mg/kg bw) for 3 days and were sacrificed 24 h after the third injection. In the chronic exposure studies, rats received lead acetate in drinking-water (50–500 ppm) from the day after conception. Acute and chronic lead exposure were found to have similar effects, causing increases in all but one GST isoform (Yb3); these increases were markedly higher under conditions of dietary calcium depletion. Lead-related increases in GSTs were partially reversed by transferring the animals to lead-free water for a 4-week period.

4.2.4 *Neurological and neurotoxic effects*

(*a*) *Humans*

(i) *Neurological symptoms of high-level exposure to lead*

Neurological and neurotoxic effects of lead are well recognized in both adults and children. High-level exposure to lead causes symptomatic lead poisoning.

Both the peripheral and the central nervous system are targets for lead, although peripheral neural effects (wrist drop and slowing of nerve conduction velocities) have, so far, been described largely in adults in occupational settings. Lead encephalopathy has been reported to occur in cases of acute symptomatic lead poisoning and its severity depends on a combination of factors, including the intensity and duration of exposure.

Children are more vulnerable than adults to the effects of lead for several reasons: a greater proportion of ingested lead is absorbed from the gastrointestinal tract of children than of adults, more lead gains access to the brain of children than of adults, and the developing nervous system is far more vulnerable to the toxic effects of lead than the mature brain (Leggett, 1993).

The symptoms of severe lead poisoning in children are typically associated with a blood lead concentration of 70 μg/dL, but can occur in some children at a concentration of 50 μg/dL (Adams & Victor, 1993). The early symptoms include lethargy, abdominal cramps, anorexia and irritability. Over a period of days or weeks, in children younger than 2 years of age, there is progression to vomiting, clumsiness and ataxia; then to alternating periods of hyperirritability and stupor; and finally coma and seizures. Children who survive are either severely cognitively compromised or frankly mentally retarded (reviewed by Lidsky & Schneider, 2003).

Rahman *et al.* (1986) described six infants, three of them neonates, diagnosed as having acute lead poisoning; four had acute encephalopathy. All had been given an indigenous preparation, 'Bint Al Zahab' (Daughter of Gold), for abdominal colic and early passage of meconium after birth. Chemical analysis of this powder revealed a lead content of 82.5%. The index case had anaemia with punctate basophilia, dense metaphysial lines on X-ray and markedly raised blood lead concentrations, arousing a strong index of suspicion for the early diagnosis of subsequent cases. Computerized axial tomography (CAT) scan in three cases showed signs of early cerebral cortical atrophy. The picture of cerebral oedema was absent in the four cases of acute lead encephalopathy.

In a later study by Al Khayat *et al.* (1997b), a group of 19 infants (mean age, 3.8 months) showed symptoms consistent with acute lead encephalopathy following the use of traditional medicines. All children presented with convulsions, and CAT scans of the brain showed oedema in four patients and atrophy in four others. Cerebrospinal fluid of nine children was analysed and showed pleocytosis in six and a high protein content in eight cases. The median lead concentration in the blood of these 19 infants was 74.5 μg/dL, and seven children had a mean lead concentration of 57 μg/dL which is below the proposed threshold (70 μg/dL) for encephalopathy. The children received chelation therapy. During follow-up 13 infants were observed to have developed brain damage. The results indicate that acute encephalopathy may occur in very young infants at lead concentrations lower than previously reported.

Blood concentrations of lead below that which produces clear clinical symptoms are also neurotoxic in children and have lasting effects on neurobehavioural function. Lead poisoning at these lower levels of exposure is far more common and is particularly insidious because of its lack of diagnostically-definitive physical signs. Some children complain of stomach pains and loss of appetite and may or may not have anaemia. Neurobehavioural deficit resulting from exposure to lead can occur in the absence of clinical symptoms (reviewed by Lidsky & Schneider, 2003).

The characteristic acute and predominantly cerebellar encephalopathy associated with high exposure to lead in neonates contrasts to the subtle, axo-dendritic disorganization shown to be associated with low-level exposure of infants to inorganic lead. In both low-level exposure to inorganic lead and exposure to organolead, there is a preferential involvement of the hippocampus, and the clinical syndromes of irritability, hyperactivity, aggression and seizures are common features of disturbed hippocampal function. Neurotransmitter system abnormalities and changes in glutamate, dopamine and/or γ-aminobutyric acid (GABA) uptake, efflux and metabolism have been described following exposure to inorganic lead. Among these effects, abnormalities of GABA and glutamate metabolism are also found after exposure to organolead. While inorganic lead produces a clinically-definable encephalopathy and neuropathy dependent upon age, route of exposure and dose, the clinical syndrome caused by organolead — i.e. triethyl lead, the neurotoxic metabolite of tetraethyl lead — is characterized by lethargy, tremors, hyperexcitability, hypermotility, aggression, convulsions, ataxia, paralysis and death (Verity, 1990).

(ii) *Impact on hearing induced by low-level exposure to lead*

Lead-induced impairment of the auditory brain and cochlea is believed to contribute substantially to the cognitive disorders and learning disabilities associated with low-level exposure to lead. However, the specific effects of elevated blood lead concentrations on central nervous system physiology and sensory systems, particularly the auditory system have not been clearly elucidated. Furthermore, earlier studies on the effects of lead intoxication on brainstem physiology and auditory sensory-neural functions have resulted in conflicting results (Otto & Fox, 1993).

Several investigations have reported that humans exposed to lead develop auditory brainstem abnormalities and significant hearing loss.

Holdstein *et al.* (1986) recorded auditory brainstem evoked potentials (ABEP; in response to 75-dBHL (decibels hearing level) clicks presented at rates of 10/sec and 55/sec) from 29 adults and children (age range, 8–56 years) (blood lead concentration range, 30–84 µg/dL) who were accidentally exposed to lead in food until approximately 1 year prior to the study. A prolonged interpeak latency difference (between peaks I and III) was the most significant recurring result, with longer intervals in lead-exposed children compared with the control group. Increasing stimulus rate, on the other hand, affected exposed adults to a greater extent than the children. The results may imply an impairment of the peripheral portion of the auditory system with axonal and myelin involvement.

Otto *et al.* (1985) evaluated 49 children aged 6–12 years for residual effects of lead exposure using the ABEP test. The initial blood lead concentration range in these children was 6–59 µg/dL, the range at the time of ABEP testing was 6–30 µg/dL. A linear relationship between blood lead concentration and slow brain wave voltage during sensory conditioning was observed at initial evaluation and at follow-up after 2 years. No significant relationship between blood lead concentration and slow wave voltage during passive conditioning was found at the 5-year follow-up. A significant linear relationship between the original blood lead concentrations and the latency of waves III and V of the ABEP was also reported. The latency of both waves increased as a function of the initial blood lead concentration, which is suggestive of subclinical pathology of the auditory pathway.

Schwartz and Otto (1987) used NHANES data to confirm the relationships previously observed between blood lead concentration and hearing threshold and found that the probability of elevated hearing thresholds at 500, 1000, 2000 and 4000 Hz increased significantly for both ears with increasing blood lead concentration. However, others have reported a lack of effects on auditory sensory-neural function.

Counter *et al.* (1997a) investigated blood lead concentrations and auditory sensory-neural function in 62 schoolchildren living in a lead-contaminated area of Ecuador and 14 children in a neighbouring area with no known lead exposure. The median blood lead concentration in the lead-exposed group was 52.6 μg/dL (range, 9.9–110.0 μg/dL) compared with 6.4 μg/dL (range, 3.9–12.0 μg/dL) in the non-exposed group ($p < 0.001$). Auditory thresholds for the lead-exposed group were normal at the pure tone frequencies of 2500–8000 Hz over the entire range of blood lead concentrations. Auditory tests in seven of the children with high blood lead concentrations showed normal absolute peak and interpeak latencies. In a more extensive neurophysiological and audiological study conducted by the same research group, the exposed children showed normal wave latencies and neural transmission times, with no statistical correlation between blood lead concentrations and interpeak latencies. Audiological tests indicated normal cochlear function and no statistical relation between auditory thresholds and blood lead concentration (Counter *et al.*, 1997b).

(iii) *Visual functions affected by low-level exposure to lead*

In 19 gun metal founders occupationally exposed to lead (initial blood lead concentrations, 16–64 μg/dL), Araki *et al.* (1987) found that the N2 latency — conduction time from the retina to the visual cortex — of the visual-evoked potential (VEP) was significantly prolonged. Twelve months later, after improvement of the work environment, the N2 latency had returned to the normal level. This change was correlated positively with absorption indicators of lead and inversely with those of zinc and copper. This suggests that lead interferes with visual function, and that this interference is antagonized by zinc and copper. In another study, an increase in P100 latency — i.e. the latency of the VEP-positive peak 100 msec after stimulus onset — was reported in 17 lead-exposed workers (non-smokers, blood lead concentrations, 25–52 μg/dL) compared with 27 unexposed controls, while the N75 latency — i.e. the latency of the VEP-negative peak 75 msec after stimulus onset — was not affected. However, no significant effects of lead were observed for the smokers or for the total subject population (31 exposed, 54 controls) (Solliway *et al.*, 1995). The results indicate that lead affects neural function even at permitted levels of exposure.

Altmann *et al.* (1998) investigated 384 children (age, 5.0–7.8 years) from lead-polluted areas for the impact of lead on the visual system. The range of blood lead concentrations in these children was 1.4–17.4 μg/dL. Statistically significant lead-related changes were found only for some of the VEP interpeak latencies after adjusting for confounding effects. All other outcome variables were not significantly related to lead concentrations.

(iv) *Peripheral nervous functions affected by low-level exposure to lead*

Nerve conduction studies have been carried out in chronically-exposed industrial workers with elevated blood lead concentrations but with no clinical evidence of neuropathy. In one of the first studies of this kind, Seppäläinen *et al.* (1975) found evidence for asymptomatic slowing of the motor nerve conduction velocity in 26 exposed workers whose blood lead concentrations had never exceeded 70 μg/dL. In a further study among 78 workers with maximal blood lead concentrations (ever recorded) in the range ≤ 40 μg/dL up to ≥ 70 μg/dL, Seppäläinen *et al.* (1979) found that ulnar nerve conduction velocity was depressed in workers whose blood lead concentrations had never exceeded 50 μg/dL. A third study reported slowing of ulnar nerve conduction velocity at blood lead concentrations just above 30 μg/dL (Seppäläinen *et al.*, 1983). Jeyaratnam *et al.* (1985) found that mean maximum motor conduction velocities of the median nerve were significantly lower in workers exposed to lead (mean blood lead concentration, 48.7 μg/dL) than in controls (mean blood lead concentration, 15.8 μg/dL). Other studies have also reported reduction in peripheral nerve conduction velocities in workers exposed to lead (Chen *et al.*, 1985; Murata *et al.*, 1987).

Triebig *et al.* (1984) studied 148 male workers exposed to lead from the manufacture of storage batteries, and 66 non-exposed controls. Statistically significant differences in nerve conduction velocities were seen only for the distal sensory fibres of the ulnar and median nerves. In contrast to the reports mentioned above, the authors concluded that at blood lead concentrations below 70 μg/dL, no functionally significant lead-induced reduction of nerve conduction velocity is to be expected. These findings repeated and confirmed the earlier results of Spivey *et al.* (1980) and Nielsen *et al.* (1982).

Schwartz *et al.* (1988) demonstrated a negative correlation between blood lead concentration and motor nerve conduction velocity in 202 asymptomatic children aged 5–9 years living near a lead smelter in Idaho, USA, whose blood lead concentrations ranged from 13–97 μg/dL. The authors found evidence for a threshold in three regression analyses: at a blood lead concentration of 30 μg/dL in 'hockey stick' regression, at 20 μg/dL in logistic regression and at 25–30 μg/dL in quadratic regression. Age, sex, socioeconomic status or duration of residence near the smelter did not significantly modify the relationship. The study confirmed that, in the absence of symptoms, increased lead absorption caused slowing of nerve conduction in children, but also indicated that measurement of maximal motor nerve conduction velocity is an insensitive screen for low-level lead toxicity.

All the above studies relate the findings on nerve conduction velocity to 'current' blood lead concentrations in humans. This practice is not ideal as the toxicity of lead to the peripheral nerves progresses over time. Chia *et al.* (1996a) studied 72 workers in a lead-battery manufacturing plant and 82 non-exposed referents. At the time of the study, mean blood lead concentrations in these groups were 36.9 (range, 7.3–68.5) and 10.5 (range, 4.4–19.8) μg/dL, respectively. Past blood lead measurements were available for 62 workers, for whom the mean cumulative blood index was 136.8 (range, 6.7–1087.0) μg-year/dL. There was a significant reduction in sensory conduction velocity of the median nerve of the dominant forearm for the group of 49 workers with mean cumulative blood lead index > 40 μg-years/dL. Current blood lead concentrations, however, did not show any trends against the nerve conduction parameters.

Ishida *et al.* (1996) studied 58 male and 70 female ceramic painters, aged 29–75 years, with lead concentrations in blood ranging from 2.1–69.5 μg/dL. They examined maximal conduction velocity in the median nerve of the forearm as a measure of motor nerve function, the variation in the cardiac cycle time in electrocardiography as a measure of parasympathetic function, and changes in finger blood-flow volume and drop velocity with change in posture from the supine to standing position as a measure of sympathetic function. No significant association was found between blood lead concentrations and the results of these neurophysiological tests.

(v) *Neurotoxicity of lead in children*

The neurotoxicity of lead was recognized as early as the 1st century AD when Dioscorides, physician to Nero, wrote that "Lead makes the mind give way." Childhood lead poisoning was first reported at the end of the 19th century (Lockhart Gibson *et al.*, 1892). Until the 20th century, it was generally thought that lead-exposed individuals who did not die during the acute illness were left without any trace of their exposure. When a study of children who had recovered from acute lead poisoning showed impaired cognition, poor school performance and increased antisocial behaviour (Byers & Lord, 1943), the long-term effects of lead toxicity were established and the modern era of lead toxicology began. Until the 1970s, it was thought that these residua were found only in children who had displayed clinical signs of encephalopathy. Among studies in the early 1970s of children in the USA who had no overt symptoms, four found lead-associated deficits in intelligence quotient (IQ) (David, 1974; Perino & Ernhart, 1974; De la Burdé & Choate, 1975; Landrigan *et al.*, 1975c), while three found no significant differences between exposed and unexposed children (Kotok, 1972; Lansdown *et al.*, 1974; Baloh *et al.*, 1975). These early studies tended to have small sample sizes and low statistical power; many used insensitive measures of cognition; covariate control was limited; and the exposure measure was lead in blood, which is a short-term storage system for lead. Later studies, using larger samples, more appropriate and sensitive outcome measures and better covariate control, tended to report impaired cognition at concentrations of lead in blood well below those associated with clinical symptoms. Not all studies reported significant effects, and the issue of silent lead exposure has continued until quite recently to be a source of contention.

Cross-sectional studies

Byers and Lord (1943) were alerted to the possibility of long-term effects of lead poisoning when two children were referred for aggressive behaviour. They were recognized as children who had in the past been treated for lead poisoning and discharged as recovered. A further 20 children with similar histories were then identified and it was found that 19 had school failure, behavioural disorders or mental retardation.

David (1974) compared blood and penicillamine-provoked urinary lead concentrations in 54 children with hyperactivity with corresponding values in 37 controls and found that the hyperactive children had increased lead concentrations in blood and urine.

Perino and Ernhart (1974) compared 30 children with blood lead concentrations > 40 μg/dL with 50 children with concentrations ranging from 10–30 μg/dL. Using multiple regression to control for age, parental intelligence and birth weight, they found a significant inverse relationship between blood lead concentrations and McCarthy intelligence scores.

De la Burdé and Choate (1975) compared 67 children who had been exposed to lead, but displayed no acute symptoms, with a group of 70 controls with no known exposure. Exposed children had deficits in global IQ and associative abilities, visual and fine motor coordination and behaviour. School failure due to learning and behavioural problems was more frequent in the lead-exposed than in the control group.

Landrigan *et al.* (1975c) compared a group of children who lived in the vicinity of a smelter and had blood lead concentrations > 40 μg/dL with children of similar socioeconomic status with blood lead concentrations < 40 μg/dL. The children with the higher lead concentrations were found to have significantly lower scores in performance and full-scale IQ tests, as well as in a finger–wrist tapping test, which measures fine motor function.

At the end of the 1970s and the beginning of the 1980s, studies were conducted with larger sample sizes, better covariate control and more sophisticated use of statistics. Needleman *et al.* (1979), using lead in shed deciduous teeth as marker of exposure, compared 58 children with high concentrations of lead in their dentine (> 24 μg/g) with 100 children with low concentrations (< 6 μg/g). After control for covariates, children with high lead concentrations had significantly lower IQ scores, impaired attention and reduced language function than those with low concentrations. Teachers' negative ratings of 2146 children on a forced-choice classroom behavioural rating scale were related to higher dentine lead concentrations (Figure 8).

Yule *et al.* (1981) classified 166 children by their blood lead concentrations (range, 7–33 μg/dL) and found significant negative associations with IQ, reading and spelling. A later study used the teachers' rating scale employed by Needleman (see Figure 8) and found the same results (Yule *et al.*, 1984).

Winneke *et al.* (1982) studied 458 school-age children whose dentine lead concentrations had been measured (range, 1.4–12.7 μg/g). From this group, two subgroups of 26 children each (mean age, 8.5 years) were chosen with low (means, 2.4 μg/g) and high (means, 9.2 μg/g) tooth lead concentrations, respectively. The groups were matched for age, sex and father's occupational status. The high-lead group scored significantly lower ($p < 0.05$) in two perceptual motor-integration tests and had a 5–7 point lower IQ (nearly significant, $p < 0.1$) than the low-lead group. In a further study (Winneke *et al.*, 1983) of 115 school-age children living in a lead-smelter area (mean tooth lead concentration, 6.2 μg/g; range, 1.9–38.5 μg/g), inverse associations — some of which were significant, $p < 0.05$ — were found between tooth lead values and outcomes of perceptual motor-integration and reaction-performance tests. After correction for confounding, there remained a tendency for children with tooth lead > 10 μg/g to have on average a 4.6-point lower IQ than children with tooth lead ≤ 4 μg/g.

Smith *et al.* (1983) measured dentine lead in 402 schoolchildren in London and reported that, after covariate adjustment, children with high lead concentrations (mean, 11 μg/g) had lower verbal IQ, performance IQ and full-scale IQ scores than those with

Figure 8. Teachers' ratings on forced-choice behavioral items classified by ascending dentine lead level

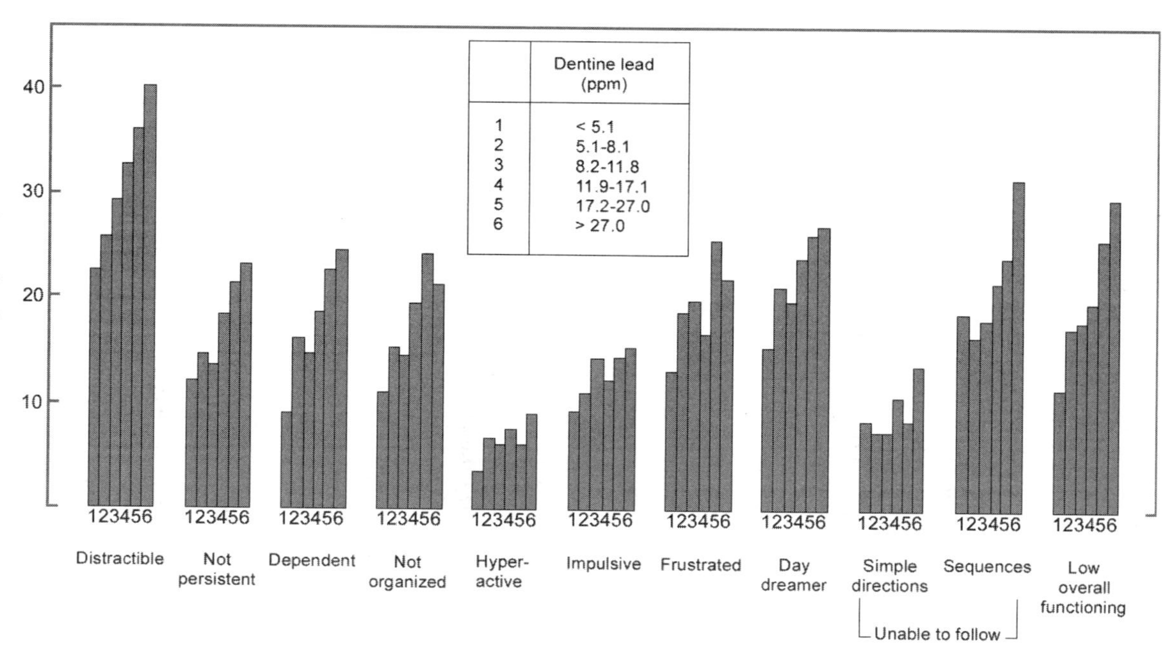

Modified from Needleman *et al.* (1979)
The group boundaries were chosen to obtain symmetrical cell sizes for the median (groups 1 and 6 = 6.8 per cent, groups 2 and 5 = 17.6 per cent, and groups 3 and 4 = 25.6 per cent).

intermediate (mean, 6 μg/g) and low dentine lead (mean, approx. 3 μg/g). The exact *p*-values were not given, and the differences were reported as 'not significant'. Children with high lead concentrations also had lower scores (also reported as 'not significant') on a word reading test.

Lansdown *et al.* (1986) found no significant associations between lead and IQ in a study of 194 children classified by blood lead concentrations in the range 7–24 μg/dL.

Fulton *et al.* (1987) evaluated 501 primary-school children aged 6–9 years in Edinburgh, United Kingdom, using the British Ability Scales combined scores. Lead burden was measured by blood lead concentrations (range, 3.3–34 μg/dL), and 33 co-variates were controlled for in the multiple regression model. A significant inverse relationship between lead and cognitive scores was found with no evidence of a threshold.

Silva *et al.* (1988) studied 579 children and found no association between blood lead concentration (mean ± SD, 11.1 ± 4.9 μg/dL; range, 4–50 μg/dL) and IQ, but a significant association with behavioural problems, including inattention and hyperactivity as reported by teachers and parents.

Hansen *et al.* (1989) studied the relationship between dentine lead concentration (average, 10.7 μg/g; range, 0.4–168.5 μg/g) and IQ in 162 schoolchildren in Denmark. After adjustment for covariates, significant inverse associations were found between lead and IQ ($p < 0.01$) and visual motor performance ($p < 0.001$).

Wang *et al.* (1989) studied 180 elementary-school children in China and found a significant inverse relationship between blood lead concentration (mean, 21.1 μg/dL; range, 4.5–52.8 μg/dL) and IQ as measured by the revised Wechsler intelligence scale for children (WISC-R).

Greene and Ernhart (1993) obtained IQ scores of 164 children aged 4 years and 10 months and measured lead concentrations in blood and in dentine of shed deciduous teeth. Using multiple regression, the association was measured with and without controlling for Home Observation for Measurement of the Environment (HOME) scores. Verbal IQ and performance IQ were inversely related ($p < 0.001$ and $p = 0.025$, respectively) to dentine lead concentration in the absence of HOME score adjustment. When HOME was entered into the model, the relationship between lead and performance IQ was no longer significant (at $p = 0.590$). An errors-in-variables analysis was applied, and verbal IQ continued to be significantly (but inversely) related with dentine lead ($p = 0.011$).

Some critics of the association between lead and intelligence have argued that the effect of lead is small and therefore inconsequential (Ernhart *et al.*, 1989). Figure 9 shows the cumulative frequency distribution of IQ scores in subjects with high and low lead concentrations in the study of Needleman *et al.* (1982). It can be seen that a median difference of six points is associated with a fourfold increased rate of severe deficit (IQ < 80). In addition, 5% of the subjects with high lead concentrations were prevented from achieving superior function (IQ > 125).

Figure 9. Cumulative frequency distribution of verbal IQ scores in subjects with low or high levels of lead

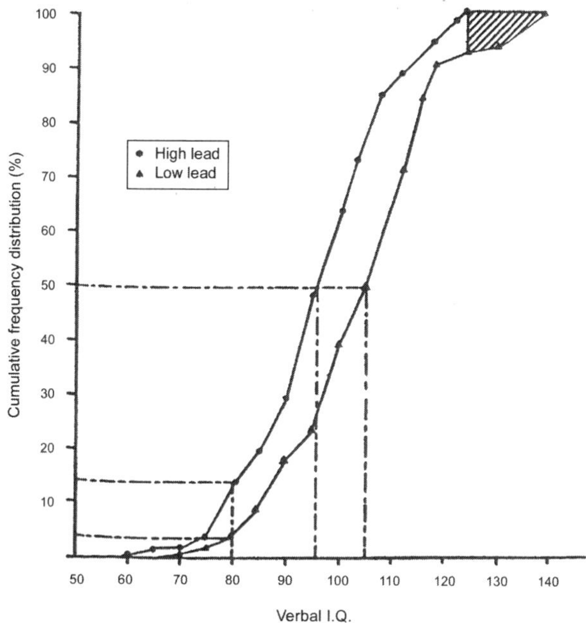

Modified from Needleman *et al.* (1982)

Prospective studies

McMichael *et al.* (1988) followed a cohort of 537 children living in the vicinity of a lead smelter in Australia from birth onwards. At 4 years of age, an inverse association was found between body lead burden and mental development, as measured according to the McCarthy Scales of Children's Abilities. At 11–13 years of age, the inverse association of blood lead concentrations with WISC scores continued to be significant (Tong *et al.*, 1996).

Ernhart *et al.* (1989) studied a group of 242 infants, and reported no significant covariate-adjusted associations between intelligence test scores of these preschool children and lead concentrations in maternal blood, umbilical cord blood or venous blood of the children up to 4 years of age. The strength of the negative inference is lessened by the use of a sample in which half of the mothers were alcohol abusers.

Needleman *et al.* (1990) followed-up 132 adolescents (mean age, 18.4 years) from the group first tested 11 years before (see above). At the time of the re-examination, blood lead concentrations were measured for 48 subjects; all were < 7 μg/dL. Subjects were grouped in quartiles according to their earlier dentine lead concentrations (< 5.9, 6.0–8.2, 8.3–22.2 and > 22.2 μg/g). Higher lead concentrations (> 20 μg/g) were associated with lower class standing in the senior year in high school, increased absenteeism, lower vocabulary and grammatical reasoning scores, poorer eye–hand coordination, longer reaction times and slower finger tapping. Having an elevated dentine lead concentration in childhood was associated with a sevenfold increased risk for failing to graduate from high school and a sixfold risk for reading disability.

Bellinger *et al.* (1992) studied a group of 148 infants at birth and at 6,12, 18, 57 and 120 months of age. Blood lead concentrations at 2 years, but not at other ages, were significantly associated with a reduced IQ score at both 57 and 120 months of age. Over the range 0–25 μg/dL, a 10-μg/dL increase in blood lead concentration at 24 months was associated with a 5.8-point decline in WISC-R score.

Fergusson *et al.* (1997) followed a birth cohort of 1265 children in New Zealand until 18 years of age. Lead burden was measured at age 6–8 years by deciduous teeth analysis. At age 18, after adjustment for confounders and errors in measurement, subjects with elevated dentine lead concentrations had significantly poorer reading scores, lower levels of success in school examinations and greater likelihood of failure to graduate.

Schnaas *et al.* (2000) followed a group of 112 children in Mexico at 6-month intervals from 6 to 60 months. After adjustment for covariates, lead was significantly related to the general cognitive index on the McCarthy scales. The postnatal lead concentrations (mean value of measurements at 6, 12 and 18 months) had a maximum effect on the cognitive index at 4–5 years of age.

Wasserman *et al.* (2000) followed 442 children in a lead-exposed and a non-exposed area in Serbia and Montenegro from before birth until 7 years of age and found that elevations in both prenatal and postnatal blood lead concentrations were related to reduced scores in cognitive ability tests (McCarthy scales; WISC).

Coscia *et al.* (2003) followed a cohort of 196 children from birth to 15 years of age, and applied growth-curve analysis to study the association between exposure to lead and cognition parameters measured at 6.5, 11 and 15 years of age. Blood was collected prenatally from the mother near the end of the first trimester of pregnancy, approximately 10 days after birth, every 3 months until the age of 5 years, at 66, 72 and 78 months, and at approximately 15 years of age. The highest mean blood lead concentration for this group of children was 17.03 ± 8.13 (SD) μg/dL, measured at 2 years of age. Children with higher lead concentrations showed lower verbal IQ scores over time, and greater decline in the rate of vocabulary development.

Recent studies

Following the removal of lead from gasoline, blood lead concentrations in the general population — first in the USA and then in Europe — began to decline. Mean blood lead concentrations in the USA were 15 μg/dL in 1975, 9 μg/dL in 1980 and 2 μg/dL in 2000 (NHANES IV). This decline has permitted investigators to compare exposed subjects to reference groups at 1 μg/dL, an opportunity that was foreclosed when the mean blood lead concentration in the general population was 15 μg/dL.

Two recent studies of the effects of extremely low concentrations of lead have been published. Lanphear *et al.* (2000b) examined data from the NHANES III on 4853 children between the ages of 6 and 16 years. The association between scores on arithmetic and reading skills, achievement scores, and blood lead concentration was measured; adjustments were made in the multiple regression analysis for age, race, sex, region of the country, parental marital status and education, poverty level and serum cotinine concentration. The geometric mean blood lead concentration was 1.9 μg/dL. Significant inverse relationships were found for arithmetic and reading tests at blood lead concentrations < 5 μg/dL, for block design at blood lead concentrations < 7.5 μg/dL and for digit span at blood lead concentrations < 10 μg/dL.

Canfield *et al.* (2003) examined the association between blood lead concentrations and Stanford-Binet Intelligence Scale (SBIS) scores in a prospective study of 172 children aged 6–60 months. A longitudinal analysis, adjusting for sex, birth weight, blood iron status, mother's IQ, education, race, tobacco use, income and HOME scores, was conducted. Mean blood lead concentrations were 3.4 μg/dL at 6 months, 9.7 μg/dL at 24 months and 6.0 μg/dL at 60 months. A significant inverse relationship between these average blood lead concentrations and SBIS scores was found.

The studies by Lanphear *et al.* (2000b) and Canfield *et al.* (2003) support the meta-analysis of Schwartz (1994) who reanalysed the data from the Boston prospective study (Bellinger *et al.*, 1992) and several others. Using non-parametric regression, Schwartz (1994) found an inverse relationship between IQ and blood lead concentrations below 5 μg/dL.

Lead and antisocial behaviour

Suggestions that lead exposure may have a role in antisocial behaviour are not new. Parents of lead-poisoned children have frequently complained that, after recovery from the acute illness, their children became oppositional, aggressive or violent. In the first follow-up study of lead-poisoned children, Byers and Lord (1943) found that 19/20 subjects had severe behavioural problems or learning disorders. Denno (1990) found that the strongest predictor of arrest of youths enrolled in the Collaborative Perinatal Disease Study in Philadelphia, USA, was a history of lead poisoning.

Needleman *et al.* (1996) studied a cohort of 301 boys in the school system in Pittsburgh, USA. Bone lead concentrations, measured by X-RF spectrometry at 12 years of age, were significantly related to parents' and teachers' child behaviour checklist ratings of aggression, attention and delinquency. The subjects' self-reports of delinquent acts were also positively associated with bone lead concentrations. Dietrich *et al.* (2001) studied 195 urban youths and found that prenatal exposure to lead was significantly related with covariate-adjusted increases in parental reports of delinquent and antisocial behaviour. Prenatal and postnatal exposure to lead was associated with self-reports of such behaviour.

Needleman *et al.* (2002) conducted a case–control study of bone lead concentrations in 194 male youths arrested and adjudicated as delinquents. Cases had significantly higher mean concentrations of lead in their bones than controls (11.0 ± 32.7 μg/g versus

1.5 ± 32.1 μg/g). Logistic regression analysis found an unadjusted odds ratio of 1.9 (95% CI, 1.1–3.2) for a lead concentration ≥ 25 μg/g versus < 25 μg/g. After adjustment for covariates and interactions, adjudicated delinquents were four times more likely to have bone lead concentrations > 25 μg/g (odds ratio, 4.0; 95% CI, 1.4–11.1). In addition, self-reports of delinquency were positively associated with bone lead concentrations.

Two recent ecological studies have reported positive associations between environmental concentrations of lead and antisocial behaviour. Stretesky and Lynch (2001) measured the association between estimated air lead concentrations for all 3111 contiguous counties in the USA (range, 0–0.17 μg/m^3) and homicide data (average over the period 1989–91) from the National Center for Health Statistics. After adjusting for 15 confounding variables, they reported a fourfold increase in homicide in the counties with the highest lead concentrations compared with those with the lowest lead concentrations.

Nevin (2000) reported a statistically significant association between sales of leaded gasoline and violent crime after adjustment for unemployment and percentage of population in the high-crime age group. Figure 10 shows the rates of violent crime in the USA by year in relation to the yearly sales of leaded gasoline.

Figure 10. Violent crime rates and sales of lead gasoline in the USA

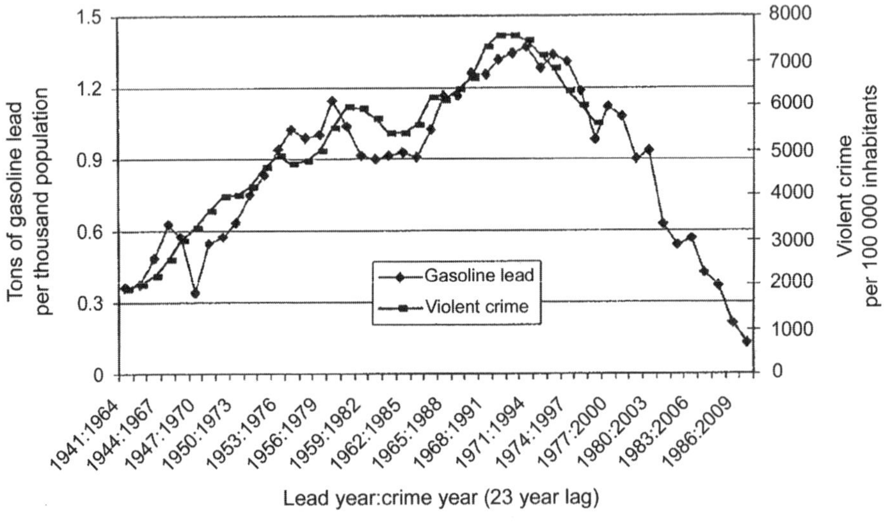

Modified from Nevin (2000)

(vi) *Other effects*

Since the late 1980s, several studies have explored the effect of lead exposure on postural stability. Motivated by a positive pilot study with 33 children (Bhattacharya *et al.*, 1988), Bhattacharya *et al.* (1990, 1993; with 63 and 109 children, respectively) confirmed an association between postural sway abnormalities and lead intoxication. There was a significant relationship between postural sway response recorded at 6 years of age and maximum blood lead concentrations during the second year of life. Chia *et al.* (1994) initially reported lead-induced postural instability among a group of workers exposed to lead compared with non-exposed workers. However, a significant relation between current blood lead concentrations and postural sway parameters could not be established. In a later study (Chia *et al.*, 1996b), there was a significant association between most of the postural sway parameters and the cumulative blood lead concentrations in the 2 years prior to the date of the postural assessment. Current blood lead concentrations were poorly correlated with most of the postural sway parameters. It was concluded that the adverse effect of lead on postural stability is the result of chronic rather than acute exposure to lead.

(vii) *Neurobehavioural effects of organic lead*

To investigate the relationship between bone lead concentration after exposure to organic lead compounds and neurobehavioural test scores, a study was conducted with 529 former organolead workers of mean age 57.6 years. The mean time since last exposure was 16 years. X-RF spectrometry of the tibia was used to estimate accumulated bone lead concentration. Lead-exposed workers had significantly lower scores on visuoconstruction tasks, verbal memory and learning. Peak tibial lead concentrations were associated with decline in verbal and visual memory, executive function and manual dexterity. These effects of lead were reported to be more pronounced in individuals who had at least one ε4 allele of the apolipoprotein E4 gene (Stewart *et al.*, 2002).

(*b*) *Experimental systems*

(i) *In-vivo studies with inorganic lead*

Several of the neurological and neurotoxic effects of lead described in humans have been investigated and confirmed in animal model systems. This section reviews a limited number of relevant studies in this area.

Acute lead encephalopathy has been induced experimentally in various animal species, such as the rat, the guinea pig, the baboon and the rhesus monkey.

Five-day-old rats that received the highest non-lethal dose of aqueous lead acetate (1 mg lead/g bw per day) on two consecutive days were found to develop haemorrhagic encephalopathy (Toews *et al.*, 1978).

Lead administered to newborn rats postnatally on days 1–15 by daily intraperitoneal injections of 10 mg lead nitrate/kg bw was found to cause haemorrhagic encephalopathy in the cerebellum at 15 days (Sundström & Karlsson, 1987).

Bouldin and Krigman (1975) induced acute lead encephalopathy in adult guinea-pigs that received 2, 3, 5 or 6 consecutive daily oral doses of lead carbonate (155 mg per dose). Clinical signs of intoxication started after 2–3 doses and became more severe with higher doses.

Lead encephalopathy in the baboon (*Papio anubis*) was reported by Hopkins and Dayan (1974). Two adult animals received 6–8 injections of lead carbonate (1 g per injection;

approx. 90 mg/kg initial weight) over a period of 8–12 months. Seizures were observed to begin at 3 and 5 months, respectively, in these two animals.

In rhesus monkeys, encephalopathy was induced by doses of 0.5 g lead subacetate, given by gastric gavage on alternate days, three times a week, for 6–18 weeks (Clasen *et al.*, 1974). Vitamin D (1000 units) was given together with each dose to enhance the alimentary absorption of lead (Sobel & Burger, 1955).

Effects on learning

Experimental studies, primarily with rodent and non-human primate models, have provided evidence that chronic low-level exposure to lead affects learning abilities and behaviour, in particular in the developing animal. The magnitude of these effects appears to be strongly dependent on the developmental period in which exposure takes place (for a review, see Cory-Slechta, 2003). Since learning requires the remodelling of synapses in the brain, lead may specifically affect synaptic transmission, and it has been proposed that the learning deficits caused by lead are due to events regulated by a calcium-dependent protein kinase C (PKC), most likely at the synapse (Bressler *et al*, 1999). However, the effects of lead on PKC studied in brain homogenates *in vitro* may not accurately reflect effects of chronic in-vivo exposure to lead (Cremin & Smith, 2002).

In a study by Altmann *et al.* (1993), rats were exposed chronically to low concentrations of lead at different stages of development, and tested with respect to active-avoidance learning and hippocampal long-term potentiation. When exposure comprised the prenatal and the early postnatal period and was continued into adulthood, both processes were impaired. However, when exposure started at 16 days after birth, neither learning nor hippocampal potentiation was affected. These results reflect the higher vulnerability of the immature hippocampus to lead-induced functional deficits compared with the mature hippocampus.

Effects on visual function

In a study by Kohler *et al.* (1997), rhesus monkeys were exposed pre- and postnatally to 0, 350 or 600 ppm lead acetate in the diet for 9 years. Lead exposure was followed by a 35-month period of lead-free diet. During this period, blood lead concentrations of the treated animals declined to nearly equal those of untreated controls. Lead exposure affected the dopaminergic amacrine cells in the retina by reducing the tyrosine hydroxylase content in these neurons. This neurotoxic effect persisted beyond the end of exposure.

Rice and Hayward (1999) exposed monkeys to lead acetate at 500 or 2000 μg lead/kg bw per day from birth onwards. Spatial and temporal contrast-sensitivity functions were assessed at adulthood and during ageing, by measuring the frequency and amplitude at peak sensitivity and the high-frequency cut-off value. Compared with controls, lead-exposed monkeys exhibited reduced temporal visual function at the first assessment but not the second. There was no evidence of an accelerated decline in contrast sensitivity as a result of exposure.

Effects on hearing

Yamamura *et al.* (1984) gave guinea-pigs intraperitoneal injections of 1% lead acetate once a week for 5 weeks. The animals were examined electrophysiologically using cochlear microphonics and action potential. There were no significant changes in the thresholds of cochlear microphonics. The thresholds of maximum voltage of N1 in the action potential of the animals injected with a total of 100 mg lead acetate were elevated by about 15 dB and increased N1 latency was also observed.

Rice (1997) determined pure tone detection thresholds in a group of six monkeys (*Macaca fascicularis*) dosed with lead acetate (2.8 mg lead/kg bw, 5 days per week) from birth until testing at 13 years of age. Blood lead concentrations at the time of testing were 60–170 μg/dL. Pure tone detection thresholds were determined at six frequencies between 0.125 and 31.5 kHz. Three lead-exposed monkeys had thresholds outside the control range at some frequencies. The findings are consistent with reports of elevated pure tone detection thresholds in lead-exposed humans, although the effect is smaller than might have been predicted given the concurrent blood lead concentrations of the monkeys in this study.

Effects on nerve conduction velocity

Conduction velocity of the optic nerve has been studied in rats that received 7.6 or 15.8 μg lead/kg bw daily by intraperitoneal injection during the first 2 weeks of postnatal life. Optic nerve conduction velocity was examined at 30 days of age in 14 rats taken from 10 different litters. The mean conduction velocities for the two faster axonal groups were 16.8 and 5.4 m/s in control rats, 10.3 and 5.8 m/s in rats given the lower dose and 9.4 and 5.2 m/s in rats given the higher dose of lead. The reduction in conduction velocity for the fastest axons was significant in both dose groups (Conradi *et al*, 1990).

Purser *et al.* (1983) maintained five cynomolgus monkeys at blood lead concentrations of 90–100 μg/dL for 9 months by daily oral dosing with lead acetate (12–15 mg lead/kg bw). The animals showed no clinical or behavioural evidence of lead poisoning at any time during the study, although there was a decrease in packed cell volume, haemoglobin and erythrocyte concentration in the blood. The maximal motor nerve conduction velocity of the ulnar nerve remained constant throughout the study, although changes were observed in the conduction velocity of slowly-conducting nerve fibres. At the end of the study, focal areas of myelin degeneration were found in the ulnar and sciatic nerves.

Effects on motor function and aggressive behaviour

Two groups of rats were given 50 ppm sodium acetate and 50 ppm lead acetate, respectively, in the drinking-water for 3 months. Ocular motor function was tested by rotating the animals on a platform at an increasing angular velocity and measuring ocular nystagmus when the rotation is abruptly stopped. The lead-exposed animals showed a reduction in post-rotatory nystagmus that was significantly related to blood lead and brain lead concentrations, while no such alterations were observed in animals treated with sodium acetate. The results show that low concentrations of lead may impair both sensory and motor functions, and indicate that these measurements provide a screening tool for neurotoxic effects of lead even in the absence of clinical signs of lead intoxication (Mameli *et al.*, 2001).

Young rats (3–4 weeks old) were treated with lead acetate (daily oral doses of 10 mg lead/kg bw) and ethanol (10% v/v in drinking-water), either alone or in combination, for 8 weeks. Motor activity, the number of fighting episodes and several lead-sensitive biochemical indices were measured. Spontaneous locomotor activity and aggressive behaviour were significantly increased in the group ingesting ethanol plus lead compared with the controls. The lead concentrations in blood, liver, kidney and brain were significantly higher in rats exposed simultaneously to lead and ethanol compared with the group treated with lead alone (Flora *et al.*, 1999).

The effects of lead exposure on a feline model of aggression were investigated by Li *et al.* (2003). Five cats were stimulated with a precisely controlled electrical current via electrodes inserted into the lateral hypothalamus. The response measure was the predatory attack threshold, i.e. the current required to elicit an attack response in 50% of the trials. Lead was mixed (as lead acetate) into cat food at doses of 50–150 mg/kg bw lead per day for 4–5 weeks. Blood lead concentrations were < 1, 21–77 and < 20 μg/dL before, during and after lead exposure, respectively. The predatory attack threshold decreased significantly during lead exposure in three of the five cats and increased after cessation of exposure in four of the five cats ($p < 0.01$). There was a significant ($p = 0.0019$) negative association between threshold current and blood lead concentration. These data show that lead exposure enhances predatory aggression in cats.

Effects on neurochemical parameters

While neurological and neurotoxic effects are difficult to define and quantify precisely, neurochemical effects are easy to define and to quantify but their interpretation remains elusive. Most neurochemical studies have been conducted since the 1970s and 1980s (see Tables 89 and 90); in this section, only the most recent and important findings are reported.

Neurochemical parameters were measured in discrete brain areas of rat pups whose mothers were intoxicated with lead in drinking-water (300 ppm) from day 1 of pregnancy until postnatal day 12. This treatment produced a significant reduction in the activity of alkaline phosphatase and ATPase in the brain, and reduced the concentration of adenine nucleotides, most notably in the striatum, but not in the hypothalamus. Lead also reduced the concentration of neurotransmitters throughout the brain, especially in the hippocampus (Antonio & Leret, 2000).

In a study to investigate the effects of lead on antioxidant enzyme activities in the developing brain, female Wistar rats were given drinking-water containing 500 ppm lead (as lead acetate) or 660 ppm sodium acetate during pregnancy and lactation. The activities of superoxide dismutase (SOD), glutathione peroxidase and glutathione reductase were determined in the hypothalamus, hippocampus and striatum of male pups at 23 or 70 days of age. In 23-day-old pups, the activity of SOD was decreased in the hypothalamus. There

Table 89. Effects of lead on catecholamines

Reference	Animal	Major results
Silbergeld & Goldberg (1975)	Mouse	Increase in norepinephrine in forebrain, midbrain, brainstem
Silbergeld & Chisolm (1976)	Mouse	Increase in VMA in whole brain
Sauerhoff & Michaelson (1973)	Rat	No change in norepinephrine, decrease in dopamine in whole brain
Golter & Michaelson (1975)	Rat	Increase in norepinephrine, no change in dopamine in whole brain
Sobotka & Cook (1974)	Rat	No change in norepinephrine in brain
Hrdina *et al.* (1976); Dubas *et al.* (1978); Jason & Kellog (1981)	Rat	Decrease in norepinephrine in hypothalamus, striatum, brainstem
Sobotka & Cook (1974)	Rat	No change in dopamine in cortex, brainstem, hypothalamus, striatum and forebrain

VMA, vanillylmandelic acid

Table 90. Cholinergic effects of lead

Reference	Animal	Cholinergic effects
Silbergeld & Goldberg (1975)	Mouse	No change in acetylcholine in whole brain
Modak *et al.* (1975); Shih & Hanin (1978)	Rat	No change in choline and acetylcholine in cerebellum, hippocampus, midbrain, pons-medulla, cortex, and striatum
Modak *et al.* (1975); Hrdina *et al.* (1976)	Rat	Increase in acetylcholine in diencephalon and cortex
Modak *et al.* (1978)	Rat	Decrease in acetylcholine in whole brain and cerebellum, medulla, diencephalon, cerebrum, striatum, and midbrain.

was no significant effect of the treatment on any of the enzymes and brain regions evaluated in adult (70-day-old) animals. Oxidative stress due to decreased antioxidant function may occur in lead-treated rats at weaning (23 days) but it is not likely to be the main mechanism involved in the neurotoxicity of lead (Moreira *et al.*, 2001).

(ii) *In-vivo studies with organic lead*

The neurotoxic properties of organic lead compounds and their neurobehavioural effects have been reviewed by Walsh and Tilson (1984). The behavioural effects produced by organic lead compounds resemble the sequelae of damage in the limbic system. Alterations in sensory responsiveness or behavioural reactivity and task-dependent changes in avoidance learning are observed following both exposure to organic lead and experimental disruption of the limbic system. In addition, the neurochemical changes induced by organic lead compounds are site-specific and restricted to the limbic forebrain and frontal cortex.

Rat pups (age, 5 days) received 15% ethanol or 3 or 6 mg/kg bw triethyl lead chloride by subcutaneous injection (LD_{50}, 13 ± 1 mg/kg bw). Controls were sham-injected with ethanol. Transient effects included reduced olfactory discrimination on day 7, decreased incidence of nipple attachment on day 9, and fine whole-body tremor on day 10. Persistent hypo-activity was observed on days 15, 22, 24, 26 and 29 in males that received the high dose. A reduction in number, but not in magnitude, of startle responses was also noted in the lead-treated animals. Thus a single postnatal injection of triethyl lead produced transient effects possibly reflecting direct pharmacological activity, as well as long-term effects suggesting potentially permanent alterations in behavioural function (Booze *et al.*, 1983).

Cragg and Rees (1984) administered tetramethyl lead dissolved in olive oil to pregnant rats by subcutaneous injection on days 7, 14 and 21 of gestation. Pups were born on day 22 and received similar injections 7 and 14 days after the last prenatal dose. The total lead concentration in the brain was about 1 μg/g at 28 days. Birth weight was unaffected, but postnatal brain growth was reduced relative to body growth, resulting in a higher body:brain weight ratio. Brain myelination, dendritic growth, granule cell production and retinal receptor development were unchanged. The body:brain weight ratio appeared to be a sensitive parameter for detecting effects on neurological development of exposure to low concentrations of tetramethyl lead, which is neurotoxic at higher concentrations.

(iii) *In-vitro studies*

Various in-vitro studies implicate second-messenger metabolism and protein kinase activation as potential pathways for the disruptive action of lead on nervous system function. These reactions could contribute to the subtle defects in brain function associated with low-level lead poisoning.

To investigate the effects of acute lead exposure on evoked responses in the hippocampus of the rat *in vitro*, field potentials in response to paired-pulse stimulation were measured in rat hippocampal slices perfused with medium containing 0.2–53 μM lead. The evoked population excitatory postsynaptic potentials and the orthodromically-evoked population spike showed a dose-dependent decrease during lead exposure, whereas the presynaptic fibre volley remained unchanged. Within 20 min after the start of exposure, the recorded responses had reached the control level again in spite of further lead perfusion. These results show that lead acts pre-synaptically in the hippocampus, and that it interferes with non-synaptic processes at the pyramidal neurons (Altmann *et al.*, 1988).

Excessive glutamate release in the brain and subsequent neuronal stimulation cause increased production of reactive oxygen species (ROS), oxidative stress, excitotoxicity and neuronal damage. The interaction between glutamate and lead may result in neuronal damage, as glutamate-induced production of ROS is greatly amplified by lead in cultured neuronal cells. Alterations in the activity of protein kinase C seem to play an important role in this process. The neurotoxic effects of lead may be amplified through glutamate-induced neuronal excitation (Savolainen *et al.*, 1998).

Lead can substitute for calcium in several intracellular regulatory events associated with neurological function. At nanomolar concentrations, lead activates calmodulin-dependent phosphodiesterase and calmodulin inhibitor-sensitive potassium channels. At picomolar concentrations it activates calmodulin-independent protein kinase C. There is evidence to support the hypothesis that activation of PKC underlies some aspects of lead neurotoxicity (Goldstein, 1993).

4.2.5 *Cardiovascular toxicity*

Cardiovascular effects of lead in humans and experimental systems have been reviewed (Victery, 1988; Goyer, 1993; Hertz-Picciotto & Croft, 1993; WHO, 1995).

(*a*) *Humans*

(i) *Blood lead concentrations and blood pressure*

The literature discussed in the reviews mentioned above can be divided into studies on the general population and occupational cohort studies. Surveys of the general population have been conducted in Belgium, Canada, Denmark, the United Kingdom and the USA. Results of most of the studies suggest positive associations between blood lead concentrations and blood pressure, but some of the studies do not show any significant association.

General population

Staessen *et al.* (1995) carried out an extensive meta-analysis including 23 studies with a total of 33 141 subjects. Among the studies were 13 surveys of the general population and 10 of occupational groups. Most studies took into account confounding factors. The association between blood pressure and blood lead was similar in men and women. For all groups and both sexes combined, a twofold increase in blood lead concentration was associated with a 1.0-mmHg rise in systolic pressure (95% CI, 0.4–1.6 mmHg; $p = 0.002$) and with a 0.6-mmHg increase in diastolic pressure (95% CI, 0.2–1.0 mmHg; $p = 0.004$). A recent update comprising 31 studies (19 surveys in the general population, 12 occupational studies) largely confirmed these results (Nawrot *et al.*, 2002).

Occupational exposure and lead poisoning

In a longitudinal study of > 500 lead-foundry workers who had been examined annually for periods of up to 14 years, Neri *et al.* (1988) found an association between short-term changes in an individual's blood lead concentration and contemporary changes in diastolic pressure. The average increase in diastolic blood pressure per 1-μg/dL increase in blood lead concentration was 0.3 mm Hg. The association remained significant after allowance for age or time trends and for effects related to changes in body weight.

Parkinson *et al.* (1987) examined the relationship between occupational exposure to lead and diastolic and systolic blood pressure in randomly-selected samples of 270 exposed and 158 non-exposed workers. After controlling for other known risk factors such as age, education, income, cigarette usage, alcohol consumption and exercise, the associations between exposure and blood pressure were small and non-significant.

(ii) *Blood pressure and renal function*

Batuman *et al.* (1983) used the EDTA lead-mobilization test to study the etiological role of lead burden in 48 men diagnosed as having essential hypertension. Patients who had hypertension and a reduced renal function (i.e. serum creatinine > 1.5 mg/dL) had significantly larger amounts of mobilizable lead than did patients who had hypertension without renal impairment. The increase in mobilizable lead was not due to the renal disease itself.

(iii) *Coronary risk of lead exposure*

Silver and Rodriguez-Torres (1968) studied electrocardiograms in 30 children (aged 17–60 months) with lead poisoning (blood lead concentration range, 60–200 μg/dL). Twenty-one patients (70%) had at least one abnormal electrocardiographic finding (mostly myocardial damage) before treatment [details of this treatment were not reported], which persisted in only four (13%) after treatment. The most significant findings were increased heart rate (six patients), and atrial arrhythmia (five patients). More frequent abnormalities were found in children with higher blood lead concentrations.

Kirkby and Gyntelberg (1985) studied the coronary risk profile in 96 heavily-exposed workers (mean ± SD blood lead concentration, 51 ± 16 μg/dL) employed at a lead smelter for 9–45 years. The reference group (mean blood lead, 11 ± 3 μg/dL) was not exposed to lead but was comparable with respect to age, sex, height, weight, social grouping, occupational status and alcohol and tobacco consumption. The exposed workers had slightly higher diastolic blood pressure, significantly more ischaemic electrocardiographic changes, and lower high-density lipoprotein levels than the reference group. The exposed workers with electrocardiographic changes had higher blood pressure than the referents with corresponding changes. These findings indicate a higher coronary risk profile for lead smelter workers, and support the hypothesis of a positive association between lead exposure and arteriosclerosis and high blood pressure.

(*b*) *Experimental systems*

(i) *Cardiovascular effects of lead*

A number of animal experiments have suggested a biphasic response of blood pressure to lead dose (Victery *et al.*, 1982; Victery, 1988; Staessen *et al.*, 1994). Rats were exposed to lead *in utero* and after birth until weaning by giving their mothers 100 or 500 ppm lead (as lead acetate) in drinking-water. This regimen was then continued for the offspring after weaning. Male rats receiving 100 ppm developed a significant elevation of systolic blood pressure at 3.5 months and remained hypertensive until sacrifice at 6 months; male rats exposed in this way to 500 ppm lead and female rats exposed to 100 or 500 ppm lead remained normotensive. At 6 months, plasma renin activity was significantly reduced in the low-dose male group but was normal in the high-dose group (Victery *et al.*, 1982).

In several experiments involving high doses of lead, hypertension was observed, but the nephrotoxicity of lead may have contributed to its development. However, in other high-dose experiments, no hypertension was seen. In contrast, the experiments conducted with lower doses of lead consistently demonstrated a hypertensive effect (Victery, 1988).

Evis *et al.* (1985) reported that chronic (3 or 12 months) low-level exposure of spontaneously hypertensive rats to lead (25 ppm lead (as lead acetate) in the drinking-water) enhanced the susceptibility of the heart to ischaemia-induced arrhythmias at 3 but not at 12 months. In contrast, chronic (3 months) high-level exposure of these rats to lead (250 or 1000 ppm in the drinking-water) resulted in slightly enhanced susceptibility of the heart to arrhythmias induced by myocardial ischaemia (Evis *et al.*, 1987).

In experiments in which rats were exposed to lead (0.25, 0.5 and 1.0% lead acetate in the drinking-water) for 90 days, Lal *et al.* (1991) found that the two higher doses of lead resulted in increased arterial blood pressure and calcium influx in atrial trabeculae and papillary muscles. No marked pathological or histochemical changes were observed in heart tissue except congestion (build-up of fluid) and a slightly reduced activity of succinic dehydrogenase in the high-dose group.

(ii) *Studies on the etiology of lead-induced hypertension*

Chai and Webb (1988) reviewed a number of animal studies on the possible role of lead in the etiology of hypertension. The main results indicate that the response of isolated vascular smooth muscle to adrenergic agonists is increased in rats with lead-induced hypertension, and that alterations in the regulation of intracellular calcium concentration may contribute to the abnormal vascular function associated with lead-induced hypertension.

Boscolo and Carmignani (1988) reported that blood pressure was increased in rats receiving 30 and 60 ppm lead (as acetate) in drinking-water for 18 months. The contractile activity of the heart was augmented only in those animals receiving the higher dose of lead, and the heart rate was not modified. Exposure to lead affected the renin-angiotensin system and induced sympathetic hyperactivity by acting on central and peripheral sympathetic junctions and by increasing the reactivity to stimulation of cardiac and vascular β-adrenergic and dopaminergic receptors.

4.2.6 *Immunological effects*

In a recent review by Singh *et al.* (2003), the immunomodulatory role of lead on cellular and humoral components of the immune system is discussed, with particular reference to effector cells such as B cells, T cells, natural killer (NK) cells and soluble mediators such as cytokines, chemokines and nitric oxide (NO).

(*a*) *Humans*

Studies in exposed workers

Ewers *et al.* (1982) examined the sera of 72 male lead-exposed workers (mean age, 36.4 years; range, 16–58 years; blood lead concentration range, 18.6–85.2 µg/dL) and of 53 reference subjects (mean age, 34.8 years; range, 21–54 years; blood lead concentration range, 6.6–20.8 µg/dL) for immunoglobulins IgM, IgG and IgA and complement C3 by radial immunodiffusion. IgA in the saliva was measured in samples from 33 workers and 40 controls. The workers had a mean duration of exposure of 10.2 years (range, 1–34 years). Lead-exposed workers had lower serum IgM ($p = 0.008$) and lower salivary IgA concentrations ($p = 0.008$) than the controls. A significant negative correlation was found between blood lead concentrations and serum concentrations of IgG and complement C3 in the lead-exposed group.

Jaremin (1990) studied the effects on the humoral immune response of exposure to lead in 77 men (mean age, 38.1 years) occupationally exposed to lead for 0.5–24 years. The ambient concentration of lead in air ranged from 0.06 to 1.6 mg/m^3. Three subgroups were distinguished: Group 1 (mean blood lead concentration, 40.1 µg/dL) without traits of lead poisoning; Group 2 (mean blood lead, 72.2 µg/dL) with biochemical features of lead poisoning; and Group 3 (mean blood lead, 106.7 µg/dL) with clinical signs of lead poisoning. Decreased concentrations of IgG and IgM in serum and reduction of the peripheral B lymphocyte pool were observed in Groups 2 and 3.

Queiroz *et al.* (1994a) examined the immunological status of 33 male lead acid–battery workers (mean age, 32.4 years; range, 18–56 years; mean exposure period, 5.8 years; range, 0.5–20 years) compared with that of 20 non-exposed, age-matched controls, all with blood lead concentrations < 10 µg/dL. The workers' blood lead concentrations ranged from 12–80 µg/dL, with 21 of them having concentrations between 40–60 µg/dL. Serum concentrations of IgG, IgA and IgM did not differ between the groups and there was no correlation between blood lead concentrations or urinary ALA concentrations and serum immunoglobulin levels. In addition, there was no difference between the groups in the capacity of peripheral blood mononuclear cells (PBMCs) to respond to the mitogen phytohaemagglutinin (PHA), a correlate of T-cell function. There was also no correlation between mitogenic response and blood lead concentration. These data suggest that chronic exposure to lead does not compromise lymphocyte function.

In a further study, Queiroz *et al.* (1994b) investigated phagocytosis and intracellular killing of *Candida albicans* and *C. pseudotropicalis* by neutrophils and splenic phagocytic function in blood samples from a similar group of lead-exposed workers (see above). The *Candida* assay is used to identify myeloperoxidase-deficient subjects who have neutrophils that are unable to kill *C. albicans*, whereas *C. pseudotropicalis* can be effectively lysed. Lysis of *C. albicans*, but not *C. pseudotropicalis*, was impaired in lead-exposed workers with blood lead concentrations and urinary ALA concentrations below 60 µg/dL and 6 mg/L, respectively, as well as in toxic ranges. This suggests that lead exposure may result in myeloperoxidase deficiency. There was no difference between the groups in any of the other parameters examined.

Ündeger *et al.* (1996) compared peripheral blood lymphocytes, serum immunoglobulins (IgG, IgA and IgM), and C3 and C4 complement protein concentrations of 25 male lead-exposed workers (mean age, 33 years; range, 22–55 years) employed in storage-battery plants (mean exposure period 6 years; range, 0.5–15 years; average blood lead concentration, 74.8 μg/dL) with those of 25 male controls with no history of lead exposure (mean age, 33 years; range, 22–56 years; average blood lead concentration, 16.7 μg/dL). The numbers and the percentage of T, T-suppressor, B, and NK cells, were not different between the groups, but the numbers of T-helper lymphocytes and the serum concentrations of IgG, IgM, C3 and C4 complement components were significantly lower in lead-exposed workers compared with controls ($p < 0.05$). These results suggest that chronic exposure to lead may be detrimental to the human immune system.

Pinkerton *et al.* (1998) evaluated a number of immune parameters in 145 lead-exposed workers (mean age, 32.9 ± 8.6 years) with a median blood lead concentration of 39 μg/dL (range, 15–55 μg/dL) and 84 unexposed workers (mean age, 30.1 ± 9.3 years; mean blood lead, < 2 μg/dL; range, < 2–12 μg/dL). After adjusting for covariates, no major differences were found between the two groups in the percentage of CD3+ cells, CD4+ T cells, CD8+ T cells, B cells, NK cells, serum immunoglobulin levels, salivary IgA, serum C3 complement levels or lymphoproliferative responses. However, among exposed workers, serum IgG was negatively associated with cumulative lead exposure, and the percentage and number of CD4+/CD45RA+ cells were positively associated with cumulative lead exposure. This study found no evidence of a marked immunotoxic effect of lead, although subtle differences in some immunological parameters were noted.

The immunological effects of occupational exposure to lead have been studied by measurement of lymphocyte proliferation, NK cell cytotoxicity and interferon (IFN)-γ production in PBMCs of three groups of lead-exposed workers: drivers of three-wheelers (30, eight of whom had blood lead > 10 μg/dL; average blood lead, 6.5 ± 4.7 μg/dL), battery workers (34, all with blood lead > 10 μg/dL; average blood lead, 128.11 ± 104 μg/dL) and silver-jewellery makers (20, 12 with blood lead > 10 μg/dL; average blood lead, 17.8 ± 18.5 μg/dL). Unexposed healthy volunteers (30, none with blood lead > 10 μg/dL; range, 1.6–9.8 μg/dL) served as controls. Lymphocyte proliferation in response to PHA stimulation was lower in lead-exposed individuals than in controls, but there was no correlation with blood lead concentrations. NK cell cytotoxicity was not different between groups. In contrast, the concentration of IFN-γ was significantly elevated in culture supernatants collected from PHA-stimulated PBMCs of lead-exposed individuals, showing a significant positive correlation with blood lead concentrations. This study demonstrates that lead can affect the immune response of exposed workers (Mishra *et al.*, 2003).

(*b*) *Experimental systems*

Swiss Webster mice that received 130 or 1300 mg/L lead as lead acetate in drinking-water for 70 days showed decreased β-lymphocyte responsiveness and humoral antibody titres (Koller & Kovacic, 1974; Koller & Brauner, 1977). Similar findings were obtained by Luster *et al.* (1978) in rats exposed to 25 or 50 mg/L lead acetate in drinking-water for 35–45 days.

In CBA mice exposed to lead in drinking-water (13–1300 mg/L, as lead acetate) for 10 weeks, the ability of the mitogens lipopolysaccharide and purified protein derivative to induce lymphocyte proliferation in the kidney was inhibited, but the response to concanavalin A was not significantly affected (Koller *et al.*, 1979).

To analyse the effect of lead on the immune system and to determine the ability of α-tocopherol to reverse lead-induced immunotoxicity, Fernandez-Cabezudo *et al.* (2003) treated groups of six TO mice intraperitoneally for 2 weeks with saline alone, lead acetate alone, lead acetate plus α-tocopherol or with α-tocopherol alone. Spleens were then analysed for (i) cellular composition by flow cytometry, (ii) cellular response to B and T cell mitogens and (iii) production of NO. The treatment with lead acetate resulted in a significant splenomegaly associated mainly with an influx of CD11b+ myeloid cells, but these cells exhibited no up-regulation of activation markers and did not produce NO. The mitogenic responses of the lymphocytes were inhibited by ≥ 70% in the lead-treated group. Concurrent treatment with lead acetate and α-tocopherol resulted in an almost complete reversal of the lead-induced splenomegaly, but the mitogenic response in this case was approximately 50% of that observed in saline-treated controls.

The effects of lead on the immune system of the developing embryo were assessed by Miller *et al.* (1998) in 9-week-old female Fischer 344 rats exposed to lead acetate (0, 100, 250 and 500 ppm lead) in their drinking-water during breeding and pregnancy. Exposure was discontinued at parturition and offspring received no additional lead treatment. At 13 weeks, tumour necrosis factor (TNF)-α and NO production were elevated in the female offspring of dams exposed to 250 ppm lead, while cell-mediated immune function was depressed, as shown by a decrease in delayed-type hypersensitivity (DTH) reactions. IFN-γ concentrations were lower in the offspring of the 500-ppm treatment group than in controls. Serum IgE levels were increased in rats exposed *in utero* to 100 ppm lead. The lead-exposed dams did not show chronic immune alterations. These results indicate that exposure of pregnant females to moderate levels of lead produces chronic immune modulation in their offspring.

Bunn *et al.* (2001) gave adult female Sprague-Dawley rats 500 ppm lead as lead acetate in the drinking-water early (days 3–9) or late in gestation (days 15–21). Significantly depressed DTH responses and elevated interleukin (IL)-10 production, higher relative monocyte numbers and increased relative thymic weights were observed when female offspring exposed during late gestation were assessed as adults. In contrast, male offspring had increased IL-12 production and decreased IL-10 production, while the DTH response, relative monocyte numbers and thymic weights were unchanged. Exposure during early gestation decreased NO production in lead-treated male, but not female offspring. These results suggest that the rat embryo may be more sensitive to lead-induced immunotoxic effects when exposed during late gestation, with the effects on DTH function being more pronounced in females.

Differential embryonic sensitivity to lead-induced immunotoxicity was studied by Lee, J.-E. *et al.* (2001) by injection of sublethal doses of lead (5–400 μg) into fertilized Cornell K Strain White Leghorn chicken eggs via the air sac on days 5, 7, 9 and 12 of incubation, designated as E5, E7, E9 and E12, respectively. In 5–6-week-old chickens, splenic lymphocyte production of IFN-γ was significantly suppressed (measured for E7 and E9 exposures only, $p < 0.05$) among lead-treated groups compared with controls. Production of NO by macrophages (measured as nitrite production) was significantly depressed ($p < 0.05$) after E5, E7 and E9 lead exposures but not following E12 lead exposure. In contrast, DTH function was unaltered following the E5, E7 and E9 exposures, but was significantly depressed ($p < 0.05$) after E12 exposure. The findings indicate that lead exposure during different stages of embryonic development results in different immunotoxic outcomes in the juvenile chicken.

In turkey poults fed 100 ppm dietary lead acetate, the concentration of arachidonic acid in macrophage phospholipids increased to twice that of controls. In-vitro production of eicosanoids by these macrophages was substantially increased, and this effect was most pronounced following lipopolysaccharide stimulation: prostaglandin F2α increased 11-fold, thromboxane B2 3-fold and prostaglandin E2 1.5-fold. The in-vitro phagocytic potential of these macrophages was only half that of control macrophages. The results show that lead influences immunological homeostasis in birds (Knowles & Donaldson, 1997).

The combined effects of a non-pathogenic immunological challenge and exposure to lead shot were investigated in three groups of 24 Japanese quail chicks (*Coturnix coturnix japonica*) that were given either one lead shot (0.05 g) or four lead shots (0.2 g) orally, at the age of 8 days. Controls did not receive lead. As immunological challenge, a third of each group of chicks was injected intraperitoneally with either 0.075 mL 10% chukar partridge (*Alectoris graeca*) red blood cells, Newcastle disease virus, or a placebo vaccine at 13 and 35 days of age. Lead did not affect antibody production or cell-mediated immune response. Granulocyte numbers were significantly higher in the lead-treated birds than in controls, and both antigen-treated groups had lower granulocyte numbers than controls. At the 0.2-g dose, lead increased haematocrit values, lowered plasma protein concentrations and increased granulocyte numbers in the quail (Fair & Ricklefs, 2002).

The effects of lead nitrate (0.1 μM–1 mM) on proliferative responses of B and T lymphocytes of mouse, rat and human origin were investigated. T cells were stimulated by PHA or by monoclonal antibodies directed at the T cell receptor/CD3 complex, while B cells were activated by T-independent mitogens (*Staphylococcus aureus* cells, *Escherichia coli* lipopolysaccharide and *Salmonella typhimurium* mitogen for human, mouse and rat lymphocytes, respectively). Large differences in proliferative responses were observed for lead nitrate across species; rat lymphocytes were very sensitive to immunomodulation by lead, whereas human cells were found to be relatively resistant (Lang *et al.*, 1993).

4.2.7 *Other toxic effects*

(*a*) *Lead-induced mitogenesis*

Endogenous DNA damage is present in every living cell and may remain relatively harmless — even when it is not, or very slowly, repaired — as long as the cell does not replicate its DNA prior to mitosis. However, when cell proliferation is induced, endogenous DNA damage may be converted into mutations, some of which may lead to disturbance of cellular growth control and, ultimately, to carcinogenesis. Stimulation of cell proliferation (mitogenesis) may, therefore, play an important role in the mode of action of carcinogens that do not directly interact with DNA (Cohen & Ellwein, 1990). The mitogenic activity of lead and lead compounds has been studied extensively.

Choie and Richter (1974a) showed that a single dose of 5 mg lead/kg bw, given as lead acetate by intracardiac injection produced a 45-fold increase in DNA synthesis in the kidney of mice, followed by a wave of mitoses. This effect was found to be preceded by a general increase in synthesis of RNA and protein (Choie & Richter, 1974b). A single intracardiac dose of lead acetate (40 mg lead/kg bw) induced a 25-fold increase in mitosis of mouse hepatocytes within 5 hours. The prompt appearance of a mitotic wave and the relatively large number of mitoses suggest that the mitotic cells were from a hepatocyte sub-population arrested in the G2 phase (Choie & Richter, 1978).

The effects of a single intraperitoneal dose of lead acetate (0.04 mg lead/kg bw) on the proliferation of the proximal tubule epithelium of the rat kidney were investigated by autoradiographic analysis of [^{3}H]thymidine incorporation, over a 3-day period after injection. Within 2 days, the labelling index increased approximately 40-fold compared with controls. Three days after injection of lead 14.5% of the proximal tubular epithelial cells were labelled (Choie & Richter, 1972c).

In a subsequent study, the same authors investigated the effects of chronic administration of lead. Rats received intraperitoneal injections once a week for 6 months, at doses of 1–7 mg lead per rat. At the end of this period, the proliferative activity of the proximal tubular epithelium was 15 times higher in treated than in untreated rats. Epithelial hyperplasia was seen in some proximal tubules, with occasional atypia. The results suggest that the renal carcinogenicity of lead (see Section 3) may be due to lead-induced stimulation of renal cell proliferation (Choie & Richter, 1972a).

Stevenson *et al.* (1977) showed that a single intraperitoneal injection of 10 mg/kg bw lead chloride into rats caused a transient twofold increase in synthesis of RNA and DNA in the kidney after 1 and 3 days, respectively; RNA synthesis in liver and lung was also increased twofold, but DNA synthesis was decreased in these organs.

Columbano *et al.* (1983, 1984) gave groups of seven male Wistar rats a single dose of lead nitrate (100 μmol/kg bw) by intravenous injection and sacrificed them 1, 2, 3, 4 and 7 days later. The treatment caused a marked enlargement of the liver, which reached a maximum of 71% at the third day after treatment. This effect was accompanied by an increase in total hepatic protein and DNA content, with a maximum at 3 and 4 days, respectively. An increase in DNA synthesis, as monitored by the incorporation of [^{3}H]labelled thymidine, was observed at 24 h, reaching a maximum at 36 h after administration of lead nitrate, with a 30-fold higher level than in control rats. DNA synthesis returned to normal within 3 days. The lead-induced stimulation of liver-cell proliferation was reflected in a significant increase in the number of parenchymal and non-parenchymal cells entering mitosis, with a peak at 48 h. No histologically detectable liver-cell necrosis was seen, which suggested that the cell proliferation induced by lead is not due to a regenerative response. The stimulatory effect of lead on liver growth was reversible; during return to normal size, cell death, morphologically similar to apoptosis, was observed in histological sections of liver from animals sacrificed 4–7 days after treatment.

A series of studies by the same research group investigated the effect of different types of cell proliferation on the development of enzyme-altered preneoplastic hepatic foci in male Wistar rats. In the first experiment, animals were given a single intraperitoneal injection of *N*-nitrosodiethylamine (NDEA; 100 mg/kg bw). After a 2-week recovery period liver cell proliferation was induced by repeated doses of carbon tetrachloride (2 mg/kg bw, by intragastric intubation), or by repeated mitogenic treatments with lead nitrate (100 μmol/kg bw, by intravenous injection). Histologically-altered hepatocytes were monitored as γ-glutamyltransferase-positive or adenosine triphosphatase-negative foci. The results indicated that compensatory cell proliferation induced by carbon tetrachloride enhanced the growth of NDEA-initiated hepatocytes to enzyme-altered foci. On the contrary, repeated waves of cell proliferation induced by lead nitrate did not result in any significant number of enzyme-altered foci (Columbano *et al.*, 1990).

In follow-up studies, the same authors determined the efficacy of different types of cell-proliferative stimuli given during several liver tumour-promoting regimens, with respect to the formation of enzyme-altered hepatocyte foci. Male Wistar rats were initiated with NDEA (150 mg/kg bw, by intravenous injection). After recovery, the animals were subjected to different promoting regimens, i.e. the resistant hepatocyte model (Solt & Farber, 1976), the phenobarbital model (Peraino *et al.*, 1971) and the orotic acid model (Laurier *et al.*, 1984). While the rats were on these regimens, they received different types of liver cell-proliferative stimuli, either a compensatory type (two-thirds partial hepatectomy or a necrogenic dose of carbon tetrachloride) or a direct hyperplastic stimulus by lead nitrate. Initiated cells thus promoted were monitored as foci of enzyme-altered hepatocytes. While compensatory cell regeneration induced by carbon tetrachloride and partial hepatectomy stimulated the promoting ability of the regimens used, direct hyperplasia induced by lead nitrate did not stimulate the formation of foci and/or nodules from initiated hepatocytes. Incorporation of [^{3}H]thymidine showed that there was no significant difference in the extent of DNA synthesis resulting from the different proliferative stimuli, irrespective of the promoting procedure used. These results suggest that the two types of cell-proliferative stimuli may involve different cell growth and signal-transduction pathways, or they may act on different cell populations (Ledda-Columbano *et al.*, 1992; Coni *et al.*, 1993a).

An enhanced susceptibility of renal tubular epithelial cells in rats to lead-induced mitogenicity was reported at doses comparable to those used in the cancer bioassay. This may contribute to the carcinogenic response seen in the kidney following exposure to lead. It is of interest to note that the liver — an organ that is not susceptible to lead-induced carcinogenicity — showed a significantly lower mitogenic response towards lead exposure (Calabrese & Baldwin, 1992).

To evaluate the effect of pre-exposure to mitogens on carbon tetrachloride-induced hepatotoxicity, Calabrese *et al.* (1995) gave male Wistar rats a single intraperitoneal injection of carbon tetrachloride (0.3 mL/kg bw in corn oil) 48 h after either a single intravenous injection of lead nitrate (0.33 mg/kg bw) or distilled water. The rats pre-treated with lead nitrate showed markedly lower serum alanine aminotransferase (ALT) and aspartate aminotransferase (AST) activities at 24, 48 and 72 h after administration of carbon tetrachloride than rats pre-treated with distilled water. However, treatment with the anti-mitotic agent colchicine did not alter the lead-induced protection. These findings suggest that the lead-induced protection is not associated with the major mitogenic response of lead, despite its strong temporal association.

Bell *et al.* (1993) tested lead nitrate and lead acetate for mitogenic effects in the liver of adult male and female rainbow trout. Groups treated with a single intraperitoneal injection of lead nitrate or lead acetate (up to 375 mg/kg bw) or a single intravenous injection of lead nitrate (up to 5 mg/kg bw) showed no statistically significant alterations in liver:body weight ratio. There was no change in hepatic DNA content of the fish that received the intraperitoneal injections. The results suggest significant interspecies differences between the mitogenic response of the liver in rainbow trout and Wistar rats exposed to lead.

(*b*) *Effects on regulatory proteins*

The steady-state levels of *c-fos* and *c-jun* messenger RNA have been investigated in rat liver tissue after various proliferative stimuli, i.e. compensatory cell regeneration induced by partial hepatectomy or carbon tetrachloride, and direct hyperplasia induced by different hepatomitogens, one of which was lead nitrate. Whereas *c-fos* and *c-jun* expression increased soon after partial hepatectomy or administration of carbon tetrachloride, an increased expression of *c-jun* in the absence of *c-fos* expression was seen during direct hyperplasia induced by lead nitrate. These results suggest that, depending on the nature of the proliferative stimulus, an increased expression of these regulatory genes may not be necessary for in-vivo induction of liver cell proliferation (Coni *et al.*, 1993b).

The influence of lead on various protein factors involved in cell signalling has been studied in relation to its neurotoxic effects. Male Long-Evans rats (aged 21 days; $n = 40$) received lead acetate (50 ppm) in drinking-water for 90 days. Control animals ($n = 40$) received sodium acetate. After this period, mean ± SD blood lead concentrations in the control and lead-exposed groups were 4 ± 0.2 and 18 ± 0.2 μg/dL, respectively. Compared with controls, the lead-exposed animals showed a significantly higher accumulation of lead in the frontal cortex, brain stem, striatum and hippocampus, as well as a three- to fourfold increase in the concentrations of NF-κB and activator protein 1, a four- to 10-fold activation of c-Jun N-terminal kinase, a five- to sixfold activation of mitogen-activated protein kinase kinase (MAPKK) and an enhanced activity of caspases in these four brain regions, which is consistent with apoptosis. These effects may contribute to the neurotoxicity of lead (Ramesh *et al.*, 2001).

To identify genes that are upregulated in PbR11 cells (a lead-resistant variant of rat glioma C6 cells), Li and Rossman (2001) applied the method of suppression subtractive hybridization between mRNAs of C6 and PbR11 cells. Three upregulated genes were identified, i.e. thrombospondin-1, heparin sulfate 6-sulfotransferase, and neuropilin-1, which play important roles in angiogenesis and axon growth during neuronal development. It is of interest to note that all these genes are functionally related to heparin sulfate. The effects of short-term lead exposure (24 h, up to 600 μM) on the expression of these genes were examined in C6 cells. While thrombospondin-1 is repressed by lead in a dose-dependent manner, neuropilin-1 and heparin sulfate 6-sulfotransferase showed low constitutive expression in C6 cells, which was not altered by exposure to lead. Since low concentrations of lead inhibit the sulfation of heparin (Fujiwara & Kaji, 1999), the results suggest that heparin sulfate 6-sulfotransferase may be the lead-sensitive enzyme responsible for this inhibition. In addition to this enzyme, neuropilin-1 and thrombospondin-1 may also be targets for lead-induced developmental neurotoxicity (Li & Rossman, 2001).

Bouton *et al.* (2001) used cDNA microarrays to analyse the effects of acute lead exposure (10 μM lead acetate, 24 h) on large-scale gene expression patterns in immortalized rat astrocytes. Control cells were treated with 10 μM sodium acetate. Many genes previously reported to be differentially regulated by lead exposure were identified in this system. In addition, novel putative targets of lead-mediated toxicity were identified, including calcium/phospholipid binding annexins, angiogenesis-inducing thrombospondins, collagens, and t-RNA synthetases. In a biochemical assay, the phospholipid binding activity of the protein annexin A_5 was shown to be induced by nanomolar concentrations of lead.

Lead acetate (100 nM–100 μM) stimulated DNA synthesis and cell-cycle progression in human astrocytoma cells through selective lead-induced activation of protein kinase Cα (PKCα) (Lu *et al.*, 2001). In a further study, the same authors investigated the ability of lead to activate the mitogen-activated protein kinase (MAPK) cascade. Exposure of these astrocytoma cells to lead acetate (1–50 μM) resulted in a concentration- and time-dependent activation of MAPK, as was evident from increased phosphorylation and increased kinase activity. This effect was significantly reduced by specific inhibition or down-regulation of PKCα. Lead also activated MAPK MEK1/2 kinase, an effect that was mediated by PKCα. Addition of specific MEK inhibitors blocked lead-induced MAPK activation and inhibited lead-induced DNA synthesis, as measured by [^{3}H]thymidine incorporation. The results of this study suggest that lead may act as a tumour promoter in transformed glial cells (Lu *et al.*, 2002).

The effect of divalent lead on protein phosphorylation in bovine adrenal chromaffin cells and human SH SY5Y cells has been examined. Cells were incubated with inorganic [^{32}P] for 1 h in the presence of lead acetate (1, 5 and 10 μM) and proteins were separated by two-dimensional polyacrylamide gel electrophoresis. Among the spots that were indicative of increased protein phosphorylation, three proteins, with an apparent molecular weight of 25 kDa and iso-electric points in the range 4.0–4.5, were immuno-identified as isoforms of the heat-shock protein 27 (Hsp27). The effect of lead on Hsp27 phosphorylation was blocked by the p38MAPK inhibitor SB203580 (1 μM) and phosphorylation of p38MAPK was increased by lead. The results were similar for both cell types studied. Thus lead can modulate the phosphorylation state of Hsp27 via activation of the p38MAPK pathway. Since Hsp27 in its non-phosphorylated form confers resistance towards oxidative stress (Rogalla *et al.*, 1999) this effect of lead may result in a higher vulnerability of cells to oxidative damage (Leal *et al.*, 2002).

The zinc finger, a major structural motif involved in protein–nucleic acid interactions, is present in the largest super-family of transcription factors (Zeng & Kagi, 1995). Zinc (Zn^{2+}) ions coordinate this finger-like structure through interaction with cysteine and histidine residues. Factors containing such motifs are potential targets for perturbation by divalent lead (Büsselberg, 1995; Guilarte *et al.*, 1995; Tomsig & Suszkiw, 1996). Lead has been shown to interfere with the DNA-binding properties of the zinc finger-containing transcription factors Sp1 and Egr-1, both *in vivo* and *in vitro*. More recently, the inhibitory effects of lead on the DNA-binding of the zinc finger protein transcription factor IIIA (TFIIIA) have been demonstrated (Hanas *et al.*, 1999). The interaction of lead with Sp1, Egr-1, and TFIIIA shows that lead can also target other cellular proteins that contain the zinc-finger motif and that this protein domain is a potential mediator for lead-induced alterations in protein function. Thus by specifically targeting zinc-finger proteins, lead is able to produce multiple responses through its action on a common site that is present in enzymes, channels and receptors (Zawia *et al.*, 2000).

(*c*) *Apoptosis*

(i) *In-vivo studies*

Apoptosis or programmed cell death is induced by various physiological or pathological stimuli. Mitochondria and a specific class of proteins, the caspases, play an important role in this process. At an early stage of apoptosis, the mitochondrial permeability transition pore is opened, which leads to depolarization of the mitochondrion and to the release of cytochrome C. Subsequently, caspases activate endonucleases that cleave the genomic DNA into the high-molecular-weight fragments that are characteristic of apoptotic cells. Although the detailed molecular mechanism of lead-induced apoptosis is still unknown, calcium overload and the generation of ROS may be important triggers. These and other mechanistic aspects of lead-induced apoptosis are discussed in recent reviews (Waalkes *et al.*, 2000; Pulido & Parrish, 2003).

Columbano *et al.* (1985) showed that in male Wistar rats, a single intravenous injection of lead nitrate (100 μmol/kg bw) caused liver enlargement associated with hepatic cell proliferation. The subsequent involution of the liver hyperplasia was studied by histological examination of liver sections prepared during regression of the liver. There was no sign of massive lytic cell necrosis, and no change in serum concentrations of glutamate pyruvate transaminase. Apoptotic bodies were observed in the involuting liver by microscopy and ultrastructural examination. A marked increase in the number of apoptotic bodies was noted 5 days after administration of lead, when the liver was already regressing, while very few were observed in control animals or in rats 2 days after lead injection, when the mitotic index reached its maximum, or at 15 days, when the liver had returned to normal. These findings suggest that the removal of excess liver tissue that follows the initial lead-induced hyperplasia is due to apoptosis.

Fox *et al.* (1998) showed that exposure to lead resulted in the selective apoptotic loss of rods and bipolar cells in the retina of rats. Lead-exposed rats were reared from dams that received 0.02% or 0.2% lead acetate in drinking-water during lactation only. At 21 days of age (weaning), the mean blood lead concentrations in the non-exposed rats and the two dose-groups were 1, 19 and 59 μg/dL, respectively. During and following lead exposure, rod/retinal cGMP phosphodiesterase expression and activity were delayed in onset and decreased, the concentration of calcium was elevated, and mitochondrial ATP synthesis was decreased in the infant rats.

(ii) *In-vitro studies*

The role of apoptosis in the effects induced by lead (lead acetate, 0.01–100 μM) and glutamate (0.1 and 1 mM) has been studied in mouse hypothalamic GT1-7 neurons. Loikkanen *et al.* (2003) found that glutamate alone had no effect on cell viability, but it enhanced neuronal cell death induced by lead (at concentrations 1–100 μM) at 72 h. Glutamate alone did not induce caspase-3-like protease activity or internucleosomal DNA fragmentation which are both biochemical hallmarks of apoptosis. However, combined exposure to lead (10 or 100 μM) and glutamate (1 mM) resulted in more prominent caspase-3-like protease activity than that caused by lead alone, with the highest activity measured at 48 h. Internucleosomal DNA fragmentation caused by lead (10 or 100 μM) was enhanced by glutamate (1 mM). Immunoblotting did not reveal any changes in p53 protein concentration in cells exposed to lead, glutamate, or their combination at any time point (3–72 h). These results suggest that lead-induced neurotoxicity may be mediated partially through p53-independent apoptosis and enhanced by glutamate.

Cultured granule cells from newborn rat cerebellum were used to study whether apoptotic or necrotic death is the major consequence of exposure to low concentrations of lead. At a dose of 1 μM, lead did not affect glutamate-induced neuronal necrosis but promoted neuronal apoptosis, as characterized by cell shrinkage and chromatin condensation, internucleosomal DNA fragmentation and by dependence on de-novo synthesis of macromolecules. The low concentrations of lead that promoted apoptosis in this study were within the range of blood lead concentrations reported to impair the cognitive function in children and to alter synaptogenesis in the neonatal rat brain. These in-vitro results suggest that the highly neurotoxic action of lead may depend on a facilitation of apoptosis (Oberto *et al.*, 1996).

In-vitro studies using rat retinas incubated in the presence of calcium or lead showed increased high molecular weight DNA fragmentation and a higher number of apoptotic rods. In addition, retinal mitochondrial ATP synthesis was decreased, mitochondrial cytochrome C was released and caspase activity was increased. These effects were additive in the presence of physiological concentrations of both calcium and lead. These results suggest that lead-induced rod and bipolar cell apoptosis is triggered by calcium and lead overload and that mitochondrial alterations play a central role in this process (Fox *et al.*, 1998).

An in-vitro model using isolated rat retinas was used to determine the mechanisms underlying retinal degeneration induced by calcium and/or lead. Confocal microscopy and histological and biochemical analyses established that elevated amounts of calcium and/or lead were concentrated around photoreceptors and produced rod-selective apoptosis. Mitochondrial depolarization, swelling and cytochrome C release were also seen, followed by activation of caspase-9 and caspase-3, but not caspase-7 or caspase-8. The effects of calcium and lead were additive. The concentrations of reduced and oxidized glutathione and pyridine nucleotides in rods were unchanged. These results show that rod mitochondria are the target sites for calcium and lead, and suggest that these metals bind to the internal binding site of the mitochondrial permeability transition pore, which then opens up, initiating the cytochrome C-caspase cascade of apoptosis (He *et al.*, 2000).

The effects of extracellular lead supplementation on the cellular lead content and on cell proliferation and survival have been studied in normal rat fibroblasts. The culture medium contained a background level of 0.060 μM lead and the normal cellular concentration of lead was 3.1 ± 0.1 ng/10^7 cells. Cells were exposed to 0.078–320 μM lead acetate, which caused a dose-dependent inhibition of cell proliferation after 48 h, which was apparent at 0.312 μM ($p = 0.122$) and became statistically significant at concentrations > 0.625 μM ($p = 0.0003$ at 5 μM). DNA fragmentation, a hallmark of apoptosis, increased significantly at lead concentrations from 2.5–10.0 μM. The occurrence of apoptosis was confirmed by flow cytometry, which showed a sub-diploid peak at 5–20 μM lead. There was a dose-dependent accumulation of cells in the G0/G1 phase, mainly compensated by a decrease in the percentage of cells in S phase. These results demonstrate that induction of apoptosis contributes to the lead-induced inhibition of cell proliferation in rat fibroblasts (Iavicoli *et al.*, 2001).

De la Fuente *et al.* (2002) incubated human peripheral blood mononuclear cells with increasing concentrations of cadmium, arsenic or lead, and determined apoptosis by flow cytometry and DNA electrophoresis. Arsenic (15 μM) induced a significant level of apoptosis after 48 h of incubation, while cadmium had a similar effect at higher concentrations (65 μM). In contrast, lead concentrations as high as 500 μM were non-toxic and did not induce a significant degree of apoptosis.

(*d*) *Effects on hepatic enzymes*

Alvares *et al.* (1975) determined metabolizing capacities in 10 normal adults and in 10 children aged 1–8 years with two test drugs, antipyrine and phenylbutazone. Eight children had biochemical evidence but no clinical expression of lead poisoning. Among the children, there were no differences in their capacities to metabolize the two drugs. The mean antipyrine half-life in the children, 6.63 h, was significantly lower than the mean half-life of 13.58 h in adults. The mean phenylbutazone half-lives in the children and adults, 1.68 and 3.16 days, respectively, also differed significantly. In two other children who showed clinical as well as biochemical manifestations of acute plumbism, antipyrine half-lives were significantly longer than normal.

Saenger *et al.* (1984) investigated the possible inhibitory effects of lead on the metabolism of 6β-hydroxycortisol (6βOHF, a highly polar metabolite of cortisol) by analysis of urinary excretion of 6βOHF in 26 children with mildly to moderately elevated blood lead concentrations (average, 44 µg/dL; range 23–60 µg/mL). The EDTA provocative test was used to assess the size of chelatable and potentially toxic lead stores in these children. Children with elevated urinary lead excretion after an EDTA provocative test, i.e. elevated tissue lead stores, had markedly decreased urinary excretion of 6βOHF (178 ± 15 µg/m^2 body surface area in 24 h) compared with children who had negative tests (333 ± 40 µg/m^2 in 24 h; $p < 0.01$); the urinary cortisol excretion in both these groups of children was not different from that of age-matched controls. These findings suggest that lead, at relatively low concentrations, may interfere with hepatic microsomal formation of a cortisol metabolite.

(*e*) *Effects on endocrine function*

(i) *Human studies*

Gustafson *et al.* (1989) carried out a study in Sweden in a group of secondary lead smelter workers and appropriately selected controls, and found a complex effect on the endocrine system induced by moderate exposure to lead, possibly mediated by changes at the hypothalamic–pituitary level. It should be noted that all the hormone values were within the normal range for the Swedish population.

The possible neuroendocrine effects of lead were studied in six children with high blood lead concentrations (range, 41–72 µg/dL) and in four children with low blood lead (0–30 µg/dL). The first group received EDTA chelation therapy. The growth rate of these children increased considerably after the chelation therapy, from 4.2 ± 0.9 cm/year before treatment to 9.0 ± 0.9 cm/year after treatment (data for 2–3-year-olds, $n = 5$). The children with low blood lead concentrations had a growth rate of 8.9 ± 1.0 cm/year (2–2.3-year-olds, $n = 3$) (Huseman *et al.*, 1992)

Thyroid function tests were performed in 58 petrol-pump workers or automobile mechanics (mean age, 31.7 ± 10.6 years; mean duration of exposure to lead, 13 ± 10 years). Their mean blood lead concentration was 51.9 ± 9.4 µg/dL, which was approximately five-fold higher than that in 35 non-exposed control subjects. There was no difference in serum concentrations of triiodothyronine (T3) or thyroxine (T4) between the groups. Interestingly, T3 was significantly lower with longer exposure times (210 versus 29 months). The mean thyroid-stimulating (TSH) concentrations were significantly higher ($p < 0.01$) in exposed workers. This was independent of exposure time, but more pronounced in individuals with higher blood lead values. However, TSH concentrations remained within the normal range. The results suggest that elevated blood lead concentrations could enhance the pituitary release of TSH without having a significant effect on circulating levels of T3 and T4 (Singh *et al.*, 2000).

The effects of lead on the endocrine system were studied in 77 lead-smelter workers (62 active, 15 retired) compared with 26 referents. Lead concentrations were determined in plasma (i.e. giving an index of recent exposure), in blood and in finger-bone (i.e. giving an index of long-term exposure). In addition, the serum concentrations of pituitary hormones, thyroid hormones and testosterone were determined. Nine exposed workers and 11 referents were challenged with gonadotrophin-releasing hormone and thyrotrophin-releasing hormone, followed by measurement of stimulated pituitary hormone concentrations in serum. Median blood lead concentrations were 33.2 μg/dL in active workers, 18.6 μg/dL in retired workers and 4.1 μg/dL in controls. Respective median bone lead concentrations were 21 μg/g, 55 μg/g and 2 μg/g. Concentrations of pituitary hormones, thyroid hormones and testosterone were similar in the three groups. In the challenge test, stimulated follicle-stimulating hormone (FSH) concentrations were significantly lower in lead workers ($p = 0.014$) than in referents, indicating an effect of lead in the pituitary. The results show that moderate exposure to lead was associated with only minor changes in male endocrine function, particularly affecting the hypothalamic–pituitary axis (Erfurth *et al.*, 2001).

(ii) *In-vitro study*

To examine the in-vitro effects of lead on cytochrome P450 aromatase and on estrogen receptor β, human ovary granulosa cells were collected from women undergoing in-vitro fertilization and cultured with 10 μM lead acetate. Lead content in these cells increased to 85 μg/g after 5 h of culture, 390 μg/g after 24 h and 1740 μg/g at 72 h. Aromatase activity was significantly reduced, as were the amounts of P450 aromatase enzyme, estrogen receptor β and their mRNAs. Inhibition of protein synthesis by cycloheximide (10 μg/mL) did not eliminate the effects of lead. The results suggest that the effects of lead on female fertility may result, in part, from the down-regulation of P450 aromatase and estrogen receptor β gene transcription in ovarian granulosa (Taupeau *et al.*, 2003).

4.3 Effects on reproduction

It is generally accepted from the older literature that lead adversely affects the reproductive process in both men and women. The evidence is however mostly qualitative and dose–effect relationships have not been established.

Most of the information is based on studies among workers with high occupational exposure to lead, while low-dose effects have been reported from occupational cohorts or groups in the general population living in polluted areas.

Some factors make it difficult to extrapolate animal data to the human situation. These difficulties are due mainly to differences among species in reproductive end-points and to the level of exposure.

4.3.1 *Humans*

(*a*) *Male fertility*

Studies have focused mainly on the quality of semen, endocrine function and birth rates in occupationally-exposed subjects, and have shown that concentrations of inorganic lead > 40 μg/dL in blood can impair male reproductive function by reducing sperm count, volume and density, and by affecting sperm motility and morphology.

Dose–response relationships, in particular at a threshold level, are poorly understood, and site, mode or mechanism of action are often unknown. Also, the effects were not always the same or associated in the same way, although the prevalent effects were on sperm count and concentration.

The classic study by Lancranjan *et al.* (1975) performed in Romania first provided some evidence of impaired spermatogenesis in men with blood lead concentrations > 40 μg/dL. The subjects were classified into four groups: 'men with lead poisoning' ($n = 23$), men with 'moderate' ($n = 42$), 'slight' ($n = 35$) or 'physiological' ($n = 50$) lead absorption. The major finding of this study was the suggestion of a dose–response relationship for the decrease in sperm count (hypospermia) and sperm motility (asthenospermia) and the increase in abnormal sperm morphology (teratospermia) with increasing lead absorption. The strengths of this study were the use of a standardized questionnaire to collect the data, the relative comparability of controls and the relatively large number of subjects involved. On the other hand, assessment of the dose–response relationship was limited by the overlap between exposure groups, by the relatively high blood lead concentrations in control subjects, by the inclusion of coitus interruptus as a means to collect semen and by lack of information on sperm counts.

Similar findings were reported by Lerda (1992) in Argentina, although no dose–response relationship was found. The result should be noted, mainly because selection of subjects and characterization of exposure to lead were well conducted, as were the collection and analysis of the semen and the statistical analyses of the results.

The cross-sectional study by Alexander *et al.* (1996) showed that blood lead concentrations > 40 μg/dL may affect spermatogenesis by reducing sperm concentration and total sperm count. No association was found between exposure to lead and sperm morphology or motility, or serum concentration of reproductive hormones. The strengths of the study were mainly the size and careful selection of the study population, availability of historical data of lead exposure, the control for all the relevant confounding factors (e.g. age, smoking, alcohol consumption, period of abstinence before semen collection, blood concentrations of other metals such as cadmium and zinc), the statistical analysis, and the validity of the semen analysis.

A study by Rodamilans *et al.* (1988) in Spain showed no clear correlation between blood lead concentrations and endocrine variables. Smelter workers were divided into three groups according to duration of exposure: < 1 year (group 1, $n = 5$), 1–5 years (group 2, $n = 8$) and > 5 years (group 3, $n = 10$). In group 3, serum testosterone was significantly lower, steroid binding globulin (SBG) was higher and there was a clear reduction in the free testosterone index (testosterone/SBG). In group 2, there was a significantly lower free testosterone index but there were no clear differences between testosterone and SBG concentrations compared to the controls. There was an increase in serum luteinizing hormone (LH) concentration in the first group, but this did not persist with longer durations of lead exposure. The authors suggested an initial testicular toxicity followed by a dysfunction in the hypothalamus or the pituitary gland, which disrupts the hypothalamic–pituitary feedback mechanism associated with prolonged exposure (Rodamilans *et al.*, 1988).

A study by McGregor and Mason (1990) suggested that lead may cause subclinical primary toxic damage to the seminiferous tubules in the testis at blood lead concentrations > 47 µg/dL. In this study, testosterone concentrations were normal, in contrast to the findings of Rodamilans *et al.* (1988).

Ng *et al.* (1991) carried out a study in Singapore and found that concentrations of LH and FSH showed a moderate increase in relation to blood lead concentrations in the range of 10–40 µg/dL, thereafter reaching a plateau or declining. An increase in concentrations of LH and FSH, with normal testosterone, was noted in subjects with < 10 years of exposure to lead whereas men exposed for 10 or more years had normal FSH and LH and low testosterone concentrations. The main conclusion was that moderate exposure to lead resulted in small changes in endocrine function in a dose-related manner, reflecting primary and secondary effects of lead on the testes and the hypothalamus–pituitary axis.

Gennart *et al.* (1992) assessed the thyroid, testes, kidney and autonomic nervous system function in 98 battery workers in Belgium (mean blood lead concentration, 51 µg/dL; range, 40–75 µg/dL) and found no abnormalities.

Several of the studies described above (Lancrajan *et al.*, 1975; Lerda, 1992; Alexander *et al.*, 1996) and that of Assennato *et al.* (1987) reported effects on testicular function in groups of men with mean blood lead concentrations above 40–50 µg/dL. These results are consistent with a likely threshold of about 45–55 µg/dL (Bonde *et al.*, 2000). In contrast, the findings of a study of semen (Robins *et al.*, 1997) in 97 men employed in a South African lead–acid battery plant, with blood lead concentrations ranging from 28–93 µg/dL, did not support an effect of lead on sperm concentration and total sperm count. However, the authors noted that their results should be interpreted with caution because of the relatively high range of current blood lead concentrations, the high prevalence of abnormalities in semen quality and the lack of a control population.

In a cross-sectional survey (Telisman *et al.*, 2000) of workers exposed to lead and non-occupationally exposed controls, a significant negative association was found between sperm count and mean blood lead concentrations in six subgroups stratified by blood lead concentration. The mean blood lead concentrations in the six subgroups ranged from 5–35 µg/dL. In contrast, in a longitudinal study (Viskum *et al.*, 1999) of battery workers in Denmark, no improvement was found in sperm concentration or in the proportion of morphological abnormalities with a decline in blood lead concentration from about 40 to 20 µg/dL.

Bonde *et al.* (2002) undertook a cross-sectional survey on some fertility parameters of 503 workers employed by 10 companies in Belgium, Italy and the United Kingdom, as part of the ASCLEPIOS project. Volume of semen and concentration of sperm were determined in a fresh semen sample according to an agreed protocol of quality assurance. Measurement of dose indicators in blood and seminal fluid and its fractions and the sperm chromatin structure assay were all performed by centralized laboratories. Abnormal chromatin structure of the spermatozoa was analysed by flow cytometric measurement of red (denaturated single stranded DNA) and green (native DNA) fluorescence in sperm cells stained with acridine, and expressed by the ratio of red to total (red + green) fluorescence (Garner *et al.*, 1986). Extraneous determinants including centre, period of sexual abstinence and age were taken into account in the statistical analysis. If appropriate, possible thresholds were examined by iterative threshold slope linear regression. The mean blood lead concentration was 31.0 μg/dL (range, 4.6–64.5 μg/dL) in 362 workers exposed to lead and 4.4 μg/dL (range, below the detection limit to 19.8 μg/dL) in 141 workers not exposed to lead. The median sperm concentration was reduced by 49% in men with blood lead concentrations > 50 μg/dL. The findings were consistent across the three centres and the sample size was larger than in earlier studies thus strengthening the findings. However, in this study and in previous ones, the authors noted that the low participation rate at two of the three sites is a major limitation conferring risk of selection bias as men who perceived themselves to be less fertile may have been more motivated to take part (Bonde *et al.*, 1996; Larsen *et al.*, 1998; Bonde *et al.*, 2002).

The concentration of inorganic lead in blood may not reflect the concentration in the target organs and therefore lead measured in seminal fluid and its fractions might be better correlated with testicular lead and histopathological alterations. Apostoli *et al.* (1999) and Bonde *et al.* (2002) found a high content of lead within spermatozoa and a low concentration in seminal fluid, indicating that lead is either taken up by spermatozoa or is incorporated into the sperm cells during spermatogenesis. The analyses based on lead in semen largely corroborated the findings based on analysis of lead concentration in blood, but men with the highest concentration of lead in spermatozoa also had higher mean αT, and a higher proportion of sperm cells outside the main population, indicating alterations of the sperm chromatin structure (Bonde *et al.*, 2002).

Zinc contributes to sperm chromatin stability and binds to protamine 2. It has recently been shown that lead competes with zinc and binds human protamine 2 (HP2) causing conformational changes in the protein (Quintanilla-Vega *et al.*, 2000). This decreases the extent of HP2-DNA binding, which probably results in alterations in sperm chromatin condensation. Alteration of sperm chromatin structure by increased in-situ denaturation is strongly correlated with the presence of sperm DNA strand breaks (Aravindan *et al.*, 1997) and is associated with reduced fecundity in humans (Spanò *et al.*, 2000).

There appears to be a direct negative correlation between seminal plasma lead concentrations and in-vitro fertilization rates (Benoff *et al.*, 2000, 2003). Lead concentrations are also negatively correlated with standard semen parameters (sperm count, motility and morphology) and sperm function biomarkers (mannose receptor expression and mannose-stimulated acrosome reaction), and positively correlated with premature acrosome breakdown.

Positive relationships between blood lead concentrations and seminal plasma lead or sperm lead concentrations have been reported after both occupational exposures (Aribarg & Shukcharoen, 1996; Telisman *et al.*, 2000; Bonde *et al.*, 2002) and environmental exposures (Telisman *et al.*, 2000) to lead.

Another way to verify the possible effect of lead on male fertility is through retrospective evaluation of time to pregnancy. A French cohort study (Coste *et al.*, 1991) of 229 workers exposed to lead (mean blood lead concentration, 46.3 µg/dL) compared with 125 unexposed subjects did not provide clear evidence of adverse effects of occupational exposure to lead on male fertility as studied by recording live births.

Apostoli *et al.* (2000) found decreased fertility among men with blood lead concentrations of at least 40 µg/dL, but this was statistically significant only in a subgroup analysis restricted to subjects with just one child. Fertility was not reduced in men with blood lead concentrations in the range 30–40 µg/dL.

Sallmén *et al.* (2000) conducted a retrospective study on time to pregnancy among the wives of men who had been monitored for lead to assess whether paternal occupational exposure to inorganic lead was associated with decreased fertility. Lead exposure was assessed by blood measurements and by questionnaires. The final study population consisted of 502 couples who did not use contraception at the beginning of the pregnancy. The fecundability density ratios, adjusted for potential confounders, were 0.92 (95% CI, 0.73–1.16), 0.89 (95% CI, 0.66–1.20), 0.58 (95% CI, 0.33–0.96) and 0.83 (95% CI, 0.50–1.32) for blood lead categories in men of 0.5–0.9, 1.0–1.4, 1.5–1.8 and ≥ 1.9 µmol/L, respectively. This study provided limited support for the hypothesis that paternal exposure to lead is associated with decreased fertility.

In a study by Joffe *et al.* (2003) as part of the ASCLEPIOS project, a total of 1104 subjects in four European countries took part, of whom 638 were occupationally exposed to lead at the relevant time. Blood lead concentrations were mainly < 50 µg/dL. No consistent association between time to pregnancy and lead exposure was found in any of the exposure models. It may be concluded from this multicentric survey that there are no detectable effects on male fertility at the levels of lead exposure currently measured in European worksites.

Lead may be determined in Leydig cells, thus in possible relation with testosterone levels in serum. Lead may also be detected in germ cells, demonstrating that it passes through the blood–testis barrier, which is functionally very similar to the blood–brain barrier, and affects the germ cells at different degrees of differentiation (spermatogonia, primary spermatocytes, spermatids or spermatozoa). In this regard, it is still an open question whether lead in cells or in fluids is a result of a breakdown of the blood–testis barrier or whether lead normally passes this barrier.

(*b*) *Effects of lead during pregnancy*

Wibberley *et al.* (1977) studied placental lead concentrations in a series of births in Birmingham, United Kingdom, classified by stillbirth, neonatal death or survival beyond one week. Average results showed higher lead concentrations in those neonates who failed to survive both birth and the neonatal period. There was no association of placental lead with impaired birth weight among survivors.

Placental transfer of lead and its effects on newborns were examined by Clark (1977). Following delivery, blood from 122 mothers and cord blood from their infants were taken to measure lead, haemoglobin, packed cell volume and mean corpuscular haemoglobin concentration. All were resident in Kasanda, Zambia, a lead mine and smelter town. The mean blood lead concentrations were 41.2 µg/dL and 37 µg/dL for maternal blood and cord blood, respectively, with a significant correlation ($r = 0.77$, $p < 0.001$). The increased lead transfer, however, did not appear to affect adversely birth weight or red cell values of the newborn.

Nordström *et al.* (1979a) investigated the frequencies of congenital malformations in the offspring of female employees at a smelter in northern Sweden and in a reference population near the smelter. In the population of the area, no significant variation in the total frequency of malformations or in any particular group of malformations was found. Among the women who worked at the smelters, the risk for malformations was about two times as high and the risk for multiple malformations about four times as high as in the reference population.

In a study of the relationship between prenatal lead exposure and congenital anomalies, Needleman *et al.* (1984) measured lead concentration in umbilical cord blood from 5183 consecutive deliveries of at least 20 weeks' gestation. The demographic and socioeconomic variables of the mothers, including exposure to lead, which were shown on univariate analysis to be associated with increased risk for congenital anomalies, were evaluated in a stepwise logistic-regression model with malformation as the outcome. Coffee, alcohol, tobacco and marijuana use, which were associated with lead concentrations, but not with risk for malformation in offspring, were also taken into account. The model was reduced in steps by eliminating the variables with the highest *p*-value, until the most parsimonious model was created. The relative risk for anomalies associated with lead was then calculated while holding other covariates constant. Lead was found to be associated, in a dose-related fashion, with an increased risk for minor anomalies, but the risk for major malformations was not increased.

Bellinger *et al.* (1991) evaluated the relationship between prenatal low-level lead exposure and fetal growth in 4354 pregnancies in which the mean lead concentration in umbilical cord blood was 7.0 µg/dL (SD, 3.3; 10th percentile, 3.4 µg/dL; 90th percentile, 10.9 µg/dL). Higher cord blood lead concentrations were significantly associated with gestations of slightly longer duration. Comparing infants with cord blood lead concentrations ≥ 15 µg/dL with those with < 5 µg/dL, adjusted risk ratios of 1.5–2.5 were observed for low birth weight (< 2500 g) and for fetal growth indices that express birth weight as a function of length of gestation (e.g. small for gestational age, intrauterine growth retardation). The 95% confidence intervals of these risk ratios included 1, but precluded rejection of the null hypothesis of no association. The authors concluded that the risk for adverse fetal growth is not increased at cord blood lead concentrations < 15 μg/dL but that modest increases in risk may be associated with concentrations ≥ 15 μg/dL.

Factor-Litvak *et al.* (1991) tested the hypothesis that exposure to lead during pregnancy is associated with reduced intrauterine growth and an increase in preterm delivery. The sample comprised women, recruited at mid-pregnancy, residing in Titova Mitrovica, a lead smelter town, or in Pristina, a non-exposed town 25 miles away, in the province of Kosovo, Serbia and Montenegro. Mean blood lead concentrations at mid-pregnancy were 0.92 μmol/L (± 0.38, n = 401) in women in the exposed town and 0.26 μmol/L (± 0.09, n = 506) in women in the comparison town. No differences were found between towns for either birth weight or length of gestation: mean birth weight was 3308 (± 566) g in Titova Mitrovica and 3361 (± 525) g in Pristina; mean length of gestation was 274 (± 18.8) days in Titova Mitrovica and 275 (± 15.6) days in Pristina. After adjustment for the effects of potential confounders, no significant relationships were found between maternal blood lead measured at mid-pregnancy, at delivery or in the umbilical cord, and either birth weight or length of gestation or preterm delivery (< 37 weeks). The authors concluded that exposure to environmental lead does not impair fetal growth or influence length of gestation.

The relation between paternal occupational exposure to lead and low birth weight/prematurity was also examined in a retrospective cohort study (Lin *et al.*, 1998). Birth weight and gestational age, obtained from New York State birth certificates (1981–92), were compared for children born to lead-exposed and non-exposed workers. The exposed group (n = 4256) consisted of births to male workers of reproductive age reported to the New York State Heavy Metals Registry. The control group (n = 2259) consisted of the offspring of a random sample of male bus drivers, frequency matched by age and residence. There were no statistically-significant differences in birth weight or gestational age between the exposed and the control groups. However, workers who had elevated blood lead concentrations for more than 5 years had a higher risk of fathering a child of low birth weight (risk ratio, 3.40; 95% CI, 1.39–8.35) or who was premature (risk ratio, 3.03; 95% CI, 1.35–6.77) than did controls after adjustment for paternal age, low maternal education, race, residence, gravidity, maternal spontaneous abortion history, perinatal complications, adequacy of prenatal care and sex of the infant.

The effect of maternal bone lead on length and head circumference of newborns and infants aged one month was evaluated by Hernandez-Avila *et al.* (2002). Birth length of newborns was found to decrease as tibia lead concentrations increased. Patella lead was positively and significantly related to the risk of a low head circumference score; this score remained unaffected by inclusion of birth weight.

(*c*) *Effects of lead on abortion*

As a whole, the literature on this topic provides consistent evidence in the form both of case series and epidemiological studies, that the risk for spontaneous abortion (defined as a pregnancy loss occurring before the 20th week of gestation, but after the stage of unrecognized, subclinical loss) is increased by maternal exposure to high concentrations of lead. The data on male exposures and spontaneous abortions in their partners are more sparse and less consistent.

Torelli (1930) provided data on pregnancies in Milan, where the printing industry was a source of lead exposure. The risk for spontaneous abortion was reported to be 4.5% in the general population, 14% in partners of men employed in the printing industry and 24% in women who themselves were so employed; these data yield relative risks of 3.1 and 5.3. The infant mortality was more than doubled among exposed women as compared with the rate in all of Italy: 320 versus 150 per 1000 livebirths (cited by Hertz-Picciotto, 2000).

Nordström *et al.* (1978a) reported an increased frequency of spontaneous abortion in women living close to a smelter in northern Sweden. In a later report, Nordström *et al.* (1979b) described the responses to a questionnaire completed by 511/662 women who had worked at the smelter and were born in 1930–59. Spontaneous abortion rates were high in those pregnancies in which the mother was employed during the pregnancy (13.9%) or had been employed before and was living close to the smelter (17%); the rate was higher (19.4%) when the father worked at the smelter. It should be noted that the smelter produced copper and lead in addition to a number of other metallurgical and chemical products (Nordström *et al.*, 1978a) and that the effects reported may not necessarily be attributable exclusively to lead.

A study of pregnancies in the centre and surrounding areas of the lead smelter town of Port Pirie, Australia, found that incidence of miscarriages (22/23) and stillbirths (10/11) was higher in women living close to the smelter (McMichael *et al.*, 1986). Two studies found a decreased length of gestation in women whose blood lead concentrations were > 0.58 μmol/L (12 μg/dL) (Dietrich *et al.*, 1986) or 0.68 μmol/L (14 μg/dL) (McMichael *et al.*, 1986). However Needleman *et al.* (1984), Bellinger *et al.*, (1984) and Factor-Litvak *et al.* (1991) did not find differences in gestational length of pregnancy in women with higher blood lead concentrations.

Murphy *et al.* (1990) analysed the rates of spontaneous abortion among women living in the vicinity of a lead smelter with those of women living in a town where exposure to lead was low. The data were taken from the obstetric histories of both groups of women when they sought prenatal care for a subsequent pregnancy. A total of 639 women (304 exposed, 335 unexposed) had at least one previous pregnancy and had lived at the same address since their first pregnancy. The geometric mean blood lead concentrations at the time of the interviews were 0.77 μmol/L [16 μg/dL] in women in the exposed town and 0.25 μmol/L [5 μg/dL] in women in the unexposed town. The rates of spontaneous abortions in first pregnancies were similar: 16.4% of women in the exposed town and 14.0% in the unexposed town . The adjusted odds ratio relating town of residence to spontaneous abortion was 1.1 (95% CI, 0.9–1.4).

A case–referent study conducted by Lindbohm *et al* (1991) focused on whether occupational exposure of men to inorganic lead is related to their partners' spontaneous abortion. The cases (213 spontaneous abortions) and referents (300 births) were identified from medical registers. Lead exposure was assessed by blood lead measurements and data obtained from a questionnaire. The results did not show a statistically-significant relationship between spontaneous abortion and paternal exposure to lead among the study subjects.

In a comparison of placental lead concentrations in 71 normal deliveries and 18 births with adverse outcomes (premature birth or premature rupture of membranes) significantly higher placental lead concentrations were found in the adverse birth groups (153.9 ± 71.7 ng/g dry weight compared with the placentas from normal deliveries (103.2 ± 49.5 ng/g dry weight) (Falcón *et al.*, 2003).

Hu (1991) provided data from Boston, MA, USA, on the pregnancies of women who themselves experienced lead poisoning during their childhood in the years 1930–44. The rationale for this study lay in the fact that lead is stored in bone tissue for decades, and the possibility that demineralization of the skeleton takes place during pregnancy. Thirty-five cases of childhood plumbism were identified from hospital records. These women were traced in the 1980s, and interviewed regarding their pregnancy histories. Matched control subjects were included for 22 of the 35 women with childhood plumbism. The proportion of pregnancies reported to have ended in spontaneous abortion or stillbirth was 22% (11/51) among cases with matched plumbism, 29% (8/28) among the cases with non-matched plumbism and 13% (6/48) among matched control subjects. The matched-pairs odds ratio was 1.6 (95% CI, 0.6–4.0) reflecting the small size of the study. Inclusion of unmatched plumbism subjects did not alter the results.

In conclusion, the studies reviewed here show that the effects of lead on fertility and abortion were not always the same either morphologically or quantitatively, neither did they always vary in the same direction. Those on sperm count and concentration were the most frequent in showing effects of lead. It is not yet clear whether the mechanism is a direct effect of lead on reproductive organs or on the endocrine control of reproduction, or both. The mechanism for inducing pregnancy loss is also not clear. Besides preconceptional chromosomal damage to the sperm or a direct teratogenic effect on the fetus, interference with the maternal–fetal hormonal environment is possible, as endocrine-disrupting activity associated with lead has been observed in rodents, primates, and humans. Vascular effects on the placenta are also plausible, given the literature on lead and hypertension (Hertz-Picciotto & Croft, 1993). Developmental toxicity to the fetus is also possible.

(*d*) *Effects on stature and growth*

The effects of low to moderate prenatal and postnatal lead exposure on children's growth in stature were studied by Shukla *et al.* (1989, 1991) in 235 subjects assessed every 3 months for lead exposure (blood lead concentration) and stature (recumbent length) up to 33 months of age. Fetal lead exposure was indexed by maternal blood lead concentration during pregnancy. Adverse effects of lead on growth during the first year of life were observed. Mean blood lead concentrations during the second and third years of life were negatively associated with attained height at 33 months of age ($p = 0.002$), but only among those children who had mean blood lead concentrations above the cohort median (> 10.77 μg/dL) during the 3–15-month period. The results suggest that the effects of lead exposure (*in utero* and during the first year of life) are transient provided that subsequent exposure to lead is not excessive. An average blood lead concentration of 25 μg/dL or higher during the second and third year of life was detrimental to the child's attained stature at 33 months of age. Approximately 15% of this cohort experienced these levels of lead exposure.

The relationship between blood lead concentration and stature was evaluated for a group of 1454 Mexican-American children (age, 5–12 years), from data sets of the 1982–84 Hispanic Health and Nutrition Examination Survey. An inverse relationship was found between blood lead concentration in the range 0.14–1.92 μmol/L [3–40 μg/dL] and stature, which suggests that growth retardation may be associated even with moderate concentrations of blood lead (Frisancho & Ryan, 1991).

Concentrations of lead, zinc and lysozyme, a factor of non-specific immunity, were determined in blood and placental tissue from 50 pregnant women with intrauterine fetal growth retardation (IUGR) and from 27 pregnant women in a control group. Statistically-significant differences in zinc and lead concentrations were found between the groups, with the IUGR group having lower zinc and higher lead concentrations. A significant negative correlation between zinc and lead concentrations was observed, as well as a statistically significant relationship between placental lead concentrations and the age of the pregnant women. Greater age was associated with higher lead concentrations in placental tissue, whereas zinc concentrations decreased. Higher lysozyme concentrations were found in placental tissues of women in the IUGR group (Richter *et al.*, 1999).

The possible role of environmental pollutants in the incidence of IUGR in India was investigated by measurement of lead and zinc concentrations in blood collected at parturition from mothers and neonates. Both maternal and cord blood lead concentrations were significantly higher in IUGR cases than in normal cases ($p < 0.05$). The mean concentration of zinc was also higher in maternal blood of IUGR cases. The mean cord blood lead concentration was > 10 μg/dL in 54% of newborns. A good correlation ($r = 0.53$; $p < 0.01$) between maternal and cord blood lead concentrations confirmed the transfer of lead from mother to fetus. There was a weak but significant inverse relationship between cord blood lead concentrations and birth weight of newborns ($r = -0.23$, $p < 0.05$) (Srivastava *et al.*, 2001).

4.3.2 *Animal studies*

(*a*) *Male fertility*

Many studies in experimental animals have generated results that are consistent with direct toxic effects of lead on seminiferous tubules or Leydig cells, but one study reported simultaneous impairment of spermatogenesis and reduced pituitary content of FSH, which points to a primary action at the extratesticular level.

The male reproductive organs of Sprague-Dawley rats and NMRI mice are apparently rather resistant to the toxicity of inorganic lead. However, several studies of other rat strains and other rodent species indicate fairly consistently that exposures to lead that result in blood lead concentrations > 30–40 μg/dL for at least 30 days are associated with impairment of spermatogenesis and reduced concentrations of circulating androgens. The great variations in hormone concentrations, whether they are circadian, age-related, seasonal, individual or even strain-related make it difficult to draw valid conclusions on hormonal effects (Lee *et al.*, 1975; Ellis & Desjardins, 1982; Heywood & James, 1985).

Age and sexual maturity of the animal may have a bearing on the results in several ways. It has been shown that prepubertal rats are less sensitive to the toxic effects of lead on testosterone and sperm production than animals exposed to lead after puberty (Sokol & Berman, 1991).

Momcilovic and Kostial (1974) found marked differences in lead distribution in suckling rats compared with adult rats. Age-related changes should also be considered: Heywood and James (1985) showed that up to 7% of rats maintained for 52 weeks showed spermatogenesis not proceeding beyond the spermatocyte stage. At 104 weeks, 20% of rats had developed atrophy of the seminiferous epithelium.

Of the 21 experimental studies reviewed by Apostoli *et al* (1998), 15 mentioned the age of the animals at the start of the experiment. However, animals were sexually mature (i.e. 90 days old) at the start of the experiment in only two studies. In four other studies, age at start was described only as ‘mature’. Descriptions of subchronic effects should be interpreted with caution when the test period is shorter than 77 days for rats, 53 days for mice, 64 days for rabbits and 57 days for monkeys. Taking this into account, about half of the animal studies reviewed by Apostoli *et al.* (1998) can be considered to assess only acute effects.

Schroeder and Mitchener (1971) have shown that mice are more vulnerable to the toxic effects of lead on reproduction than rats. Exposure of sexually-mature animals to lead caused varying degrees of impaired spermatogenesis (Chowdhury *et al.*, 1984; Barratt *et al.*, 1989), premature acrosome reaction and reduction of fertility (Johansson, 1989) or hormonal disorders (Sokol & Berman, 1991) at widely varying (30–187 μg/dL) blood lead concentrations (Apostoli *et al.*, 1998).

Ivanova-Cemišanska *et al.* (1980) reported changes in levels of enzymatic activity and ATP in testicular homogenate of rats given 0.2 and 20 mg/kg bw solutions of lead acetate, over a 4-month period.

Chowdhury *et al.* (1984) found testicular atrophy and cellular degeneration in rats with blood lead concentrations > 70 μg/dL, but not in rats with blood lead concentrations of 54.0 μg/dL.

A comprehensive study in rabbits (Moorman *et al.*, 1998) estimated a threshold for effects on total sperm count of 23.7 μg/dL lead in blood.

Groups of cynomolgus monkeys with mean blood lead concentrations of 10 ± 3 μg/dL ($n = 4$) and 56 ± 49 μg/dL ($n = 7$) after treatment with lead acetate from birth to the age of 15–20 years had increased abnormal sperm chromatin as expressed by the αT distribution (shift from green to red fluorescence) with a larger SD αT when compared with a reference group with blood lead < 1 μg/dL. However, there were no effects of treatment on parameters of semen quality such as sperm count, viability, motility (Foster *et al.*, 1996).

The results of studies on the lead content of testicular or seminal fluid are inconclusive (Hilderbrand *et al.*, 1973; Der *et al.*, 1976; Chowhury *et al.*, 1984; Sokol *et al.*, 1985; Saxena *et al.*, 1987; Boscolo *et al.*, 1988; Barratt *et al.*, 1989; Saxena *et al.*, 1990; Sokol & Berman, 1991; Nathan *et al.*, 1992; Pinon-Lataillade *et al.*, 1993; Thoreux-Manlay *et al.*, 1995). Although a relation between testicular lead content and histopathological changes has been noted, the lack of uniformity regarding age of the animals, duration of exposure, assessment of internal doses, identification of reproductive end-points, and methods to measure effect indicators, makes it impossible to draw any clear conclusions on mechanisms and dose–response relationships.

(*b*) *Effects on pregnancy, fertility and growth and development in animals*

Many early studies identified effects on spermatogenesis in rats exposed to lead and also indicated that high exposure of dams to lead can reduce numbers and size of offspring. There may also be paternally-transmitted effects resulting in reductions of litter size, weights of offspring and survival rate (for references, see WHO, 1995). Other important topics are the exposure periods, the sites of action, and growth and development.

Lead (as lead acetate) was administered to mouse dams via the drinking-water (at 10 mg/mL) during three periods: (1) when target mice were born (postnatal); (2) after conception of target mice (gestational); or (3) during the mothers' own pre-weaning age (pre-mating). These experiments showed variable effects of lead exposure on brain weight, DNA per brain and protein per brain (Epstein *et al.*, 1999).

Exposure of female rats to lead produced irregular estrous cycles at blood lead concentrations of 30 μg/dL and morphological changes in ovaries including follicular cysts and reduction in numbers of corpora lutea at blood lead concentrations of 53 μg/dL (Hilderbrand *et al.*, 1973).

Grant *et al.* (1980) reported delayed vaginal opening in rats whose mothers were given 25, 50 and 250 ppm lead in drinking-water. The vaginal opening delays in the 25-ppm group occurred in the absence of any growth retardation or other developmental delays and were associated with median blood lead concentrations of 18–29 μg/dL.

Testicular homogenates from 2–3-week-old male offspring of lead-exposed female rats (mean blood lead concentration in the pups, 6.3 μg/dL) showed decreased ability to metabolize progesterone (Wiebe *et al.*, 1982).

In a study by McGivern *et al.* (1991), Sprague-Dawley dams were given lead acetate (0.1%) in drinking-water from day 14 of gestation until parturition to determine whether exposure of the fetus to elevated lead concentrations during a period of rapid differentiation of the hypothalamic–pituitary–gonadal (HPG) axis would disrupt HPG function in adulthood. Female offspring from lead-treated dams were found to have a significant delay in the day of vaginal opening and prolonged and irregular periods of diestrous accompanied by an absence of observable corpora lutea at 83 days of age. Male offspring from these dams were found to have decreased sperm counts at 70 and 165 days of age, exhibit enlarged prostates at 165 days and ~35% reduction in the volume of the sexually dimorphic nucleus of the preoptic area of the hypothalamus. Pulsatile release of gonadotropins, measured in castrated male and female adult animals, revealed irregular release patterns of both FSH and LH in some lead-treated animals which were not observed in controls. The overall pattern of data suggested to the authors that multiple functional aspects of the HPG axis can be affected by exposure to lead during a period of gestation when structures related to the HPG axis are undergoing rapid proliferation.

The reproductive toxicity and growth effects of lead exposure in developing rats have also been assessed by Ronis *et al.* (1996). Lead exposure was initiated *in utero*, prepubertally, or postpubertally. In male animals, weights of testis and all secondary sex organs were significantly decreased in animals exposed prepubertally. Serum testosterone levels were significantly suppressed, most severely in animals exposed *in utero*. In female animals exposed prepubertally, delayed vaginal opening and disrupted estrous cycling was observed in 50% of the animals. The group treated *in utero* had suppression of circulating estradiol accompanied by significant decreases in both circulating LH concentrations and pituitary LH protein concentration, but no effect on LHβ mRNA was observed. These findings suggested to the authors a dual site of action for lead: (a) at the level of the hypothalamic pituitary unit; and (b) at the level of gonadal steroid biosynthesis. Prepubertal growth in both sexes was suppressed by 25% in the group exposed *in utero*. The effects of lead on growth are possibly due to a delay in the development of sex-specific pituitary growth hormone secretion rather than a persistent developmental defect.

Studies on female monkeys have shown that pre- and/or postnatal exposure to lead can affect pubertal progression and hypothalamic–pituitary–ovarian–uterine functions. Chronic exposure to lead of nulliparous female monkeys, resulting in blood concentrations of approximately 35 μg/dL, induced subclinical suppression of circulating LH, FSH and estradiol without producing overt effects on general health and menstrual function (Foster, 1992).

4.4 Genetic and related effects

4.4.1 *Human studies* (see Table 91)

In human genotoxicity studies, co-exposures to lead and other compounds could not be discounted and thus it is difficult to attribute genetic and other related effects to lead alone. A general description of lead concentrations in air and blood in various exposure situations is given in Section 1.

The single-cell gel electrophoresis assay (Comet assay) provides data that are indicative of DNA damage; either direct strand breaks or alkali-labile sites. Five studies of DNA damage using the Comet assay on blood leukocytes in lead-exposed workers gave positive results. In workers in a secondary lead smelter in India with blood lead concentrations of 24.8 ± 14.7 μg/dL, there was a significant increase in the percentage of leukocytes showing

Table 91. Genetic and related effects in humans occupationally or non-occupationally exposed to lead

Subjects	No. of exposed/controls	End-point Result[a]	Air lead concentration (µg/m^3)	Mean blood lead concentration (µg/dL)	Reference
Occupationally exposed					
		DNA damage (SCGE (Comet) assay)			
Secondary lead smelter workers, Hyderabad, India	45 exposed	% of cells with tail length increased, 44.6 ± 8.5 ($p < 0.05$);	4.2	24.8 ± 14.7	Danadevi *et al.* (2003)
	36 controls	21.1 ± 11.7		2.75 ± 1.52	
Secondary lead smelter workers, China	46 exposed 28 controls	Significant increase in tail length, dose-related ($p < 0.05$)	–	Range of medians in different subgroups, < 13–> 37; median in controls, 9	Ye *et al.* (1999)
Battery plant workers, Italy	37 exposed 29 controls	Significant increase in tail moment ($p = 0.011$), dose-related	–	39.6 ± 7.6 4.4 ± 1.7	Fracasso *et al.* (2002)
Battery plant workers, Colombia	43 exposed 13 controls	Significant increase in tail length, no dose–response ($p < 0.05$)	–	98.5 ± 25.3 5.4 ± 3.6	De Restrepo *et al.* (2000)
Battery plant workers, Poland	44 exposed	% of cells with tail length increased, 15.6 ± 4.1 ($p < 0.05$)	–	50.4 ± 9.2	Palus *et al.* (2003)
	40 controls	11.3 ± 5.0		5.6 ± 2.8	
		Other DNA damage			
		DNA–protein crosslinks			
Battery plant workers, Taiwan, China	23 high exposed 34 low exposed 30 controls	1.8 ± 0.7%^{S}; 1.4 ± 0.5^{NS} ($p < 0.05$) 1.2 ± 0.4^{S}; 1.1 ± 0.5^{NS} 1.0 ± 0.2^{S}; 1.0 ± 0.3^{NS}	0.2–10.3	32.5 ± 14.5 9.3 ± 2.9 4.2 ± 1.4	Wu *et al.* (2002)
		DNA single strand break			
Workers exposed at 10 facilities in Hessen, Germany (Cd and Co co-exposed)	78 exposed 22 controls	No significant effects	1.6–50 Median, 3	2.8–13.7 Median, 4.41	Hengstler *et al.* (2003)
		Micronuclei (% of cells with micronuclei)			
Battery plant workers, Bulgaria	73 exposed 23 controls	38.6 ± 16.8% ($p < 0.05$) 19.1 ± 16.2%	193–700 60	67 ± 23 25 ± 6	Vaglenov *et al.* (1997)

Table 91 (contd)

Subjects	No. of exposed/controls	End-point Result[a]	Air lead concentration ($\mu g/m^3$)	Mean blood lead concentration ($\mu g/dL$)	Reference
Battery plant workers, Pazardzik, Bulgaria	22 exposed 19 external controls 19 internal controls	62 ± 3% ($p < 0.001$) 20 ± 2% 26 ± 3%	447 ± 52 73 ± 22 58 ± 5	61 ± 3 (SE) 18 ± 0.6 (SE) 2.8 ± 1.6 (SE)	Vaglenov *et al.* (1998)
Metal powder factory (exposure to Pb, Zn, Cd), Turkey	31 exposed 20 controls	0.65/cell ($p < 0.01$) 0.24/cell	–	40 ± 18 12 ± 4	Hamurcu *et al.* (2001)
Battery plant workers (may include some subjects from previous study), Pazardzik, Bulgaria	103 workers 78 controls (43 internal, 35 external combined)	43 ± 2% ($p < 0.001$) 22 ± 1%	–	56 ± 2 19 ± 0.8	Vaglenov *et al.* (2001)
Battery plant workers, Poland	30 exposed 42 controls	18.6 ± 5.0% ($p < 0.01$) 6.6 ± 3.9%	–	50.4 ± 9.2 5.6 ± 2.8	Palus *et al.* (2003)
		Chromosomal aberrations			
Lead oxide workers, Germany	8 exposed[b] 14 controls	Significant increase in various types of chromosome damage ($p < 0.01$)	–	74.7 ± 9.4 14.9 ± 4	Schwanitz *et al.* (1970)
Lead manufacturing workers, Germany	32 exposed 20 controls	No significant effect	–	NR (3 with lead intoxication)	Schmid *et al.* (1972)
Ship-breaking workers, UK	 35 exposed 31 controls 285 other survey controls	Chromatid abs[c] / Chromosomal abs[c] 5.16% / 0.69% 4.46% / 0.42% 2.18% / 1.16%	–	 Range, 40–> 120 < 40	O'Riordan & Evans (1974)
Steel plant workers, Germany	105 exposed no control group	No significant correlation with blood lead or urine ALA	–	37.7 ± 20.7	Schwanitz *et al.* (1975)
Battery plant workers (prospective study), Italy	11 exposed (same subjects, pre-employment)	Significant increase in chromosomal aberrations ($p < 0.05$)	< 800	After 1 month: 45 ± 17.3 Pre-employment: 34 ± 12.6	Forni *et al.* (1976)

Table 91 (contd)

Subjects	No. of exposed/controls	End-point Result[a]	Air lead concentration (µg/m³)	Mean blood lead concentration (µg/dL)	Reference
Lead smelter workers, Finland	18 exposed 12 controls	1.3% 1.8% no significant effect	50–500	48.7 ± 1.7 < 10	Mäki-Paakkanen *et al.* (1981)
Smelter workers (exposed to Pb, As), Rönnskär, Sweden	26 exposed Historical controls	Chromatid abs/cell — Chromosomal abs/cell 0.023 — 0.027 ($p < 0.001$) 0.019 — 0.004 0.006 — 0.000 0.004 — 0.001	–	High: 64.77 ± 10.95 Medium: 39.19 ± 7.13 Low: 22.48 ± 1.77	Nordenson *et al.* (1978)
Battery plant workers, Baghdad, Iraq	19 exposed 9 controls	Chromatid abs — Chromosomal abs 3.4 ± 2.4% — 3.3 ± 2.3% 1.5 ± 3.0% — 2.0 ± 2.3%	–	NR	Al-Hakkak *et al.* (1986)
Battery plant workers, China	7 high exposed 7 medium exposed 7 low exposed 7 controls	3.71 ($p < 0.01$) 2.71 1.43 1.14	–	86.9 ± 16.5 52.1 ± 7.3 33.7 ± 5.9 7.8 ± 2.3	Huang, X.-P. *et al.* (1988)
		Sister chromatid exchange			
Lead smelter workers, Finland	18 exposed 12 controls	11.7 ± 0.4[S]; 9.8 ± 0.7[NS] ($p < 0.05$ in smokers only) 10.4 ± 0.4[S]; 9.2 ± 0.4[NS]	50–500	48.7 ± 1.7 < 10	Mäki-Paakkanen *et al.* (1981)
Battery plant workers, Denmark	10 long-term exposed 18 new employees	Long-term exposed: lower frequency after a 4-wk vacation New employees: no significant increase after 2–4 months employment	–	29.0–74.5 6.2–29.0	Grandjean *et al.* (1983)
Battery plant workers, Monterrey, Mexico	54 exposed 13 controls	7.9 ± 1.5 7.0 ± 1.2	–	45.2 ± 16.6 25.5 ± 6.4	Leal-Garza *et al.* (1986)
Battery plant workers, China	7 high exposed 7 medium exposed 7 low exposed 7 controls	7.06 ± 0.39 ($p < 0.001$) 4.48 ± 0.75 3.93 ± 0.53 4.04 ± 0.33	–	86.9 ± 16.5 52.1 ± 7.3 33.7 ± 5.9 7.8 ± 2.3	Huang, X.-P. *et al.* (1988)
Printers, India	13 exposed 16 controls	No increase	–	NR	Rajah & Ahuja (1995)

Table 91 (contd)

Subjects	No. of exposed/controls	End-point Result[a]	Air lead concentration ($\mu g/m^3$)	Mean blood lead concentration ($\mu g/dL$)	Reference
Metal-powder factory workers, Turkey	32 exposed 20 controls	8.9 ± 1.4^{S}; 8.2 ± 0.9^{NS} ($p < 0.01$ in nonsmokers only) 8.7 ± 1.0^{S}; 7.2 ± 0.6^{NS}	–	13.8 ± 9.2 2.4 ± 0.9	Donmez *et al.* (1998)
Battery plant workers, Taiwan, China	23 high exposed 34 low exposed 30 controls	6.4 ± 0.5^{S}; 5.9 ± 0.7^{NS} ($p < 0.05$) 5.8 ± 0.4^{S}; 5.5 ± 0.7^{NS} 5.7 ± 0.3^{S}; 4.9 ± 0.4^{NS}	0.2–10.3	32.5 ± 14.5 9.3 ± 2.9 4.2 ± 1.4	Wu *et al.* (2002)
Battery plant workers, Ankara, Turkey	71 exposed 20 controls	Significant increase in group with blood lead > 50 μg/dL ($p < 0.05$)	–	34.5 ± 1.5 10.4 ± 0.4	Duydu & Süzen (2003)
Battery plant workers, Poland	30 exposed 43 controls	7.6 ± 0.9^{S}; 7.1 ± 0.9^{NS} ($p < 0.05$) 6.5 ± 1.1^{S}; 5.9 ± 0.8^{NS}	–	50.4 ± 9.2 5.6 ± 2.8	Palus *et al.* (2003)
Non-occupationally exposed					
		Oxidative DNA damage			
Citizens of Bremen, Germany	141	No increase in oxidative DNA damage (Fpg-sensitive sites)	–	Median, 4.6	Merzenich *et al.* (2001)
		Sister chromatid exchange			
Children living near a lead smelter, Milan, Italy	19 exposed 12 controls	No effect	–	29.3–62.7 10.0–21.0	Dalpra *et al.* (1983)
		Chromosomal aberrations			
Male volunteers, Netherlands	11 ingested[d] 10 controls	No significant effect	–	$40 \pm 5 \times 7$ wks	Bijlsma & de France (1976)
Children living near lead smelter, Germany	20 exposed 20 controls	No significant effect	–	> 30 7–19	Bauchinger *et al.* (1977)

–, No data; S, smoker; NS, nonsmoker; SE, standard error; NR, not reported; ALA, δ-aminolevulinic acid; Fpg, formamidopyrimidine-DNA glycosylase

[a] Dose–response refers to blood lead concentrations.

[b] Exposed workers have significantly increased mitotic index.

[c] Chromatid/chromosomal abnormalities

[d] Daily ingested lead acetate to give mean blood lead concentration of 40 ± 5 μg/dL for 7 wks

DNA damage and increased Comet tail length compared with controls (non-exposed). Blood lead was positively associated with the percentage of DNA-damaged cells (Danadevi *et al.*, 2003). [The Working Group noted that the air lead level was unexpectedly low.] Significantly increased percentages of DNA-damaged leukocytes and tail length, as well as increased malondialdehyde concentrations were also seen in workers in a secondary lead smelter in China. The effects were dose-related, with minimal blood lead concentrations of 27–37 μg/dL being associated with genotoxicity (Ye *et al.*, 1999). Similar results were seen in workers in battery plants in Italy, Columbia and China, Province of Taiwan (De Restrepo *et al.*, 2000; Fracasso *et al.*, 2002; Wu, F.-Y. *et al.*, 2002) where significant increases in tail moment, tail length and/or DNA in the tail were observed in workers' lymphocytes. In one study, the Comet assay results were correlated with blood lead concentrations, and with decreased concentrations of reduced glutathione (GSH) in blood (Fracasso *et al.*, 2002). The DNA damage occurred at blood lead concentrations > 40 μg/dL in the workers in Columbia and sister chromatid exchange occurred at blood lead concentrations > 15 μg/dL in workers in China, Province of Taiwan.

In a single study, evidence for increased DNA–protein crosslinks was seen at high blood lead concentrations in the highly-exposed group (blood lead, 32.5 ± 14.5 μg/dL) of battery plant workers (Wu, F.-Y. *et al.*, 2002). DNA single-strand breaks (measured with the alkaline elution assay) were not increased in lymphocytes of workers with median blood lead concentrations of 4.41 μg/dL (Hengstler *et al.*, 2003). [The Working Group noted that the air lead level was unexpectedly low.] However, in the latter study, lead exposure increased the effects of cadmium in inducing DNA strand breaks.

All of five studies of micronuclei in blood lymphocytes of exposed workers found increases. These occurred in battery plant workers exposed to at least 193 μg/m^3 lead in air (resulting in 3.16 μM [65.5 μg/dL] in blood) (Vaglenov *et al.*, 1997). A second study confirmed these results and demonstrated a reduction in micronucleus frequency in workers given a vitamin and mineral supplement (Vaglenov *et al.*, 1998). The authors suggested that oxidative DNA damage may be responsible for the micronuclei. Battery plant workers in Poland were shown to have increased micronuclei in both centromere-positive and centromere-negative classes, indicating both a clastogenic and aneugenic effect of lead (Palus *et al.*, 2003).

Studies of chromosomal aberrations in lead-exposed workers gave mixed results. Chromosomal aberrations were evaluated in 105 lead-exposed workers in Germany and found to be slightly but not significantly increased (Schwanitz *et al.*, 1975). In an earlier report from this group with a small number of subjects, chromosomal aberrations were positively correlated to excretion of ALA (Schwanitz *et al.*, 1970), but a higher mitotic index in lymphocytes from workers was noted. Negative results for chromosomal aberrations were reported by Schmid *et al.* (1972) and O'Riordan and Evans (1974) for workers in lead manufacturing and ship breaking, respectively. In a prospective study in which 11 battery plant workers acted as their own controls, a doubling of chromosomal aberrations (mostly chromatid and one-break aberrations) was seen after 1 month of employment. There was a further increase in the second month, but then the level remained the same for at least 7 months. The increased frequency of chromosomal aberrations was correlated to inhibition of ALAD in red blood cells (Forni *et al.*, 1976). The authors speculated that culture conditions may have been responsible for the DNA damage, whose repair is inhibited by lead because, in a previous study in which the bone-marrow cells were not cultured, exposure to lead did not result in increased chromosomal aberrations (Forni & Secchi, 1972). Mäki-Paakkanen *et al.* (1981) also found evidence of 'culture-born aberrations', and noted that these may have influenced the outcome of the study.

In a study in which primary copper and lead smelter workers were stratified by blood lead concentrations, increased frequencies of chromatid-type aberrations were seen in the intermediate group (mean blood lead, 39.19 μg/dL); and chromosome-type aberrations were seen only in the 'high' group (mean blood lead, 64.77 μg/dL) (Nordenson *et al.*, 1978). The authors estimated that a blood lead concentration of 25 μg/dL is the minimum required to produce any chromosomal effects. Huang *et al.* (1988) only saw an increased frequency of chromosomal aberrations in their intermediate group (mean blood lead, 52.1 μg/dL).

The results of studies measuring sister chromatid exchange in workers exposed to lead are mostly positive but, in some studies, positive responses were seen only in smokers. For example, a small increase in sister chromatid exchange was seen only in lead smelter workers who smoked (Mäki-Paakkanen *et al.*, 1981). No significant increase in sister chromatid exchange was seen in printers (confounded by smoking) (Rajah & Ahuja, 1995), whereas there was a significant increase in battery plant workers after controlling for smoking (Duydu & Süzen, 2003). In these studies, there was also inconsistency in the correlations with blood lead concentrations. In one study, the level of sister chromatid exchange decreased in battery plant workers after a 4-week vacation (Grandjean *et al.*, 1983). The same authors also monitored newly-employed workers and found no increases in sister chromatid exchange after 2–4 months of employment.

In general, studies in which a variety of genotoxic end-points were measured in non-occupationally exposed subjects (children living near plants, volunteers, general population) gave negative results (Table 91).

4.4.2 *Effects in animals* (see Table 92)

DNA damage was assessed in kidney cells of male rats by use of the Comet assay (single-cell gel electrophoresis). In cells isolated from the kidneys of rats that had received three doses of lead acetate by oral administration, a larger Comet tail was seen than in cells from animals that had been given the same amount of lead in a single dose. The same study also showed an increased level of sister chromatid exchange in kidney cells, with the single high dose being more effective (Robbiano *et al.*, 1999). When mice were exposed for three generations to lead acetate in the drinking-water, Comet tail length increased in blood cells in the F_1 and F_2 generations, but not in the dams (Yuan & Tang, 2001). With an inhalation protocol in mice, DNA damage was detected in the liver and lung after a single exposure to lead acetate, whereas kidney, brain, nasal cells, bone

Table 92. Genetic and related effects of lead compounds in animals *in vivo*

Test system	Result	Dose[a] (LED or HID)	Reference
Lead acetate			
DNA damage, female Kunming mouse leukocytes (SCGE)	–	1 µg/mL water approx. 3–4 mo	Yuan & Tang (2001)
DNA damage, Kunming mouse leukocytes (SCGE), 2nd and 3rd generations of multigeneration study	+	1 µg/mL water *in utero* to sexual maturity	Yuan & Tang (2001)
DNA damage, male CD-1 mouse liver, kidney, nasal cavity, brain, bone-marrow cells (SCGE)	w+	6800 µg/m^3, inhal., 60 min × 2/wk, 4 wk	Valverde *et al.* (2002)
DNA damage, male CD-1 mouse testicle cells, leukocytes (SCGE)	–	6800 µg/m^3, inhal., 60 min × 2/wk, 4 wk	Valverde *et al.* (2002)
DNA damage, male CD-1 mouse lung cells (SCGE)	?*	6800 µg/m^3, inhal., 60 min × 2/wk, 4 wk	Valverde *et al.* (2002)
DNA damage, unilaterally nephrectomized Sprague-Dawley rat kidney (SCGE)	+	78 mg/kg bw po × 3	Robbiano *et al.* (1999)
Sister chromatid exchange, rabbit lymphocytes	–	0.5 mg/kg bw sc 3×/wk, 14 wk	Willems *et al.* (1982)
Micronucleus formation, female C57BL mouse bone marrow	–	25 mg/kg bw ip × 2	Jacquet *et al.* (1977)
Micronucleus formation, female C57BL/6 × C3H/He F_1 mouse bone marrow	–	1000 mg/kg bw ip	Bruce & Heddle (1979)
Micronucleus formation, male and female Sprague-Dawley rat bone marrow	w+	104 mg/kg bw ip	Tachi *et al.* (1985)
Micronucleus formation, rabbit bone marrow erythrocytes	–	0.5 mg/kg bw sc 3×/wk, 14 wk	Willems *et al.* (1982)
Micronucleus formation, unilaterally nephrectomized Sprague-Dawley rat kidney	+	78 mg/kg bw po × 3	Robbiano *et al.* (1999)
Chromosomal aberrations, female C57B1 mouse bone marrow	–	0.5% diet × 1 mo	Jacquet *et al.* (1977)
Chromosomal aberrations, male C57B1 mouse bone marrow	–	Normal diet + 0.5% × 1 mo	Deknudt & Gerber (1979)
Chromosomal aberrations, male C57B1 mouse bone marrow	+	Low Ca diet + 0.5% × 1 mo	Deknudt & Gerber (1979)
Chromosomal aberrations, female Sprague-Dawley rat bone marrow	+	104 mg/kg bw ip	Tachi *et al.* (1985)
Chromosomal aberrations, male Sprague-Dawley rat bone marrow	–	104 mg/kg bw ip	Tachi *et al.* (1985)
Chromosomal aberrations, female Sprague-Dawley rat bone marrow	–	104 mg/kg bw ip × 5	Tachi *et al.* (1985)
Chromosomal aberrations, male Sprague-Dawley rat bone marrow	w+	104 mg/kg bw ip × 5	Tachi *et al.* (1985)
Chromosomal aberrations, Wistar rat bone marrow	–	10 mg/kg bw po 5×/wk, 4 wk	Nehéz *et al.* (2000)
Chromosomal aberrations, male and female A/sw mouse leukocytes	+	1% diet × 2 wk	Muro & Goyer (1969)
Chromosomal aberrations, cynomolgus monkey lymphocytes	±	6 mg/d po × 10 mo	Deknudt *et al.* (1977)
Chromosomal aberrations, cynomolgus monkey leukocytes	–	5 mg/kg bw po/d × 12 mo	Jacquet & Tachon (1981)
Aneuploidy, Wistar rat bone marrow	+	10 mg/kg bw po 5×/wk, 4 wk	Nehéz *et al.* (2000)
Aneuploidy, cynomolgus monkey lymphocytes	±	6 mg/d po × 10 mo	Deknudt *et al.* (1977)
Sperm morphology, C57BL/6 F_1 × C3H/He F_1 mice	+	125 mg/kg bw ip	Bruce & Heddle (1979)
Sperm morphology, rabbits	–	0.5 mg/kg bw sc 3×/wk, 14 wk	Willems *et al.* (1982)
Sperm abnormality, cynomolgus monkey (acid denaturation of DNA)	+	50 µg/kg bw/d for 100–200 d[b]	Foster *et al.* (1996)

Table 92 (contd)

Test system	Result	Dose[a] (LED or HID)	Reference
Lead chloride			
Dominant lethal mutations, NMRI mice	–	1.33 g/L dw	Kristensen *et al.* (1993)
Lead nitrate			
Sister chromatid exchange, pregnant female Swiss Webster mouse bone marrow	+	150 mg/kg bw iv	Nayak *et al.* (1989)
Sister chromatid exchange, liver and/or lung of fetus of maternal Swiss Webster mice	–	200 mg/kg bw iv	Nayak *et al.* (1989)
Sister chromatid exchange, male Swiss albino mouse bone marrow	+	10 mg/kg bw ip	Dhir *et al.* (1993)
Micronucleus test, male and female Swiss albino mouse bone marrow	?	80 mg/kg bw ip	Jagetia & Aruna (1998)
Chromosomal aberrations, maternal bone marrow and fetal liver cells of Swiss Webster mouse	+	100 mg/kg bw iv	Nayak *et al.* (1989)
Aneuploidy, maternal bone marrow and fetal liver cells of Swiss Webster mouse	+	100 mg/kg bw iv	Nayak *et al.* (1989)
Induction of nondisjunction, *Drosophila melanogaster*	–	200 ppm feed	Ramel & Magnusson (1979)

+, positive; –, negative; ±, equivocal; w+, weak positive; ?, significant variation from dose to dose, no clear dose–response relationship; ?*, significant variation from week to week; po, oral; inhal., inhalation; dw, drinking-water; sc, subcutaneous; iv, intravenous; d, day; wk, week; mo, month; SCGE, single-cell gel electrophoresis; bw, body weight

[a] Lowest effective dose or highest ineffective dose

[b] Dose resulted in blood lead concentrations of 6–20 μg/dL.

marrow and leukocytes required more than one exposure before DNA damage was seen. No damage to testicular cells was seen after 4 weeks (Valverde *et al.*, 2002).

No increases in sister chromatid exchange in rabbit lymphocytes were seen after subcutaneous injections of lead acetate (Willems *et al.*, 1982). The same treatment also failed to cause sperm abnormalities or micronucleus formation in bone-marrow erythrocytes. However, intravenous injection of lead nitrate on day 9 of gestation increased sister chromatid exchange frequency in the bone marrow of F_1 mice, but not in fetal liver and/or fetal lung cells, although the lead was shown to cross the placenta (Nayak *et al.*, 1989). In this study, lead nitrate caused chromosomal aberrations, mostly deletions, in both dams and fetal cells, as well as aneuploidy, increased embryonic resorptions and reduced placental weights. Dhir *et al.* (1993) showed that intraperitoneal injection of low doses of lead nitrate caused a significant increase in sister chromatid exchange in bone marrow in male Swiss albino mice. The lowest dose that caused micronucleus formation in bone marrow (but without a dose–response relationship) was 0.63 mg/kg bw lead nitrate. Male mice were found to be more sensitive than females (Jagetia & Aruna, 1998).

Feeding mice a diet containing lead acetate resulted in increased frequencies of chromosomal aberrations in leukocytes, particularly involving single chromatids (Muro & Goyer, 1969). Similar results were seen in a study in female C57BL mice (Jacquet *et al.*, 1977) but, in a further study, only when mice were given a low-calcium diet (Deknudt & Gerber, 1979).

Female (but not male) rats given a single intraperitoneal injection of lead acetate had increased chromosomal aberrations (mostly gaps) (Tachi *et al.*, 1985). In the same study, both male and female rats showed an increased frequency of micronuclei following treatment with lead acetate. The nature of the micronuclei was not determined, but lead acetate-induced chromatid gaps may reflect mostly clastogenicity rather than aneuploidy. Aneuploidy was induced in pregnant mice and their offspring (maternal bone marrow and fetal liver cells) by intravenous administration of lead nitrate on day 9 of gestation (Nayak *et al.*, 1989) and in rats (bone marrow) given lead acetate orally (Nehéz *et al.*, 2000), but nondisjunction did not increase in *Drosophila* given lead acetate in feed (Ramel & Magnusson, 1979).

Increased frequencies of chromosomal aberrations (gaps and fragments) and enhanced aneuploidy were seen in lymphocytes of monkeys given lead acetate orally or by intubation in one study (Deknudt *et al.*, 1977) but not in another (Jacquet & Tachon, 1981).

In a single in-vivo mutagenesis study, lead chloride in the drinking-water had no effect in the dominant lethal assay in mice (Kristensen *et al.*, 1993).

Increased abnormal sperm morphology was seen in mice given lead acetate intraperitoneally (Bruce & Heddle, 1978). Increased sperm abnormality (analysed by sperm chromatin structure assay) was seen in monkeys given lead acetate resulting in blood lead concentrations of up to 20 μg/dL (Foster *et al.*, 1976). However, subcutaneous administration of lead acetate did not induce sperm abnormalities in rabbits (Willems *et al.*, 1982).

4.4.3 *Mammalian cells* in vitro (for references, see Table 93)

The genetic effects of lead compounds have been reviewed (Hartwig, 1994; Silbergeld *et al.*, 2000). Equivocal results have been published with respect to the mutagenicity of water-soluble lead compounds in mammalian cells in culture; in most classical test systems, the effects were rather weak and/or restricted to toxic doses. Nevertheless, in AS52 Chinese hamster ovary cells carrying a single copy of an *Escherichia coli gpt* gene, lead chloride induced mutations in a dose-dependent manner at non-cytotoxic concentrations of < 1 μM (Ariza & Williams, 1996, 1999; Ariza *et al.*, 1998). More detailed studies revealed predominantly point mutations with increasing frequencies of partial and complete deletions, in the dose range 0.5–1.0 μM (Ariza & Williams, 1999). Increased mutant frequencies in the *Hprt* gene were also observed in a study in Chinese hamster ovary K1 cells, but at higher, although still not cytotoxic concentrations of lead acetate, starting at 0.5 mM. Analysis of mutation spectra revealed base substitutions predominantly at G-C sites, as well as small and large deletions resulting from DNA damage induced by ROS (Yang *et al.*, 1996). Furthermore, two studies revealed an increase in mutation frequency in combination with ultraviolet (UV) C irradiation or treatment with *N*-methyl-*N*-nitro-*N*-nitrosoguanidine (MNNG) (Roy & Rossman, 1992). One potential mechanism may be the interaction with DNA repair processes; although results are equivocal, different outcomes may depend on incubation conditions. Thus, in human HeLa cell lines, two independent studies showed repair inhibition of X-ray-induced or UVC-induced DNA damage after 24 and 20 h preincubation, respectively (Skreb & Habazin-Novak, 1977; Hartwig *et al.*, 1990), while one study did not show an effect after 30 min preincubation (Snyder *et al.*, 1989).

With respect to the induction of chromosomal aberrations by lead acetate, treatment of human leukocytes showed clearly elevated frequencies of achromatic lesions, chromatid breaks and isochromatid breaks in 72-h cultures but not 48-h cultures (Beek & Obe, 1975); other studies with lead nitrate and lead glutamate were mostly negative. However, consistently positive results were obtained with lead chromate, which the authors related to the probable action of chromate (Wise *et al.*, 1994). Concerning the induction of micronuclei, a recent study reported a dose-dependent increase starting at concentrations of 1.1 μM lead chloride or 0.05 μM lead acetate. Both positive and negative results have been reported for the induction of sister chromatid exchange; nevertheless, similar to the enhancement of UVC-induced mutagenicity noted above, lead acetate also increased the UVC-induced frequency of sister chromatid exchange. More consistently, lead acetate as well as particulate lead chromate induced cell transformation in several studies; in the case of lead chromate, the effect was thought by the authors to be not due solely to the action of chromate (Elias *et al.*, 1989; Sidhu *et al.*, 1991). The induction of DNA damage in mammalian cells by lead acetate and lead nitrate has been investigated repeatedly, yielding negative or (mostly weakly) positive results for DNA strand breaks; one study did not find 8-OH-deoxyguanosine (8-OH-dG) in nuclear DNA, and one suggested the induction of DNA–protein crosslinks. Besides genotoxic effects, there is growing evidence for altered gene

Table 93. Genetic and related effects of lead and lead compounds; in-vitro studies

Test system	Result		Dose[a] (LED or HID)	Reference
	Without exogenous metabolic system	With exogenous metabolic system		
Lead acetate				
DNA strand breaks, isolated plasmid DNA	+[b]	NT	1 mM	Roy & Rossman (1992)
DNA strand breaks, isolated plasmid DNA	+	NT	0.1 mM	Yang *et al.* (1999)
8-OH-dG, calf thymus DNA	+[b]	NT	0.5 mM	Yang *et al.* (1999)
Escherichia coli WP2, rec-assay	–	NT	50 mM	Nishioka (1975)
Salmonella typhimurium TA100, TA1535, TA1537, TA1538, TA98, reverse mutation	–	NT	333 μg/plate	Dunkel *et al.* (1984)
Salmonella typhimurium TA1535, TA1538, reverse mutation	–	–	250 μg/plate	Rosenkranz & Poirier (1979)
Escherichia coli WP-2 *uvr*A, reverse mutation	–	NT	333 μg/plate	Dunkel *et al.* (1984)
Saccharomyces cerevisiae D3, mitotic recombination	–	–	50 000 μg/mL	Simmon (1979)
Plant cuttings of *Tradescantia* clone 4430 (exposed to lead tetraacetate), micronucleus formation	+		0.44 ppm	Sandhu *et al.* (1989)
DNA strand breaks, primary rat kidney cells *in vitro*	+	NT	560 μM	Robbiano *et al.* (1999)
DNA strand breaks, Chinese hamster ovary (CHO) cells *in vitro*	(+)	NT	1 mM	Robison *et al.* (1984)
DNA strand breaks, transgenic cell lines G12 from Chinese hamster V79 cells *in vitro*	+		1.7 mM	Roy & Rossman (1992)
8-OHdG in nuclear DNA, Chinese hamster ovary (CHO K1) cells *in vitro*	–	NT	100 μg/mL	Yusof *et al.* (1999)
Gene mutation, Chinese hamster ovary (CHO K1) cells, *Hprt* locus *in vitro*	+	NT	0.5 mM	Yang *et al.* (1996)
Gene mutation, Chinese hamster V79 cells, *Hprt* locus *in vitro*	–		5 μM	Hartwig *et al.* (1990)
Gene mutation, transgenic cell lines G12 from Chinese hamster V79 cells, *Gpt* locus *in vitro*	(+)		1.7 mM	Roy & Rossman (1992)
Sister chromatid exchange, Chinese hamster V79 cells *in vitro*	–		10 μM	Hartwig *et al.* (1990)
Enhancement of UVC-induced sister chromatid exchange, Chinese hamster V79 cells *in vitro*	+		1 μM	Hartwig *et al.* (1990)
Micronucleus formation, Chinese hamster V79 cells *in vitro*	+		0.05 μM	Thier *et al.* (2003)
Chromosomal (structural) aberrations, Chinese hamster ovary (CHO) cells *in vitro*	–		1 mM	Bauchinger & Schmid (1972)
Cell transformation, Syrian hamster embryo (SHE) cells	+		10 μM	Zelikoff *et al.* (1988)
DNA strand breaks, human kidney cells *in vitro*	+		1.8 mM	Robbiano *et al.* (1999)
DNA strand breaks, human HeLa cells *in vitro*	–		500 μM	Hartwig *et al.* (1990)
DNA single- and double-strand breaks, human lymphocytes *in vitro*	(+)		1 μM	Wozniak & Blasiak (2003)
DNA-protein cross-links, human lymphocytes *in vitro*	+		100 μM	Wozniak & Blasiak (2003)
Effect on the resealing of X-ray induced DNA single-strand breaks, human HeLa cells *in vitro*	–		100 μM	Snyder *et al.* (1989)

Table 93 (contd)

Test system	Result: Without exogenous metabolic system	Result: With exogenous metabolic system	Dose[a] (LED or HID)	Reference
Effect of pyrimidine dimer removal induced by UVC, human	–		10 mM	Snyder *et al.* (1989)
Inhibition of UVC-induced DNA repair, human HeLa cells *in vitro*	+		500 µM	Hartwig *et al.* (1990)
Gene mutation, diploid human fibroblasts, *HPRT* locus *in vitro*	–		2 mM	Hwua & Yang (1998)
Sister chromatid exchange, human leukocytes *in vitro*	–		10 µM	Beek & Obe (1975)
Chromosomal aberrations, human lymphocytes *in vitro*	–		1 mM	Schmid *et al.* (1972)
Chromosomal aberrations, human lymphocytes *in vitro*	?		1 mM	Deknudt & Deminatti (1978)
Chromosomal aberrations, human lymphocytes *in vitro*	–		1 mM	Gasiorek & Bauchinger (1981)
Achromatic lesions, chromatid breaks and isochromatid breaks, human leukocytes *in vitro*	+		10 µM	Beek & Obe (1974)
Cell transformation, diploid human fibroblasts (anchorage-independent growth)	+		0.5 mM	Hwua & Yang (1998)
Lead bromide				
Salmonella typhimurium TA1535, reverse mutation	+		9.0 µg/plate	Maslat & Haas (1989)
Salmonella typhimurium TA1537, reverse mutation	–		68.0 µg/plate	Maslat & Haas (1989)
Serratia marcescens, reverse mutation	+		1.91 mM	Maslat & Haas (1989)
Escherichia coli KMBL 1851, reverse mutation, met[+] and his[+]	+		3.27 mM	Maslat & Haas (1989)
Lead chloride				
Escherichia coli WP2, rec-assay	–		50 mM	Nishioka (1975)
Escherichia coli K12, Trp[+] reversion plate test	–		1 mM	Nestmann *et al.* (1979)
Salmonella typhimurium TA98, TA100 reverse mutation	–	–	580 µg/plate	Nestmann *et al.* (1979)
Saccharomyces cerevisiae D7, mitotic cross-over	+		0.3 mM	Fukunaga *et al.* (1982)
Gene mutation, Chinese hamster ovary AS52 cells, *Gpt* locus *in vitro*	+		0.1 µM	Ariza & Williams (1996); Ariza *et al.* (1998); Ariza & Williams (1999)
Micronucleus formation, Chinese hamster V79 cells *in vitro*	+		1.1 µM	Thier *et al.* (2003)
Inhibition of X-ray-induced DNA repair, human HeLa cells *in vitro*	+[c]		250 µM [70 µg/mL]	Skreb & Habazin-Novak (1977)
Lead chromate				
Escherichia coli K12 Gal[+] forward mutation	–		100 µg/mL	Nestmann *et al.* (1979)
Escherichia coli Trp[+] reversion plate test	–		1 mM	Nestmann *et al.* (1979)
Escherichia coli WP2 Uvr[–] Trp[+] reversion fluctuation assay	+		5 µM	Nestmann *et al.* (1979)

Table 93 (contd)

Test system	Result		Dose[a] (LED or HID)	Reference
	Without exogenous metabolic system	With exogenous metabolic system		
Salmonella typhimurium TA100, reverse mutation	–	–	200 µg/plate	Nestmann *et al.* (1979)
Salmonella typhimurium TA1535, reverse mutation	–	–	100 µg/plate	Nestmann *et al.* (1979)
Salmonella typhimurium TA1537, reverse mutation	+	–	200 µg/plate	Nestmann *et al.* (1979)
Salmonella typhimurium TA1538, TA98, reverse mutation	+	+	200 µg/plate	Nestmann *et al.* (1979)
Saccharomyces cerevisiae D5, mitotic recombination	+	–	63 µg/mL	Nestmann *et al.* (1979)
DNA strand breaks, DNA–protein crosslinks, Chinese hamster ovary (CHO) cells *in vitro*	+		0.08 µg/cm^2 (1 µM)	Xu *et al.* (1992)
Gene mutation, C3H 10T1/2 mouse cells, ouabain resistance *in vitro*	–		100 µM	Patierno *et al.* (1988)
Gene mutation, Chinese hamster ovary (CHO) cells, 6-thioguanine resistance and ouabain resistance *in vitro*	–		100 µM	Patierno & Landolph (1989); Patierno *et al.* (1988)
Chromosomal aberrations, Chinese hamster ovary (CHO) cells *in vitro*	+		0.4 µg/cm^2 (5 µM)	Xu *et al.* (1992)
Chromosomal aberrations, Chinese hamster ovary (CHO) cells *in vitro*	+		0.4 µg/cm^2 (5 µM)	Wise *et al.* (1992); Wise *et al.* (1994)
Cell transformation, C3H 10T1/2 mouse cells	+		25 µM	Patierno & Landolph (1989); Patierno *et al.* (1988)
Cell transformation, Syrian hamster embryo (SHE) cells, simian adenovirus SA7 viral enhancement	+		80 µM	Schechtman *et al.* (1986)
Cell transformation, Syrian hamster embryo (SHE) cells	+		~0.8 µg/mL	Elias *et al.* (1989)
Chromosomal aberrations, human foreskin fibroblasts *in vitro*	+		0.08 µg/cm^2 (1 µM)	Wise *et al.* (1992)
Cell transformation, nontumorigenic human osteosarcoma (HOS) TE85 cells	+		2 µg/mL	Sidhu *et al.* (1991)
Lead glutamate				
Chromosomal aberrations, Chinese hamster ovary (CHO) cells *in vitro*	?		1 mM	Wise *et al.* (1994)
Lead nitrate				
Saccharomyces cerevisiae D7, mitotic gene conversion, reverse mutation	–		60 µg/mL	Kharab & Singh (1985)
Allium cepa L, chromosomal aberrations	+		10 ppm	Lerda (1992)
Drosophila melanogaster, non-disjunction	–		200 ppm	Ramel & Magnusson (1979)
Gene mutation, Chinese hamster V79 cells, *Hprt* locus *in vitro*	+		500 µM	Zelikoff *et al.* (1988)
Gene mutation, transgenic cell lines G12 from Chinese hamster V79, *Gpt* locus *in vitro*	–		1.7 mM	Roy & Rossman (1992)
Sister chromatid exchange, Chinese hamster V79 cells *in vitro*	–		3 mM	Zelikoff *et al.* (1988)

Table 93 (contd)

Test system	Result		Dose[a] (LED or HID)	Reference
	Without exogenous metabolic system	With exogenous metabolic system		
Sister chromatid exchange, Chinese hamster ovary (CHO) cells *in vitro*	+		3 μM	Lin *et al.* (1994)
Sister chromatid exchange, Chinese hamster ovary (CHO) cells *in vitro*	+		100 nM	Cai & Arenaz (1998)
Micronucleus formation, Chinese hamster ovary (CHO) cells *in vitro*	–		30 μM	Lin *et al.* (1994)
Chromosomal aberrations, Chinese hamster ovary (CHO) cells *in vitro*	–		30 μM	Lin *et al.* (1994)
Chromosomal aberrations, Chinese hamster ovary (CHO) cells *in vitro*	–		2 mM	Wise *et al.* (1994)
DNA strand breaks, transgenic cell lines G12 from Chinese hamster V79 cells *in vitro*	+		1.7 mM	Roy & Rossman (1992)
Lead sulfide				
Gene mutation, Chinese hamster V79 cells, *Hprt* locus *in vitro*	+		376 μM	Zelikoff *et al.* (1988)
Sister chromatid exchange, Chinese hamster V79 cells *in vitro*	–		938 μM	Zelikoff *et al.* (1988)
Lead, diethyl dichloride				
Drosophila melanogaster, non-disjunction	+		16 ppm	Ramel & Magnusson (1979)
Lead, triethyl chloride				
Drosophila melanogaster, non-disjunction	+		8 ppm	Ramel & Magnusson (1979)

SCGE, Single-cell gel electrophoresis
+, positive; (+), weakly positive; –, negative; ?, inconclusive; NT, not tested
[a] LED, lowest effective dose; HID, highest ineffective dose unless otherwise stated; in-vitro tests, μg/mL; in-vivo tests, mg/kg bw/day; ip, intraperitoneal; po, oral; NG, not given
[b] In the presence of H_2O_2
[c] Incorporation of [^{3}H]thymidine or [^{3}H]uridine triphosphate

expression resulting from low-level exposure to lead (Bouton *et al.*, 2001; Li & Rossman, 2001).

4.4.4 *Prokaryotic systems* (for references, see Table 93)

Lead acetate and lead chloride were not mutagenic in bacterial test systems. In contrast, lead chromate was mutagenic in *E. coli* and *Salmonella typhimurium*, indicating that chromate may be the active component. Furthermore, one study demonstrated lead bromide to be mutagenic which may be due to bromination of uracil subsequently incorporated into DNA (Maslat & Haas, 1989).

4.4.5 *Yeast and plants* (for references, see Table 93)

In yeast, lead acetate and lead nitrate usually gave negative results in test systems assessing mitotic recombination. One study demonstrated a limited number of mitotic gene conversions at growth inhibitory concentrations; however, among the convertants there were significantly higher frequencies of mitotic crossing-over. Chromosomal aberrations and micronuclei were observed in plants after exposure of roots to lead nitrate or cuttings to lead tetraacetate, respectively.

4.4.6 *Cell-free systems* (for references, see Table 93)

The effect of lead acetate on isolated DNA has been investigated in detail. A dose-dependent increase in DNA strand breaks was observed in plasmid DNA as well as an increase in 8-OH-dG in calf thymus DNA in the presence of hydrogen peroxide as determined by HPLC-electrochemical detection. Studies with different radical scavengers suggested the participation of singlet oxygen ($^1O_2$) and hydrogen peroxide in DNA damage induction. A Fenton-like reaction, involving the reduction of Pb^{2+} to Pb^{1+} and/or lead-oxygen or lead-peroxide complexes, has been proposed to play a role in this process (Yang *et al.*, 1999). One other mode of action with potential relevance for genetic stability consists of interactions with zinc-binding motifs in DNA-binding proteins. In this context, zinc finger 3 of transcription factor TFIIIA exerts a higher binding constant for Pb^{2+} than for Zn^{2+}, and lead chloride has been shown to inhibit DNA binding of transcription factor TFIIIA and Sp1 (Petering *et al.*, 2000; Razmiafshari *et al.*, 2001). However, the zinc finger-containing repair proteins XPA and Fpg were not inhibited by lead (Asmuss *et al.*, 2000).

4.5 Mechanistic considerations

4.5.1 *Introduction*

A considerable number of experiments have been conducted to elucidate the toxicokinetic and toxicodynamic mechanisms by which exposure to lead may result in cancer. Chemical form and route, patterns and magnitude of exposure are important factors in evaluating the toxicokinetic mechanisms relevant to the carcinogenic potential of lead. Issues such as mode of action, genotoxicity and the mitogenic and/or cytotoxic potential of lead must be considered in describing the toxicodynamics of lead carcinogenicity.

4.5.2 *Toxicokinetics and metabolism of lead*

(*a*) *Inorganic lead*

(i) *Absorption*

Lead absorption from the gastrointestinal tract in both humans and experimental animals is strongly influenced by age (neonates and the young absorb a larger fraction than do adults), fasting/fed status (fasting experimental animals and humans absorb much greater fractions), nutritional status (fat and caloric intakes, and phosphorus, copper, zinc and especially iron and calcium status all affect absorption), solubility (soluble compounds are better absorbed) and particle size (in controlled studies in rats, lead absorption from mining wastes was shown to be inversely proportional to particle size).

The fraction of lead absorbed from an inhalation exposure is not known to be dependent on the amount of lead in the lung. Patterns and rates of deposition are highly dependent on particle size and ventilation rate, but all lead deposited deep in the lung is eventually absorbed.

Limited studies indicate that dermal absorption of inorganic lead is negligible, although slightly enhanced by high perspiration rates.

Intravenous, intraperitoneal or subcutaneous administration of lead salts gives no useful information about the kinetics of lead, because metal salts administered by these routes are distributed and excreted very differently from the same salts absorbed by a more physiological or natural route.

(ii) *Distribution*

In both experimental animals and humans, absorbed lead is distributed from blood plasma rapidly and simultaneously into erythrocytes, soft tissues, and bone. Once the lead in soft tissues has reached an approximate equilibrium with that in blood, the concentration of lead in blood is determined almost entirely by the balance among absorption, elimination, and transfers to and from bone. Initially, however, distribution into soft tissues dominates the shape of the blood lead concentration–time curve, with a half-life of 20–130 days in adult humans and 3.5 days in rats. In both humans and rats, the highest soft-tissue concentrations of lead are found in the liver and kidney, with considerably lower concentrations in the brain.

After equilibration with soft tissues and in the absence of continuing exposure, the blood lead concentration–time profile mirrors the return of lead from bone. Because of the nature of the several processes that mediate bone lead uptake and release, loss of lead from bone is not a first-order process, and in principle neither return of lead from bone nor whole-body loss can be characterized by a single half-life. Nonetheless, half-lives are commonly used for this purpose. While the bone can be a significant source of endogenous lead, exposures must be both moderately high and extended in time to load the bone with lead.

Plasma, rather than whole blood, is generally accepted as the source of lead available for distribution and excretion processes. The fraction of whole blood lead that is in the plasma is substantially larger at high blood lead concentrations than at low blood lead concentrations. Although the relationship of plasma lead to whole blood lead is curvilinear at all points, it can be approximated by a straight line at low blood lead concentrations. In one group of 73 adult women, it has been established that the slope of the plasma lead to whole blood lead regression line is 0.00246 at whole blood lead concentrations below about 6 μg/dL; up to this concentration, the relationship between plasma lead and whole blood lead can be approximated by a straight line, and the mean plasma lead concentration is 0.24% of the whole blood lead concentration. The most marked outlier in this group of women had a plasma lead concentration of 0.017 μg/dL at a whole blood lead concentration of about 3 μg/dL (0.56%). At whole blood lead concentrations exceeding about 40 μg/dL, the fraction of blood lead found in the plasma increases. For example, at a whole blood lead concentration of 60 μg/dL, plasma lead concentration is about 0.8 μg/dL (1.3%); at 80 μg/dL in whole blood, it is about 1.5 μg/dL (nearly 2%); and at 100 μg/dL in whole blood, it may be as high as 3 μg/dL (3%) (Manton *et al.*, 2001).

In certain physiological states, such as pregnancy, lactation and the period just after menopause in women, an increase in bone resorption rate takes place without a fully compensatory increase in bone formation rate. In general, it appears that whenever any of these situations has been studied, significant increases in markers of bone resorption have been observed along with comparable increases in that fraction of blood lead coming from bone.

(iii) *Excretion*

Absorbed lead is excreted both in the urine and in faeces (by secretion in the bile). Excretion in the urine is by filtration and reabsorption, and the rate of excretion is proportional to the concentration of lead in plasma. Excretion in bile is highly variable among experimental animal species. In humans, biliary excretion has been reported to be between 25% and 50% of urinary excretion.

Absorbed inorganic lead is not exhaled from the lung.

(*b*) *Organic lead*

(i) *Absorption*

Organic lead compounds, such as tetraethyl lead and tetramethyl lead, behave as gases in the respiratory tract, and are absorbed to a greater extent than are inorganic lead particles. Organic lead compounds are also absorbed through the skin in both humans and experimental animals.

(ii) *Distribution and metabolism*

Tetraethyl lead and tetramethyl lead are oxidatively dealkylated in the body. Any inorganic lead produced endogenously is distributed in the same pattern as administered inorganic lead, but the parent compounds and the intermediate dealkylated products are distributed quite differently and in accordance with their lipophilicity. In humans exposed to tetraethyl lead, concentrations of the parent compound and its metabolites, including inorganic lead, are highest in the liver and kidneys followed by the brain and heart. The rates of metabolite production are not known in detail for either humans or experimental animals. In rats, however, production of the toxic metabolite triethyl lead appears to be fairly rapid (in the order of hours), while production of subsequent metabolites is much slower (in the order of weeks). The highest concentrations of total lead in rats after exposure to alkyl leads are found in the kidney and liver, followed by the brain.

(iii) *Excretion*

In humans, tetraethyl lead was found to be excreted in the urine as diethyl lead and inorganic lead. In rats and rabbits, dialkyl lead is the major metabolite found in urine. Tetraalkyl leads would also be excreted in the faeces as inorganic lead, the end product of metabolism.

In humans, exhalation of tetraethyl lead and tetramethyl lead from the lung is a major route of excretion, accounting for 40% (tetramethyl lead) and 20% (tetraethyl lead) of the inhaled dose at 48 h after inhalation.

4.5.3 *Toxicodynamics and mode of action of lead*

(*a*) *Genotoxic mechanisms*

In considering the possible mechanisms whereby lead compounds could be mutagenic, it is important to keep in mind the doses at which different biological responses are seen. Since those mechanisms that occur only at highly toxic doses are not relevant carcinogenesis, the mechanisms discussed below emphasize findings at lower doses.

In most commonly-used test systems, effects were rather weak and/or restricted to toxic lead doses. In two published studies, in Chinese hamster ovary AS52 cells carrying a single copy of an *Escherichia coli gpt* gene, lead chloride induced mutations in a dose-dependent manner, at concentrations less than 1.0 μM. High mutant frequencies after exposure to lead were also observed in a different study in Chinese hamster ovary CHO K1 cells at higher but non-cytotoxic concentrations of lead starting at 0.5 mM. The mutation spectrum included base substitutions predominantly at G-C sites, as well as small and large deletions similar to DNA damage induced by ROS. Furthermore, two studies revealed an increase in mutant frequency when non-mutagenic concentrations of lead were used in combination with UVC irradiation or MNNG. One potential mechanism may be the interference with DNA repair processes. Two independent studies revealed an inhibition by lead of repair of UVC-induced or X-ray-induced DNA damage.

In addition to inducing gene mutations, lead appears to be an effective clastogen *in vivo* (although not consistently) and *in vitro*. Human studies are mostly confounded by the presence of other genotoxic compounds. Lead can induce aneuploidy, chromosomal aberrations, micronuclei, sister chromatid exchange and DNA damage (as measured most frequently with the Comet assay).

There is some evidence to suggest that one of the mechanisms of the genotoxicity seen after exposure to lead may be mediated by ROS. Lead appears to stimulate lipid peroxidation *in vivo*. ROS can be increased in cells through a number of mechanisms. For example, ALA, the haeme precursor whose levels are increased by lead exposure as a result of inhibition of the enzyme ALAD, can generate free radicals in cells and cause the formation of oxidative DNA lesions. Another mechanism may be depletion of cellular antioxidants such as glutathione. The loss of protection against ROS generated by other events may result in increased free radical and oxidative damage to DNA. Another aspect of lead that will result in oxidative DNA damage is the ability of lead to undergo Fenton-type reactions in the presence of hydrogen peroxide, leading to DNA strand breaks. One study suggested that singlet oxygen may be involved, since singlet oxygen quenchers, but not hydrogen peroxide or hydroxyl radical quenchers, blocked the reaction.

Dose considerations

As indicated earlier (see Distribution, above), the usual concentration of lead measured in blood is almost entirely accounted for by the fraction present within and bound to erythrocytes. Only a small fraction of blood lead is present in plasma, the precise proportion depending on the concentration in whole blood. In people heavily exposed to lead, with blood lead concentrations of about 100 μg/dL, plasma lead may be as high as 3 μg/dL (about 140 nM), whereas human populations in less contaminated environments may have whole blood lead concentrations of about 10 μg/dL, which corresponds to 0.024 μg/dL (about 1 nM) in plasma. These values are important in considering the human and non-human applicability of genetic toxicity data obtained from in-vitro experiments (see Tables 92 and 93).

(*b*) *Cell proliferation by mitogenic and regenerative mechanisms*

Cell proliferation can occur either as a regenerative response to cytotoxicity or by a process termed mitogenesis which does not involve cytotoxicity. Lead can increase proliferation of rat and mouse kidney cells, rat liver cells, vascular smooth muscle cells and spleen cells as well as cultured human astrocytoma cells. Often, these proliferative effects occur in the absence of cytotoxicity, although, at higher doses, lead is clearly causing cell death. Thus, tritiated thymidine incorporation was significantly increased in human astrocytoma cells at 1 μM lead concentrations, while lactate dehydrogenase activity in the medium (a measure of cytotoxicity) was not significantly increased until a concentration of 20 μM lead was reached (10 μM having no effect). In the kidneys of mice treated with intracardiac doses of lead acetate, there was a dose-related increase in tritiated thymidine incorporation into DNA that was evident at 1 mg/kg bw lead and maximal at 5 mg/kg bw lead in the absence of tubular necrosis. It is therefore plausible that lead exposure can induce proliferation by both mechanisms and could act as a tumour promoter. It is also plausible, given the demonstration of lead-induced proliferation in such a wide variety of cells, that any cell capable of replication in any tissue could be stimulated to do so by lead.

Lead has been shown to activate PKC, which comprises a large family of isozymes. Activation of PKC has multiple consequences, including neurotransmitter release and the induction of cell proliferation or differentiation and apoptosis. In human astrocytoma cells specifically, lead induces the translocation of the PKCα isoform from the cytosolic to the membrane fraction and stimulates DNA synthesis by a signal transduction cascade of the form PKCα → Raf-1 → MEK1/2 → ERK1/2 → $p90^{RSK}$, a protein that stimulates DNA synthesis. The authors of the study stress, however, that this mechanism might not be applicable to other cell types.

In rat kidneys, the early toxic effects of lead appear to be localized primarily in cells of the proximal tubule, where lead is taken up by extensive membrane binding and possibly by a passive transport mechanism. Studies in rats have demonstrated proximal tubular damage, which is characterized by the development of intranuclear inclusion bodies in cells that remain capable of division. Renal tumours have been observed in rodents after high-dose exposure to lead. The inclusion bodies, which mainly consist of lead and lead-binding proteins (PbBPs), are thought to act as intracellular depots of non-diffusible lead. A number of high-affinity renal PbBPs have been identified, one of which is a cleavage product of α_{2u}-globulin, a male rat-specific protein. A cytolethal mechanism in the development of tumours after lead exposure that involves α_{2u}-globulin is, however, unlikely, since lead induces tumours in male and female mice as well as male and female rats. Several other cytosolic PbBPs have been found in kidneys from environmentally exposed humans. These include thymosin β_4 and the 9-kDa acyl-coenzyme A binding protein. Other similar low molecular weight proteins bind lead in brain and analogous proteins exist in several species. A common feature seems to be that they are rich in aspartic and glutamic dicarboxylic acid residues. In-vitro studies using rat cells have shown that the renal PbBP facilitate the intranuclear transport of lead and provide evidence of chromatin binding of the lead binding complex. It has been suggested that this could lead to the altered gene expression associated with the mitogenic effects of lead in the kidney.

Lead can induce significant functional impairments *in vivo* in major target organs at doses below those associated with cytotoxicity. Significant increases in proliferative lesions of the kidneys, including tubular cell carcinomas, were observed after lead acetate exposures that did not result in pathological changes in adjacent tissues. Chronic nephropathy was not observed in any of the studies at doses that produced tumours. Thus, non-specific target organ toxicity, resulting in cell death, does not appear to be responsible for the production of tumours due to lead exposure. On the other hand, other evidence suggests that some form of cytotoxicity might play a role in renal carcinogenesis.

Cystic hyperplasia, a late morphological manifestation of chronic lead nephropathy, is a risk factor for renal cancer. Renal adenocarcinoma in experimental animals occurs against a background of proximal tubular cell hyperplasia, cytomegaly and cellular dysplasia. Cystic hyperplasia was reported to occur prior to adenoma formation in animals treated with renal carcinogens. One hypothesis regarding the progression from hyperplasia to cancer is that cells lining cysts become transformed and proliferate abnormally in response to increased volumes of intracystic fluid. Both human and experimental studies suggest that renal cyst formation contributes to an increased incidence of renal adenocarcinomas. In the case of lead, adenocarcinoma may be a consequence of the cystic change in the renal cortex that follows chronic lead-induced nephropathy.

More subtle types of cytotoxicity may also play roles in the carcinogenic process. Oxidative stress may contribute to some aspects of the cellular toxicity of lead by disrupting the pro-oxidant–antioxidant balance that exists within cells. For example, lipid oxidation is significantly elevated in animals exposed to inorganic lead. These results suggest that lead exerts its toxic effects by enhancing peroxidative damage to the membranes, thus compromising cellular functions.

(c) *Molecular mechanisms of action*

The main mutagenic mechanisms of lead at non-cytotoxic concentrations demonstrated to date are: (1) those involving ROS; and (2) interference with DNA repair processes. It has been shown in many systems that exposure to lead results in altered ROS levels and species. The mechanisms by which this can occur include inhibition of antioxidant defence systems, catalysis of Fenton-type reactions, and via accummulation of ALA. Nucleotide excision repair has been shown to be blocked by exposure to lead. This type of inhibition would be expected to enhance the mutagenicity of agents such as polycyclic aromatic hydrocarbons, UV and other agents causing bulky lesions in DNA. The co-mutagenicity of lead with UVC or MNNG is consistent with the hypothesis that both nucleotide excision repair and base excision repair may be affected by lead.

One mechanism for lead interaction with proteins could be via displacement of metals, such as zinc or calcium, from their respective binding sites. In cell-free systems, lead has been shown to reduce DNA binding of transcription factors TFIIIA and Sp1, presumably by replacing zinc in zinc fingers. However, the zinc finger-containing repair proteins XPA and Fpg were not inhibited by lead. Thus, zinc finger proteins cannot be considered as a general target, but interactions depend on the specific protein. Furthermore, these interactions have not yet been demonstrated in intact cells.

Another mechanism that may be relevant for carcinogenesis by lead is its ability to alter gene expression. One pathway by which this could occur is via activation of PKC, which occurs at low concentrations of lead. PKC activation starts a signaling pathway that leads to upregulation of 'immediate early response' genes, which ultimately results in a proliferative response.

In conclusion, lead is a toxic metal and one expression of this property is genetic toxicity. There is, however, little evidence that it interacts directly with DNA at normally encountered concentrations. The genetic toxicity of lead appears to be modified in part by increases in and modulation of ROS. In addition, lead itself can interact with proteins, including those involved in DNA repair. This latter mechanism might be responsible for the enhancement of genotoxicity caused by other agents. These properties could result in mutation, changes in gene expression and cell proliferation, all of which would contribute to a carcinogenic response if exposure is sustained.

5. Summary of Data Reported and Evaluation

5.1 Exposure data

Lead is found at low concentrations in the earth's crust predominantly as lead sulfide (*galena*), but the widespread occurrence of lead in the environment is largely the result of anthropogenic activity. The utility of lead and lead compounds was discovered in prehistoric times. Lead has been used in plumbing and tableware since the time of the Roman Empire. Lead usage increased progressively with industrialization and rose dramatically with the widespread use of the automobile in the twentieth century. Lead has found major uses in pipes and plumbing, pigments and paints, gasoline additives, construction materials and lead–acid batteries. The uses of lead in pipes, paints and gasoline additives have resulted in substantial introductions of lead into the environment and human exposure, and are being phased out in many countries. The predominant use of lead is now in lead–acid batteries and, to a lesser extent, in construction materials and lead-based chemicals.

As a result of anthropogenic activity, lead can enter the environment at any stage from its mining to its final use, including during recycling, and it contaminates crops, soil, water, food, air and dust. Once lead is introduced, it persists. The important routes of human exposure from these sources are inhalation or ingestion. The dispersion of lead throughout the global environment and consequent human exposure has arisen predominantly from the widespread use of leaded gasoline. Some geographic areas, for instance near lead mines and smelters, have high environmental concentrations of lead. The past and present use of lead-based paints can result in substantial risk for localized exposure to lead-contaminated dust. Small industries (e.g. jewellery-making, ceramics, soldering, leaded glass) and individual activities (smoking, home renovations, use of herbal remedies and cosmetics, certain crafts and hobbies, and unregulated recycling) can lead to high exposure. Occupations in which the highest potential exposure exists include mining, primary and secondary smelting, production of lead–acid batteries, pigment production, construction and demolition.

Efforts to reduce environmental concentrations of lead, predominantly through the decreased use of leaded gasoline, have resulted in substantial decreases in the introduction of lead into the environment. In contaminated environments, dust control and hygienic measures can considerably decrease exposure. In spite of the persistence of lead in the environment, human exposure has decreased substantially in countries where control measures have been implemented over the past 10–30 years.

5.2 Human carcinogenicity data

Occupational studies

For lung cancer, six occupational cohort studies of highly exposed workers are particularly informative (battery workers in the USA, battery workers in the United Kingdom, primary smelter workers in Italy, Sweden and the USA (two studies)). Potentially confounding exposures to other known occupational lung carcinogens were largely absent in the battery workers. Several of the cohorts of smelter workers had low documented exposures to arsenic, the principal occupational potential confounder of interest; the smelter workers in Sweden had potentially high exposures to arsenic. Overall, with the exception of the smelter workers in Sweden, these studies were consistent in showing no or a slight excess of lung cancer compared with external reference populations. Observed excesses were quite small and well within the range that might be explained by chance or confounding by smoking. Few or no data for dose–response analyses and no smoking data were available for these cohorts. The Swedish study of smelter workers showed a statistically significant twofold excess of lung cancer but this excess may well have been caused by exposure to arsenic. A Finnish study of workers across many industries, whose blood lead concentrations were sampled as part of a surveillance programme, was judged to be moderately informative. Exposure to lead in this study was lower than in the six cohorts of highly exposed workers but higher than in the general population. There was a modest trend of increasing lung cancer with increasing levels of exposure in the Finnish cohort; this trend was not statistically significant.

For stomach cancer, five (battery workers in the UK and the USA, primary smelter workers in Italy and the USA (two studies)) of the six occupational cohort studies used for the evaluation of lung cancer were judged to be particularly informative. In four of these five studies, there was a fairly consistent excess of 30–50% of stomach cancer compared with external reference populations. Exposure to arsenic is not considered to be a cause of stomach cancer and any potential confounding by smoking is likely to be small. Some analyses of limited exposure surrogates were carried out, but these did not implicate lead exposure as the cause of the stomach cancer excess. However, little or no data for quantitative dose–response analysis were available in these cohorts. It is possible that ethnicity, dietary habits, prevalence of *Helicobacter pylori* infections or socioeconomic status played a role in the stomach cancer excesses.

Five of the six cohort studies of highly exposed workers reported findings for kidney cancer. In one study, there was a twofold statistically significant excess of kidney cancer, based on comparison with an external reference population. In the remaining four studies, mortality was either close to, or below, expected values. All five studies were based on small numbers of deaths.

Four of the six cohort studies of highly exposed workers reported findings for tumours of the brain and nervous system. On the basis of comparisons with external reference populations, mortality showed no consistent pattern. In addition, in a nested case–control study, the cohort of workers from Finland showed a statistically significant positive dose–response relationship between blood lead concentrations and the risk for glioma. The cohort in the Finnish study had lower exposures to lead than the other occupational cohorts; all studies were based on small numbers of deaths.

Environmental studies

Among the general population studies, the most informative are the two follow-up studies on the US NHANES II population. A limitation of these two studies is the reliance on one blood lead measurement per subject to define exposure. Both studies, analysing essentially the same population, found a positive dose–response relationship between blood lead concentrations and lung cancer, which approached or attained statistical significance. However, these results within a low-dose population are not consistent with those for lung cancer in more highly exposed occupational populations, for whom no consistent lung cancer excess is apparent. At least some of the reported dose–response relationships for lung cancer in these two studies may be due to residual confounding from smoking, which was correlated with blood lead concentrations. Higher concentrations of blood lead were apparent in those with lower income, so it is also possible that residual confounding from occupational exposure to lung carcinogens may have contributed to positive dose–response trends.

5.3 Animal carcinogenicity data

Lead acetate

Oral exposure to lead acetate has been shown to be carcinogenic in the rat kidney in seven separate studies, producing adenomas and adenocarcinomas after chronic exposure in males and/or females. Both of the studies that allowed assessment of a dose–response relationship showed that such a relationship existed. In another experiment the offspring of female mice exposed to oral lead acetate during pregnancy and lactation showed dose-related increases in renal tumours as adults in the absence of chronic lead-induced nephropathy.

Brain gliomas were observed after oral exposure to lead acetate in rats in two separate studies.

One study in rats indicated that oral exposure to lead acetate was associated with tumours of the adrenal gland, testes and prostate in males and adrenal gland in females. In a study of a mixed population of male and female rats, oral exposure to lead acetate was associated with tumours of the lung, pituitary, prostate, mammary gland and adrenal gland.

Lead subacetate

One experiment in male and female mice and six experiments in male and/or female rats showed that oral exposure to lead subacetate induced renal cancer. One of these studies showed a dose–response relationship. Brain gliomas were observed in rats after oral administration of lead subacetate in one study. Three studies show that repeated intraperitoneal injections of lead subacetate increased lung tumour multiplicity in strain A mice. One study of oral exposure to lead subacetate in strain A mice was negative for lung tumours. In one study, hamsters exposed orally to lead subacetate did not develop tumours.

Lead powder

Two studies in rats exposed to lead powder orally or by intramuscular injection and one study on intrarenal injection of lead powder in rats did not produce tumours.

Lead oxide

In one experiment, inhalation of lead oxide did not produce tumours in male rats.

Lead chromate

One study showed that injection-site sarcomas were induced by a single subcutaneous injection of lead chromate in rats. One study of intramuscular injection of lead chromate in rats produced renal tumours. One study of intramuscular injection of lead chromate in mice and one study of intrabronchiolar implantation of different lead chromates in rats were negative. The role of chromium in the carcinogenic response of lead chromate in these studies cannot be excluded.

Lead phosphate

In four separate studies, injection of lead phosphate subcutaneously, or combined subcutaneously and intraperitoneally, was shown to produce renal cancers in rats.

Lead arsenate

One study of oral administration of lead arsenate in male and female rats was negative.

Tetraethyl lead

One experiment with repeated subcutaneous injections of tetraethyl lead was found to be inadequate for evaluation.

Administration of lead compounds with known carcinogens or modifiers

Three experiments showed that oral exposure to lead subacetate enhanced *N*-ethyl-*N*-hydroxyethylnitrosamine-induced renal carcinogenesis in male rats. One study showed that oral lead subacetate-induced renal tumours in rats were increased by concomitant oral administration of calcium acetate. One study in strain A mice showed that calcium acetate and magnesium acetate inhibited lung adenomas induced by intraperitoneal injection of lead subacetate. Intratracheal instillations of combinations of lead oxide and benzo[*a*]-pyrene in hamsters produced lung tumours not observed with either agent alone. Oral exposure to lead nitrate increased the incidence of *N*-nitrosodimethylamine-induced renal tumours in male rats while intraperitoneal injections of lead subacetate enhanced *N*-nitrosodimethylamine-induced lung tumour multiplicity in mice.

Overall, extensive experimental evidence shows that various water-soluble and -insoluble lead compounds can induce kidney tumours in rodents. In addition, one study showed that renal tumours can occur in the absence of lead-induced nephropathy. It is also noteworthy that the induction of brain gliomas, which are rarely spontaneous, occurred after oral exposure to lead in rats. Lead proved to be an effective renal tumour carcinogen/promoter in rats and mice exposed to various organic renal carcinogens.

5.4 Other relevant data

Toxicokinetics and metabolism of lead

Inorganic lead

Lead absorption from the gastrointestinal tract in both humans and experimental animals is strongly influenced by age (neonates and the young absorb a larger fraction than adults), fasting/fed status (fasting humans and experimental animals absorb much larger fractions than their fed counterparts), nutrition (fat and caloric intakes; phosphorus, copper, zinc and especially iron and calcium status, all affect lead absorption), solubility (soluble lead compounds are better absorbed) and particle size (in controlled studies in rats, lead absorption from ingested mining wastes was shown to be inversely proportional to particle size). There are no data indicating that the fraction of lead absorbed from an inhalation exposure is dependent on the amount of lead in the lung. Patterns and rates of particle deposition are highly dependent on particle size and ventilation rate, but all lead deposited deep in the lung is eventually absorbed. Limited studies indicate that dermal absorption of inorganic lead is negligible, although slightly increased by high perspiration rates in humans.

In both humans and experimental animals, absorbed lead is rapidly distributed from blood plasma simultaneously into erythrocytes, soft tissues, and bone. The half-life of lead in blood and soft tissues is 20–30 days in adult humans and 3–5 days in adult rats. In both humans and rats, the soft-tissue concentrations of lead are highest in liver and kidney and much lower in brain. Plasma, rather than whole blood, is generally accepted as the source of lead available for distribution and excretion, although plasma lead comprises only 0.2–0.3% of whole blood lead concentrations when these are < 6 µg/dL. The fraction of whole blood lead in plasma is substantially larger at high blood lead concentrations than at low blood lead concentrations.

The majority of lead is stored in bone (in adults $> 90\%$) and is partitioned mainly into trabecular and cortical bone. The higher rate of remodelling in trabecular bone is reflected in a shorter half-life of lead in trabecular bone (2–8 years) compared with that in cortical bone (> 20 years). Bone can be a significant source of endogenous lead, in particular when the bone resorption rate is increased, such as during pregnancy, lactation, the period just after menopause, and during weightlessness.

After oral ingestion, inorganic lead that has not been absorbed in the gastrointestinal tract is excreted in the faeces. Absorbed lead is excreted in the urine and, via the bile, in the faeces. Excretion of lead through sweat is of minor importance.

Organic lead

Organic lead compounds, such as tetraethyl lead and tetramethyl lead, behave as gases in the respiratory tract and are absorbed to a greater extent than are inorganic lead particles. Organic lead compounds are also absorbed through the skin of both humans and experimental animals.

Tetraethyl lead and tetramethyl lead are oxidatively dealkylated in the body. Any inorganic lead produced from these reactions is distributed in the same way as administered inorganic lead. In humans and rats exposed to alkyl lead, concentrations of lead are highest in the liver and kidneys followed by the brain and heart. The rates of metabolite production are not known in detail for either humans or experimental animals.

In humans, tetraethyl lead is excreted in the urine as diethyl lead, ethyl lead, and inorganic lead. In rats and rabbits, dialkyl lead is the major metabolite found in urine. One of the end-products of metabolism of tetraalkyl leads is inorganic lead, which is also excreted in the faeces.

In humans, exhalation of unmetabolized tetraethyl lead and tetramethyl lead from the lung is a major route of excretion.

Toxic effects of inorganic lead

Typical clinical manifestations of lead poisoning include weakness, irritability, asthenia, nausea, abdominal pain with constipation, and anaemia.

Lead interferes with numerous physiological processes. In the haeme biosynthetic pathway, it inhibits δ-aminolevulinic acid dehydratase (also known as porphobilinogen synthase), probably through its high affinity for the zinc-binding site in the enzyme. Although lead displaces zinc more readily in one of the alloenzymes of the protein, the relationship between δ-aminolevulinic acid dehydratase genotype and sensitivity to lead at different blood lead concentrations is at present unclear. Lead also causes an increase in zinc protoporphyrin, by a mechanism which is not fully established. Lead inhibits pyrimidine-5′-nucleotidase, resulting in accumulation of nucleotides, and subsequent haemolysis and anaemia.

Renal manifestations of acute lead poisoning include glycosuria, aminoaciduria and phosphaturia. Chronic exposure to low concentrations of lead is associated with increased urinary excretion of low-molecular-weight proteins and lysosomal enzymes. Chronic exposure to high concentrations of lead results in interstitial fibrosis, glomerular sclerosis, tubular dysfunction and, ultimately, in chronic renal failure. Lead has also been implicated in the development of hypertension secondary to nephropathy.

A considerable body of evidence suggests that children are more sensitive than adults to the neurotoxic properties of lead. Although clinical symptoms of toxicity generally become apparent at blood lead concentrations of 70 μg/dL, many important disturbances occur at much lower concentrations. These include electrophysiological anomalies of evoked brain potential in response to auditory stimuli and reduced peripheral nerve conduction. Both cross-sectional and prospective studies of children have found impairments in cognition, attention, and language function at concentrations of lead previously thought to be harmless. In studies with larger samples, better measures of lead burden and neurobehavioural function, and more advanced statistical techniques, effects are detectable at blood lead concentrations below 10 μg/dL. The relative effect is greater below 10 μg/dL than above this level. Recently, attention has shifted from the impact of lead on cognition to its effects on behaviour. Exposure to lead has been found to be associated with attentional dysfunction, aggression and delinquency.

Exposure to lead is associated with cardiovascular effects and with changes in endocrine and immune functions.

Many of the effects of lead exposure in humans have been confirmed in experimental systems. At the cellular level, lead has mitogenic properties; it affects various regulatory proteins, including those that depend on the presence of zinc.

Studies on the reproductive and developmental toxicity of lead did not show consistent effects, morphologically or quantitatively, on markers of male fertility. It is not clear whether the effects are caused by a direct interaction of lead with the reproductive organs, or by modulation of the endocrine control of reproduction, or both.

There is consistent evidence in humans, in the form of case series and epidemiological studies, that the risk for spontaneous abortion (pregnancy loss before the 20th week of gestation, but after the stage of unrecognized, sub-clinical loss) is increased by maternal exposure to high concentrations of lead.

In humans, prenatal lead exposure is associated with an increased risk for minor malformations, low birth weight and reduced postnatal growth rate. The effect on postnatal growth rate is apparent only in those children with continuing postnatal lead exposure.

Differences in reproductive end-points between species make it unlikely that useful conclusions can be extrapolated from animals to humans.

Genotoxicity of inorganic lead compounds

Human studies

Humans occupationally exposed to lead show evidence of genotoxicity as measured in a variety of assays. In some studies, these effects were correlated with blood lead concentrations. However, all the human genotoxicity studies involved co-exposure to lead and other compounds, making it difficult to attribute genetic and other effects to lead alone.

In a limited number of studies on non-occupationally exposed individuals, no genotoxic effects were found that were correlated with blood lead concentrations.

Studies in experimental systems

Mutations were not induced in bacteria by either lead acetate or lead chloride, but were induced by both lead chromate and lead bromide. In these last two cases, however, the activity appeared to be due to the anions. In cultures of various mammalian cells, lead acetate, lead chromate and lead nitrate induced DNA strand breaks. Furthermore, most studies revealed positive mutagenic responses even though the extent of mutagenicity and the lead concentrations at which the responses were observed varied considerably, depending on cell type and experimental conditions. Tests for sister chromatid exchange and chromosomal aberrations showed variable responses. Micronucleus formation has been shown to occur at low concentrations of lead. In a single study, lead sulfide induced micronuclei, gene mutations and sister chromatid exchanges. Organo-lead compounds do not appear to have been tested *in vitro*.

Studies of genetic toxicity in animals have been conducted by the oral, inhalation, subcutaneous, intraperitoneal and intravenous routes. It should be noted that blood lead concentrations were not available in these studies, except in a single study in cynomolgus monkeys, and that the exposure concentrations were generally far higher than those reported in human occupational studies. DNA strand breakage has been demonstrated in lead-exposed animals, and variable results have been found in tests for induction of sister chromatid exchange. Micronucleus induction in bone-marrow cells of lead-exposed animals has been demonstrated in some studies. Most studies of chromosomal aberrations have demonstrated increased frequencies in mice, rats and in the one study in cynomolgus monkeys reported. Aneuploidy has been demonstrated in lead-exposed rats and mice. Increases in the proportion of morphologically abnormal sperm have also been found in mice and cynomolgus monkeys, but not in rabbits. Dominant lethal effects were not observed in male mice exposed to lead in a single study.

In conclusion, lead is a toxic metal and one expression of this property is genetic toxicity. There is, however, little evidence that it interacts directly with DNA at normally encountered blood lead concentrations. The genetic toxicity of lead appears to be mediated in part by increases in, and modulation of, reactive oxygen species. In addition, lead interacts with proteins, including those involved in DNA repair. This latter mechanism might be responsible for enhancing the genotoxicity of other agents. These properties could result in mutation, changes in gene expression and cell proliferation, all of which would contribute to a carcinogenic response if exposure is sustained.

5.5 Evaluation

There is *limited evidence* in humans for the carcinogenicity of inorganic lead compounds.

There is *inadequate evidence* in humans for the carcinogenicity of organic lead compounds.

There is *sufficient evidence* in experimental animals for the carcinogenicity of inorganic lead compounds.

There is *sufficient evidence* in experimental animals for the carcinogenicity of lead acetate, lead subacetate, lead chromate, and lead phosphate.

There is *inadequate evidence* in experimental animals for the carcinogenicity of lead oxide and lead arsenate.

There is *inadequate evidence* in experimental animals for the carcinogenicity of organic lead compounds.

There is *inadequate evidence* in experimental animals for the carcinogenicity of tetraethyl lead.

There is *inadequate evidence* in experimental animals for the carcinogenicity of lead powder.

Overall evaluation

Inorganic lead compounds are *probably carcinogenic to humans (Group 2A)*.

Organic lead compounds are *not classifiable as to their carcinogenicity to humans (Group 3)*.

The Working Group noted that organic lead compounds are metabolized, at least in part, to ionic lead both in humans and animals. To the extent that ionic lead, generated from organic lead, is present in the body, it will be expected to exert the toxicities associated with inorganic lead.

6. References

Abdel-Moati, A.R. & Atta, M.M. (1991) *Patella vulgata, Mytilus minimus* and *Hyale prevosti* as bioindicators for Pb and Se enrichment in Alexandria coastal waters. *Marine Pollut. Bull.*, **22**, 148–150

Abu Melha, A., Ahmed, N.A.M. & El Hassan, A.Y. (1987) Traditional remedies and lead intoxication. *Trop. geogr. Med.*, **39**, 100–103

ACGIH (2001) *Lead, Elemental and Inorganic (BEI)*, Cincinnati, OH

ACGIH® Worldwide (2003) *Documentation of the TLVs® and BEIs® with Other Worldwide Occupational Exposure Values — 2003 CD-ROM*, Cincinnati, OH

Adams, R.D. & Victor, M. (1993) *Principles of Neurology*, 5th Ed., New York, McGraw-Hill

Adeniyi, F.A.A. & Anetor, J.I. (1999) Lead-poisoning in two distant states of Nigeria: An indication of the real size of the problem. *Afr. J. Med. med. Sci.*, **28**, 107–112

Ades, A.E. & Kazantzis, G. (1988) Lung cancer in a non-ferrous smelter: The role of cadmium. *Br. J. ind. Med.*, **45**, 435–442

Agarwal, V., Nath, S.P. & Bhavyesh, G. (2002) Chronic low level lead exposure vis-a-vis some biophysiological variants. *Indian J. occup. environ. Med.*, **6**, 183–185

Ahlgren, L., Lidén, K., Mattsson, L.S. & Tejning, S. (1976) X-ray fluorescence analysis of lead in human skeleton in vivo. *Scand. J. Work Environ. Health*, **2**, 82–86

Ahmed, N.S., El-Gendy, K.S., El-Refaie, A.K., Marzouk, S.A., Bakry, N.S., El-Sebae, A.H. & Solimar, S.A. (1987) Assessment of lead toxicity in traffic controllers of Alexandria, Egypt, road intersections. *Arch. environ. Health*, **42**, 92–95

Ahner, B.A., Price, N.M. & Morel, F.M.M. (1994) Phytochelatin production by marine phytoplankton at low free metal ion concentrations: Laboratory studies and field data from Massachussets Bay. *Proc. natl Acad. Sci. USA*, **91**, 8433–8436

Aitchinson, L. (1960) *A History of Metals*, London, MacDonald and Evans

Ajayi, A. & Kamson, O.F. (1983) Determination of lead in roadside dust in Lagos City by atomic absorption spectrophotometry. *Environ. Intern.*, **9**, 397–400

Albalak, R., Noonan, G., Buchanan, S., Flanders, W.D., Gotway-Crawford, C., Kim, D., Jones, R.L., Sulaiman, R., Blumenthal, W., Tan, R., Curtis, G. & McGeehin, M.A. (2003) Blood lead levels and risk factors for lead poisoning among children in Jakarta, Indonesia. *Sci. total Environ.*, **301**, 75–85

Albert, L.A. & Badillo, F. (1991) Environmental lead in Mexico. *Rev. environ. Contam. Toxicol.*, **117**, 1–49

Alessio, L., Bertazzi, P.A., Monelli, O. & Foa, V. (1976) Free erythrocyte protoporphyrin as an indicator of the biological effect of lead in adult males. II. Comparison between erythrocyte protoporphyrin and other indicators of effect. *Int. Arch. occup. environ. Health*, **37**, 89–105

Alexander, F.W., Clayton, B.E. & Delves, H.T. (1974) Mineral and trace-metal balances in children receiving normal and synthetic diets. *Q. J. Med.*, **43**, 89–111

Alexander, B.H., Checkoway, H., van Netten, C., Muller, C.H., Ewers, T.G., Kaufman, J.D., Mueller, B.A., Vaughan, T.L. & Faustman, E.M. (1996) Semen quality of men employed at a lead smeller. *Occup. environ. Med.*, **53**, 411–416

Alexander, B.H., Checkoway, H., Costa-Mallen, P., Faustman, E.M., Woods, J.S., Kelsey, K.T., van Netten, C. & Costa, L.G. (1998) Interaction of blood lead and δ-aminolevulinic acid dehydratase genotype on markers of heme synthesis and sperm production in lead smelter workers. *Environ. Health Perspect.*, **106**, 213–216

Al-Hakkak, Z.S., Hamamy, H.A., Murad, A.M.B. & Hussain, A.F. (1986) Chromosome aberrations in workers at a storage battery plant in Iraq. *Mutat. Res.*, **171**, 53–60

Ali, A.R., Smales, O.R.C. & Aslam, M. (1978) Surma and lead poisoning. *Br. med. J.*, **2**, 915–916

Ali, E.A., Nasralla, M.M. & Shakour, A.A. (1986) Spatial and seasonal variation of lead in Cairo atmosphere. *Environ. Pollut. (Series B)*, **11**, 205–210

Ali, M.B., Tripathi, R.D., Rai, U.N. & Singh, S.P. (1999) Physico-chemical characteristics and pollution level in lake Nainital (V.P., India): Role of macrophytes and phytoplankton in biomonitoring phytoremediation of toxic metal ions. *Chemosphere*, **39**, 2171–2182

Al Khayat, A., Habibullah, J., Koutouby, A., Ridha, A. & Almchdi, A.M. (1997a) Correlation between maternal and cord blood lead levels. *Int. J. environ. Health Res.*, **7**, 323–328

Al Khayat, A., Menon, N.S. & Alidina, M.R. (1997b) Acute lead encephalopathy in early infancy — Clinical presentation and outcome. *Ann. trop. Paediatr.*, **17**, 39–44

Allen, J.R., McWey, P.J. & Suomi, S.J. (1974) Pathobiological and behavioral effects of lead intoxication in the infant rhesus monkey. *Environ. Health Perspect.*, **7**, 239–246

van Alphen, M. (1999) Lead in paints and water in India. In: *Lead Poisoning Prevention and Treatment: Implementing a National Programme in Developing Countries, February 8–10, Bangalore, India*, pp. 265–272 [http://www.leadpoison.net/environment/paints.htm; accessed 09/02/2004]

Al-Saleh, I. (1998) Sources of lead in Saudi Arabia: A review. *J. environ. Pathol. Toxicol. Oncol.*, **17**, 17–35

Al-Saleh, I. & Shinwari, N. (2001a) Report on the levels of cadmium, lead, and mercury in imported rice grain samples. *Biol. trace Elem. Res.*, **83**, 91–96

Al-Saleh, I. & Shinwari, N. (2001b) Levels of cadmium, lead, and mercury in human brain tumors. *Biol. trace Elem. Res.*, **79**, 197–203

Al-Saleh, I., Khalil, M.A. & Taylor, A. (1995) Lead, erythrocyte protoporphyrin, and hematological parameters in normal maternal and umbilical cord blood from subjects of the Riyadh region, Saudi Arabia. *Arch. environ. Health*, **50**, 66–73

Al-Saleh, I., Nester, M., DeVol, E., Shinwari, N., Munchari, L. & Al-Shahria, S. (2001) Relationships between blood lead concentrations, intelligence, and academic achievement of Saudi Arabian schoolgirls. *Int. J. Hyg. environ. Health*, **204**,165–174

Altmann, L., Lohmann, H. & Wiegand, H. (1988) Acute lead exposure transiently inhibits hippocampal neuronal activities in vitro. *Brain Res.*, **455**, 254–261

Altmann, L., Weinsberg, F., Sveinsson, K., Lilienthal, H., Wiegand, H. & Winneke, G. (1993) Impairment of long-term potentiation and learning following chronic lead exposure. *Toxicol. Lett.*, **66**, 105–112

Altmann, L., Sveinsson, K., Krämer, U., Weishoff-Houben, M., Turfeld, M., Winneke, G. & Wiegand, H. (1998) Visual functions in 6-year-old children in relation to lead and mercury levels. *Neurotoxicol. Teratol.*, **20**, 9–17

Alvares, A.P., Kapelner, S., Sassa, S. & Kappas, A. (1975) Drug metabolism in normal children, lead-poisoned children, and normal adults. *Clin. Pharmacol. Ther.*, **17**, 179–183

American Academy of Pediatrics (1998) Screening for elevated blood lead levels. Policy statement. Committee on Environmental Health. *Pediatrics*, **101**, 1072–1078

Amici, A., Emanuelli, M., Raffaelli, N., Ruggieri, S., Saccucci, F. & Magni, G. (2000) Human erythrocyte pyrimidine 5′-nucleotidase, PN-I, is identical to p36, a protein associated to lupus inclusion formation in response to alpha-interferon. *Blood*, **96**, 1596–1598

Angle, C.R. & McIntire, M.S. (1978) Low level lead inhibition of erythrocyte pyrimidine nucleotidase. *Environ. Res.*, **17**, 296–302

Ankrah, N.A., Kamiya, Y., Appiah-Opong, R., Akyeampon, Y.A. & Addae, M.M. (1996) Lead levels and related biochemical findings occurring in Ghanaian subjects occupationally exposed to lead. *East Afr. med. J.*, **73**, 375–379

Annest, J.L., Pirkle, J.L., Makuc, D., Neese, J.W., Bayse, D.D. & Kovar, M.G. (1983) Chronological trend in blood lead levels between 1976 and 1980. *New Engl. J. Med.*, **308**, 1373–1377

Antonio, M.T. & Leret, M.L. (2000) Study of the neurochemical alterations produced in discrete brain areas by perinatal low-level lead exposure. *Life Sci.*, **67**, 635–642

Anttila, A. (1994) Occupational exposure to lead and risk of cancer. *Acta Universitatis Tamperensis* (Tampere, Finland, University of Tampere), **A417**, 1–86

Anttila, A., Heikkilä, P., Pukkala, E., Nykyri, E., Kauppinen, T., Hernberg, S. & Hemminki, K. (1995) Excess lung cancer among workers exposed to lead. *Scand. J. Work Environ. Health*, **21**, 460–469

Anttila, A., Heikkilä, P., Nykyri, E., Kauppinen, T., Pukkala, E., Hernberg, S. & Hemminki, K. (1996) Risk of nervous system cancer among workers exposed to lead. *J. occup. environ. Med.*, **38**, 131–136

APEC (1997) *Urbanization and Environment in Malaysia: Managing the Impact, Institute of Developing Economics*, APEC Study Center, Report of Commissioned Studies No. 1, pp. 74–90

Apol, A.G. (1981) Health Hazard Evaluation Report, HETA 81-0036-1023, Alaska Smelting & Refining Co., Wisilla, AK, USA, NIOSH

Apostoli, P. & Maranelli, G. (1986) The erythrocyte zinc protoporphyrin test in biological monitoring of workers exposed to lead. *Med. Lav.*, **77**, 529–537 (in Italian)

Apostoli, P., Kiss, P., Porru, S., Bonde, J.P., Vanhoorne, M. & the ASCLEPIOS Study Group (1998) Male reproductive toxicity of lead in animals and humans. *Occup. environ. Med.*, **55**, 364–374

Apostoli, P., Porru, S. & Bisanti, L. (1999) Critical aspects of male fertility in the assessment of exposure lo lead. *Scand. J. Work Environ. Health*, **25** (Suppl. 1), 40–43

Apostoli, P., Bellini, A., Porru, S. & Bisanti, L. (2000) The effect of lead on male fertility: A time to pregnancy (TTP) study. *Am. J. ind. Med.*, **38**, 310–315

Arai, F. & Yamamura, Y. (1990) Excretion of tetramethyllead, trimethyllead, dimethyllead and inorganic lead after injection of tetramethyllead to rabbits. *Ind. Health*, **28**, 63–76

Arai, F., Yamamura, Y., Yoshida, M. & Kishimoto, T. (1994) Blood and urinary levels of metals (Pb, Cr, Cd, Mn, Sb, Co and Cu) in cloisonne workers. *Ind. Health*, **32**, 67–78

Arai, F., Yamauchi, H., Chiba, K. & Yoshida, K. (1998) Excretion of triethyllead, diethyllead and inorganic lead in rabbits after injection of triethyl neopentoxy lead. *Ind. Health*, **36**, 331–336

Araki, S., Murata, K. & Aono, H. (1987) Central and peripheral nervous system dysfunction in workers exposed to lead, zinc and copper: A follow-up study of visual and somatosensory evoked potentials. *Int. Arch. occup. environ. Health*, **59**, 177–187

Aravindan, G.R., Bjordahl, J., Jost, L.K. & Evenson, D.P. (1997) Susceptibility of human sperm to *in situ* DNA denaturation is strongly correlated with DNA strand breaks identified by single-cell electrophoresis. *Exper. Cell Res.*, **236**, 231–237

Aribarg, A. & Sukcharoen, N. (1996) Effects of occupational lead exposure on spermatogenesis. *J. med. Assoc. Thai.*, **79**, 91–97

Ariza, M.E. & Williams, M.V. (1996) Mutagenesis of AS52 cells by low concentrations of lead(II) and mercury(II). *Environ. mol. Mutag.*, **27**, 30–33

Ariza, M.E. & Williams, M.V. (1999) Lead and mercury mutagenesis: Type of mutation dependent upon metal concentration. *J. Biochem. mol. Toxicol.*, **13**, 107–112

Ariza, M.E., Bijur, G.N. & Williams, M.V. (1998) Lead and mercury mutagenesis: Role of H_2O_2, superoxide dismutase, and xanthine oxidase. *Environ. mol. Mutag.*, **31**, 352–361

Artaxo, P., Maenhaut, W., Storms, H. & Van Grieken, R. (1990) Aerosol characteristics and sources for the Amazon basin during the wet season. *J. geophys. Res.*, **95**, 16971–16985

Aschengrau, A., Beiser, A., Bellinger, D., Copenhafer, D. & Weitzman, M. (1994) The impact of soil lead abatement on urban children's blood lead levels: Phase II results from the Boston lead-in-soil demonstration project. *Environ. Res.*, **67**, 125–148

Asmuss, M., Mullenders, L.H.F., Eker, A. & Hartwig, A. (2000) Differential effects of toxic metal compounds on the activities of Fpg and XPA, two zinc finger proteins involved in DNA repair. *Carcinogenesis*, **21**, 2097–2104

Assennato, G., Paci, C., Baser, M.E., Molinini, R., Candela, R.G., Altamura, B.M. & Giorgino, R. (1987) Sperm count suppression without endocrine dysfunction in lead-exposed men. *Arch. environ. Health*, **42**, 124–127

Association of Official Analytical Chemists (1994) AOAC official method 994.02, lead in edible oils and fats — Direct graphite furnace — Atomic absorption spectrophotometric method. *J. AOAC Int.*

Association of Official Analytical Chemists (2000a) AOAC official method 999.10, lead, cadmium, zinc, copper, and iron in foods. Atomic absorption spectrophotometry after microwave digestion. *J. AOAC Int.*

Association of Official Analytical Chemists (2000b) AOAC official method 972.25, lead in foods. Atomic absorption spectrophotometric method. *J. AOAC Int.*

Association of Official Analytical Chemists (2000c) AOAC official method 979.17, lead in evaporated milk and fruit juice. Anodic stripping voltammetric method. *J. AOAC Int.*

Association of Official Analytical Chemists (2000d) AOAC official method 997.15, lead in sugars and syrups. Graphite furnace atomic absorption method. *J. AOAC Int.*

ASTM (1999) *Standard Test Method for Determination of Lead by Inductively Coupled Plasma Atomic Emission Spectrometry (ICP-AES), Flame Atomic Absorption Spectrometry (FAAS), or Graphite Furnace Atomic Absorption Spectrometry (GFAAS) Techniques, Designation: E1613-99*, West Conshohocken, PA, USA, ASTM International

ASTM (2002) *Standard Test Method for Elements in Water by Inductively-Coupled Argon Plasma Atomic Emission Spectroscopy, Designation: D1976-02*, West Conshohocken, PA, USA, ASTM International

ASTM (2003a) *Standard Test Method for Elements in Water by Inductively-Coupled Plasma — Mass Spectrometry, Designation: D5673-03*, West Conshohocken, PA, USA, ASTM International

ASTM (2003b) *Standard Test Method for On-Line Measurement of Low Level Particulate and Dissolved Metals in Water by X-Ray Fluorescence (XRF), Designation D6502-99 (Reapproved 2003)*, West Conshohocken, PA, USA, ASTM International

ATSDR (1999) *Toxicological Profile for Lead*, Washington DC, US Department of Health and Human Services, Public Health Service, Agency for Toxic Substances and Disease Registry

Aufderheide, A.C. & Wittmers, L.E., Jr (1992) Selected aspects of the spatial distribution of lead in bone. *Neurotoxicology*, **13**, 809–819

Aungst, B.J. & Fung, H.-L. (1981) Intestinal lead absorption in rats: Effects of circadian rhythm, food, undernourishment, and drugs which alter gastric emptying and GI motility. *Res. Commun. chem. Pathol. Pharmacol.*, **34**, 515–530

Aungst, B.J. & Fung, H.-L. (1985) The effects of dietary calcium on lead absorption, distribution, and elimination kinetics in rats. *J. Toxicol. environ. Health*, **16**, 147–159

Aungst, B.J., Dolce, J.A. & Fung, H.-L. (1981) The effect of dose on the disposition of lead in rats after intravenous and oral administration. *Toxicol. appl. Pharmacol.*, **61**, 48–57

Awad el Karim, M.A., Hamed, A.S., Elhaimi, Y.A. & Osman, Y. (1986) Effects of exposure to lead among lead–acid battery factory workers in Sudan. *Arch. environ. Health*, **41**, 261–265

Awasthi, S., Awasthi, R., Pande, V.K., Srivastav, R.C. & Frumkin, H. (1996) Blood lead in pregnant women in the urban slums of Lucknow, India. *Occup. environ. Med.*, **53**, 836–840

Awasthi, S., Awasthi, R. & Srivastav, R.C. (2002) Maternal blood lead level and outcomes of pregnancy in Lucknow, North India. *Indian Pediatr.*, **39**, 855–860

Azar, A., Trochimowicz, H.J. & Maxfield, M.E. (1973) Review of lead studies in animals carried out at Haskell Laboratory: Two-year feeding study and response to hemorrhage study. In: Environmental health aspects of lead. In: *Proceedings of an International Symposium, October 2–6 1972 Amsterdam*, pp. 199–210

Baer, R.D., Garcia de Alba, J., Cueto, L.M., Ackerman, A. & Davison, S. (1989) Lead based remedies for empacho: Patterns and consequences. *Soc. Sci. Med.*, **29**, 1373–1379

Baker, E.L., Folland, D., Taylor, T.A., Frank, M., Peterson, W., Lovejoy, G., Cox, D., Housworth, J. & Landrigan, P.J. (1977) Lead poisoning in children of lead workers. Home contamination with industrial dust. *New Engl. J. Med.*, **296**, 260–261

Baker, E.L., Jr, Landrigan, P.J., Barbour, A.G., Cox, D.H., Folland, D.S., Ligo, R.N. & Throckmorton, J. (1979) Occupational lead poisoning in the United States: Clinical and biochemical findings related to blood lead levels. *Br. J. ind. Med.*, **36**, 314–322

Balachandran, S., Meena, B.R. & Khillare, P.S. (2000) Particle size distribution and its elemental composition in the ambient air of Delhi. *Environ. int.*, **26**, 49–54

Baldwin, R.W., Cunningham, G.J. & Pratt, D. (1964) Carcinogenic action of motor engine oil additives. *Br. J. Cancer*, **18**, 503–507

Baló, J., Bajtai, A. & Szende, B. (1965) [Experimental afenoms of the kidney produced by chronic administration of lead phosphate.] *Skagyar Onkol.*, **9**, 144–151 (in Hungarian)

Baloh, R., Sturm, R., Green, B. & Gleser, G. (1975) Neuropsychological effects of chronic asymptomatic increased lead absorption. A controlled study. *Arch. Neurol.*, **32**, 326–330

Bannon, D.I., Portnoy, M.E., Olivi, L., Lees, P.S.J., Culotta, V.C. & Bressler, J.P. (2002) Uptake of lead and iron by divalent metal transporter 1 in yeast and mammalian cells. *Biochem. biophys. Res. Commun.*, **295**, 978–984

Barltrop, D. (1969) Transfer of lead to the human foetus. In: Barltrop, D. & Burland, W.L., eds, *Mineral Metabolism in Pediatrics*, Blackwell Scientific Publications, Oxford, pp. 135–151

Barltrop, D. & Khoo, H.E. (1976) The influence of dietary minerals and fat on the absorption of lead. *Sci. total Environ.*, **6**, 265–273

Barltrop, D. & Meek, F. (1975) Absorption of different lead compounds. *Postgrad. med. J.*, **51**, 805–809

Barltrop, D. & Meek, F. (1979) Effect of particle size on lead absorption from the gut. *Arch. environ. Health*, **34**, 280–285

Barltrop, D. & Strehlow, C.D. (1978) The absorption of lead by children. In: Kirchgessner, M., ed., *Trace Element Metabolism in Man and Animals III*, Technische Universität Munchen, Germany, Freising-Weihenstephan, pp. 332–334

Barratt, C.L.R., Davies, A.G., Bansal, M.R. & Williams, M.E. (1989) The effects of lead on the male rat reproductive system. *Andrologia*, **21**, 161–166

Barregård, L., Svalander, C., Schütz, A., Westberg, G., Sallsten, G., Blohmé, I., Mölne, J., Attman, P.-O. & Haglind, P. (1999) Cadmium, mercury, and lead in kidney cortex of the general Swedish population: A study of biopsies from living kidney donors. *Environ. Health Perspect.*, **107**, 867–871

Barry, P.S.I. (1975) A comparison of concentrations of lead in human tissues. *Br. J. ind. Med.*, **32**, 119–139

Barsan, M.E. & Miller, A. (1996) Health Hazard Evaluation Report, HETA 91-0346-2572, FBI Academy, Quantico, VA, USA, NIOSH

Barton, J.C. & Conrad, M.E. (1981) Effect of phosphate on the absorption and retention of lead in the rat. *Am. J. clin. Nutr.*, **34**, 2192–2198

Barton, J.C., Conrad, M.E., Harrison, L. & Nuby, S. (1978a) Effects of calcium on the absorption and retention of lead. *J. Lab. clin. Med.*, **91**, 366–376

Barton, J.C., Conrad, M.E., Nuby, S. & Harrison, L. (1978b) Effects of iron on the absorption and retention of lead. *J. Lab. clin. Med.*, **92**, 536–547

Barton, J.C., Conrad, M.E., Harrison, L. & Nuby, S. (1980) Effects of vitamin D on the absorption and retention of lead. *Am. J. Physiol.*, **238**, G124–130

Barton, J.C., Patton, M.A., Edwards, C.Q., Griffen, L.M., Kushner, J.P., Meeks, R.G. & Leggett, R.W. (1994) Blood lead concentrations in hereditary hemochromatosis. *J. lab. clin. Med.*, **124**, 193–198

Battistuzzi, G., Petrucci, R., Silvagni, L., Urbani, F.R. & Caiola, S. (1981) δ-Aminolevulinate dehydrase: A new genetic polymorphism in man. *Ann. hum. Genet.*, **45**, 223–229

Batuman, V., Maesaka, J.K., Haddad, B., Tepper, E., Landy, E. & Wedeen, R.P. (1981) The role of lead in gout nephropathy. *New Engl. J. Med.*, **304**, 520–523

Batuman, V., Landy, E., Maesaka, J.K. & Wedeen, R.P. (1983) Contribution of lead to hypertension with renal impairment. *New Engl. J. Med.*, **309**, 17–21

Bauchinger, M. & Schmid, E. (1972) [Chromosome analysis of cultures of Chinese hamster cells after treatment with lead acetate.] *Mutat. Res.*, **14**, 95–100 (in German)

Bauchinger, M., Dresp, J., Schmid, E., Englert, N. & Krause, C. (1977) Chromosome analyses of children after ecological lead exposure. *Mutat. Res.*, **56**, 75–80

Baum, C.R. & Shannon, M.W. (1997) The lead concentration of reconstituted infant formula. *Clin. Toxicol.*, **35**, 371–375

Bearer, C.F., O'Riordan, M.A. & Powers, R. (2000) Lead exposure from blood transfusion to premature infants. *J. Pediatr.*, **137**, 549–554

Bearer, C.F., Linsalata, N., Yomtovian, R., Walsh, M. & Singer, L. (2003) Blood transfusions: A hidden source of lead exposure. *Lancet*, **362**, 332

Beckett, P.H., Davis, R.D. & Brindley, P. (1979) The disposal of sewage sludge onto farmland: The scope of the problem of toxic elements. *Water Pollut. Control*, **78**, 419–436

Beek, B. & Obe, G. (1974) Effect of lead acetate on human leukocyte chromosomes *in vitro*. *Experientia*, **30**, 1006–1007

Beek, B. & Obe, G. (1975) The human leukocyte test system. VI. The use of sister chromatid exchanges as possible indicators for mutagenic activities. *Humangenetik*, **29**, 127–134

Behari, J.R., Singh, S. & Tandon, S.K. (1983) Lead poisoning among Indian silver jewellery makers. *Ann. occup. Hyg.*, **27**, 107–109

Bell, C.E., Baldwin, L.A., Kostecki, P.T. & Calabrese, E.J. (1993) Comparative response of rainbow trout and rat to the liver mitogen, lead. *Ecotoxicol. environ. Saf.*, **26**, 280–284

Bellinger, D.C., Needleman, H.L., Leviton, A., Waternaux, C., Rabinowitz, M.R. & Nichols, M.L. (1984) Early sensory-motor development and prenatal exposure to lead. Neurobehav. *Toxicol. Teratol.*, **6**, 387–402

Bellinger, D., Leviton, A., Rabinowitz, M., Allred, E., Needleman, H. & Schoenbaum, S. (1991) Weight gain and maturity in fetuses exposed to low levels of lead. *Environ. Res.*, **54**, 151–158

Bellinger, D.C., Stiles, K.M. & Needleman, H.L. (1992) Low-level lead exposure, intelligence and academic achievement: A long-term follow-up study. *Pediatrics*, **90**, 855–861

Bener, A., Almehdi, AM., Alwash, R. & Al-Neamy, F.R.M. (2001) A pilot survey of blood lead levels in various types of workers in the United Arab Emirates. *Environ. int.*, **27**, 311–314

Benkmann, H.-G., Bogdanski, P. & Goedde, H.W. (1983) Polymorphism of delta-aminolevulinic acid dehydratase in various populations. *Hum. Hered.*, **33**, 62–64

Benoff, S., Cooper, G.W., Centola, G.M., Jacob, A., Hershlag, A. & Hurley, I.R. (2000) Metal ions and human sperm mannose receptors. *Andrologia*, **32**, 317–319

Benoff, S., Centola, G.M., Millan, C., Napolitano, B., Marmar, J.L. & Hurley, I.R. (2003) Increased seminal plasma lead levels adversely affect the fertility potential of sperm in IVF. *Hum. Reprod.*, **18**, 374–383

Benson, G.I., George, W.H.S., Litchfield, M.H. & Seaborn, D.J. (1976) Biochemical changes during the initial stages of industrial lead exposure. *Br. J. ind. Med.*, **33**, 29–35

Berg, J.W. & Burbank, F. (1972) Correlations between carcinogenic trace metals in water supplies and cancer mortality. *Ann. N. Y. Acad. Sci.*, **199**, 249–264

Bergdahl, I.A. & Skerfving, S. (1997) Partition of circulating lead between plasma and red cells does not seem to be different for internal and external sources of lead. *Am. J. ind. Med.*, **32**, 317–318

Bergdahl, I.A., Schütz, A., Gerhardsson, L., Jensen, A. & Skerfving, S. (1997a) Lead concentrations in human plasma, urine and whole blood. *Scand. J. Work Environ. Health*, **23**, 359–363

Bergdahl, I.A., Grubb, A., Schütz, A., Desnick, R.J., Wetmur, J.G., Sassa, S. & Skerfving, S. (1997b) Lead binding to δ-aminolevulinic acid dehydratase (ALAD) in human erythrocytes. *Pharmacol. Toxicol.*, **81**, 153–158

Bergdahl, I.A., Gerhardsson, L., Schütz, A., Desnick, R.J., Wetmur, J.G. & Skerfving, S. (1997c) delta-Aminolevulinic acid dehydratase polymorphism: Influence on lead levels and kidney function in humans. *Arch. environ. Health*, **52**, 91–96

Bergdahl, I.A., Sheveleva, M., Schütz, A., Artamonova, V.G. & Skerfving, S. (1998a) Plasma and blood lead in humans: Capacity-limited binding to δ-aminolevulinic acid dehydratase and other lead-binding components. *Toxicol. Sci.*, **46**, 247–253

Bergdahl, I.A., Strömberg, U., Gerhardsson, L., Schütz, A., Chettle, D.R. & Skerfving, S. (1998b) Lead concentrations in tibial and calcaneal bone in relation to the history of occupational lead exposure. *Scand. J. Work environ. Health*, **24**, 38–45

Bergdahl, I.A., Vahter, M., Counter, S.A., Schutz, A., Buchanan, L.H., Ortega, F., Laurell, G. & Skerfving, S. (1999) Lead in plasma and whole blood from lead-exposed children. *Environ. Res.*, **80**, 25–33

Berglund, M., Åkesson, A., Bjellerup, P. & Vahter, M. (2000) Metal-bone interactions. *Toxicol. Lett.*, **112–113**, 219–225

Berlin, A. & Schaller, K.H. (1974) European standardized method for the determination of δ-aminolevulinic acid dehydratase activity in blood. *Z. klin. Chem. klin. Biochem.*, **12**, 389–390

Bernard, S.M. (2003) Should the Centers for Disease Control and Prevention's childhood lead poisoning intervention level be lowered? *Am. J. publ. Health*, **93**, 1253–1260

Bertazzi, P.A. & Zocchetti, C. (1980) A mortality study of newspaper printing workers. *Am. J. ind. Med.*, **1**, 85–97

Bhattacharya, A., Shukla, R., Bornshein, R., Dietrich, K. & Kopke, J.E. (1988) Postural disequilibrium quantification in children with chronic lead exposure: A pilot study. *NeuroToxicology*, **9**, 327–340

Bhattacharya, A., Shukla, R. & Bornshein, R.L., Dietrich, K.N. & Keith, R. (1990) Lead effects on postural balance of children. *Environ. Health. Perspect.*, **89**, 35–42

Bhattacharya, A., Shukla, R., Kietrich, K.N., Miller, J., Bagchee, A., Bornschein, R.L., Cox, C. & Mitchell, T. (1993) Functional implications of postural disequilibrium due to lead exposure. *Neurotoxicology*, **14**, 179–189

Biagini, G., Misciattelli, M.E., Contri Baccarani, M., Vangelista, A., Raffi, G.B. & Caudarella, R. (1977) [Electron microscopy features of renal changes in chronic lead poisoning.] *Lav. Um.*, **29**, 179–187 (in Italian)

Bicknell, R.J. (1982) Health Hazard Evaluation Report, HETA 82-0255-1193, Firing Range — Police Dept., Cape Girardeau, MO, USA, NIOSH

Bijlsma, J.B. & de France, H.F. (1976) Cytogenetic investigations in volunteers ingesting inorganic lead. *Int. Arch. occup. environ. Health*, **38**, 145–148

Birch, J., Harrison, R.M. & Laxen, D.P.H. (1980) A specific method for 24–48 hour analysis of tetraalkyl lead in air. *Sci. tot. Environ.*, **14**, 31–42

Blade, L.M. & Bresler, F.T. (1994) Health Hazard Evaluation Report, HETA 91-0292-2467, Magnetics Division of Spang & Co., Butler, PA, USA, NIOSH

Blake, K.C.H. (1976) Absorption of ^{203}Pb from gastrointestinal tract of man. *Environ. Res.*, **11**, 1–4

Blake, K.C. & Mann, M. (1983) Effect of calcium and phosphorus on the gastrointestinal absorption of ^{203}Pb in man. *Environ. Res.*, **30**, 188–194

Blakley, B.R. (1987) The effect of lead on chemical- and viral-induced tumor production in mice. *J. appl. Toxicol.*, **7**, 167–172

Blank, E. & Howieson, J. (1983) Lead poisoning from a curtain weight. *J. Am. med. Assoc.*, **249**, 2176–2177

Blaylock, M.J., Salt, D.E., Dushenkov, S., Zakharova, O., Gussman, C., Kapulnik, Y., Ensley, B.D. & Raskin, I. (1997) Enhanced accumulation of Pb in Indian mustard by soil-applied chelating agents. *Environ. Sci. Technol.,* **31**, 860–865

Bloom, N.S. & Crecelius, E.A. (1987) Distribution of silver, mercury, lead, copper and cadmium in Central Puget Sound sediments. *Marine Chem.*, **21**, 377–390

Bloomer, J.R., Reuter, R.J., Morton, K.O. & Wehner, J.M. (1983) Enzymatic formation of zinc-protoporphyrin by rat liver and its potential effect on hepatic heme metabolism. *Gastroentero-logy*, **85**, 663–668

Boerngen, J.G. & Shacklette, H.T. (1981) *Chemical Analyses of Soils and Other Surficial Materials of the Conterminous United States*, US Geological Survey, Open-File Report 81–197, Denver, CO, US Geological Survey

Bogden, J.D., Gertner, S.B., Kemp, F.W., McLeod, R., Bruening, K.S. & Chung, H.R. (1991) Dietary lead and calcium: Effects on blood pressure and renal neoplasia in Wistar rats. *J. Nutr.*, **121**, 718–728

Bolanowska, W. (1968) Distribution and excretion of triethyllead in rats. *Br. J. ind. Med.*, **25**, 203–208

Bolanowska, W., Piotrowski, J. & Garczynski, H. (1967) Triethyllead in the biological material in cases of acute tetraethyllead poisoning. *Arch. Toxikol.*, **22**, 278–282

Bolger, P.M., Carrington, C.D., Capar, S.G. & Adams, M.A. (1991) Reductions in dietary lead exposure in the United States. *Chem. Spec. Bioavail.*, **3**, 31–36

Bonanno, J., Robson, M.G., Buckley, B. & Modica, M. (2002) Lead exposure at a covered outdoor firing range. *Bull. Environ. Contam. Toxicol.*, **68**, 315–323

Bonde, J.P., Giwercman, A. & Ernst, E. (1996) Identifying environmental risk to male reproductive function by occupational sperm studies: Logistics and design options. *Occup. environ. Med.*, **53**, 511–519

Bonde, J.P., Joffe, M., Apostoli, P., Dale, A., Kiss, P., Spano, M., Caruso, F., Giwercman, A., Bisanti, L., Porru, S., Vanhoorne, M., Camhaire, F. & Zschiesche, W. (2002) Sperm count and chromatin structure in men exposed to inorganic lead: Lowest adverse effect levels. *Occup. environ. Med.*, **59**, 234–242

Bono, R., Pignata, C., Scursatone, E., Rovere, R., Natale, P. & Gilli, G. (1995) Updating about reductions of air and blood lead concentrations in Turin, Italy, following reductions in the lead content of gasoline. *Environ. Res.*, **70**, 30–34

Booze, R.M., Mactutus, C.F., Annau, Z. & Tilson, H.A. (1983) Neonatal triethyl lead neurotoxicity in rat pups: Initial behavioral observations and quantification. *Neurobehav. Toxicol. Teratol.*, **5**, 367–375

Börjesson, J., Mattsson, S., Strömberg, U., Gerhardsson, L., Schütz, A. & Skerfving, S. (1997) Lead in fingerbone: A tool for retrospective exposure assessment. *Arch. environ. Health*, **52**, 104–112

Boscolo, P. & Carmignani, M. (1988) Neurohumoral blood pressure regulation in lead exposure. *Environ. Health Perspect.*, **78**, 101–106

Boscolo, P., Carmignani, M., Sacchettoni-Logroscino, G., Rannelletti, F.O., Artese, L. & Preziosi P. (1988) Ultrastructure of the testis in rats with blood hypertension induced by long-term lead exposure. *Toxicol. Lett.*, **41**, 129–137

Boudene, C., Malet, D. & Masse, R. (1977) Fate of ^{210}Pb inhaled by rats. *Toxicol. appl. Pharmacol.*, **41**, 271–276

Bouldin, T.W. & Krigman, M.R. (1975) Acute lead encephalopathy in the guinea pig. *Acta neuropathol.*, **33**, 185–190

Boulos, B.M. & von Smolinski, A. (1988) Alert to users of calcium supplements as antihypertensive agents due to trace metal contaminants. *Am. J. Hypertension*, **1**, 137S–142S

Bourgoin, B.P., Evans, D.R., Cornett, J.R., Lingard, S.M. & Quattrone, A.J. (1993) Lead content in 70 brands of dietary calcium supplements. *Am. J. public Health*, **83**, 1155–1160

Bouton, C.M., Hossain, M.A., Frelin, L.P., Laterra, J. & Pevsner, J. (2001) Microarray analysis of differential gene expression in lead-exposed astrocytes. *Toxicol. appl. Pharmacol.*, **176**, 34–53

Boyland, E., Dukes, C.E., Grover, P.L. & Mitchley, B.C.V. (1962). The induction of renal tumours by feeding lead acetate to rats. *Br. J. Cancer*, **16**, 283–288

Bradbury, M.W.B. & Deane, R. (1993) Permeability of the blood-brain barrier to lead. *Neurotoxicology*, **14**, 131–136

Bress, W.C. & Bidanset, J.H. (1991) Percutaneous in vivo and in vitro absorption of lead. *Vet. hum. Toxicol.*, **33**, 212–214

Bressler, J., Kim, K., Chakraborti, T. & Goldstein, G. (1999) Molecular mechanisms of lead neurotoxicity. *Neurochem. Res.*, **24**, 595–600

Brito, J.A.A., McNeill, F.E., Stronach, I., Webber, C.E., Wells, S., Richard, N. & Chettle, D.R. (2001) Longitudinal changes in bone lead concentration: Implications for modelling of human bone lead metabolism. *J. environ. Monit.*, **3**, 343–351

Brody, D.J., Pirkle, J.L., Kramer, R.A., Flegal, K.M., Matte, T.D., Gunter, E.W. & Pashal, D.C. (1994) Blood lead levels in the US population. Phase 1 of the Third National Health and Nutrition Examination Survey (NHANES III, 1988 to 1991). *J. Am. med. Assoc.*, **272**, 277–283

Brown, J.R. (1983) A survey of the effects of lead on gunners. *J. R. Army med. Corps*, **129**, 75–81

Brown, A. & Tompsett, S.L. (1945) Poisoning due to mobilization of lead from the skeleton by leucaemic hyperplasia of bone marrow. *Br. med. J.*, **11**, 764–765

Brown, M.J., Hu, H., Gonzales-Cossio, T., Peterson, K.E., Sanin, L.-H., de Luz Kageyama, M., Palazuelos, E., Aro, A., Schnaas, L. & Hernandez-Avila, M. (2000) Determinants of bone and blood lead concentrations in the early postpartum period. *Occup. environ. Med.*, **57**, 535–541

Browne, D.R., Husni, A. & Risk, M.J. (1999) Airborne lead and particulate levels in Semarang, Indonesia and potential health impacts. *Sci. total Environ.*, **227**, 145–154

Bruaux, P. & Svartengren, M., eds (1985) *Assessment of Human Exposure to Lead: Comparison between Belgium, Malta, Mexico and Sweden*, National Swedish Institute of Environmental

Medicine, Department of Environmental Hygiene, Karolinska Institute, Stockholm and Institute of Hygiene and Epidemiology, Ministry of Health, Brussels
Bruce, W.R. & Heddle, J.A. (1979) The mutagenic activity of 61 agents as determined by the micronucleus, *Salmonella*, and sperm abnormality assays. *Can. J. Genet. Cytol.*, **21**, 319–334
Bruyneel, M., De Caluwe, J.P., des Grottes, J.M. & Collart, F. (2002) [Use of kohl and severe lead poisoning in Brussels.] *Rev. méd. Brux.*, **23**, 519–522 (in French)
Buchet, J.P., Lauwerys, R., Roels, H. & Hubermont, G. (1977) Mobilization of lead during pregnancy in rats. *Int. Arch. occup. environ. Health*, **40**, 33–36
Buchet, J.P., Roels, H., Bernard, A. & Lauwerys, R. (1980) Assessment of renal function of workers exposed to inorganic lead, calcium or mercury vapor. *J. occup. Med.*, **22**, 741–750
Buchet, J.P., Lauwerys, R., Vandevoorde, A. & Pycke, J.M. (1983) Oral daily intake of cadmium, lead, manganese, copper, chromium, mercury, calcium, zinc and arsenic in Belgium: A duplicate meal study. *Food chem. Toxicol.*, **21**, 19–24
Buckley, J.D., Robison, L.L., Swotinsky, R., Garabrant, D.H., LeBeau, M., Manchester, P., Nesbit, M.E., Odom, L., Peters, J.M., Woods, W.G. & Hammond, G.D. (1989) Occupational exposures of parents of children with acute nonlymphocytic leukemia: A report from the Childrens Cancer Study Group. *Cancer Res.*, **49**, 4030–4037
Bull, R.J., McCauley, P.T., Taylor, D.H. & Croften, K.M. (1983) The effects of lead on the developing central nervous system of the rat. *NeuroToxicology*, **4**, 1–18
Bull, R.J., Robinson, M. & Laurie, R.D. (1986) Association of carcinoma yield with early papilloma development in SENCAR mice. *Environ. Health Perspect.*, **68**, 11–17
Bunn, T.L., Parsons, P.J., Kao, E. & Dietert, R.R. (2001) Exposure to lead during critical windows of embryonic development: Differential immunotoxic outcome based on stage of exposure and gender. *Toxicol. Sci.*, **64**, 57–66
Bu-Olayan, A.H. & Al-Yakoob, S. (1998) Lead, nickel and vanadium in seafood: An exposure assessment for Kuwaiti consumers. *Sci. total Environ.*, **223**, 81–86
Burger, J., Kennamer, R.A., Brisbin, I.L., Jr & Gochfeld, M. (1997) Metal levels in mourning doves from South Carolina: Potential hazards to doves and hunters. *Environ. Res.*, **75**, 173–186
Burger, J., Kennamer, R.A., Brisbin, I.L., Jr & Gochfeld, M. (1998) A risk assessment for consumers of mourning doves. *Risk Anal.*, **18**, 563–573
Burmaa, B., Dorogova, V.B., Enhtsetseg, S., Erdenechtsmeg, E. & Enkhzhargal, A. (2002) [Impact of lead-induced environmental pollution on children's health in Mongolia.] *Gig. Sanit.*, **3**, 21–23 (in Russian)
Burns, C.B. & Currie, B. (1995) The efficacy of chelation therapy and factors influencing mortality in lead intoxicated petrol sniffers. *Aust. N.Z. J. Med.*, **25**, 197–203
Buscema, I., Prieto, A., Araujo, L. & Gonzalez, G. (1997) Determination of lead and cadmium content in the rice consumed in Maracaibo, Venezuela. *Bull. environ. Contam. Toxicol.*, **59**, 94–98
Bush, V.J., Moyer, T.P., Batts, K.P. & Parisi, J.E. (1995) Essential and toxic element concentrations in fresh and formalin-fixed human autopsy tissues. *Clin. Chem.*, **41**, 284–294
Bushnell, P.J. & DeLuca, H.F. (1983) The effects of lactose on the absorption and retention of dietary lead. *J. Nutr.*, **113**, 365–378
Büsselberg, D. (1995) Calcium channels as target sites of heavy metals. *Toxicol. Lett.*, **82–83**, 255–261
Byers, R.K. & Lord, E.E. (1943) Late effects of lead poisoning on mental development. *Am. J. Dis. Child.*, **66**, 471–494

Cai, M.-Y. & Arenaz, P. (1998) Antimutagenic effect of crown ethers on heavy metal-induced sister chromatid exchanges. *Mutagenesis*, **13**, 27–32

Cake, K.M., Bowins, R.J., Vaillancourt, C., Gordon, C.L., McNutt, R.H., Laporte, R., Webber, C.E. & Chettle, D.R. (1996) Partition of circulating lead between serum and red cells is different for internal and external sources of lead. *Am. J. ind. Med.*, **29**, 440–445

Calabrese, E.J. & Baldwin, L.A. (1992) Lead-induced cell proliferation and organ-specific tumorigenicity. *Drug Metab. Rev.*, **24**, 409–416

Calabrese, E.J., Baldwin, L.A., Leonard, D.A. & Zhao, X.Q. (1995) Decrease in hepatotoxicity by lead exposure is not explained by its mitogenic response. *J. appl. Toxicol.*, **15**, 129–132

Calder, I.C., Roder, D.M., Esterman, A.J., Lewis, M.J., Harrison, M.C. & Oldfield, R.K. (1986) Blood lead levels in children in the north-west of Adelaide. *Med. J. Aust.*, **144**, 509–512

Campbell, B.C., Beattie, A.D., Moore, M.R., Goldberg, A. & Reid, A.G. (1977) Renal insufficiency associated with excessive lead exposure. *Br. med. J.*, **1**, 482–485

Campbell, B.C., Meredith, P.A., Moore, M.R. & Watson, W.S. (1984) Kinetics of lead following intravenous administration in man. *Toxicol. Lett.*, **21**, 231–235

Canfield, R.L., Henderson, C.R., Jr, Cory-Slechta, D.A., Cox, C., Jusko, T.A. & Lanphear, B.P. (2003) Intellectual impairment in children with blood lead concentrations below 10 micrograms per deciliter. *New Engl. J. Med.*, **348**, 1517–1526

Capar, S.G. & Gould, J.H. (1979) Lead, fluoride, and other elements in bonemeal supplements. *J. Assoc. off. anal. Chem.*, **62**, 1054–1061

Capar, S.G. & Rigsby, E.J. (1989) Survey of lead in canned evaporated milk. *J. Assoc. off. anal. Chem.*, **72**, 416–417

Cárdenas, A., Roels, H., Bernard, A.M., Barbon, R., Buchet, J.P., Lauwerys, R.R., Roselló, J., Ramis, I., Mutti, A., Franchini, I., Fels, L.M., Stolte, H., de Broe, M.E., Nuyts, G.D., Taylor, S.A. & Price, R.G. (1993) Markers of early renal changes induced by industrial pollutants. II. Application to workers exposed to lead. *Br. J. ind. Med.*, **50**, 28–36

Carney, J.K. & Garbarino, K.M. (1997) Childhood lead poisoning from apple cider. *Pediatrics*, **100**, 1048–1049

Caroli, S., Alimonti, A., Coni, E., Petrucci, F., Senofonte, O. & Violante, N. (1994). The assessment of reference values for elements in human biological tissues and fluids: A systematic review. *Crit. Rev. anal. Chem.*, **24**, 363–398

Carta, P., Cocco, P. & Picchiri, G. (1994) Lung cancer mortality and airways obstruction among metal miners exposed to silica and low levels of radon daughters. *Am. J. ind. Med.*, **25**, 489–506

Carvalho, F.M., Barreto, M.L., Silvany-Neto, A.M., Waldron, H.A. & Tavares, T.M. (1984) Multiple causes of anaemia amongst children living near a lead smelter in Brazil. *Sci. total Environ.*, **35**, 71–84

Carvalho, F.M., Silvany-Neto, A.M., Tavares, T.M., Lima, M.E.C. & Waldron, H.A. (1985a) Lead poisoning among children from Santo Amaro, Brazil. *Bull. PAHO*, **19**, 165–175

Carvalho, F.M., Silvany-Neto, A.M., Lima, M.E.C., Tavares, T.M. & Alt, F. (1985b) [Lead and cadmium poisoning among workers in small establishments for repairing batteries in Salvador, Brazil.] *Rev. Saúde pública*, **19**, 411–420 (in Portuguese)

Carvalho, F.M., Silvany-Neto, A.M., Chaves, M.E.C., de Melo, A.M.C., Galvão, A.L. & Tavares, T.M. (1989) [Lead and cadmium contents in hair of children from Santo Amaro da Purificação, Bahia.] *Ciê. Cultura*, **41**, 646–651 (in Portuguese)

Carvalho, F.M., Silvany-Neto, A.M., Peres, M.F.T., Gonçalves, H.R., Guimarães, G.C., de Amorin, C.J.B., Silva, J.A.S., Jr & Tavares, T.M. (1996) [Lead poisoning: Zinc protoporphyrin in blood of children from Santo Amaro da Purificação and Salvador, Bahia. Brazil.] *J. Pediatr.*, **72**, 295–298 (in Portuguese)

Carvalho, F.M., Neto, A.M.S., Peres, M.F.T., Gonçalves, H.R., Guimarães, G.C., de Amorin, C.J.B., Silva, J.A.S., Jr & Tavares, T.M. (1997) Lead poisoning: Zinc protoporphyrin in blood of children from Santo Amaro da Purificação and Salvador, Bahia, Brazil. *J. pediatr.*, **73** (Suppl. 1), 11–14

Carvalho, F.M., Silvany Neto, A.M., Tavares, T.M., Costa, A.C.A., Chaves, C.R., Nascimento, L.D. & Reis, M.A. (2003) [Blood lead levels in children and environmental legacy of a lead foundry in Brazil.] *Rev. panam. Salud publica*, **13**, 19–23 (in Portuguese)

Case, J.M., Reif, C.B. & Timko, A. (1989) Lead in the bottom sediments of Lake Nuangola and fourteen other bodies of water in Luzerne County, Pennsylvania. *J. Pennsylvania Acad. Sci.*, **63**, 67–72

Casteel, S.W., Cowart, R.P., Weis, C.P., Henningsen, G.M., Hoffman, E., Brattin, W.J., Guzman, R.E., Starost, M.F., Payne, J.T., Stockham, S.L., Becker, S.V., Drexler, J.W. & Turk, J.R. (1997) Bioavailability of lead to juvenile swine dosed with soil from the Smuggler Mountain NPL Site of Aspen, Colorado. *Fundam. appl. Toxicol.*, **36**, 177–187

Castellino, N., Lamanna, P. & Grieco, B. (1966) Biliary excretion of lead in the rat. *Br. J. ind. Med.*, **23**, 237–239

Cavalleri, A. & Minoia, C. (1987) Lead level of whole blood and plasma in workers exposed to lead stearate. *Scand. J. Work Environ. Health*, **13**, 218–220

CDC (1975) *Increased Lead Absorption and Lead Poisoning in Young Children. A Statement by the Center for Disease Control*, Atlanta, GA, Centers for Disease Control, US Department of Health, Education and Welfare

CDC (1981) Use of lead tetroxide as a folk remedy for gastrointestinal illness. *Mortal. Morbid. Wkly Rep.*, **30**, 546–547

CDC (1983) Folk remedy-associated lead poisoning in Hmong children — Minnesota. *Mortal. Morbid. Wkly Rep.*, **32**, 555–556

CDC (1985) *Preventing Lead Poisoning in Young Children* (Publication No. 99-2230), Atlanta, GA, Centers for Disease Control

CDC (1991) *Preventing Lead Poisoning in Young Children*, Atlanta, GA, Centers for Disease Control

CDC (1993) Lead poisoning associated with use of traditional ethnic remedies — California, 1991–1992. *Mortal. Morbid. Wkly Rep.*, **42**, 521–524

CDC (1997a) Children with elevated blood lead levels attributed to home renovation and remodeling activities — New York, 1993–1994. *Mortal. Morbid. Wkly Rep.*, **45**, 1120–1123

CDC (1997b) Update: Blood lead levels — United States, 1991–1994. *Morbid. Mortal. Wkly Rep.*, **46**, 141–146

CDC (1998) Lead poisoning associated with imported candy and powdered food coloring — California and Michigan. *Mortal. Morbid. Wkly Rep.*, **47**, 1041–1043

CDC (1999) Adult lead poisoning from an Asian remedy for menstrual cramps — Connecticut, 1997. *Mortal. Morbid. Wkly Rep.*, **48**, 27–29

CDC (2001) Public health dispatch: Potential risk for lead exposure in dental offices. *Mortal. Morbid. Wkly Rep.*, **50**, 873–874

CDC (2002) Childhood lead poisoning associated with tamarind candy and folk remedies — California, 1999–2000. *Mortal. Morbid. Wkly Rep.*, **51**, 684-686

CDC (2003a) *Second National Report on Human Exposure to Environmental Chemicals, NCEH Pub. No. 02-0716*, Atlanta, GA, National Center for Environmental Health, pp. 9–12

CDC (2003b) Surveillance for elevated blood lead levels among children — United States, 1997–2001. *Mortal. Morbid. Wkly Rep.*, **52**, SS-10

Cedeño, A.L., Arrocha, A. & Lombardi, C. (1990) *Comparative Study of the Levels of Lead in the Air and Blood Part II* (Technical Report), Los Teques, Intevep SA

Central Pollution Control Board (1998–99) *Annual Report 1998–1999*, New Delhi, Central Pollution Control Board

Central Pollution Control Board (2001–02) *Annual Report (2001–2002)*, New Delhi, Central Pollution Control Board [http://www.cpcb.delhi.nic.in/ar2002/ar1-2content.htm; accessed 31/12/2003]

Chai, S. & Webb, R.C. (1988) Effects of lead on vascular reactivity. *Environ. Health Perspect.*, **78**, 85–89

Chakraborti, D., De Jonghe, W.R.A., Van Mol, W.E., Van Cleuvenbergen, R.J.A. & Adams, F.C. (1984) Determination of ionic alkyllead compounds in water by gas chromatography/atomic absorption spectrometry. *Anal. Chem.*, **56**, 2692–2697

Chamberlain, A.C., Heard. M.J., Little, P., Newton, D., Wells, A.C. & Wiffen, R.D. (1978) *Investigations into Lead from Motor Vehicles* (Rep. AERE-R9198), Harwell, United Kingdom Atomic Energy Authority

Chandra, P., Tripathi, R.D., Rai, U.N., Sinha, S. & Garg, P. (1993) Biomonitoring and amelioration of nonpoint source pollution in some aquatic bodies. *Water Sci. Technol.*, **28**, 323–326

Chaney, R.L., Malik, M., Li, Y.M., Brown, S.L., Brewer, E.P., Angle, J.S. & Baker, A.J.M. (1997) Phytoremediation of soil metals. *Curr. Opin. Biotechnol.*, **8**, 279–284

Chartsias, B., Colombo, A., Hatzichristidis, D. & Leyendecker, W. (1986) The impact of gasoline lead on man blood lead: First results of the Athens lead experiment. *Sci. total Environ.*, **55**, 275–283

Chatterjee, A. & Banerjee, R.N. (1999) Determination of lead and other metals in a residential area of greater Calcutta. *Sci. total Environ.*, **227**, 175–185

Chau, T.T., Chen, W.Y., Hsiao, T.M. & Liu, H.W. (1995) Chronic lead intoxication at an indoor firing range in Taiwan. *Clin. Toxicol.*, **33**, 371–372

Chemical Information Services (2003) *Directory of World Chemical Producers (Online Version)*, Dallas, TX [www.chemicalinfo.com; accessed 12/12/2003]

Chen, Z.-Q., Chan, Q.-I., Par, C.-C. & Qu, J.-Y. (1985) Peripheral nerve conduction velocity in workers occupationally exposed to lead. *Scand. J. Work Environ. Health.*, **11** (Suppl. 4), 26–28

Cheng, Y., Willett, W.C., Schwartz, J., Sparrow, D., Weiss, S. & Hu, H. (1998) Relation of nutrition to bone lead and blood lead levels in middle-aged to elderly men. The Normative Aging Study. *Am. J. Epidemiol.*, **147**, 1162–1174

Cheng, Y., Schwartz, J., Sparrow, D., Aro, A., Weiss, S.T. & Hu, H. (2001) Bone lead and blood lead levels in relation to baseline blood pressure and the prospective development of hypertension: The Normative Aging Study. *Am. J. Epidemiol.*, **153**, 164–171

Chettle, D.R., Fleming, D.E., McNeill, F.E. & Webber, C.E. (1997) Serum (plasma) lead, blood lead, and bone lead. *Am. J. ind. Med.*, **32**, 319–320

Chia, S.E., Chia, K.S. & Ong, C.N. (1991) Ethnic differences in blood lead concentration among workers in a battery manufacturing factory. *Ann. Acad. Med. Singapore*, **20**, 758–761

Chia, S.E., Phoon, W.H., Lee, H.S., Tan, K.T. & Jeyaratnam, J. (1993) Exposure to neurotoxic metals among workers in Singapore: An overview. *Occup. Med.*, **43**, 18–22

Chia, S.E., Chua, L.H., Ng, T.P., Foo, S.C. & Jeyaratnam, J. (1994) Postural stability of workers exposed to lead. *Occup. environ. Med.*, **51**, 768–771

Chia, K.S., Jeyaratnam, J., Lee, J., Tan, C., Ong, H.Y., Ong, C.N. & Lee, E. (1995) Lead-induced nephropathy: Relationship between various biological exposure indices and early markers of nephrotoxicity. *Am. J. ind. Med.*, **27**, 883–895

Chia, S.E., Chia, H.P., Ong, C.N. & Jeyaratnam, J. (1996a) Cumulative blood lead levels and nerve conduction parameters. *Occup. Med.*, **46**, 59–64

Chia, S.E., Chia, H.P., Ong, C.N. & Jeyaratnam, J. (1996b) Cumulative concentrations of blood lead and postural stability. *Occup. environ. Med.*, **53**, 264–268

Chiaradia, M., Gulson, B.L. & MacDonald, K. (1997) Contamination of houses by workers occupationally exposed in a lead-zinc-copper mine and impact on blood lead concentrations in the families. *Occup. environ. Med.*, **54**, 117–124

Chiba, M. (1976) Activity of erythrocyte δ-aminolevulinic acid dehydrase and its change by heat treatment as indices of lead exposure. *Br. J. ind. Med.*, **33**, 36–42

Chisholm, J.J., Jr (1962) Aminoaciduria as a manifestation of renal tubular injury in lead intoxication and a comparison with patterns of aminoaciduria seen in other diseases. *J. Pediatr.*, **60**, 1–17

Chisolm, J.J., Jr (1964) Disturbances in the biosynthesis of heme in lead intoxication. *J. Pediatr.*, **64**, 174–187

Chisolm, J.J., Jr (1986) Removal of lead paint from old housing: The need for a new approach. *Am. J. public Health*, **76**, 236–237

Cho, H.Y., Moon, D.H., Jun, J.H., Lee, C.U. & Kim, S.C. (1992) The level of ambient heavy metal pollution in Pusan area. *Inje Med. J.*, **13**, 177–190

Choie, D.D. & Richter, G.W. (1972a) Cell proliferation in rat kidneys after prolonged treatment with lead. *Am. J. Pathol.*, **68**, 359–370

Choie, D.D. & Richter, G.W. (1972b) Lead poisoning: Rapid formation of intranuclear inclusions. *Science*, **177**, 1194–1195

Choie, D.D. & Richter, G.W. (1972c) Cell proliferation in rat kidney induced by lead acetate and effects of uninephrectomy on the proliferation. *Am. J. Pathol.*, **66**, 265–275

Choie, D.D. & Richter, G.W. (1974a) Cell proliferation in mouse kidney induced by lead. I. Synthesis of deoxyribonucleic acid. *Lab. Invest.*, **30**, 647–651

Choie, D.D. & Richter, G.W. (1974b) Cell proliferation in mouse kidney induced by lead. II. Synthesis of ribonucleic acid and protein. *Lab. Invest.*, **30**, 652–656

Choie, D.D. & Richter, G.W. (1978) G2 sub-population in mouse liver induced into mitosis by lead acetate. *Cell Tissue Kinet.*, **11**, 235–239

Chowdhury, A.R., Dewan, A. & Gandhi, D.N. (1984) Toxic effect of lead on the testes of rat. *Biomed. biochim. Acta*, **43**, 95–100

Christoffersson, J.O., Ahlgren, L., Schütz, A., Skerfving, S. & Mattsson, S. (1986) Decrease of skeletal lead levels in man after end of occupational exposure. *Arch. environ. Health*, **41**, 312–318

Chu, N.F., Liou, S.H., Wu, T.N., Ko, K.N. & Chang, P.Y. (1998) Risk factors for high blood lead levels among the general population in Taiwan. *Eur. J. Epidemiol.*, **14**, 775–781

Chuang, H.-Y., Lee, M-.L.T., Chao, K.-Y., Wang, J.-D., Hu, H. (1999) Relationship of blood lead levels to personal hygiene habits in lead battery workers: Taiwan, 1991–1997. *Am. J. ind. Med.*, **35**, 595–603

Cikrt, M. (1972) Biliary excretion of ^{203}Hg, ^{64}Cu, ^{52}Mn, and ^{210}Pb in the rat. *Brit. J. ind. Med.*, **29**, 74–80

Cikrt, M. & Tichy, M. (1975) Role of bile in intestinal absorption of ^{203}Pb in rats. *Experientia*, **31**, 1320–1321

Cikrt, M., Lepši, P. & Tichy, M. (1983) Biliary excretion of lead in rats drinking lead-containing water. *Toxicol. Lett.*, **16**, 139–143

Cilliers, L. & Retief, F.P. (2000) Poisons, poisoning and the drug trade in ancient Rome. *Akroterion*, **45**, 88–100

Clark, A.R.L. (1977) Placental transfer of lead and its effects on the newborn. *Postgrad. med. J.*, **53**, 674–678

Clark, M., Royal, J. & Seeler, R. (1988) Interaction of iron deficiency and lead and hematologic findings in children with severe lead poisining. *Paediatrics*, **81**, 247–254

Clark, N.J., Montopoli, M., Burr, G.A. & Rubin, C. (1991) Health Hazard Evaluation Report, HETA 91-0077-2160, Pilot Industrial Batteries, Kankakee, IL, USA, NIOSH

Clark, N.J., O'Brien, D.M., Edmonds, M.A. & Gressel, M.G. (1992) Health Hazard Evaluation Report, HETA 91-0092-2190, William Powell, Co., Cincinnati, OH, USA, NIOSH

Clasen, R.A., Hartmann, J.F., Coogan, P.S., Pandolfi, S., Laing, I. & Becker, R.A. (1974) Experimental acute lead encephalopathy in the juvenile rhesus monkey. *Environ. Health Perspect.*, **7**, 175–185

Clausen, J. & Rastogi, S.C. (1977) Heavy metal pollution among autoworkers. I. Lead. *Br. J. ind. Med.*, **34**, 208–215

Cocco, P.L., Carta, P., Belli, S., Picchiri, G.F. & Flore, M.V. (1994a) Mortality of Sardinian lead and zinc miners: 1960–88. *Occup. environ. Med.*, **51**, 674–682

Cocco, P.L., Carta, P., Flore, V., Picchiri, G.F. & Zucca, C. (1994b) Lung cancer mortality among female mine workers exposed to silica. *J. occup. Med.*, **36**, 894–898

Cocco, P., Carta, P., Flore, C., Congia, P., Manca, M.B., Saba, G. & Salis, S. (1996) Mortality of lead smelter workers with the glucose-6-phosphate dehydrogenase-deficient phenotype. *Cancer Epidemiol. Biomarkers Prev.*, **5**, 223–225

Cocco, P., Hua, F., Boffetta, P., Carta, P., Flore, C., Flore, V., Onnis, A., Picchiri, G.F. & Colin, D. (1997) Mortality of Italian lead smelter workers. *Scand. J. Work Environ. Health*, **23**, 15–23

Cocco, P., Dosemeci, M. & Heineman, E.F. (1998a) Brain cancer and occupational exposure to lead. *J. occup. environ. Med.*, **40**, 937–942

Cocco, P., Ward, M.H. & Dosemeci, M. (1998b) Occupational risk factors for cancer of the gastric cardia. Analysis of death certificates from 24 US states. *J. occup. environ. Med.*, **40**, 855–861

Cocco, P., Heineman, E.F. & Dosemeci, M. (1999a) Occupational risk factors for cancer of the central nervous system (CNS) among US women. *Am. J. ind. Med.*, **36**, 70–74

Cocco, P., Ward, M.H. & Dosemeci, M. (1999b) Risk of stomach cancer associated with 12 workplace hazards: Analysis of death certificates from 24 states of the United States with the aid of job exposure matrices. *Occup. environ. Med.*, **56**, 781–787

Cohen, S.M. & Ellwein, L.B. (1990) Cell proliferation in carcinogenesis. *Science*, **249**, 972–975

Cohen, A.J. & Roe, F.J.C. (1991) Review of lead toxicology relevant to the safety assessment of lead acetate as a hair colouring. *Food chem. Toxicol.*, **29**, 485–507

Columbano, A., Ledda, G.M., Sirigu, P., Perra, T. & Pani, P. (1983) Liver cell proliferation induced by a single dose of lead nitrate. *Am. J. Pathol.*, **110**, 83–88

Columbano, A., Ledda-Columbano, G.M., Coni, P.P., Vargiu, M., Faa, G. & Pani, P. (1984) Liver hyperplasia and regression after lead nitrate administration. *Toxicol. Pathol.*, **12**, 89–95

Columbano, A., Ledda-Columbano, G.M., Coni, P.P., Faa, G., Liguori, C., Santa Cruz, G. & Pani, P. (1985) Occurrence of cell death (apoptosis) during the involution of liver hyperplasia. *Lab. Invest.*, **52**, 670–675

Columbano, A., Ledda-Columbano, G.M., Ennas, M.G., Curto, M., Chelo, A. & Pani, P. (1990) Cell proliferation and promotion of rat liver carcinogenesis: Different effect of hepatic regeneration and mitogen induced hyperplasia on the development of enzyme-altered foci. *Carcinogenesis*, **11**, 771–776

Coni, P., Pichiri-Coni, G., Curto, M., Simbula, G., Giacomini, L., Sarma, D.S.R., Ledda-Columbano, G.M. & Columbano, A. (1993a) Different effects of regenerative and direct mitogenic stimuli on the growth of initiated cells in the resistant hepatocyte model. *Jpn J. Cancer Res.*, **84**, 501–507

Coni, P., Simbula, G., Carceriri de Prati, A., Menegazzi, M., Suzuki, H., Sarma, D.S.R., Ledda-Columbano, G.M. & Columbano, A. (1993b) Differences in the steady-state levels of c-*fos*, c-*jun* and c-*myc* messenger RNA during mitogen-induced liver growth and compensatory regeneration. *Hepatology*, **17**, 1109–1116

Conrad, M.E. & Barton, J.C. (1978) Factors affecting the absorption and excretion of lead in the rat. *Gastroenterology*, **74**, 731–740

Conradi, N.G., Sjostrom, A., Gustafsson, B. & Wigstrom, H. (1990) Decreased nerve conduction velocity in optic nerve following early post-natal low-dose lead exposure. *Acta physiol. scand.*, **140**, 515–519

Consumer Product Safety Commission (1977) *CPSC Announces Final Ban on Lead-containing Paint*, Washington DC, US Consumer Product Safety Commission

Consumer Product Safety Commission (1996) *CPSC Finds Lead Poisoning Hazard for Young Children in Imported Vinyl Miniblinds*, Washington DC, US Consumer Product Safety Commission [http://www.cpsc.gov/cpscpub/prerel/prhtml/96150.html; accessed 10/02/2004]

Cook, L., Schafer-Mitchell, M., Angle, C. & Stohs, S. (1985) Assay of human erythrocyte pyrimidine and deoxypyrimidine 5′-nucleotidase by isocratic reversed-phase high-performance liquid chromatography. *J. Chromatogr.*, **339**, 293–301

Cook, L.R., Angle, C.R. & Stohs, S.J. (1986) Erythrocyte arginase, pyrimidine 5′-nucleotidase (P5N), and deoxypyrimidine 5′-nucleotidase (dP5N) as indices of lead exposure. *Br. J. ind. Med.*, **43**, 387–390

Cook, C.K., Tubbs, R.L. & Klein, M.K. (1993) Health Hazard Evaluation Report, HETA 92-0034-2356, Saint Bernard Police Dept., Saint Bernard, OH, USA, NIOSH

Cooper, W.C. (1976) Cancer mortality patterns in the lead industry. *Ann. N.Y. Acad. Sci.*, **271**, 250–259

Cooper, W.C. (1981) Mortality in employees of lead production facilities and lead battery plants, 1971–1975. In: *Environmental Lead: Proceedings of the Second International Symposium on Environmental Lead Research, Cincinnati, Ohio, December 1978*, Academic Press, New York, London, San Francisco, pp. 111–143

Cooper, W.C. (1988) Deaths from chronic renal disease in US battery and lead production workers. *Environ. Health Perspect.*, **78**, 61–63

Cooper, W.C. & Gaffey, W.R. (1975) Mortality of lead workers. *J. occup. Med.*, **17**, 100–107

Cooper, W.C., Wong, O. & Kheifets, L. (1985) Mortality among employees of lead battery plants and lead-producing plants, 1947–1980. *Scand. J. Work Environ. Health*, **11**, 331–345

Cordioli, G., Cuoghi, L., Solari, P.L., Berrino, F., Crosignani, P. & Riboli, E. (1987) [Mortality from tumors in a cohort of workers in the glass industry.] *Epidemiol. Prev.*, **30**, 16–18 (in Italian)

Cory-Slechta, D.A. (1990) Lead exposure during advanced age: Alterations in kinetics and biochemical effects. *Toxicol. appl. Pharmacol.*, **104**, 67–78

Cory-Slechta, D.A. (2003) Lead-induced impairments in complex cognitive function: Offerings from experimental studies. *Neuropsychol. Dev. Cogn. Sect. C Child Neuropsychol.*, **9**, 54–75

Cory-Slechta, D.A., Weiss, B. & Cox, C. (1989) Tissue distribution of Pb in adult vs. old rats: A pilot study. *Toxicology*, **59**, 139–150

Coscia, J.M., Ris, M.D., Succop, P.A. & Dietrich, K.N. (2003) Cognitive development of lead exposed children from ages 6 to 15 years: An application of growth curve analysis. *Neuropsychol. Dev. Cogn. Sect. C Child Neurophsycol.*, **9**, 10–21

Costa, L.G. (2003) Correspondence re: Navas-Acien *et al.*, Interactive effect of chemical substances and occupational electromagnetic field exposure on the risk of gliomas and meningiomas in Swedish men. *Cancer Epidemiol. Biomarkers Prev.*, **12**, 950

Coste, J., Mandereau, L., Pessione, F., Bregu, M., Faye, C., Hemon, D. & Spira, A (1991) Lead-exposed workmen and fertility: A cohort study on 354 subjects. *Eur. J. Epidemiol.*, **7**, 154–158

Counter, S.A., Vahter, M., Laurell, G., Buchanan, L.H., Ortega, F. & Skerfving, S. (1997a) High lead exposure and auditory sensory-neural function in Andean children. *Environ. Health Perspect.*, **105**, 522–526

Counter, S.A., Buchanan, L.H., Ortega, F. & Laurell, G. (1997b) Normal auditory brainstem and cochlear function in extreme pediatric plumbism. *J. Neurol. Sci.*, **152**, 85–92

Counter, S.A., Buchanan, L.H., Ortega, F., Amarasiriwardena, C. & Hu, H. (2000) Environmental lead contamination and pediatric lead intoxication in an Andean Ecuadorian village. *Int. J. occup. environ. Health*, **75**, 169–176

Cragg, B. & Rees, S. (1984) Increased body:brain weight ratio in developing rats after low exposure to organic lead. *Exp. Neurol.*, **86**, 113–121

Cramér, K., Goyer, R.A., Jagenburg, R. & Wilson, M.H. (1974) Renal ultrastructure, renal function, and parameters of lead toxicity in workers with different periods of lead exposure. *Br. J. ind. Med.*, **31**, 113–127

Cremin, J.D., Jr & Smith, D.R. (2002) In vitro vs in vivo Pb effects on brain protein kinase C activity. *Environ. Res.*, **90**, 191–199

Cremin, J.D., Jr, Luck, M.L., Laughlin, N.K. & Smith, D.R. (2001) Oral succimer decreases the gastrointestinal absorption of lead in juvenile monkeys. *Environ. Health Perspect.*, **109**, 613–619

Crowe, A. & Morgan, E.H. (1996) Interactions between tissue uptake of lead and iron in normal and iron-deficient rats during development. *Biol. trace Elem. Res.*, **52**, 249–261

Crowne, H., Lim, C.K. & Samson, D. (1981) Determination of 5-aminolaevulinic acid dehydrase activity in erythrocytes by high-performance liquid chromatography. *J. Chromatogr.*, **223**, 421–425

Cueto, L.M., Baer, R.D. & Montano Gonzalez, E. (1989) Three cases of unusual lead poisoning. *Am. J. Gastroenterol.*, **84**, 1460

Cunningham, S.D. & Ow, D.W. (1996) Promises and prospects for phytoremediation. *Plant Physiol.*, **110**, 715–719

Dabeka, R.W. & McKenzie, A.D. (1987) Lead, cadmium, and fluoride levels in market milk and infant formulas in Canada. *J. Assoc. off. anal. Chem.*, **70**, 754–757

Dabeka, R.W. & McKenzie, A.D. (1988) Lead and cadmium levels in commercial infant foods and dietary intake by infants 0–1 year old. *Food Addit. Contam.*, **5**, 333–342

Dabeka, R.W., McKenzie, A.D. & Lacroix, G.M.A. (1987) Dietary intakes of lead, cadmium, arsenic and fluoride by Canadian adults: A 24-hour duplicate diet study. *Food Addit. Contam.*, **4**, 89–102

Dabeka, R.W., Karpinski, K.F., McKenzie, A.D. & Badjik, C.D. (1988) Survey of lead and cadmium in human milk and correlation of levels with environmental and food factors. *Sci. total Environ.*, **71**, 65–66

Dalpra, L., Tibiletti, M.G., Nocera, G., Giulotto, P., Auriti, L., Carnelli, V. & Simoni, G. (1983) SCE analysis in children exposed to lead emission from a smelting plant. *Mutat. Res.*, **120**, 249–256

Dalton, C.B., McCammon, J.B., Hoffman, R.E. & Baron, R.C. (1997) Blood lead levels in radiator repair workers in Colorado. *J. occup. environ. Med.*, **39**, 58–62

Dams, R., Vandecasteele, C., Desmet, B., Helsen, M., Nagels, M., Vermeir, G. & Yu, Z.Q. (1988) Element concentrations in the air of an indoor shooting range. *Sci. total Environ.*, **77**, 1–13

Danadevi, K., Rozati, R., Saleha Banu, B., Hanumanth Rao, P. & Grover, P. (2003) DNA damage in workers exposed to lead using comet assay. *Toxicology*, **187**, 183–193

Daniels, W.J. (1988) Health Hazard Evaluation Report, HETA 88-0031-1894, Camp Bird Ventures, Ouray, CO, USA, NIOSH

Daniels, W.J. & Hales, T.R. (1989) Health Hazard Evaluation Report, HETA 89-0136-1991, Blue Range Mining Co., Lewistown, MT, USA, NIOSH

Daniels, W.J., Hales, T.R. & Gunter, B.J. (1989) Health Hazard Evaluation Report, HETA 89-0213-1992, Blue Range Engineering Co., Butte, MT, USA, NIOSH

David, O.J. (1974) Association between lower level lead concentrations and hyperactivity in children. *Environ. Health Perspect.*, **7**, 17–25

Davies, B.E. (1983) A graphical estimation of the normal lead content of some British soils. *Geoderma*, **29**, 67–75

Davies, J.M. (1984a) Lung cancer mortality among workers making lead chromate and zinc chromate pigments at three English factories. *Br. J. ind. Med.*, **41**, 158–169

Davies, J.M. (1984b) Long term mortality study of chromate pigment workers who suffered lead poisoning. *Br. J. ind. Med.*, **41**, 170–178

Davies, B.E., Elwood, P.C., Gallacher, J. & Ginnever, R.C. (1985) The relationships between heavy metals in garden soils and house dusts in an old lead mining area of North Wales, Great Britain. *Environ. Pollut.*, **B9**, 255–266

Davies, D.J.A., Watt, J.M. & Thornton, I. (1987) Air lead concentration in Birmingham, England — A comparison between levels inside and outside inner-city homes. *Environ. Geochem. Health*, **9**, 3–7

Davis, A., Ruby, M.V. & Bergstrom, P.D. (1992) Bioavailability of arsenic and lead in soils from the Butte, Montana, mining district. *Environ. Sci. Technol.*, **26**, 461–468

Davis, A., Ruby, M.V. & Bergstrom, P.D. (1994) Factors controlling lead bioavailability in the Butte mining district, Montana, USA. *Environ. Geochem. Health*, **16**, 147–157

Decker, J. & Galson, S. (1991) Health Hazard Evaluation Report, HETA 91-0073-2165, Carbonnaire Co. Palmerton, PA, USA, NIOSH

De Jonghe, W.R.A., Chakraborti, D. & Adams, F.C. (1981) Identification and determination of individual tetraalkyllead species in air. *Env. Sci. Technol.*, **15**, 1217–1222

Deknudt, G. & Deminatti, M. (1978) Chromosome studies in human lymphocytes after in vitro exposure to metal salts. *Toxicology*, **10**, 67–75

Deknudt, G. & Gerber, G.B. (1979) Chromosomal aberrations in bone-marrow cells of mice given a normal or a calcium-deficient diet supplemented with various heavy metals. *Mutat. Res.*, **68**, 163–168

Deknudt, G., Colle, A. & Gerber, G.B. (1977) Chromosomal abnormalities in lymphocytes from monkeys poisoned with lead. *Mutat. Res.*, **45**, 77–83

De la Burdé, B. & Choate, M.S. (1975) Early asymptomatic lead exposure and development at school age. *J. Pediatr.*, **87**, 638–642

De la Fuente, H., Portales-Pérez, D., Baranda, L., Díaz-Barriga, F., Saavedra-Alanís, V., Layseca, E. & González-Amaro, R. (2002) Effect of arsenic, cadmium and lead on the induction of apoptosis of normal human mononuclear cells. *Clin. exp. Immunol.*, **129**, 69–77

De Leacy, E. (1991) Lead crystal. *Lancet*, **337**, 858–859

Delves, H.T., Diaper, S.J., Oppert, S., Prescott-Clarke, P., Periam, J., Dong, W., Colhoun, H. & Gompertz, D. (1996) Blood lead concentrations in United Kingdom have fallen substantially since 1984. *Br. med. J.*, **313**, 883–884

Denno, D.W. (1990) *Biology and Violence*, New York, Cambridge University Press

Der, R., Fahim, Z., Yousef, M. & Fahim, M. (1976) Environmental interaction of lead and cadmium on reproduction and metabolism of male rats. *Res. Comm. chem. Pathol. Pharmacol.*, **14**, 689–713

De Restrepo, H.G., Sicard, D. & Torres, M.M. (2000) DNA damage and repair in cells of lead exposed people. *Am. J. ind. Med.*, **38**, 330–334

DeSilva, P.E. (1981) Determination of lead in plasma and studies on its relationship to lead in erythrocytes. *Br. J. ind. Med.*, **38**, 209–217

Dhir, H., Roy, A.K. & Sharma, A. (1993) Relative efficiency of *Phyllanthus emblica* fruit extract and ascorbic acid in modifying lead and aluminium-induced sister-chromatid exchanges in mouse bone marrow. *Environ. mol. Mutag.*, **21**, 229–236

Díaz, C., Galindo, L., Montelongo, F.G., Lerrechi, M.S. & Rius, F.X. (1990) Metals in coastal waters of Santa Cruz de Tenerife, Canary Islands. *Marine Pollut. Bull.*, **21**, 91–95

Dickinson, L., Reichert, E.L., Ho, R.C.S., Rivers, J.B. & Kominami, N. (1972) Lead poisoning in a family due to cocktail glasses. *Am. J. Med.*, **52**, 391–394

Diemel, J.A.L., Brunekreef, B., Boleij, J.S.M., Biersteker, K. & Veenstra, S.J. (1981) The Arnhem lead study. II. Indoor pollution, and indoor/outdoor relationships. *Environ. Res.*, **25**, 449–456

Dieter, M.P., Matthews, H.B., Jeffcoat, R.A. & Moseman, R.F. (1993) Comparison of lead bioavailability in F344 rats fed lead acetate, lead oxide, lead sulfide, or lead ore concentrate from Skagway, Alaska. *J. Toxicol. environ. Health*, **39**, 79–93

Dietrich, K., Krafft, K., Bier, M., Succop, P., Berger, O. & Bornschein, R. (1986) Early effects of fetal lead exposure: Neurobehavioural findings at six months. *Int. J. Biosoc. Res.*, **8**, 151–168

Dietrich, K.N., Ris, M.D., Succop, P.A., Berger, O.G. & Bornschein, R.L. (2001) Early exposure to lead and juvenile delinquency. *Neurotoxicol. Teratol.*, **23**, 511–518

Dillman, R.O., Crumb, C.K. & Lidsky, M.J. (1979) Lead poisoning from a gunshot wound: Report of a case and review of the literature. *Am. J. Med.*, **66**, 509–514

Dingwall-Fordyce, I. & Lane, R.E. (1963) A follow-up study of lead workers. *Br. J. ind. Med.*, **20**, 313–315

Djuric, D., Kerin, Z., Graovac-Leposavic, L., Novak, L. & Kop, M. (1971) Environmental contamination by lead from a mine and smelter — A preliminary report. *Arch. environ. Health*, **23**, 275–279

Donald, J.M., Cutler, M.G. & Moore, M.R. (1986) Effects of lead in the laboratory mouse. 1. Influence of pregnancy upon absorption, retention, and tissue distribution of radio-labeled lead. *Environ. Res.*, **41**, 420–431

Donmez, H., Dursun, N., Ozkul, Y. & Demirtas, H. (1998) Increased sister chromatid exchanges in workers exposed to occupational lead and zinc. *Biol. trace Elem. Res.*, **61**, 105–109

Donovan, B.A. (1994) Health Hazard Evaluation Report, HETA 92-0029-2392, Kessler Studios, Loveland, OH, USA, NIOSH

Drasch, G.A. (1982) Lead burden in prehistorical, historical and modern human bone. *Sci. total Environ.*, **24**, 199–231

Drasch, G.A., Böhm, J. & Baur, C. (1987) Lead in human bones. Investigations on an occupationally non-exposed population in southern Bavaria (F.R.G.). I. Adults. *Sci. total Environ.*, **64**, 303–315

Drasch, G.A., Wanghofer, E. & Roider, G. (1997) Are blood, urine, hair, and muscle valid biomonitors for the internal burden of men with the heavy metals mercury, lead and cadmium? *Trace Elem. Electrolytes*, **14**, 116–123

Driscoll, R.J. & Elliott, L.J. (1990) Health Hazard Evaluation Report, HETA 87-0126-2019, Chrysler Chemical Division, Trenton, MI, USA, NIOSH

Driscoll, W., Mushak, P., Garfias, J. & Rothenberg, S.J. (1992) Reducing lead in gasoline — Mexico's experience. *Environ. Sci. Technol.*, **26**, 1702–1705

Dubas, T.C., Stevenson, A., Singhal, R.L. & Hrdina, P.D. (1978) Regional alterations in brain biogenic amines in young rats following chronic lead exposure. *Toxicology*, **9**, 185–190

Ducoffre, G., Claeys, F. & Bruaux, P. (1990) Lowering time trend of blood lead levels in Belgium since 1978. *Environ. Res.*, **51**, 25–34

Dunbabin, D.W., Tallis, G.A., Popplewell, P.Y. & Lee, R.A. (1992) Lead poisoning from Indian herbal medicine (Ayurveda). *Med. J. Austr.*, **157**, 835–836

Dunkel, V.C., Zeiger, E., Brusick, D., McCoy, E., McGregor, D., Mortelmans, K., Rosenkranz, H.S. & Simmon, V.F. (1984) Reproducibility of microbial mutagenicity assays: I. Tests with Salmonella typhimurium and Escherichia coli using a standardized protocol. *Environ. Mutag.*, **6**, 1–254

Duraisamy, V.P., Subramaniam, K.S., Chitdeshwari, T. & Singh, M.V. (2003) Seasonal and temporal changes in heavy metal pollution in sewage and their impacts on soil quality. In: Singh, V.P. & Yadava, R.N., eds, *Environmental Pollution: Proceedings of the International Conference on Water and Environment (WE-2003)*, New Delhi, Allied Publishers Pvt. Ltd., pp. 108–121

Dussias, V., Stefos, T., Stefanidis, K., Paraskevaidis, E., Karabini, F. & Lolis, D. [originally cited as Vasilios, D., Theodor, S., Konstantinos, S., Evangelos, P., Fotini, K., Dimitrios, L.] (1997) Lead concentrations in maternal and umbilical cord blood in areas with high and low air pollution. *Clin. exp. Obstet. Gynecol.*, **24**, 187–189

DuVal, G. & Fowler, B.A. (1989) Preliminary purification and characterization studies of a low molecular weight, high affinity cytosolic lead-binding protein in rat brain. *Biochem. biophys. Res. Commun.*, **159**, 177–184

Duydu, Y. & Süzen, H. S. (2003) Influence of δ-aminolevulinic acid dehydratase (ALAD) polymorphism on the frequency of sister chromatid exchange (SCE) and the number of high-frequency cells (HFCs) in lymphocytes from lead-exposed workers. *Mutat. Res.*, **540**, 79–88

Dwivedi, S.K. & Dey, S. (2002) Medicinal herbs: A potential source of toxic metal exposure for man and animals in India. *Arch. environ. Health*, **57**, 229–231

Dwivedi, S.K., Swarup, D., Dey, S. & Patra, R.C. (2001) Lead poisoning in cattle and buffalo near primary lead-zinc smelter in India. *Vet. hum. Toxicol.*, **43**, 93–94

Dykeman, R., Aguilar-Madrid, G., Smith, T., Juárez-Pérez, C.A., Piacitelli, G.M., Hu, H. & Hernandez-Avila, M. (2002) Lead exposure in Mexican radiator repair workers. *Am. J. ind. Med.*, **41**, 179–187

Eades, L.J., Farmer, J.G., MacKenzie, A.B., Kirika, A. & Bailey-Watts, A.E. (2002) Stable lead isotopic characterisation of the historical record of environmental lead contamination in dated freshwater lake sediment cores from northern and central Scotland. *Sci. total Environ.*, **292**, 55–67

Eastwell, H.D., Thomas, B.J. & Thomas, B.W. (1983) Skeletal lead burden in Aborigine petrol sniffers. *Lancet*, **ii**, 524–525

Eaton, DL., Kalman, D., Garvey, D., Morgan, M. & Omenn, G.S. (1984) Biological availability of lead in a paint aerosol. 2. Absorption, distribution and excretion of intratracheally instilled lead paint particles in the rat. *Toxicol. Lett.*, **22**, 307–313

Echt, A., Klein, M. & Reh, C.M. (1992) Health Hazard Evaluation Report, HETA 91-0124-2192, U.S. Park Police, Washington, DC, USA, NIOSH

Eckel, W.P. & Jacob, T.A. (1988) Ambient levels of 24 dissolved metals in U.S. surface and ground waters. In: *Proceedings of the 196th Meeting of the American Chemical Society, Division of Environmental Chemistry*, **28**, 371–372

Edelstein, S., Fullmer, C.S. & Wasserman, R.H. (1984) Gastrointestinal absorption of lead in chicks: Involvement of the cholecalciferol endocrine system. *J. Nutr.*, **114**, 692–700

Edminster, S.C. & Bayer, M.J. (1985) Recreational gasoline sniffing: Acute gasoline intoxication and latent organolead poisoning. Case reports and literature review. *J. Emerg. Med.*, **3**, 365–370

Ehrlich, R., Robins, T., Jordaan, E., Miller, S., Mbuli, S., Selby, P., Wynchank, S., Cantrell, A., De Broe, M., D'Haese, P., Todd, A. & Landrigan, P. (1998) Lead absorption and renal dysfunction in a South African battery factory. *Occup. environ. Med.*, **55**, 453–460

Eldred, R.A. & Cahill, T.A. (1994) Trends in elemental concentrations of fine particles at remote sites in the United States of America. *Atmos. Environ.*, **28**, 1009–1019

Elias, R.W. (1985) Lead exposures in the human environment. In: Mahaffey, K.R., ed., *Dietary and Environmental Lead: Human Health Effects*, Amsterdam, Elsevier Science Publisher B.V., pp. 79–107

Elias, Z., Poirot, O., Pezerat, H., Suquet, H., Schneider, O., Danière, M.C., Terzetti, F., Baruthio, F., Fournier, M. & Cavelier, C. (1989) Cytotoxic and neoplastic transforming effects of industrial hexavalent chromium pigments in Syrian hamster embryo cells. *Carcinogenesis*, **10**, 2043–2052

Elinder, C.-G., Friberg, L., Lind, B., Nilsson, B., Svartengren, M. & Övermark, I. (1986) Decreased blood lead levels in residents of Stockholm for the period 1980–1984. *Scand. J. Work Environ. Health*, **12**, 114–120

Ellis, G.B. & Desjardins, C. (1982) Male rats secrete luteinizing hormone and testosterone episodically. *Endocrinology*, **110**, 1618–1627

Elmarsafawy, S.F., Tsaih, S.-W., Korrick, S., Dickey, J.H., Sparrow, D., Aro, A. & Hu, H. (2002) Occupational determinants of bone and blood lead levels in middle aged and elderly men from the general community: The Normative Aging Study. *Am. J. ind. Med.*, **42**, 38–49

Englyst, V., Lundstrom, N., Gerhardsson, L., Rylander, L. & Nordberg, G. (1999) Determinants of lung cancer risks among lead exposed smelter workers (Abstract). In: *Proceedings of the International Conference on Lead Exposure, Reproductive Toxicity, and Carcinogenicity, June 7–9, 1999, Gargano, Italy*

Englyst, V., Lundström, N.-G., Gerhardsson, L., Rylander, L. & Nordberg, G. (2001) Lung cancer risks among lead smelter workers also exposed to arsenic. *Sci. total Environ.*, **273**, 77–82

Enterline, P.E., Marsh, G.M., Esmen, N.N., Henderson, V.L., Callahan, C.M. & Paik, M. (1987) Some effects of cigarette smoking, arsenic, and SO_2 on mortality among US copper smelter workers. *J. occup. Med.*, **29**, 831–838

Environment Agency, Japan (1997) [*Air Pollution in Japan, 1996*], The Government of Japan, Tokyo, Gyosei Publishers (in Japanese)

Environmental Management Bureau (1996) *Philippine Environmental Quality Report 1990–1995*, Manila, Environmental Management Bureau, Department of Environmental and Natural Resources, the Government of the Philippines, p. 9

Environment Protection Administration ROC (1991) [*Domestic Environmental Information and Statistics of Taiwan Area ROC, 1990*], Taipei, Environmental Protection Administration Printing Office, p. 480 (in Chinese)

Epstein, S.S. & Mantel, N. (1968) Carcinogenicity of tetraethyl lead. *Experientia*, **24**, 580–581

Epstein, H.T., Newton, J.T. & Fenton, K. (1999) Lead effects on offspring depend on when mouse mothers were exposed to lead. *Biol. Neonate*, **75**, 272–278

Erfurth, E.M., Gerhardsson, L., Nilsson, A., Rylander, L., Schütz, A., Skerfving, S. & Börjesson, J. (2001) Effects of lead on the endocrine system in lead smelter workers. *Arch. environ. Health*, **56**, 449–455

Erkkilä, J., Armstrong, R., Riihimaki, V., Chettle, D.R., Paakkari, A., Scott, M., Somervaille, L., Starck, J., Kock, B. & Aitio, A. (1992) In vivo measurements of lead in bone at four anatomical sites: Long term occupational and consequent endogenous exposure. *Br. J. Ind. Med.*, **49**, 631–644

Ernhart, C., Morrow-Tlucak, M., Wolf, A.W., Super, D. & Drotar, D. (1989) Low level lead exposure in the prenatal and early preschool periods: Intelligence prior to school entry. *Neurotoxicol. Teratol.*, **11**, 161–170

Esernio-Jenssen, D., Donatelli-Guagenti, A. & Mofenson, H.C. (1996) Severe lead poisoning from an imported clothing accessory: 'Watch' out for lead. *Clin. Toxicol.*, **34**, 329–333

ESPI Corp. (2002) *Technical Data Sheets: Lead*, Ashland, OR, USA, pp. 169–174

Esswein, E.J., Boeniger, M.F., Hall, R.M. & Mead, K. (1996) Health Hazard Evaluation Report, HETA 94-0268-2618, Standard Industries, San Antonio, TX, USA, NIOSH

European Commission (1998) Council Directive 98/24/EC of 7 April 1998 on the protection of the health and safety of workers from the risks related to chemical agents at work (fourteenth individual Directive within the meaning of Article 16(1) of Directive 89/391/EEC), *Official Journal of the European Communities*, **L131**, 11–23

Everson, J. & Patterson, C.C. (1980) 'Ultra-clean' isotope dilution/mass spectrometric analyses for lead in human blood plasma indicate that most reported values are artificially high. *Clin. Chem.*, **26**, 1603–1607

Evis, M.J., Kane, K.A., Moore, M.R. & Parratt, J.R. (1985) The effects of chronic low lead treatment and hypertension on the severity of cardiac arrhythmias induced by coronary artery ligation in anesthetized rats. *Toxicol. appl. Pharmacol.*, **80**, 235–242

Evis, M.J., Dhaliwal, K., Kane, K.A., Moore, M.R. & Parratt, J.R. (1987) The effects of chronic lead treatment and hypertension on the severity of cardiac arrhythmias induced by coronary artery occlusion or by noradrenaline in anaesthetised rats. *Arch. Toxicol.*, **59**, 336–340

Ewers, U., Stiller-Winkler, R. & Idel. H. (1982) Serum immunoglobulin, complement C3, and salivary IgA levels in lead workers. *Environ. Res.*, **29**, 351–357

Ewers, L.M., Piacitelli, G.M. & Whelan, E.A. (1995) Health Hazard Evaluation Report, HETA 93-0502-2503, George Campbell Painting Co., Groton, CT, USA, NIOSH

Facchetti, S. (1989) Lead in petrol. The isotopic lead experiment. *Acc. Chem. Res.*, **22**, 370–374

Factor-Litvak, P., Graziano, J.H., Kline, J.K., Popovac, D., Mehmeti, A., Ahmedi, G., Shrout, P., Murphy, M.J., Gashi, E., Haxhiu, R., Rajovic, L., Nenezic, D.U. & Stein, Z.A. (1991) A prospective study of birthweight and length of gestation in a population surrounding a lead smelter in Kosovo, Yugoslavia. *Int. J. Epidemiol.*, **20**, 722–728

Fair, J.M. & Ricklefs, R.E. (2002) Physiological, growth, and immune responses of Japanese quail chicks to the multiple stressors of immunological challenge and lead shot. *Arch. environ. Contam. Toxicol.*, **42**, 77–87

Fairhall, L.T. & Miller, J.W. (1941) A study of the relative toxicity of the molecular components of lead arsenate. *Publ. Health Rep.*, **56**, 1610–1625

Falcón, M., Viñas, P. & Luna, A. (2003) Placental lead and outcome of pregnancy. *Toxicology*, **185**, 59–66

Fanning, D. (1988) A mortality study of lead workers, 1926–1985. *Arch. environ. Health*, **43**, 247–251

FAO/WHO (1993) *Evaluation of Certain Food Additives and Contaminants*, Forty-first Report of the Joint FAO/WHO Expert Committee on Food Additives (Technical Report Series 837), Geneva, World Health Organization

Farias, P., Borja-Aburto, V.H., Rios, C., Hertz-Picciotto, I., Rojas-Lopez, M. & Chavez-Ayala, R. (1996) Blood lead levels in pregnant women of high and low socioeconomic status in Mexico City. *Environ. Health Perspect.*, **104**, 1070–1074

Farmer, A.A. & Farmer, A.M. (2000) Concentrations of cadmium, lead and zinc in livestock feed and organs around a metal production centre in eastern Kazakhstan. *Sci. total Environ.*, **257**, 53–60

Fayerweather, W.E., Karns, M.E., Nuwayhid, I.A. & Nelson, T.J. (1997) Case–control study of cancer risk in tetraethyl lead manufacturing. *Am. J. ind. Med.*, **31**, 28–35

Fears, T.R., Elashoff, R.M. & Schneiderman, M.A. (1989) The statistical analysis of carcinogen mixture experiment. III Carcinogens with different target systems, aflatoxins B1, *N*-butyl-*N*-(4-hydroxybutyl)nitrosamine, lead acetate, and thiouracil. *Toxicol. ind. Health*, **5**, 1–23

Fergusson, D.M., Horwood, L.J. & Lynskey, M.T. (1997) Early dentine lead levels and educational outcomes at 18 years. *J. Child Psychol. Psychiat.*, **38**, 471–478

Fernández, R., Morales, F. & Benzo, Z. (2003) Lead exposure in day care centres in the Caracas Valley — Venezuela. *Int. J. environ. Health Res.*, **13**, 3–9

Fernandez-Cabezudo, M.J., Hasan, M.Y., Mustafa, N., El-Sharkawy, R.T., Fahim, M.A. & Al-Ramadi, B.K. (2003) Alpha tocopherol protects against immunosuppressive and immunotoxic effects of lead. *Free Radic. Res.*, **37**, 437–445

Fernando, N.P., Healy, M.A., Aslam, M., Davis, S.S. & Hussein, A. (1981) Lead poisoning and traditional practices: The consequences for world health. A study in Kuwait. *Public Health (London)*, **95**, 250–260

Fett, M.J., Mira, M., Smith, J., Alperstein, G., Causer, J., Brokenshire, T., Gulson, B. & Cannata, S. (1992) Community prevalence survey of children's blood lead levels and environmental lead contamination in inner Sidney. *Med. J. Aust.*, **157**, 441–445

Fischbein, A., Rice, C., Sarkozi, L., Kon, S.H., Petrocci, M. & Selikoff, I.J. (1979) Exposure to lead in firing ranges. *JAMA*, **241**, 1141–1144

Fischbein, A., Wallace, J., Sassa, S., Kappas, A., Butts, G., Rohl, A. & Kaul, B. (1992) Lead poisoning from art restoration and pottery work: Unusual exposure source and household risk. *J. environ. Pathol. Toxicol. Oncol.*, **11**, 7–11

Fischer, A.B., Georgieva, R., Nikolova, V., Halkova, J., Bainova, A., Hristeva, V., Penkov, D. & Alandjiisk, D. (2003) Health risk for children from lead and cadmium near a non-ferrous smelter in Bulgaria. *Int. J. Hyg. environ. Health*, **206**, 25–38

Fitch, A. (1998) Lead analysis: Past and present. *Crit. Rev. anal. Chem.*, **28**, 267–345

Fitchko, J. & Hutchinson, T.C. (1975) A comparative study of heavy metal concentrations in river mouth sediments around the Great Lakes. *J. Great Lakes Res.*, **1**, 46–78

Flanagan, P.R., Hamilton, D.L., Haist, J. & Valberg, L.S. (1979) Interrelationships between iron and lead absorption in iron-deficient mice. *Gastroenterology*, **77**, 1074–1081

Fleming, D.E.B., Boulay, D., Richard, N.S., Robin, J.-P., Gordon, C.L., Webber, C.E. & Chettle, D.R. (1997) Accumulated body burden and endogenous release of lead in employees of a lead smelter. *Environ. Health Perspect.*, **105**, 224–233

Fleming, D.E.B., Chettle, D.R., Wetmur, J.G., Desnick, R.J., Robin, J.-P., Boulay, D., Richard, N.S., Gordon, C.L. & Webber, C.E. (1998) Effect of the δ-aminolevulinate dehydratase polymorphism on the accumulation of lead in bone and blood in lead smelter workers. *Environ. Res.*, **77**, 49–61

Fleming, D.E., Chettle, D.R., Webber, C.E. & O'Flaherty, E.J. (1999) The O'Flaherty model of lead kinetics: An evaluation using data from a lead smelter population. *Toxicol. appl. Pharmacol.*, **161**, 100–109

Flora, S.J.S. & Tandon, S.K. (1986) Preventive and therapeutic effects of thiamine, ascorbic acid and their combination in lead intoxication. *Acta pharmacol. toxicol.*, **58**, 374–378

Flora, G.J.S., Khanna, V.K. & Seth, P.K. (1999) Changes in neurotransmitter receptors and neurobehavioral variables in rats co-exposed to lead and ethanol. *Toxicol. Lett.*, **109**, 43–49

Florence, T.M., Lilley, S.G. & Stauber, J.L. (1988) Skin absorption of lead. *Lancet*, **ii**, 157–158

Florence, T.M., Stauber, J.L., Dale, L.S., Henderson, D., Izard, B.E. & Belbin, K. (1998) The absorption of ionic lead compounds through the skin of mice. *J. nutr. environ. Med.*, **8**, 19–23

Forbes, G.B. & Reina, J.C. (1972) Effect of age on gastrointestinal absorption (Fe, Sr, Pb) in the rat. *J. Nutr.*, **102**, 647–652

Forni, A. & Secchi, G.C. (1972) Chromosome changes in preclinical and clinical lead poisoning and correlation with biochemical findings. In: *Proceedings of the International Symposium 'Environmental Health Aspects of Lead', Amsterdam, Oct 2–6*, pp. 473–485

Forni, A., Cambiaghi, G. & Secchi, G.C. (1976) Initial occupational exposure to lead. Chromosome and biochemical findings. *Arch. environ. Health*, **31**, 73–78

Foster, W.G. (1992) Reproductive toxicity of chronic lead exposure in the female cynomolgus monkeys. *J. reprod. Toxicol.*, **6**, 123–131

Foster, W.G., McMahon, A. & Rice, D.C. (1996) Sperm chromatin structure is altered in cynomolgus monkeys with environmentally relevant blood lead levels. *Toxicol. ind. Health*, **12**, 723–735

Fouassin, A. & Fondu, M. (1980) Evaluation of the daily intake of lead and cadmium from food in Belgium. *Arch. Belg. Méd. Soc. Hyg. Méd. Trav. Méd. Lég.*, **38**, 453–467

Fowler, B.A. (1998) Roles of lead-binding proteins in mediating lead bioavailability. *Environ. Health Perspect.*, **106** (Suppl. 6), 1585–1587

Fowler, B.A. & DuVal, G. (1991) Effects of lead on the kidney: Roles of high-affinity lead-binding proteins. *Environ. Health Perspect.*, **91**, 77–80

Fowler, B.A., Kimmel, C.A., Woods, J.S., McConnell, E.E. & Grant, L.D. (1980) Chronic low-level lead toxicity in the rat. III. An integrated assessment of long-term toxicity with special reference to the kidney. *Toxicol. appl. Pharmacol.*, **56**, 59–77

Fowler, B.A., Kahng, M.W., Smith, D.R., Conner, E.A. & Laughlin, N.K. (1993) Implications of lead binding proteins for risk assessment of lead exposure. *J. Exp. Anal. environ. Epidemiol.*, **3**, 441–448

Fox, D.A., He, L., Poblenz, A.T., Medrano, C.J., Blocker, Y.S. & Srivastava, D. (1998) Lead-induced alterations in retinal cGMP phosphodiesterase trigger calcium overload, mitochondrial dysfunction and rod photoreceptor apoptosis. *Toxicol. Lett.*, **102–103**, 359–361

Fracasso, M.E., Perbellini, L., Solda, S., Talamini, G. & Franceschetti, P. (2002) Lead induced DNA strand breaks in lymphocytes of exposed workers: Role of reactive oxygen species and protein kinase C. *Mutat. Res.*, **515**, 159–169

Franco, G., Cottica, D. & Minoia, C. (1994) Chewing electric wire coatings: An unusual source of lead poisoning. *Am. J. ind. Med.*, **25**, 291–296

Franklin, C.A., Inskip, M.J., Baccanale, C.L., Edwards, C.M., Manton, W.I., Edwards, E. & O'Flaherty, E.J. (1997) Use of sequentially administered stable lead isotopes to investigate changes in blood lead during pregnancy in a nonhuman primate (*Macaca fascicularis*). *Fundam. appl. Toxicol.*, **39**, 109–119

Freeman, G.B., Johnson, J.D., Killinger, J.M., Liao, S.C., Feder, P.I., Davis, A.O., Ruby, M.V., Chaney, R.L., Lovre, S.C. & Bergstrom, P.D. (1992) Relative bioavailability of lead from mining waste soil in rats. *Fundam. appl. Toxicol.*, **19**, 388–398

Freeman, G.B., Johnson, J.D., Liao, S.C., Feder, P.I., Davis, A.O., Ruby, M.V., Schoof, R.A., Chaney, R.L. & Bergstrom, P.D. (1994) Absolute bioavailability of lead acetate and mining waste lead in rats. *Toxicology*, **91**, 151–163

Freeman, G.B., Dill, J.A., Johnson, J.D., Kurtz, P.J., Parham, F. & Matthews, H.B. (1996) Comparative absorption of lead from contaminated soil and lead salts by weanling Fischer 344 rats. *Fundam. appl. Toxicol.*, **33**, 109–119

Frenz, P.Y., Vega, J.M., Marchetti, N.P., Torres, J.P., Kopplin, E.I., Delgado, I.B. & Vega, F.A. (1997) [Chronic exposure to environmental lead in Chilean nursing infants.] *Rev. méd. Chile*, **125**, 1137–1144 (in Spanish)

Friberg, L. & Vahter, M. (1983) Assessment of exposure to lead and cadmium through biological monitoring: Results of UNEP/WHO global study. *Environ. Res.*, **30**, 95–128

Frisancho, A.R. & Ryan, A.S. (1991) Decreased stature associated with moderate blood lead concentrations in Mexican-American children. *Am. J. clin. Nutr.*, **54**, 516–519

Froom, P., Kristal-Boneh, E., Benbassat, J., Ashkanazi, R. & Ribak, J. (1998) Predective value of determinations of zinc protoporphyrin for increased blood lead concentrations. *Clim. Chem.*, **44**, 1283–1288

Fu, H. & Boffetta, P. (1995) Cancer and occupational exposure to inorganic lead compounds: A meta-analysis of published data. *Occup. environ. Med.*, **52**, 73–81

Fujiwara, Y. & Kaji, T. (1999) Possible mechanism for lead inhibition of vascular endothelial cell proliferation: A lower response to basic fibroblast growth factor through inhibition of heparan sulfate synthesis. *Toxicology*, **133**, 147–157

Fukui, Y., Miki, M., Ukai, H., Okamoto, S., Takada, S., Higashikawa, K. & Ikeda, M. (1999) Urinary lead as a possible surrogate of blood lead among workers occupationally exposed to lead. *Int. Arch. occup. environ. Health*, **72**, 516–20

Fukunaga, M., Kurachi, Y. & Mizuguchi, Y. (1982) Action of some metal ions on yeast chromosomes. *Chem. pharm. Bull.*, **30**, 3017–3019

Fullmer, C.S. (1990) Intestinal lead and calcium absorption: Effect of 1,25-dihydroxycholecalciferol and lead status. *Proc. Soc. exp. Biol. Med.*, **194**, 258–264

Fullmer, C.S. (1991) Intestinal calcium and lead absorption: Effects of dietary lead and calcium. *Environ. Res.*, **54**, 159–169

Fullmer, C.S. (1997) Lead–calcium interactions: Involvement of 1,25-dihydroxyvitamin D. *Environ. Res.*, **72**, 45–55

Fullmer, C.S., Edelstein, S. & Wasserman, R.H. (1985) Lead-binding properties of intestinal calcium-binding proteins. *J. biol. Chem.*, **260**, 6816–6819

Fulton, M., Thomson, G., Hunter, R., Raab, G., Laxen, D. & Hepburn, W. (1987) Influence of blood lead on the ability and attainment of children in Edinburgh. *Lancet*, **i**, 1221–1226

Fuortes, L. & Bauer, E. (2000) Lead contamination of imported candy wrappers. *Vet. hum. Toxicol.*, **42**, 41–42

Furst, A., Schlauder, M. & Sasmore, D.P. (1976) Tumorigenic activity of lead chromate. *Cancer Res.*, **36**, 1779–1783

Galal-Gorchev, H. (1991a) Dietary intake of pesticide residues, cadmium, mercury and lead. *Food addit. Contam.*, **8**, 793–806

Galal-Gorchev, H. (1991b) Global overview of dietary lead exposure. *Chem. Speciation Bioavailab.*, **3**, 5–11

Galke, W., Clark, S., Wilson, J., Jacobs, D., Succop, P., Dixon, S., Bornschein, B., McLaine, P. & Chen, M. (2001) Evaluation of the HUD Lead Hazard Control grant program: Early overall findings. *Environ. Res.*, **A86**, 149–156

Gallicchio, L., Scherer, R.W. & Sexton, M. (2002) Influence of nutrient intake on blood lead levels of young children at risk for lead poisoning. *Environ. Health Perspect.*, **110**, A767–A772

Garber, B.T. & Wei, E. (1974) Influence of dietary factors on the gastrointestinal absorption of lead. *Toxicol. appl. Pharmacol.*, **27**, 685–691

Garrido Latorre, F., Hernandez-Avila, M., Tamayo Orozco, J., Albores Medina, C.A., Aro, A., Palazuelos, E. & Hu, H. (2003) Relationship of blood and bone lead to menopause and bone mineral density among middle-age women in Mexico City. *Environ. Health Perspect.*, **111**, 631–636

Garner, D.L., Pinkel, D., Johnson, L.A. & Pace, M.M. (1986) Assessment of spermatozoal function using dual fluorescent staining and flow cytometric analyses. *Biol. Reprod.*, **34**, 127–138

Gartrell, M.J., Craun, J.C., Podrebarac, D.S. & Gunderson, E.L. (1985a) Pesticides, selected elements, and other chemicals in adult total diet samples, October 1979–September 1980. *J. Assoc. Off. Anal. Chem.*, **68**, 1184–1197

Gartrell, M.J., Craun, J.C., Podrebarac, D.S. & Gunderson, E.L. (1985b) Pesticides, selected elements, and other chemicals in infant and toddler total diet samples, October 1979–September 1980. *J. Assoc. Off. Anal. Chem.*, **68**, 1163–1183

Gasiorek, K. & Bauchinger, M. (1981) Chromosome changes in human lymphocytes after separate and combined treatment with divalent salts of lead, cadmium, and zinc. *Environ. Mutag.*, **3**, 513–518

Gélinas, Y., Lafond, J. & Schmit, J.-P. (1998) Multielemental Analysis of Human Fetal Tissues using Inductively Coupled Plasma-Mass Spectrometry. *Biol. Trace Elem. Res.*, **59**, 63–74

Gennart, J.P., Bernard, A. & Lauwerys, R. (1992) Assessment of thyroid, testes, kidney and autonomic nervous system function in lead-exposed workers. *Int. Arch. occup. environ. Health*, **64**, 49–57

George, P.M., Walmsley, T.A., Currie, D. & Wells, J.E. (1993) Lead exposure during recreational use of small bore rifle ranges. *N.Z. Med. J.*, **106**, 422–424

Gerhardsson, L., Lundström, N.-G., Nordberg, G. & Wall, S. (1986) Mortality and lead exposure: A retrospective cohort study of Swedish smelter workers. *Br. J. ind. Med.*, **43**, 707–712

Gerhardsson, L., Chettle, D.R., Englyst, V., Nordberg, G.F., Nyhlin, H., Scott, M.C., Todd, A.C. & Vesterberg, O. (1992) Kidney effects in long term exposed lead smelter workers. *Br. J. ind. Med.*, **49**, 186–192

Gerhardsson, L., Attewell, R., Chettle, D.R., Englyst, V., Lundström, N.G., Nordberg, G.F., Nyhlin, H., Scott, M.C. & Todd, A.C. (1993) In vivo measurements of lead in bone in long-term exposed lead smelter workers. *Arch. environ. Health*, **48**, 147–156

Gerhardsson, L., Hagmar, L., Rylander, L. & Skerfving, S. (1995a) Mortality and cancer incidence among secondary lead smelter workers. *Occup. environ. Med.*, **52**, 667–672

Gerhardsson, L., Englyst, V., Lundström, N.-G., Nordberg, G., Sandberg, S. & Steinvall, F. (1995b) Lead in tissues of deceased lead smelter workers. *J. trace Elem. Med. Biol.*, **9**, 136–143

Gerhardt, R.E., Crecelius, E.A. & Hudson, J.B. (1980) Trace element content of moonshine. *Arch. environ. Health*, **35**, 332–334

Gerr, F., Letz, R., Stokes, L., Chettle, D., McNeill, F. & Kaye, W. (2002) Association between bone lead concentration and blood pressure among young adults. *Am. J. ind. Med.*, **42**, 98–106

Gersberg, R.M., Gaynor, K., Tenczar, D., Bartzen, M., Ginsberg, M., Gresham, L.S. & Molgaard, C. (1997) Quantitative modeling of lead exposure from glazed ceramic pottery in childhood lead poisoning cases. *Int. J. environ. Health Res.*, **7**, 193–202

Gerson, M., Van Den Eeden, S.K. & Gahagan, P. (1996) Take-home lead poisoning in a child from his father's occupational exposure. *Am. J. ind. Med.*, **29**, 507–508

Gething, J. (1975) Tetramethyl lead absorption : A report of human exposure to a high level of tetramethyl lead. *Br. J. ind. Med.*, **32**, 329–333

Gisbert, C., Ros, R., De Haro, A., Walker, D.J., Bernal, M.P., Serrano, R. & Navarro-Aviñó, J. (2003) A plant genetically modified that accumulates Pb is especially promising for phyto-remediation. *Biochem. biophys. Res. Commun.*, **303**, 440–445

Gittleman, J. Estacio, P., O'Brien, D. & Montopoli, M. (1991) Health Hazard Evaluation Report, HETA 91-0213-2123, G.T. Jones Tire & Battery Distributing Inc., Birmingham, AL, USA, NIOSH

Giuffré de López Camelo, L., Ratto de Miguez, S. & Marbán, L. (1997) Heavy metals input with phosphate fertilizers used in Argentina. *Sci. total Environ.*, **204**, 245–250

Godwin, H.A. (2001) The biological chemistry of lead. *Curr. Opin. chem. Biol.*, **5**, 223–227

Goering, P.L. (1993) Lead-protein interactions as a basis for lead toxicity. *Neurotoxicology*, **14**, 45–60

Gogte, S.T., Basu, N., Sinclair, S., Ghai, O.P. & Bhide, N.K. (1991) Blood lead levels of children with pica and surma use. *Indian J. Pediatr.*, **58**, 513–519

Goldberg, A., Doyle, D., Yeung-Laiwah, A., Moore, M.R. & McColl, K.E.L. (1985) Relevance of cytochrome C oxidase deficiency to pathogenesis of acute porphyria. *Q. J. Med.*, **57**, 799 (Abstract)

Goldberg, R.L., Hicks, A.M., O'Leary, L.M. & London, S. (1991) Lead exposure at uncovered out-door firing ranges. *J. occup. Med.*, **33**, 718–719

Goldman, R.H., Baker, E.L., Hannan, M. & Kamerow, D. (1987) Lead poisoning in automobile radiator mechanics. *New Engl. J. Med.*, **317**, 214–218

Goldstein, G.W. (1993) Evidence that lead acts as a calcium substitute in second messenger meta-bolism. *Neurotoxicology*, **14**, 97–101

Goldstein, D.H., Benoit, J.N. & Tyroler, H.A. (1970) An epidemiologic study of an oil mist expo-sure. *Arch. environ. Health*, **21**, 600–603

Golter, M. & Michaelson, I.A. (1975) Growth, behavior and brain catecholamines in lead exposed neonatal rats: A reappraisal. *Science*, **187**, 359–361

González-Cossio, T., Peterson, K.E., Sanín, L.-H., Fishbein, E., Palazuelos, E., Aro, A., Hernández-Avila, M. & Hu, H. (1997) Decrease in birth weight in relation to maternal bone-lead burden. *Pediatrics*, **100**, 856–862

Gordon, J.N., Taylor, A. & Bennett, P.N. (2002) Lead poisoning: Case studies. *Br. J. clin. Pharma-col.*, **53**, 451–458

Goyer, R.A. (1989) Mechanisms of lead and cadmium nephrotoxicity. *Toxicol. Lett.*, **46**, 153–162

Goyer, R.A. (1990a) Transplacental transport of lead. *Environ. Health Perspect.*, **89**, 101–105

Goyer, R.A. (1990b) Lead toxicity: From overt to subclinical to subtle health effects. *Environ. Health Perspect.*, **86**, 177–181

Goyer, R.A. (1993) Lead toxicity: Current concerns. *Environ. Health Perspect.*, **100**, 177–187

Goyer, R.A. & Wilson, M.H. (1975) Lead-induced inclusion bodies: Results of ethylenediamine-tetraacetic acid treatment. *Lab. Invest.*, **32**, 149–156

Goyer, R.A., Leonard, D.L., Moore, J.F., Rhyne, B. & Krigman, M.R. (1970) Lead dosage and the role of the intranuclear inclusion body: An experimental study. *Arch. environ. Health*, **20**, 705–711

Grandjean, P. & Bach, E. (1986) Indirect exposures: The significance of bystanders at work and at home. *Am. ind. Hyg. Assoc. J.*, **47**, 819–824

Grandjean, P., Wulf, H.C. & Niebuhr, E. (1983) Sister chromatid exchange in response to variations in occupational lead exposure. *Environ. Res.*, **32**, 199–204

Granick, J.L., Sassa, S., Granick, S., Levere, R.D. & Kappas, A. (1973) Studies in lead poisoning. II. Correlation between the ratio of activated to inactivated δ-aminolevulinic acid dehydratase of whole blood and the blood lead level. *Biochem. Med.*, **8**, 149–159

Grant, L.D., Kimmel, C.A., West, G.L., Martinez-Vargas, C.M. & Howard, J.L. (1980) Chronic low-level toxicity in the rat. II. Effects on postnatal physical and behavioral development. *Toxicol. appl. Pharmacol.*, **56**, 42–58

Grant, S., Walmsley, T.A. & George, P.M. (1992) Industrial blood lead levels in the South Island during 1988 and 1989: Trends and follow up patterns. *N.Z. med. J.*, **105**, 323–326

Graziano, J.H. & Blum, C. (1991) Lead exposure from lead crystal. *Lancet*, **337**, 141–142

Graziano, J.H., Popovac, D., Factor-Litvak, P., Shrout, P., Kline, J., Murphy, M.J., Zhao, Y.H., Mehmeti, A., Ahmedi, X., Rajovic, B., Zvicer, Z., Nenezic, D.U., Lolacono, N.J. & Stein, Z. (1990) Determinants of elevated blood lead during pregnancy in a population surrounding a lead smelter in Kosovo, Yugoslavia. *Environ. Health Perspect.*, **89**, 95–100

Graziano, J.H., Slavkovic, V., Factor-Litvak, P., Popovac, D., Ahmedi, X. & Mehmeti, A. (1991) Depressed serum erythropoietin in pregnant women with elevated blood lead. *Arch. environ. Health*, **46**, 347–350

Graziano, J.H., Blum, C.B., Lolacono, N.J., Slavkovich, V., Manton, W.I., Pond, S. & Moore, M.R. (1996) A human *in vivo* model for the determination of lead bioavailability using stable isotope dilution. *Environ. Health Perspect.*, **104**, 176–179

Greene, T. & Ernhart, C.B. (1993) Dentine lead and intelligence prior to school entry: A statistical sensitivity analysis. *J. clin. Epidemiol.*, **46**, 323–339

Gregus, Z. & Klaassen, C.D. (1986) Disposition of metals in rats: A comparative study of fecal, urinary, and biliary excretion and tissue distribution of eighteen metals. *Toxicol. appl. Pharmacol.*, **85**, 24–38

Griffin, T.B., Coulston, F., Wills, H., Russel, J.C. & Knelson, J.H. (1975a) Clinical studies on men continuously exposed to airborne particulate lead. *Environ. Qual. Saf.*, **Suppl. 2**, 221–240

Griffin, T.B., Coulston, F., Wills, H. & Russell, J.C. (1975b) Biologic effects of airborne particulate lead on continuously exposed rats and rhesus monkeys. *Environ. Qual. Saf.*, **Suppl. 2**, 202–220

Grill, E., Winnacker, E.-L. & Zenk, M.H. (1985) Phytochelatins: The principal heavy-metal complexing peptides of higher plants. *Science*, **230**, 674–676

Grill, E., Gekeler, W., Winnacker, E.-L. & Zenk, H.H. (1986) Homo-phytochelatins are heavy metal-binding peptides of homo-glutathione containing Fabales. *FEBS Letters*, **205**, 47–50

Grill, E., Winnacker, E.-L. & Zenk, M.H. (1987) Phytochelatins, a class of heavy-metal-binding peptides from plants, are functionally analogous to metallothioneins. *Proc. natl Acad. Sci. USA*, **84**, 439–443

Grill, E., Löffler, S., Winnacker, E.-L. & Zenk, M.H. (1989) Phytochelatins, the heavy-metal-binding peptides of plants, are synthesized from glutathione by a specific γ-glutamylcysteine dipeptidyl transpeptidase (phytochelatin synthetase). *Proc. natl Acad. Sci. USA*, **86**, 6838–6842

Grill, E., Winnacker, E.L. & Zenk, M.H. (1991) Phytochelatins. *Meth. Enzymol.*, **205**, 333–341

Grobler, S.R., Rossouw, R.J. & Maresky, L.S. (1985) Blood lead levels in a remote, unpolluted rural area in South Africa. *S. Afr. Med. J.*, **68**, 323–324

Grobler, S.R., Rossouw, R.J. & Kotze, D. (1988) Effect of airborne lead on the blood lead levels of rats. *S. Afr. J. Sci.*, **84**, 260–262

Grobler, S.R., Rossouw, R.J., Kotze, T.J.V.W. & Stander, I.A. (1991) The effect of airborne lead on lead levels of blood, incisors and alveolar bone of rats. *Arch. oral Biol.*, **36**, 357–360

Gross, S.B., Pfitzer, E.A., Yeager, D.W. & Kehoe, R.A. (1975) Lead in human tissues. *Toxicol. appl. Pharmacol.*, **32**, 638–651

Guilarte, T.R., Miceli, R.C. & Jett, D.A. (1995) Biochemical evidence of an interaction of lead at the zinc allosteric sites of the NMDA receptor complex: Effects of neuronal development. *Neurotoxicology*, **16**, 63–71

Gulson, B.L. (1986) *Lead Isotopes in Mineral Exploration. Developments in Economic Geology*, Vol. 23, Amsterdam, Elsevier

Gulson, B.L. (1996a) Tooth analyses of sources and intensity of lead exposure in children. *Environ. Health Perspect.*, **104**, 306–312

Gulson, B.L. (1996b) Nails: Concern over their use in lead exposure assessment. *Sci. total Environ.*, **177**, 323–327

Gulson, B.L., Mizon, K.J., Law, A.J., Korsch, M.J. & Davis, J.J. (1994) Source and pathways of lead in humans from the Broken Hill mining community — An alternative use of exploration methods. *Econom. Geol.*, **89**, 889–908

Gulson, B.L., Mahaffey, K.R., Mizon, K.J., Korsch, M.J., Cameron, M.A. & Vimpani, G. (1995) Contribution of tissue lead to blood lead in adult female subjects based on stable lead isotope methods. *J. Lab. clin. Med.*, **125**, 703–712

Gulson, B.L., James, M., Giblin, A.M., Sheehan, A. & Mitchell, P. (1997a) Maintenance of elevated lead levels in drinking water from occasional use and potential impact on blood leads in children. *Sci. total Environ.*, **205**, 271–275

Gulson, B.L., Mahaffey, K.R., Vidal, M., Jameson, C.W., Vidal, M., Law, A.J., Mizon, K.J., Smith, A.J.M. & Korsch, M.J. (1997b) Dietary lead intakes for mother/child pairs and relevance to pharmacokinetic models. *Environ Health Perspect.*, **105**, 1334–1342

Gulson, B.L., Jameson, C.W., Mahaffey, K.R., Mizon, K.J., Korsch, M.J. & Vimpani, G. (1997c) Pregnancy increases mobilization of lead from maternal skeleton. *J. Lab. Clin. Med.*, **130**, 51–62

Gulson, B.L., Jameson, C.W., Mahaffey, K.R., Mizon, K.J., Patison, N., Law, A.J., Korsch, M.J. & Salter, M.A. (1998a) Relationships of lead in breast milk to lead in blood, urine, and diet of the infant and mother. *Environ. Health Perspect.*, **106**, 667–674

Gulson, B.L., Cameron, M.A., Smith, A.J., Mizon, K.J., Korsch, M.J., Vimpani, G., McMichael, A.J., Pisaniello, D., Jameson, C.W. & Mahaffey, K.R. (1998b) Blood lead-urine lead relationships in adults and children. *Environ. Res.*, **78**, 152–160

Gulson, B.L., Stockley, C.S., Lee T.H., Gray, B., Mizon, K.J. & Patison, N. (1998c) Contribution of lead in wine to the total dietary intake of lead in humans with and without a meal: A pilot study. *J. Wine Res.*, **9**, 5–14

Gulson, B.L., Mahaffey, K.R., Jameson, C.W., Mizon, K.J., Korsch, M.J., Cameron, M.A. & Eisman, J.A. (1998d) Mobilization of lead from the skeleton during the postnatal period is larger than during pregnancy. *J. Lab. clin. Med.*, **131**, 324–329

Gulson, B.L., Gray, B., Mahaffey, K.R., Jameson, C.W., Mizon, K.J., Patison, N. & Korsch, M.J. (1999) Comparison of the rates of exchange of lead in the blood of newly born infants and their mothers with lead from their current environment. *J. Lab. clin. Med.*, **133**, 171–178

Gulson, B.L., Mizon, K.J., Palmer, J.M., Korsch, M.J., Patison, N., Jameson, C.W. & Donnelly, J.B. (2000) Urinary lead isotopes during pregnancy and postpartum indicate no preferential partitioning of endogenous lead into plasma. *J. Lab. clin. Med.*, **136**, 236–242

Gulson, B.L., Mizon, K.J., Palmer, J.M., Patison, N., Law, A.J., Korsch, M.J., Mahaffey, K.R. & Donnelly, J.B. (2001a) Longitudinal study of daily intake and excretion of lead in newly born infants. *Environ. Res.*, **85**, 232–245

Gulson, B.L., Mizon, K.J., Palmer, J.M., Korsch, M.J. & Taylor, A.J. (2001b) Contribution of lead from calcium supplements to blood lead. *Environ. Health Perspect.*, **109**, 283–288

Gulson, B., Mizon, K., Smith, H., Eisman, J., Palmer, J., Korsch, M., Donnelly, J. & Waite, K. (2002) Skeletal lead release during bone resorption: Effect of bisphosphonate treatment in a pilot study. *Environ. Health Perspect.*, **110**, 1017–1023

Gulson, B.L., Mizon, K.J., Korsch, M.J., Palmer, J.M. & Donnelly, J.B. (2003) Mobilization of lead from human bone tissue during pregnancy and lactation — A summary of long-term research. *Sci. total Environ.*, **303**, 79–104

Gulson, B.L., Mizon, K.J., Palmer, J.M., Korsch, M.J., Taylor, A.J. & Mahaffey, K.R. (2004) Blood lead changes during pregnancy and postpartum with calcium supplementation. *Environ. Health Perspect.*, **112**, 1499–1507

Gunshin, H., Mackenzie, B., Berger, U.V., Gunshin, Y., Romero, M.F., Boron, W.F., Nussberger, S., Gollan, J.L. & Hediger, M.A. (1997) Cloning and characterization of a mammalian proton-coupled metal-ion transporter. *Nature*, **388**, 482–488

Gunter, B.J. (1985) Health Hazard Evaluation Report, HETA 85-0170-1643, C.F. & I. Steel, Pueblo, CO, USA, NIOSH

Gunter, B.J. (1987) Health Hazard Evaluation Report, HETA 86-0070-1774, Silver Deer Spectrum, Boulder, CO, USA, NIOSH

Gunter, B.J. & Daniels, W. (1990) Health Hazard Evaluation Report, HETA 89-0295-2007, Peerless Alloy Inc., Denver, CO, USA, NIOSH

Gunter, B.J. & Hales, T.R. (1990a) Health Hazard Evaluation Report, HETA 89-0231-2016, Sims Radiator Shop, Decatur, GA, USA, NIOSH

Gunter, B.J. & Hales, T.R. (1990b) Health Hazard Evaluation Report, HETA 89-0234-2014, Sims Radiator Shop, Decatur, GA, USA, NIOSH

Gunter, B.J. & Hales, T.R. (1990c) Health Hazard Evaluation Report, HETA 89-0232-2015, Sims Radiator Shop, Chamblee, GA, USA, NIOSH

Gunter, B.J. & Hales, T.R. (1990d) Health Hazard Evaluation Report, HETA 89-0233-2013, Sims Radiator Shop, Lawrenceville, GA, USA, NIOSH

Gunter, B.J. & Hammel, R. (1989) Health Hazard Evaluation Report, HETA 88-0354-1955, Lakewood Radiator Shop, Denver, CO, USA, NIOSH

Gunter, B.J. & Seligman, P.J. (1984) Health Hazard Evaluation Report, HETA 84-0038-1513, Kennecott Smelter, Hurley, NM, USA, NIOSH

Gunter, B.J. & Thoburn, T.W. (1984) Health Hazard Evaluation Report, HETA 84-0099-1514, C.F. & I. Steel, Pueblo, CO, USA, NIOSH

Gunter, B.J. & Thoburn, T.W. (1985) Health Hazard Evaluation Report, HETA 84-0384-1580, Crystal Zoo, Boulder, CO, USA, NIOSH

Gunter, B.J. & Thoburn, T.W. (1986a) Health Hazard Evaluation Report, HETA 86-0348-1756, J'Leen Ltd., Boulder, CO, USA, NIOSH

Gunter, B.J. & Thoburn, T.W. (1986b) Health Hazard Evaluation Report, HETA 86-0087-1686, TAC Radiator, Minot, ND, USA, NIOSH

Gunter, B.J., Richardson, F. & Anderson, K.E. (1986) Health Hazard Evaluation Report, HETA 86-0438,0534-1795, Bondar-Clegg, Lakewood, CO & Sparks, NV, USA, NIOSH

Guo, H.R., Ballard, T.J., Madar, S., Piacitelli, G.M. & Seligman, P.J. (1994) Health Hazard Evaluation Report, HETA 93-0955-2390, United Seal Co., Columbus, OH, USA, NIOSH

Gupta, S. & Dogra, T.D. (2002) Air pollution and human health hazards. *Indian J. occup. environ. Med.*, **6**, 89–93

Gustafson, A., Hedner, P., Schütz, A. & Skjerfving, S. (1989) Occupational lead exposure and pituitary function. *Int. Arch. occup. environ. Health*, **61**, 277–281

Hackett, P.L., Hess, J.O. & Sikov, M.R. (1982a) Effect of dose level and pregnancy on the distribution and toxicity of intravenous lead in rats. *J. Toxicol. environ. Health*, **9**, 1007–1020

Hackett, P.L., Hess, J.O. & Sikov, M.R. (1982b) Distribution and effects of intravenous lead in the fetoplacental unit of the rat. *J. Toxicol. environ. Health*, **9**, 1021–1032

Hadi, D.A., Chowdhury, A.H. & Akhter, S. (1996) Status of lead and cadmium in poly(vinyl chloride) pipes. *Bangladesh J. sci. ind. Res.*, **31**, 39–42

Haeger-Aronsen, B., Abdulla, M. & Fristedt, B.I. (1974) Effect of lead on δ-aminolevulinic acid dehydratase activity in red blood cells. *Arch. environ. Health*, **29**, 150–153

Hales, T.R. & Gunter, B.J. (1990) Health Hazard Evaluation Report, HETA 89-0196-2023, Hazen Research Inc., Golden, CO, USA, NIOSH

Hales, T.R., Kiefer, M., Mitchell, C. & Salisbury, S. (1991) Health Hazard Evaluation Report, HETA 91-0393-2171, Georgia Metals, Inc., Powder Springs, GA, USA, NIOSH

Hall, R.M., Page, E., Mattorano, D. & Roegner, K. (1998) Health Hazard Evaluation Report, HETA 97-0292-2678, General Electric — Bridgeville Glass Plant, Bridgeville, PA, USA, NIOSH

Hamilton, J.W., Bement, W.J., Sinclair, P.R., Sinclair, J.F., Alcedo, J.A. & Wetterhahn, K.E. (1991) Heme regulates hepatic 5-aminolevulinate synthase mRNA expression by decreasing mRNA half-life and not by altering its rate of transcription. *Arch. Biochem. Biophys.*, **289**, 387–392

Hammad, T.A., Sexton, M. & Langenberg, P. (1996) Relationship between blood lead and dietary iron intake in preschool children. A cross-sectional study. *Ann. Epidemiol.*, **6**, 30–33

Hamurcu, Z., Donmez, H., Saraymen, R. & Demirtas, H. (2001) Micronucleus frequencies in workers exposed to lead, zinc, and cadmium. *Biol. trace Elem. Res.*, **83**, 97–102

Hanas, J.S., Rodgers, J.S., Bantle, J.A. & Cheng, Y.-G. (1999) Lead inhibition of DNA-binding mechanism of Cys_2His_2 zinc finger proteins. *Mol. Pharmacol.*, **56**, 982–988

Hansen, O.N., Trillingsgaard, A., Beese, I., Lyngbye, T. & Grandjean, P. (1989) A neuropsychological study of children with elevated dentine lead level: Assessment of the effect of lead in different socio-economic groups. *Neurotoxicol. Teratol.*, **11**, 205–213

Harney, J.M. & Barsan, M.E. (1999) Health Hazard Evaluation Report, HETA 97-0255-2735, Forest Park Police Department, Forest Park, OH, USA, NIOSH

Harper, C.C., Mathee, A., von Schirnding, Y., De Rosa, C.T. & Falk, H. (2003) The health impact of environmental pollutants: A special focus on lead exposure in South Africa. *Int. J. Hyg. environ. Health*, **206**, 315–322

Hart, C. (1987) Art hazards: An overview for sanitarians and hygienists. *J. environ. Health*, **49**, 282–287

Hart, M.H. & Smith, J.L. (1981) Effect of vitamin D and low dietary calcium on lead uptake and retention in rats. *J. Nutr.*, **111**, 694–698

Hartwig, A. (1994) Role of DNA repair inhibition in lead- and cadmium-induced genotoxicity: A review. *Environ. Health Perspect.*, **102** (Suppl. 3), 45–50

Hartwig, A., Schlepegrell, R. & Beyersmann, D. (1990) Indirect mechanism of lead-induced genotoxicity in cultured mammalian cells. *Mutat. Res.*, **241**, 75–82

Hashim, J.H., Hashim, Z., Omar, A. & Shamsudin, S.B. (2000) Blood lead levels of urban and rural Malaysian primary school children. *Asia Pac. J. public Health*, **12**, 65–70

Hass, G.M., Brown, D.V.L., Eisenstein, R. & Hemmens, A. (1964) Relations between lead poisoning in rabbit and man. *Am. J. Pathol.*, **45**, 691–727

Hass, G.M., McDonald, J.H., Oyasu, R., Battifora, H.A. & Paloucek, J.T. (1967) Renal neoplasia induced by combinations of dietary lead subacetate and N-2-fluorenylacetamide. In: *Renal Neoplasia*, pp. 377–412

Hayakawa, K. (1972) Microdetermination and dynamic aspects of in vivo alkyl lead compounds. II. Studies on the dynamic aspects of alkyl lead compounds in vivo. *Nippon Eiseigaku Zasshi*, **26**, 526–535

He, L., Poblenz, A.T., Medrano, C.J. & Fox, D.A. (2000) Lead and calcium produce rod photoreceptor cell apoptosis by opening the mitochondrial permeability transition pore. *J. biol. Chem.*, **275**, 12175–12184

Healy, M.A., Harrison, P.G., Aslam, M., Davis, S.S. & Wilson, C.G. (1982) Lead sulphide and traditional preparations: Routes for ingestion, and solubility and reactions in gastric fluid. *J. clin. Hosp. Pharm.*, **7**, 169–173

Heard, M.J. & Chamberlain, A.C. (1982) Effect of minerals and food on uptake of lead from the gastrointestinal tract in humans. *Hum. Toxicol.*, **1**, 411–415

Heard, M.J. & Chamberlain, A.C. (1984) Uptake of Pb by human skeleton and comparative metabolism of Pb and alkaline earth elements. *Health Phys.*, **47**, 857–865

Heard, M.J., Wells, A.C., Newton, D. & Chamberlain, A.C. (1979) Human uptake and metabolism of tetra ethyl and tetramethyl lead vapour labelled with ^{203}Pb. In: *Proceedings of an International Conference on Management and Control of Heavy Metals in the Environment, London, England, September*, Edinburgh, CEP Consultants, pp. 103–108

Heard, M.J., Chamberlain, A.C. & Sherlock, J.C. (1983) Uptake of lead by humans and effect of minerals and food. *Sci. total Environ.*, **30**, 245–253

Hengstler, J.G., Bolm-Audorff, U., Faldum, A., Janssen, K., Reifenrath, M., Gotte, W., Jung, D., Mayer-Popken, O., Fuchs, J., Gebhard, S., Bienfait, H.G., Schlink, K., Dietrich, C., Faust, D., Epe, B. & Oesch, F. (2003) Occupational exposure to heavy metals: DNA damage induction and DNA repair inhibition prove co-exposures to cadmium, cobalt and lead as more dangerous than hitherto expected. *Carcinogenesis*, **24** , 63–73

Henning, S.J. & Leeper, L.L. (1984) Duodenal uptake of lead by suckling and weanling rats. *Biol. Neonate*, **46**, 27–35

Hernández, E., Gutiérrez-Ruiz, M.C. & García Vargas, G. (1998) Effect of acute lead treatment on coproporphyrinogen oxidase activity in HepG2 cells. *Toxicology*, **126**, 163–171

Hernandez-Avila, M., Gonzalez-Cossio, T., Palazuelos, E., Romieu, I., Aro, A., Fishbein, E., Peterson, K.E. & Hu, H. (1996) Dietary and environmental determinants of blood and bone lead levels in lactating postpartum women living in Mexico City. *Environ. Health Perspect.*, **104**, 1076–1082

Hernandez-Avila, M., Smith, D., Meneses, F., Sanin, L.H. & Hu, H. (1998) The influence of bone and blood lead on plasma lead levels in environmentally exposed adults. *Environ. Health Perspect.*, **106**, 473–477

Hernandez-Avila, M., Villalpando, C.G., Palazuelos, E., Hu, H., Villalpando, M.E. & Martinez, D.R. (2000) Dcterminants of blood lead levels across the menopausal transition. *Arch. environ. Health*, **55**, 355–360

Hernandez-Avila, M., Peterson, K.E., Gonzalez-Cossio, T., Sanin, L.H., Aro, A., Schnaas, L. & Hu, H. (2002) Effect of maternal bone lead on length and head circumference of newborns and 1-month-old infants. *Arch. environ. Health*, **57**, 482–488

Hernandez-Avila, M., Gonzalez-Cossio, T., Hernandez-Avila, J.E., Romieu, I., Peterson, K.E., Aro, A., Palazuelos, E. & Hu, H. (2003) Dietary calcium supplements to lower blood lead levels in lactating women: A randomized placebo-controlled trial. *Epidemiology*, **14**, 206–212

Hernberg, S. (2000) Lead poisoning in a historical perspective. *Am. J. ind. Med.*, **38**, 244–254

Hershko, C., Eisenberg, A., Avni, A., Grauer, F., Acker, C., Hamdallah, M., Shahin, S., Moreb, J., Richter, E. & Weissenberg, E. (1989) Lead poisoning by contaminated flour. *Rev. environ. Health*, **8**, 17–23

Hertz-Picciotto, I. (2000) The evidence that lead increases the risk for spontaneous abortion. *Am. J. ind. Med.*, **38**, 300–309

Hertz-Picciotto, I. & Croft, J. (1993) Review of the relation between blood lead and blood pressure. *Epidemiol. Rev.*, **15**, 352–373

Hertz-Picciotto, I., Schramm, M., Watt-Morse, M., Chantala, K., Anderson, J. & Osterloh, J. (2000) Patterns and determinants of blood lead during pregnancy. *Am. J. Epidemiol.*, **152**, 829–837

Heywood, R. & James, R.W. (1985) Current laboratory approaches for assessing male reproductive toxicity: Testicular toxicity in laboratory animals. In: Dixon, R.L., ed., *Reproductive Toxicology* (Target Organ Toxicology Series), New York, Raven Press, pp. 147–160

Hiasa, Y., Ohshima, M., Kitahori, Y., Fujita, T., Yuasa, T. & Miyashiro, A. (1983) Basic lead acetate: Promoting effect on the development of renal tubular cell tumors in rats treated with N-ethyl-N-hydroxyethylnitrosamine. *J. natl Cancer Inst.*, **70**, 761–765

Hiasa, Y., Konishi, N., Nakaoka, S., Nakamura, M., Nishii, S., Kitahori, Y. & Ohshima, M. (1991) Possible application to medium-term organ bioassays for renal carcinogenesis modifiers in rats treated with N-ethyl-N-hydroxyethylnitrosamine and unilateral nephrectomy. *Jpn. J. Cancer Res.*, **82**, 1385–1390

Hilderbrand, D.C., Der, R., Griffin, W.T. & Fahim, M.S. (1973) Effect of lead acetate on reproduction. *Am. J. Obstet. Gynecol.*, **115**, 1058–1065

Hill, G.J. & Hill, S. (1995) Lead poisoning due to *hai ge fen*. *J. Am. med. Assoc.*, **273**, 24–25

Hills, B. & Savery, H. (1988) Health Hazard Evaluation Report, HETA 87-0410-1868, Klotz Brothers, Inc., Staunton, VA, USA, NIOSH

Hindy, K.T., Farag, S.A., El-Taieb, N.M., Rizk, H.F. & Ibrahim, J.M. (1987) Spectrographic study of heavy metals in an industrial area in North Cairo. In: *Proceedings, International Conference on Heavy Metals in the Environment*, New Orleans, Vol. 1, pp. 134–136

Hinton, D.E., Lipsky, M.M., Heatfield, B.M. & Trump, B.F. (1979) Opposite effects of lead on chemical carcinogenesis in kidney and liver of rats. *Bull. environ. Contam. Toxicol.*, **23**, 464–469

Hinton, D., Coope, P.A., Malpress, W.A. & Janus, E.D. (1986) Trends in blood lead levels in Christchurch (NZ) and environs 1978–85. *J. Epidemiol. Community Health*, **40**, 244–248

Hirata, M., Yoshida, T., Miyajima, K., Kosaka, H. & Tabuchi, T. (1995) Correlation between lead in plasma and other indicators of lead exposure among lead-exposed workers. *Int. Arch. occup. environ. Health*, **68**, 58–63

Hisham, J. & Pertanika, Z.H. (1995) Lead and cadmium content of total suspended particulates in the atmosphere over the Klang valley. *J. Sci. Technol.*, **3**, 57–65

Ho, S.F., Sam, C,T. & Embi, G.B. (1998) Lead exposure in the lead–acid storage battery manufacturing and PVC compounding industries. *Occup. Med.*, **48**, 369–373

Hoar, S.K., Morrison, A.S., Cole, P. & Silverman, D.T. (1980) An occupation and exposure linkage system for the study of occupational carcinogenesis. *J. occup. Med.*, **22**, 722–726

Hodgkins, D.G., Robins, T.G., Hinkamp, D.L., Schork, M.A., Levine, S.P. & Krebs, W.H. (1991) The effect of airborne lead particle size on worker blood-lead levels: An empirical study of battery workers. *J. occup. Med.*, **33**, 1265–1273

Holdstein, Y., Pratt, H., Goldsher, M., Rosen, G., Shenhav, R., Linn, S., Mor, A. & Barkai, A. (1986) Auditory brainstem evoked potentials in asymptomatic lead-exposed subjects. *J. Laryngol. Otol.*, **100**, 1031–1036

Hollett, B. & Moody, P.L. (1984) Health Hazard Evaluation Report, HETA 80-0115-1401, U.S. Steel, Lorain-Cayahoga Works, Lorain, OH, USA, NIOSH

Hopkins, A.P. & Dayan, A.D. (1974) The pathology of experimental lead encephalopathy in the baboon (*Papio anubis*). *Br. J. ind. Med.*, **31**, 128–133

Hoppin, J.A., Aro, A., Hu, H. & Ryan, P.B. (1997) In vivo bone lead measurement in suburban teenagers. *Pediatrics*, **100**, 365–370

Hoppin, J.A., Aro, A., Hu, H. & Ryan, P.B. (2000) Measurement variability associated with KXRF bone lead measurement in young adults. *Environ. Health Perspect.*, **108**, 239–242

Horiguchi, S., Teramoto, K., Kiyota, I., Shinagawa, K., Nakano, H., Karai, I. & Matsuda, F. (1981) Relationships among the parameters of lead absorption and lead effects especially on the hematopoietic system. *Osaka City med. J.*, **27**, 35–45

Houston, D.K. & Johnson, M.A. (2000) Does vitamin C intake protect against lead toxicity? *Nutr. Rev.*, **58**, 73–75

Hrdina, P.D., Peters, D.A.V. & Singhal, R.L. (1976) Effects of chronic exposure to cadmium, lead and mercury on brain biogenic amines in the rat. *Res. Commun. chem. Pathol. Pharmacol.*, **15**, 483–493

Hryhorczuk, D.O., Rabinowitz, M.B., Hessl, S.M., Hoffman, D., Hogan, M.M., Mallin, K., Finch, H., Orris, P. & Berman, E. (1985) Elimination kinetics of blood lead in workers with chronic lead intoxication. *Am. J. ind. Med.*, **8**, 33–42

Hsiao, C.Y., Wu, H.D.I., Lai, J.S. & Kuo, H.W. (2001) A longitudinal study of the effects of long-term exposure to lead among lead battery factory workers in Taiwan (1989–1999). *Sci. total Environ.*, **279**, 151–158

Hu, H. (1991) Knowledge of diagnosis and reproductive history among survivors of childhood plumbism. *Am. J. pub. Health*, **81**, 1070–1072

Hu, H., Pepper, L & Goldman, R. (1991) Effect of repeated occupational exposure to lead, cessation of exposure, and chelation on levels of lead in bone. *Am. J. ind. Med.*, **20**, 723–735

Hu, H., Aro, A. & Rotnitzky, A. (1995) Bone lead measured by X-ray fluorescence: Epidemiologic methods. *Environ. Health Perspect.*, **103** (Suppl. 1), 105–110

Hu, H., Hashimoto, D. & Besser, M. (1996a) Levels of lead in blood and bone of women giving birth in a Boston hospital. *Arch. environ. Health*, **51**, 52–58

Hu, H., Aro, A., Payton, M., Korrick, S., Sparrow, D., Weiss, S.T. & Rotnitzky, A. (1996b) The relationship of bone and blood lead to hypertension. The Normative Aging Study. *J. Am. med. Assoc.*, **275**, 1171–1176

Hu, H., Payton, M., Korrick, S., Aro, A., Sparrow, D., Weiss, S.T. & Rotnitzky, A. (1996c) Determinants of bone and blood lead levels among community-exposed middle-aged to elderly men. The Normative Aging Study. *Am. J. Epidemiol.*, **144**, 749–759

Hu, H., Rabinowitz, M. & Smith, D. (1998) Bone lead as a biological marker in epidemiologic studies of chronic toxicity: Conceptual paradigms. *Environ. Health Perspect.*, **106**, 1–8

Hu, H., Wu, M.-T., Cheng, Y., Sparrow, D., Weiss, S. & Kelsey, K. (2001) The δ-aminolevulinic acid dehydratase (ALAD) polymorphism and bone and blood lead levels in community-exposed men: The Normative Aging Study. *Environ. Health Perspect.*, **109**, 827–832

Hu, J., Johnson, K.C., Mao, Y., Guo, L., Zhao, X., Jia, X., Bi, D., Huang, G. & Liu, R. (1998) Risk factors for glioma in adults: A case–control study in northeast China. *Cancer Detect. Prev.*, **22**, 100–108

Hu, J., Little, J., Xu, T., Zhao, X., Guo, L., Jia, X., Huang, G., Bi, D. & Liu, R. (1999) Risk factors for meningioma in adults: A case–control study in northeast China. *Int. J. Cancer*, **83**, 299–304

Huang, J.W. & Cunningham, S.D. (1996) Lead phytoextraction: Species variation in lead uptake and translocation. *New Phytol.*, **134**, 75–84

Huang, J.X., He, F.S., Wu, Y.G. & Zhang, S.C. (1988) Observations on renal function in workers exposed to lead. *Sci. total Environ.*, **71**, 535–537

Huang, X.-P., Feng, Z.-Y., Zhai, W.-L. & Xu, J.-H. (1988) Chromosomal aberrations and sister chromatid exchanges in workers exposed to lead. *Biomed. environ. Sci.*, **1**, 382–387

Huang, J.W., Chen, J., Berti, W.R. & Cunningham, S.D. (1997) Phytoremediation of lead-contaminated soils: Role of synthetic chelates in lead phytoextraction. *Environ. Sci. Technol.*, **31**, 800–805

Hueper, W.C. (1961) Environmental carcinogenesis and cancers. *Cancer Res.*, **21**, 842–857

Huguet, J.M., Braun, J.P., Burgat-Sacaze, V., Bernard, P. & Rico, A.G. (1982) Acute kidney disturbances by lead acetate in the rat. *Toxicol. Lett.*, **10**, 395–398

Hunaiti, A., Soud, M. & Khalil, A. (1995) Lead concentration and the level of glutathione, glutathione *S*-transferase, reductase and peroxidase in the blood of some occupational workers from Irbid City, Jordan. *Sci. total Environ.*, **170**, 95–100

Hunter, D. (1978) The ancient metals. In: *The Diseases of Occupations*, 6th Ed., London, Hodder & Stroughton

Hursh, J.B. (1973) Retention of ^{210}Pb in beagle dogs. *Health Phys.*, **25**, 29–35

Hursh, J.B. & Suomela, J. (1968) Absorption of ^{212}Pb from the gastrointestinal tract of man. *Acta radiol. ther. phys. biol.*, **7**, 108–120

Huseman, C.A., Varma, M.M. & Angle, C.R. (1992) Neuroendocrine effects of toxic and low blood lead levels in children. *Pediatrics*, **90**, 186–189

Hussain, T., Khan, I.H. & Ali Khan, M. (1990) Study of environmental pollutants in and around the city of Lahore. I. Determination of lead in blood of various population groups. *Sci. total Environ.*, **99**, 137–143

Hwang, Y.-H., Chao, K.-Y., Chang, C.-W., Hsiao, F.-T., Chang, H.-L. & Han, H.-Z. (2000) Lip lead as an alternative measure for lead exposure assessment of lead battery assembly workers. *Am. ind. Hyg. Assoc. J.*, **61**, 825–831

Hwang, K.-Y., Schwartz, B.-S., Lee, B.-K., Strickland, P.T., Todd, A.C. & Bressler, J.P. (2001) Associations of lead exposure and dose measures with erythrocyte protein kinase C activity in 212 current Korean lead workers. *Toxicol. Sci.*, **62**, 280–288

Hwua, Y.-S. & Yang, J.-L. (1998) Effect of 3-aminotriazole on anchorage independence and mutagenicity in cadmium- and lead-treated diploid human fibroblasts. *Carcinogenesis*, **19**, 881–888

Hytten, F. (1985) Blood volume changes in normal pregnancy. *Clin. Haematol.*, **14**, 601–612

IAEA (1987) Co-ordinated research programme on human daily dietary intakes of nutritionally important trace elements as measured by nuclear and other techniques. *IAEA Newl.*, **2**, 6–15

IARC (1972) *IARC Monographs on the Evaluation of Carcinogenic Risk of Chemicals to Man*, Vol. 1, *Some Inorganic Substances, Chlorinated Hydrocarbons, Aromatic Amines, N-Nitroso Compounds, and Natural Products*, Lyon

IARC (1973) *IARC Monographs on the Evaluation of Carcinogenic Risk of Chemicals to Man*, Vol. 2, *Some Inorganic and Organometallic Compounds*, Lyon

IARC (1976) *IARC Monographs on the Evaluation of Carcinogenic Risk of Chemicals to Man*, Vol. 12, *Some Carbamates, Thiocarbamates and Carbazides*, Lyon

IARC (1980) *IARC Monographs on the Evaluation of the Carcinogenic Risk of Chemicals to Humans*, Vol 23, *Some Metals and Metallic Compounds*, Lyon

IARC (1987) *IARC Monographs on the Evaluation of Carcinogenic Risks to Humans*, Suppl. 7, *Overall Evaluations of Carcinogenicity: An Updating of IARC Monographs Volumes 1 to 42*, Lyon

IARC (1989) *IARC Monographs on the Evaluation of Carcinogenic Risks to Humans*, Vol. 46, *Diesel and Gasoline Engine Exhausts and Some Nitroarenes*, Lyon, pp. 153

IARC (1990) *IARC Monographs on the Evaluation of Carcinogenic Risks to Humans*, Vol. 49, *Chromium, Nickel and Welding*, Lyon

IARC (1994) *IARC Monographs on the Evaluation of Carcinogenic Risks to Humans*, Vol. 58, *Beryllium, Cadmium, Mercury, and Exposures in the Glass Manufacturing Industry*, Lyon, pp. 371

IARC (1999) *IARC Monographs on the Evaluation of Carcinogenic Risks to Humans*, Vol. 74, *Surgical Implants and Other Foreign Bodies*, Lyon

IARC (2004a) *IARC Monographs on the Evaluation of Carcinogenic Risks to Humans*, Vol. 83, *Tobacco Smoke and Involuntary Smoking*, Lyon

IARC (2004b) *IARC Monographs on the Evaluation of Carcinogenic Risks to Humans*, Vol. 84, *Some Drinking-water Disinfectants and Contaminants, including Arsenic*, Lyon

Iavicoli, I., Sgambato, A., Carelli, G., Ardito, R., Cittadini, A. & Castellino, N. (2001) Lead-related effects on rat fibroblasts. *Mol. cell. Biochem.*, **222**, 35–40

Iavicoli, I., Carelli, G., Stanek, E.J. III, Castellino, N. & Calabrese, E.J. (2003) Effects of low doses of dietary lead on red blood cell production in male and female mice. *Toxicol. Lett.*, **137**, 193–199

Ikeda, M., Zhang, Z.W., Shimbo, S., Watanabe, T., Nakatsuka, H., Moon, C.-S., Matsuda-Inoguchi, N. & Higashikawa, K. (2000a) Exposure of women in general populations to lead via food and air in East and Southeast Asia. *Am. J. intern. Med.*, **38**, 271–280

Ikeda, M., Zhang, Z.-W., Shimbo, S., Watanabe, T., Nakatsuka, H., Moon, C.-S., Matsuda-Inoguchi, N. & Higashikawa, K. (2000b) Urban population exposure to lead and cadmium in East and South-East Asia. *Sci. total Environ.*, **249**, 373–384

Industrias Deriplom SA (2003) *Our Products: Pure Lead and Alloys; Lead Oxides; Lead Shot Pellets; Lead Sheets*, Buenos Aires

Inskip, M.J., Franklin, C.A., Baccanale, C.L., Manton, W.I., O'Flaherty, E.J., Edwards, C.M.H., Blenkinsop, J.B. & Edwards, E.B. (1996) Measurement of the flux of lead from bone to blood in a nonhuman primate (*Macaca fascicularis*) by sequential administration of stable lead isotopes. *Fundam. appl. Toxicol.*, **33**, 235–245

International Lead and Zinc Study Group (1990) *Lead and Zinc Statistics — 1960–1988*, London, pp. 9–56

International Lead and Zinc Study Group (1992) *Principal Uses of Lead and Zinc, 1960–1990*, London, pp. 32–51, 63–86

International Lead and Zinc Study Group (2000) *Environmental and Health Controls on Lead*, London

International Lead and Zinc Study Group (2003) *Principal Uses of Lead and Zinc*, London, pp. 5, 7

International Lead and Zinc Study Group (2004) *Interactive Statistical Database*, London [http://www.ilzsg.org; accessed 03/02/2004]

International Lead Management Center (ILMC) (1999) *Lead in Gasoline Phase-Out Report Card*, Washington DC [http://www.ilmc.org; accessed 10/02/2004]

IOMC (1998) Lead exposure and human health. In: *Global Opportunities for Reducing the Use of Leaded Gasoline*, United Nations, Inter-organization Programme for the sound Management of Chemicals, pp. 7–16

Ishida, M., Ishizaki, M. & Yamada, Y. (1996) Decreases in postural change of finger blood flow in ceramic painters chronically exposed to low level lead. *Am. J. ind. Med.*, **29**, 547–553

Israili, A.W. (1991) Occurrence of heavy metals in Ganga river water and sediments of western Uttar Pradesh. *Pollut. Res.*, **10**, 103–109

Israili, A.W. & Khurshid, S. (1991) Distribution of heavy metals in Yamuna river water and sediments from Delhi to Allahabad. *Poll. Res.*, **10**, 215–222

Ito, N. (1973) Experimental studies on tumors of the urinary system of rats induced by chemical carcinogens. *Acta pathol. Jpn*, **23**, 87–109

Ito, N., Hiasa, Y., Kamamoto, Y., Makiura, S., Sugihara, S. & Marugami, M. (1971) Histopathological analysis of kidney tumors in rats induced by chemical carcinogens. *Gann*, **62**, 435–444

Ivanova-Cemišanska, L., Antov, G., Hinkova, L., Valceva, V. & Hristeva, V. (1980) Lead acetate effect upon reproduction in male Albino rats. *Hig. Zdraveopazvane*, **23**, 304–308

Jacobson, J.L. & Snowdon, C.T. (1976) Increased lead ingestion in calcium-deficient monkeys. *Nature*, **262**, 51–52

Jacquet, P. & Tachon, P. (1981) Effects of long-term lead exposure on monkey leucocyte chromosomes. *Toxicol. Lett.*, **8**, 165–169

Jacquet, P., Léonard, A. & Gerber, G.B. (1977) Cytogenetic investigations on mice treated with lead. *J. Toxicol. Environ. Health*, **2**, 619–624

Jaffe, E.K., Bagla, S. & Michini, P.A. (1991) Reevaluation of a sensitive indicator of early lead exposure. Measurement of porphobilinogen synthase in blood. *Biol. trace Elem. Res.*, **28**, 223–231

Jaffe, E.K., Volin, M., Bronson-Mullins, C.R., Dunbrack, R.L., Jr, Kervinen, J., Martins, J., Quinlan, J.F., Jr, Sazinsky, M.H., Steinhouse, E.M. & Yeung, A.T. (2000) An artificial gene for human porphobilinogen synthetase allows comparison of an allelic variation implicated in susceptibility to lead poisoning. *J. biol. Chem.*, **275**, 2619–2626

Jaffe, E.K., Martins, J., Li, J., Kervinen, J. & Dunbrack, R.L., Jr (2001) The molecular mechanism of lead inhibition of human porphobilinogen synthase. *J. biol. Chem.*, **276**, 1531–1537

Jagetia, G.C. & Aruna, R. (1998) Effect of various concentrations of lead nitrate on the induction of micronuclei in mouse bone marrow. *Mutat. Res.*, **415**, 131–137

James, H.M., Hilburn, M.E. & Blair, J.A. (1985) Effects of meals and meal times on uptake of lead from the gastrointestinal tract in humans. *Hum. Toxicol.*, **4**, 401–407

Janakiraman, V., Ettinger, A., Mercado-Garcia, A., Hu, H. & Hernandez-Avila, M. (2003) Calcium supplements and bone resorption in pregnancy. A randomized crossover trial. *Am. J. prev. Med.*, **24**, 260–264

Janin, Y., Couinaud, C., Stone, A. & Wise, L. (1985) The 'lead-induced colic' syndrome in lead intoxication. *Surg. Annu.*, **17**, 287–307

Jaremin, B. (1990) Immunological humoral responsiveness in men occupationally exposed to lead. *Bull. Inst. marit. trop. Med. Gdynia*, **41**, 27–36

Jasmin, G. & Riopelle, J.L. (1976) Renal carcinomas and erythrocytosis in rats following intrarenal injection of nickel subsulfide. *Lab. Invest.*, **35**, 71–78

Jason, K.M. & Kellog, C.K. (1981) Neonatal lead exposure: Effects of development of behavior and striatal dopamine neurons. *Pharmacol. Biochem. Behav.*, **15**, 641–649

JECFA (2002) *Summary of Evaluations Performed by the Joint FAO/WHO Expert Committee on Food Additives*, Geneva, International Programme on Chemical Safety, World Health Organization

Jemal, A., Graubard, B.I., Devesa, S.S. & Flegal, KM. (2002) The association of blood lead level and cancer mortality among whites in the United States. *Environ. Health Perspect.*, **110**, 325–329

Jeyaratnam, J., Devathasan, G., Ong, C.N., Phoon, W.O. & Wong, P.K. (1985) Neurophysiological studies on workers exposed to lead. *Br. J. ind. Med.*, **42**, 173–177

Jiang, X., Liang, Y. & Wang, Y. (1992) Studies of lead exposure on reproductive system: A review of work in China. *Biomed. environ. Sci.*, **5**, 266–275

Jin, Y.-P., Kobayashi, E., Okubo, Y., Suwazono, Y., Nogawa, K. & Nakagawa, H. (2000) Changes of lead levels in 24-h urine from 1985 to 1998 in Japanese adults. *Toxicol. Lett.*, **114**, 91–99

Johansson, L. (1989) Premature acrosome reaction in spermatozoa from lead-exposed mice. *Toxicology*, **54**, 151–162

Joffe, M., Bisanti, L., Apostoli, P., Kiss, P., Dale, A., Roeleveld, N., Lindbohm, M.-L., Sallmén, M., Vanhoorne, M. & Bonde, J.P. & the ASCLEPIOS Study Group (2003) Time to pregnancy and occupational lead exposure. *Occup. environ. Med.*, **60**, 752–758

Jorhem, L., Mattsson, P. & Slorach, S. (1988) Lead in table wines on the Swedish market. *Food addit. Contam.*, **5**, 645–649

Jowsey, J., Kelly, P.J., Riggs, B.L., Bianco, A.J., Jr, Scholz, D.A. & Gershon-Cohen, J. (1965) Quantitative microradiographic studies of normal and osteoporotic bone. *J. Bone Joint Surg.*, **47A**, 785–806

Kachru, D.N., Tandon, S.K., Misra, U.K. & Nag, D. (1989) Occupational lead poisoning among silver jewellery workers. *Indian J. med. Sci.*, **43**, 89–91

Kaiser, R., Henderson, H.A.K., Daley, W.R., Naughton, M., Khan, M.H., Rahman, M., Kieszak, S. & Rubin, C.H. (2001) Blood lead levels of primary school children in Dhaka, Bangladesh. *Environ. Health Perspect.*, **109**, 563–566

Kákosy, T., Hudák, A. & Náray, M. (1996) Lead intoxication epidemic caused by ingestion of contaminated ground paprika. *Clin. Toxicol.*, **34**, 507–511

Kalra, V., Chitralekha, K.T., Dua, T., Pandey, R.M. & Gupta, Y. (2003) Blood lead levels and risk factors for lead toxicity in children from schools and an urban slum in Delhi. *J. trop. Pediatr.*, **49**, 121–123

Kamal, A.-A., Eldamaty, S.E. & Faris, R. (1991) Blood lead level of Cairo traffic policemen. *Sci. tot. Environ.*, **105**, 165–170

Kamaraj, S., Muthuvel, P., Dhakshinamoorthy, M. & Singh, M.V. (2003) Heavy metal accumulation in a swell-shrink soil environment as influenced by long term fertilization. In: Singh, V.P. & Yadava, R.N., eds, *Environmental Pollution: Water and Environment*, New Delhi, Allied Publishers, pp. 236–242

Kampe, W. (1983) [Lead and cadmium in food — A current danger?] *Forum Städte-Hyg.*, **34**, 236–241 (in German)

Kandiloros, D.C., Goletsos, G.A., Nikolopoulos, T.P., Ferekidis, E.A., Tsomis, A.S. & Adamopoulos, G.K. (1997) Effect of subclinical lead intoxication on laryngeal cancer. *Br. J. clin. Pract.*, **51**, 69–70

Kang, H.K., Infante, P.F. & Carra, J.S. (1980) Occupational lead exposure and cancer. *Science*, **207**, 935–936

Kanisawa, M. & Schroeder, H. A. (1969) Life term studies on the effect of trace elements on spontaneous tumors in mice and rats. *Cancer Res.*, **29**, 892–895

Kantor, A.F., Curnen, M.G., Meigs, J.W. & Flannery J.T. (1979) Occupations of fathers of patients with Wilms's tumour. *J. Epidemiol. Community Health*, **33**, 253–256

Kapaki, E.N., Varelas, P.N., Syrigou, A.I., Spanaki, M.V., Andreadou, E., Kakami, A.E. & Papageorgiou, C.T. (1998) Blood lead levels of traffic- and gasoline-exposed professionals in the city of Athens. *Arch. environ. Health*, **53**, 287–291

Kaphalia, B.S., Chandra, H., Bhargava, S.K., Seth, T.D. & Gupta, B.N. (1981) Lead in drinking water. *Indian J. environ. Prot.*, **1**, 92–96

Karita, K., Shinozaki, T., Yano, E. & Amari, N. (2000) Blood lead levels in copper smelter workers in Japan. *Ind. Health*, **38**, 57–61

Kasprzak, K.S., Hoover, K.L. & Poirier, L.A. (1985) Effects of dietary calcium acetate on lead subacetate carcinogenicity in kidneys of male Sprague-Dawley rats. *Carcinogenesis*, **6**, 279–282

Kastori, R., Plesnicar, M., Sakac, Z., Pankovic, D. & Arsenijevic-Maksimovic, I. (1998) Effect of excess lead on sunflower growth and photosynthesis. *J. Plant Nutr.*, **21**, 75–85

Kaul, B. (1999) Lead exposure and iron deficiency among Jammu and New Delhi children. *Indian J. Pediatr.*, **66**, 27–35

Kaul, P.S. & Kaul, B. (1986) Blood lead and erythrocyte protoporphyrin levels among papier-mâché workers in Kashmir. *Mount Sinai J. Med.*, **53**, 145–148

Kaul, B., Rasmuson, J.O., Olsen, R.L., Chanda, C.R., Slazhneva, T.I., Granovsky, E.L. & Korchevsky, A.A. (2000) Blood lead and erythrocyte protoporphyrin levels in Kazakhstan. *Indian J. Pediatr.*, **67**, 87–91

Kauppinen, T., Riala, R., Seitsamo, J. & Hernberg, S. (1992) Primary liver cancer and occupational exposure. *Scand. J. Work Environ. Health*, **18**, 18–25

Kaye, W.E., Novotny, T.E. & Tucker, M. (1987) New ceramics-related industry implicated in elevated blood lead levels in children. *Arch. environ. Health*, **42**, 161–164

KCM SA (2003) *Product Data Sheet: Lead*, Plovdiv

Kehoe, R.A. (1987) Studies of lead administration and elimination in adult volunteers under natural and experimentally induced conditions over extended periods of time. *Food chem. Toxicol.*, **25**, 421–493

Kelada, S.N., Shelton, E., Kaufmann, R.B. & Khoury, M.J. (2001) δ-aminolevulinic acid dehydratase genotype and lead toxicity: A HuGE review. *Am. J. Epidemiol.*, **154**, 1–13

Keller, C.A. & Doherty, R.A. (1980a) Lead and calcium distributions in blood, plasma and milk of the lactating mouse. *J. Lab. clin. Med.*, **95**, 81–89

Keller, C.A. & Doherty, R.A. (1980b) Distribution and excretion of lead in young and adult female mice. *Environ. Res.*, **21**, 217–228

Kello, D. & Kostial, K. (1973) The effect of milk diet on lead metabolism in rats. *Environ. Res.*, **6**, 355–360

Kemper, A.R., Bordley, W.C. & Downs, S.M. (1998) Cost-effectiveness analysis of lead poisoning screening strategies following the 1997 guidelines of the Centers for Disease Control and Prevention. *Arch. pediatr. adoles. Med.*, **152**, 1202–1208

Kerr, M.A., Nasca, P.C., Mundt, K.A., Michalek, A.M., Baptiste, M.S. & Mahoney, M.C. (2000) Parental occupational exposures and risk of neuroblastoma: A case–control study (United States). *Cancer Causes Control*, **11**, 635–643

Kessler, M., Durand, P.Y., Huu, T.C., Royer-Morot, M.J., Chanliau, J., Netter, P. and Duc, M. (1999) Mobilization of lead from bone in end-stage renal failure patients with secondary hyperparathyroidism. *Nephrol. Dial. Transplant.*, **14**, 2731–2733

Khalil-Manesh, F., Gonick, H.C., Cohen, A.H., Alinovi, R., Bergamaschi, E., Mutti, A. & Rosen, V.J. (1992a) Experimental model of lead nephropathy. I. Continuous high-dose lead administration. *Kidney int.*, **41**, 1192–1203

Khalil-Manesh, F., Gonick, H.C., Cohen, A., Bergamaschi, E. & Mutti, A. (1992b) Experimental model of lead nephropathy. II. Effect of removal from lead exposure and chelation treatment with dimercaptosuccinic acid (DMSA). *Environ. Res.*, **58**, 35–54

Khalil-Manesh, F., Tartaglia-Erler, J. & Gonick, H.C. (1994) Experimental model of lead nephropathy. IV. Correlation between renal functional changes and hematological indices of lead toxicity. *J. trace Elem. Electrolytes Health Dis.*, **8**, 13–19

Khan, M.H., Khan, I., Shah, S.H. & Rashid, Q. (1995) Lead poisoning — A hazard of traffic and industries in Pakistan. *J. environ. Pathol. Toxicol. Oncol.*, **14**, 117–120

Khandekar, R.N., Mishra, U.C. & Vohra, K.G. (1984) Environmental lead exposure of an urban Indian population. *Sci. total Environ.*, **40**, 269–278

Kharab, P. & Singh, I. (1985) Genotoxic effects of potassium dichromate, sodium arsenite, cobalt chloride and lead nitrate in diploid yeast. *Mutat. Res.*, **155**, 117–120

Kiefer, M., Trout, D. & Wallace, M.E. (1998) Health Hazard Evaluation Report, HETA 97-0260-2716, Avondale Shipyards, Avondale, LA, USA, NIOSH

Kies, C & Ip, S.W. (1991) Lead bioavailability to humans from diets containing constant amounts of lead: Impact of supplemental copper, zinc and iron. In: Hemphill, D.H.C. & Cothern, C.R., eds, *Trace Substances in Environmental Health*, Vol. XXIV, University of Missouri, Columbia, pp. 177–184

Kim, Y., Harada, K., Ohmori, S., Lee, B.K., Miura, H. & Ueda, A. (1995a) Evaluation of lead exposure in workers at a lead-acid battery factory in Korea: With focus on activity of erythrocyte pyrimidine 5′-nucleotidase (P5N). *Occup. environ. Med.*, **52**, 484–488

Kim, R., Aro, A., Rotnitzky, A., Amarasiriwardena, C. & Hu, H. (1995b) K X-ray fluorescence measurements of bone lead concentration: The analysis of low-level data. *Phys. med. Biol.*, **40**, 1475–1485

Kim, R., Hu, H., Rotnitzky, A., Bellinger, D. & Needleman, H. (1996a) Longitudinal relationship between dentin lead levels in childhood and bone lead levels in young adulthood. *Arch. environ. Health*, **51**, 375–382

Kim, R., Rotnitsky, A., Sparrow, D., Weiss, S.T., Wager, C. & Hu, H. (1996b) A longitudinal study of low-level lead exposure and impairment of renal function. The Normative Aging Study. *J. Am. med. Assoc.*, **275**, 1177–1181

Kim, Y., Lee, H., Lee, C.R., Park, D.U., Yang, J.S., Park, I.J., Lee, K.Y., Lee, M.Y., Kim, T.-K., Sohn, N.-S., Cho, Y.S., Lee, N.R. & Chung, H.K. (2002) Evaluation of lead exposure in workers at secondary lead smelters in South Korea: With focus on activity of erythrocyte pyrimidine 5′-nucleotidase (P5N). *Sci. total Environ.*, **286**, 181–189

Kimmel, E.C., Fish, R.H., & Casida, J.E. (1977) Bioorganotin chemistry: Metabolism of organotin compounds in microsomal monoxygenase systems and in mammals. *J. agric. Food Chem.*, **25**, 1–9

Kinnes, G.M. & Hammel, R.R. (1990) Health Hazard Evaluation Report, HETA 88-0357-2042, A.W. Cash Valve Manufacturing Corp., Decatur, IL, USA, NIOSH

Kirkby, H. & Gyntelberg, F. (1985) Blood pressure and other cardiovascular risk factors of long-term exposure to lead. *Scand. J. Work Environ. Health*, **11**, 15–19

Klaassen, C.D. & Shoeman, D.W. (1974) Biliary excretion of lead in rats, rabbits, and dogs. *Toxicol. appl. Pharmacol.*, **29**, 434–446

Klein, M., Namer, R., Harpur, E. & Corbin, R. (1970) Earthenware containers as a source of fatal lead poisoning. *New Engl. J. Med.*, **283**, 669–672

Knowles, S.O. & Donaldson, W.E. (1997) Lead disrupts eicosanoid metabolism, macrophage function, and disease resistance in birds. *Biol. trace Elem. Res.*, **60**, 13–26

Kobayashi, N. & Okamoto, T. (1974) Effects of lead oxide on the induction of lung tumors in Syrian hamsters. *J. natl Cancer Inst.*, **52**, 1605–1610

Koh, D., Ng, V., Chua, L.H., Yang, Y., Ong, H.Y. & Chia, S.E. (2003) Can salivary lead be used for biological monitoring of lead exposed individuals? *Occup. environ. Med.*, **60**, 696–698

Kohler, K., Lilienthal, H., Guenther, E., Winneke, G. & Zrenner, E. (1997) Persistent decrease of the dopamine-synthesizing enzyme tyrosine hydroxylase in the rhesus monkey retina after chronic lead exposure. *NeuroToxicology*, **18**, 623–632

Koller, L.D. & Brauner, J.A. (1977) Decreased B-lymphocyte response after exposure to lead and cadmium. *Toxicol. appl. Pharmacol.*, **42**, 621–624

Koller, L.D. & Kovacic, S. (1974) Decreased antibody formation in mice exposed to lead. *Nature*, **250**, 148–150

Koller, L.D., Roan, J.G. & Isaacson Kerkvliet, N. (1979) Mitogen stimulation of lymphocytes in CBA mice exposed to lead and cadmium. *Environ. Res.*, **19**, 177–188

Koller, L.D., Kerkvliet, N.I. & Exon, J.H. (1985) Neoplasia induced in male rats fed lead acetate, ethyl urea, and sodium nitrite. *Toxicol. Pathol.*, **13**, 50–57

Kopito, L., Byers, R.K. & Shwachman, H. (1967) Lead in hair of children with chronic lead poisoning. *New Engl. J. Med.*, **276**, 949–953

Korea Zinc Co. (2003) *Product Data Sheet: Lead*, Seoul

Korrick, S.A., Hunter, D.J., Rotniszky, A., Hu, H. & Speizer, F.E. (1999) Lead and hypertension in a sample of middle-aged women. *Am. J. pub. Health*, **89**, 330–335

Korrick, S.A., Schwartz, J., Tsaih, S.-W., Hunter, D.J., Aro, A., Rosner, B., Speizer, F.E. & Hu, H. (2002) Correlates of bone and blood lead levels among middle-aged and elderly women. *Am. J. Epidemiol.*, **156**, 335–343

Kosnett, M.J., Becker, C.E., Osterloh, J.D., Kelly, T.J. & Pasta, D.J. (1994) Factors influencing bone lead concentration in a suburban community assessed by noninvasive K X-ray fluorescence. *J. Am. med. Assoc.*, **271**, 197–203

Kostial, K. & Kello, D. (1979) Bioavailability of lead in rats fed 'human' diets. *Bull. environ. Contam. Toxicol.*, **21**, 312–314

Kostial, K. & Momcilovic, B. (1972) The effect of lactation on the absorption of ^{203}Pb and ^{47}Ca in rats. *Health Phys.*, **23**, 383

Kostial, K. & Momcilovic, B. (1974) Transport of lead 203 and calcium 47 from mother to offspring. *Arch. environ. Health*, **29**, 28–30

Kostial, K., Kello, D., Jugo, S., Rabar, I. & Maljkovic, T. (1978) Influence of age on metal metabolism and toxicity. *Environ. Health Perspect.*, **25**, 81–86

Kotok, D. (1972) Development of children with elevated blood lead levels: A controlled study. *J. Pediatr.*, **80**, 57–61

Kovar, I.Z., Strehlow, C.D., Richmond, J. & Thompson, M.G. (1984) Perinatal lead and cadmium burden in a British urban population. *Arch. Dis. Child*, **59**, 36–39

Kozarzewska, Z. & Chmielnicka, J. (1987) Dynamics of diethyllead excretion in the urine of rabbits after tetraethyllead administration. *Br. J. ind. Med.*, **44**, 417–421

Kristensen, P. & Andersen, A. (1992) A cohort study on cancer incidence in offspring of male printing workers. *Epidemiology*, **3**, 6–10

Kristensen, P., Eilertsen, E., Einarsdóttir, E., Øvrebø, S. & Haugen, A. (1993) Effect modification by inorganic lead in the dominant lethal assay. *Mutat. Res.*, **302**, 33–38

Kroes, R., van Logten, M.J., Berkvens, J.M., de Vries, T. & van Esch, G.J. (1974) Study on the carcinogenicity of lead arsenate and sodium arsenate and on the possible synergistic effect of diethylnitrosamine. *Food Cosmet. Toxicol.*, **12**, 671–679

Krueger, J.A. & Duguay, K.M. (1989) Comparative analysis of lead in Maine urban soils. *Bull. environ. Contam. Toxicol.*, **42**, 574–581

Krugner-Higby, L.A., Gendron, A., Laughlin, N.K., Luck, M., Scheffler, J. & Phillips, B. (2001) Chronic myelocytic leukemia in a juvenile rhesus macaque (Macaca mulatta). *Contemp. top. Lab. Anim. Sci.*, **40**, 44–48

Ku, Y., Alvarez, G.H. & Mahaffey, K.R. (1978) Comparative effects of feeding lead acetate and phospholipid-bound lead on blood and tissue lead concentrations in young and adult rats. *Bull. environ. Contam. Toxicol.*, **20**, 561–567

Kumar, B.D. & Krishnaswamy, K. (1995a) Detection of sub-clinical lead toxicity in monocasters. *Bull. environ. Contam. Toxicol.*, **54**, 863–869

Kumar, B.D. & Krishnaswamy, K. (1995b) Detection of occupational lead nephropathy using early renal markers. *Clin. Toxicol.*, **33**, 331–335

Kumar, R.K. & Kesaree, N. (1999) Blood lead levels in urban and rural Indian children. *Indian Pediatr.*, **36**, 303–306

Kurasaki, M., Hartoto, D.I., Saito. T., Suzuki-Kurasaki, M. & Iwakuma, T. (2000) Metals in water in the central Kalimantan, Indonesia. *Bull. environ. Contam. Toxicol.*, **65**, 591–597

Labbé, R.F., Vreman, H.J. & Stevenson, D.K. (1999) Zinc protoporphyrin: A metabolite with a mission. *Clin. Chem.*, **45**, 2060–2072

Lagerkvist, B.J., Sandberg, S., Frech, W., Jin, T. & Nordberg, G.F. (1996a) Is placenta a good indicator of cadmium and lead exposure? *Arch. environ. Health*, **51**, 389–394

Lagerkvist, B.J., Ekesrydh, S., Englyst, V., Nordberg, G.F., Söderberg, H.-A. & Wiklund, D.-E. (1996b) Increased blood lead and decreased calcium levels during pregnancy: A prospective study of Swedish women living near a smelter. *Am. J. public Health*, **86**, 1247–1252

LaGoy, P.K. (1987) Estimated soil ingestion rates for use in risk assessment. *Risk Anal.*, **7**, 355–359

Lai, C.S. (1972) Lead poisoning as an occupational hazard in Chinese opera actors — A case report. *Singap. Med. J.*, **13**, 115–117

Lai, J.S., Wu, T.N., Liou, S.H., Shen, C.Y., Guu, C.F., Ko, K.N., Chi, H.Y. & Chang, P.Y. (1997) A study of the relationship between ambient lead and blood lead among lead battery workers. *Int. Arch. occup. environ. Health*, **69**, 295–300

Lal, B., Murthy, R.C., Anand, M., Chandra, S.V., Kumar, R., Tripathi, O. & Srimal, R.C. (1991) Cardiotoxicity and hypertension in rats after oral lead exposure. *Drug chem. Toxicol.*, **14**, 305–318

Lalor, G., Rattray, R., Vutchkov, M., Campbell, B. & Lewis-Bell, K. (2001) Blood lead levels in Jamaican school children. *Sci. total Environ.*, **269**, 171–181

Lamola, A.A. & Yamane, T. (1974) Zinc protoporphyrin in the erythrocytes of patients with lead intoxication and iron deficiency anemia. *Science*, **186**, 936–938

Lancranjan, I., Popescu, H.I., Gavanescu, O., Klepsch, I. & Serbanescu, M. (1975) Reproductive ability of workmen occupationally exposed lo lead. *Arch. environ. Health*, **30**, 396–401

Landrigan, P.J. & Straub, W.E. (1985) Health Hazard Evaluation Report, HETA 85-0132-1598, Mystic Seaport, Mystic, CT, USA, NIOSH

Landrigan, P.J., Gehlbach, S.H., Rosenblum, B.F., Shoults, J.M., Candelaria, R.M., Barthel, W.F., Liddle, J.A., Smrek, A.L., Staehling, N.W. & Sanders, J.F. (1975a) Epidemic lead absorption near an ore smelter — The role of particulate lead. *N. Engl. J. Med.*, **292**, 123–129

Landrigan, P.J., McKinney, A.S., Hopkins, L.C., Rhodes, W.W., Jr, Price, W.A. & Cox, D.H. (1975b) Chronic lead absorption: Result of poor ventilation in an indoor pistol range. *JAMA*, **234**, 394–397

Landrigan, P.J., Baloh, R.W., Barthel, W.F., Whitworth, R.H., Staehling, N.W. & Rosenblum, B.F. (1975c) Neuropsychological dysfunction in children with chronic low-level lead absorption. *Lancet*, **i**, 708–712

Landrigan, P.J., Straub, W., McManus, K., Stein, G.F., Baker, E.L. & Himmelstein, J.S. (1980) Technical Assistance Report, TA 80-099-859, Tobin-Mystic River Bridge, Boston, MA, USA, NIOSH

Landrigan, P.J., Albrecht, W.N., Watanabe, A. & Lee, S. (1982) Health Hazard Evaluation Report, HETA 80-0116-1034, Ferro Corp., Cleveland, OH, USA, NIOSH

Lang, D.S., Meier, K.L. & Luster, M.I. (1993) Comparative effects of immunotoxic chemicals on *in vitro* proliferative responses of human and rodent lymphocytes. *Fundam. appl. Toxicol.*, **21**, 535–545

Langlois, P., Smith, L., Fleming, S., Gould, R., Goel, V. & Gibson, B. (1996) Blood lead levels in Toronto children and abatement of lead-contaminated soil and house dust. *Arch. environ. Health*, **51**, 59–67

Lanphear, B.P., Matte, T.D., Rogers, J., Clickner, R.P., Dietz, B., Bornschein, R.L., Succop, P., Mahaffey, K.R., Dixon, S., Galke, W., Rabinowitz, M., Farfel, M., Rohde, C., Schwartz, J., Ashley, P. & Jacobs, D.E. (1998) The contribution of lead-contaminated house dust and residential soil to children's blood lead levels — A pooled analysis of 12 epidemiologic studies. *Environ. Res.*, **79**, 51–68

Lanphear, B.P., Eberly, S. & Howard, C.R. (2000a) Long-term effect of dust control on blood lead concentrations. *Pediatrics*, **106**, 48–51

Lanphear, B.P., Dietrich, K., Auinger, P. & Cox, C. (2000b) Cognitive deficits associated with blood lead concentrations < 10 microg/dL in US children and adolescents. *Public Health Rep.*, **115**, 521–529

Lanphear, B.P., Hornung, R., Ho, M., Howard, C.R., Eberle, S. & Knauf, K. (2002) Environmental lead exposure during early childhood. *J. Pediatr.*, **140**, 40–47

Lansdown, R.G., Sheperd, J., Clayton, B.E., Delves, H.T., Graham P.J. & Turner, W.C. (1974) Blood lead levels, behaviour and intelligence: A population study. *Lancet*, **i**, 538–541

Lansdown, R., Yule, W., Urbanowicz, M.-A. & Hunter, J. (1986) The relationship between blood-lead concentrations, intelligence, attainment and behaviour in a school population: The second London study. *Int. Arch. occup. environ. Health*, **57**, 225–235

Larsen, S.B., Abell, A. & Bonde, J.P. (1998) Selection bias in occupational sperm studies. *Am. J. Epidemiol.*, **147**, 681–685

Larson, J.K., Buchan, R.M., Blehm, K.D. & Smith, C.W. (1989) Characterization of lead fume exposure during gas metal arc welding on carbon steel. *Appl. ind. Hyg.*, **4**, 330–333

Larsson, B., Slorach, S.A., Hagman, U. & Hofvander, Y. (1981) WHO collaborative breast feeding study. II. Levels of lead and cadmium in Swedish human milk, 1978–1979. *Acta paediatr. scand.*, **70**, 281–284

Lasheen, M.R. (1987) The distribution of trace metals in Aswan High Dam Reservoir and River Nile ecosystems. In: Hutchinson, T.C. & Meema, K.M., eds, *Lead, Mercury, Cadmium and Arsenic in the Environment*, New York, Wiley, pp. 235–253

Laurier, C., Tatematsu, M., Rao, P.M., Rajalakshmi, S. & Sarma, D.S.R. (1984) Promotion by orotic acid of liver carcinogenesis in rats initiated by 1,2-dimethylhydrazine. *Cancer Res.*, **44**, 2186–2191

Lauwerys, R.R., Buchet, J.-P. & Roels, H.A. (1973) Comparative study of effect of inorganic lead and cadmium on blood δ-aminolevulinate dehydratase in man. *Br. J. ind. Med.*, **30**, 359–364

Lauwerys, R.R., Bernard, A., Roels, H. & Buchet, J.P. (1995) Health risk assessment of long-term exposure to non-genotoxic chemicals: Application of biological indices. *Toxicol. Lett.*, **77**, 39–44

Lead Development Association International (2003a) *Technical Note: Primary Extraction of Lead*, London [www.ldaint.org/default.htm; accessed 01/02/2004]

Lead Development Association International (2003b) *Lead Information*, London [www.ldaint.org/default.htm; accessed 01/02/2004]

Lead Development Association International (2003c) *Technical Note: Primary Lead Refining*, London [www.ldaint.org/default.htm; accessed 01/02/2004]

Lead Development Association International (2003d) *Technical Note: Secondary lead production*, London [www.ldaint.org/default.htm; accessed 01/02/2004]

Lead Development Association International (2003e) *Technical Note: Lead Products and Their Uses*, London [www.ldaint.org/default.htm; accessed 01/02/2004]

Leal, R.B., Cordova, F.M., Herd, L., Bobrovskaya, L. & Dunkley, P.R. (2002) Lead-stimulated p38MAPK-dependent Hsp27 phosphorylation. *Toxicol. appl. Pharmacol.*, **178**, 44–51

Leal-Garza, C., Montes de Oca, R., Cerda-Flores, R.M., Garcia-Martinez, E. & Garza-Chapa, R. (1986) Frequency of sister chromatid exchange (SCE) in lead exposed workers. *Arch. invest. Med.*, **17**, 267–276

Ledda-Columbano, G.M., Coni, P., Curto, M., Giacomini, L., Faa, G., Sarma, D.S.R. & Columbano, A. (1992) Mitogen-induced liver hyperplasia does not substitute for compensatory regeneration during promotion of chemical hepatocarcinogenesis. *Carcinogenesis*, **13**, 379–383

Lee, S.A. (1987) Health Hazard Evaluation Report, HETA 87-0262-1852, Artistic Awards, Colorado Springs, CO, USA, NIOSH

Lee, S.A. (1991) Health Hazard Evaluation Report, HETA 91-0076-2164, Silver Deer, Boulder, CO, USA, NIOSH

Lee, B.K. (1999) The role of biological monitoring in the health management of lead-exposed workers. *Toxicol. Lett.*, **108**, 149–160

Lee, S.A. & McCammon, C.S. (1992) Health Hazard Evaluation Report, HETA 91-0161-2225, Denver Police Dept., Denver, CO, USA, NIOSH

Lee, V.W.K., De Kretser, D.M., Hudson, B. & Wang, C. (1975) Variations in serum FSH, LH, and testosterone levels in male rats from birth to sexual maturity. *J. Reprod. Fertil.*, **42**, 121–126

Lee, R.G., Becker, W.C. & Collins, D.W. (1989) Lead at the tap: Sources and control. *J. Am. Water Works Assoc.*, **81**, 52–62

Lee, S.A., Goldfield, J., Hales, T.R. & Gunter, B.J. (1990a) Health Hazard Evaluation Report, HETA 89-0052-2006, Alma American Labs, Fairplay, CO, USA, NIOSH

Lee, S.A., Hales, T.R. & Daniels, W.J. (1990b) Health Hazard Evaluation Report, HETA 89-0139-2025, Tamco, Etiwanda, CA, USA, NIOSH

Lee, D.-S., Lee, Y.-K., Huh, J.-W., Lee, S.-I., Sohn, D.-H. & Kim, M.-G. (1994) [Annual variation of atmospheric lead concentration in Seoul (1984–1993).] *J. Kor. Air Pollut. Res. Assoc.*, **10**, 170–174 (in Korean with English Abstract)

Lee, J.-E., Chen, S., Golemboski, K.A., Parsons, P.J. & Dietert, R.R. (2001) Developmental windows of differential lead-induced immunotoxicity in chickens. *Toxicology*, **156**, 161–170

Lee, S.-S., Lee, B.-K., Lee, G.-S., Stewart, W.F., Simon, D., Kelsey, K., Todd, A.C. & Schwartz, B.S. (2001) Associations of lead biomarkers and delta-aminolevulinic acid dehydratase and vitamin D receptor genotypes with hematopoietic outcomes in Korean lead workers. *Scand. J. Work Environ. Health*, **27**, 402–411

Lee, C.R., Lee, J.H., Yoo, C.I. & Kim, S.-R. (2002) Trend of blood lead levels in children in an industrial complex and its suburban area in Ulsan, Korea. *Int. Arch. occup. environ. Health*, **75**, 507–510

Leggett, R.W. (1993) An age-specific kinetic model of lead metabolism in humans. *Environ. Health Perspect.*, **101**, 598–616

Leighton, J., Klitzman, S., Sedlar, S., Matte, T. & Cohen, N.L. (2003) The effect of lead-based paint hazard remediation on blood lead levels of lead poisoned children in New York City. *Environ. Res.*, **92**, 182–190

Lerda, D. (1992) Study of sperm characteristics in persons occupationally exposed lo lead. *Am. J. ind. Med.*, **22**, 567–571

Leroyer, A., Hemon, D., Nisse, C., Bazerques, J., Salomez, J.L. & Haguenoer, J.M. (2001) Environmental exposure to lead in a population of adults living in northern France: Lead burden levels and their determinants. *Sci. total Environ.*, **267**, 87–99

Leung, F.Y., Bradley, C. & Pellar, T.G. (1993) Reference intervals for blood lead and evaluation of zinc protoporphyrin as a screening test for lead toxicity. *Clin. Biochem.*, **26**, 491–496

Levin, L., Zheng, W., Blot, W.J., Yu-tang, G. & Fraumeni, J.F., Jr (1988) Occupation and lung cancer in Shanghai: A case–control study. *Br. J. ind. Med.*, **45**, 450–458

Levy, L.S. & Venitt, S. (1986) Carcinogenicity and mutagenicity of chromium compounds: The association between bronchial metaplasia and neoplasia. *Carcinogenesis*, **7**, 831–836

Levy, L.S., Martin, P.A. & Bidstrup, P.L. (1986) Investigation of the potential carcinogenicity of a range of chromium containing materials on rat lung. *Br. J. ind. Med.*, **43**, 243–256

Li, P. & Rossman, T.G. (2001) Genes upregulated in lead-resistant glioma cells reveal possible targets for lead-induced developmental neurotoxicity. *Toxicol. Sci.*, **64**, 90–99

Li, W., Han, S., Gregg, T.R., Kemp, F.W., Davidow, A.L., Louria, D.B., Siegel, A. & Bogden, J.D. (2003) Lead exposure potentiates predatory attack behavior in the cat. *Environ. Res.*, **92**, 197–206

Lide, D.R., ed. (2003) *CRC Handbook of Chemistry and Physics on CD-ROM, Version 2004*, 84th Ed., Boca Raton, FL, pp. 4-17–4-18; 4-64–4-65

Lidsky, T.I. & Schneider, J.S. (2003) Lead neurotoxicity in children: Basic mechanisms and clinical correlates. *Brain*, **126**, 5–19

Lilley, S.G., Florence, T.M. & Stauber, J.L. (1988) The use of sweat to monitor lead absorption through the skin. *Sci. total Environ.*, **76**, 267–278

Lin, R.H., Lee, C.H., Chen, W.K. & Lin-Shiau, S.Y. (1994) Studies on cytotoxic and genotoxic effects of cadmium nitrate and lead nitrate in Chinese hamster ovary cells. *Environ. mol. Mutag.*, **23**, 143–149

Lin, S., Hwang, S.-A., Marshall, E.G. & Marion, D. (1998) Does paternal occupational lead exposure increase the risks of low birth weight or prematurity? *Am. J. Epidemiol.*, **148**, 173–181

Lindblad, B., Lindstedt, S. & Steen, G. (1977) On the enzymic defects in hereditary tyrosinemia. *Proc. natl Acad. Sci. USA*, **74**, 4641–4645

Lindbohm, M.L., Sallmén, M., Anttila, A., Taskinen, H. & Hemminki, K. (1991) Paternal occupational lead exposure and spontaneous abortion. *Scand. J. Work Environ. Health*, **17**, 95–103

Linden, M.A., Manton, W.I., Stewart, R.M., Thal, E.R. & Feit, H. (1982) Lead poisoning from retained bullets: Pathogenesis, diagnosis, and management. *Ann. Surg.*, **195**, 305–313

Lin-Fu, J.S. (1992) Modern history of lead poisoning: A century of discovery and rediscovery. In: Needleman, H.L., ed., *Human Lead Exposure*, Boca Raton, FL, CFRC Press, pp. 23–43

Liou, S.H., Wu, T.N., Chiang, H.C., Yang, T., Yang, G.Y., Wu, Y.Q., Lai, J.S., Ho, S.T., Guo, Y.L., Ko, Y.C., Ko, K.N. & Chang, P.Y. (1996) Three-year survey of blood lead levels in 8828 Taiwanese adults. *Int. arch. Occup. Environ. Health*, **68**, 80–87

Little, P., Fleming, R.G. & Heard, M.J. (1981) Uptake of lead by vegetable foodstuffs during cooking. *Sci. total Environ.*, **17**, 111–131

Litvinov, N.N., Voronin, V.M. & Kazachkov, V.I. (1982) [Experimental study of aniline, lead nitrate and sodium alkylsulfate as modifiers of chemical blastomogenesis] *Vopr. Onkol.*, **28**, 56–59 (in Russian)

Litvinov, N.N., Voronin, V.M. & Kazachkov, V.I. (1984) [Characteristics of aniline, lead nitrate, carbon tetrachloride and formaldehyde as modifiers of chemical carcinogenesis] *Vopr. Onkol.*, **30**, 56–60 (in Russian)

Lloyd, R.D., Mays, C.W., Atherton, D.R. & Bruenger, F.W. (1975) ^{210}Pb studies in beagles. *Health Phys.*, **28**, 575–583

Lockhart Gibson, J., Love, W., Hardie, D., Bancroft, P. & Jefferis Turner, A. (1892) Notes on lead-poisoning as observed among children in Brisbane. In: *Transactions of the Intercolonial Medical Congress of Australia*, Sydney, pp. 78–83

Lockitch, G., Berry, B., Roland, E., Wadsworth, L., Kaikov, Y. & Mirhady, F. (1991) Seizures in a 10-week-old infant: Lead poisoning from an unexpected source. *Can. med. Assoc. J.*, **145**, 1465–1468

Löfstedt, H., Seldén, A., Storéus, L. & Bodin, L. (1999) Blood lead in Swedish police officers. *Am. J. Ind. Med.*, **35**, 519–522

Loghman-Adham, M. (1997) Renal effects of environmental and occupational lead exposure: A review. *Environ. Health Perspect.*, **105**, 928–938

Loikkanen, J., Chvalova, K., Naarala, J., Vähäkangas, K.H. & Savolainen, K.M. (2003) Pb^{2+}-induced toxicity is associated with p53-independent apoptosis and enhanced by glutamate in GT1-7 neurons. *Toxicol. Lett.*, **144**, 235–246

Lokhande, R.S. & Kelkar, N. (1999) Studies on heavy metals in water of Vasai Creek, Maharashtra. *Indian J. environ. Prot.*, **19**, 664–668

Loranger, S. & Zayed, J. (1994) Manganese and lead concentrations in ambient air and emission rates from unleaded and leaded gasoline between 1981 and 1992 in Canada: A comparative study. *Atmos. Environ.*, **28**, 1645–1651

Lu, H., Guizzetti, M. & Costa, L.G. (2001) Inorganic lead stimulates DNA synthesis in human astrocytoma cells: Role of protein kinase C alpha. *J. Neurochem.*, **78**, 590–599

Lu, H., Guizzetti, M. & Costa, L.G. (2002) Inorganic lead activates the mitogen-activated protein kinase kinase-mitogen-activated protein kinase-p90(RSK) signaling pathway in human astrocytoma cells via a protein kinase C-dependent mechanism. *J. Pharmacol. exp. Ther.*, **300**, 818–823

Lubin, J.H., Pottern, L.M., Stone, B.J. & Fraumeni, J.F., Jr (2000) Respiratory cancer in a cohort of copper smelter workers: Results from more than 50 years of follow-up. *Am. J. Epidemiol.*, **151**, 554–565

Lucas, S.R., Sexton, M. & Langenberg, P. (1996) Relationship between blood lead and nutritional factors in preschool children: A cross-sectional study. *Pediatrics*, **97**, 74–78

Lundström, N.-G., Nordberg, G., Englyst, V., Gerhardsson, L., Hagmar, L., Jin, T., Rylander, L. & Wall, S. (1997) Cumulative lead exposure in relation to mortality and lung cancer morbidity in a cohort of primary smelter workers. *Scand. J. Work Environ. Health*, **23**, 24–30

Luo, W., Zhang, Y. & Li, H. (2003) Children's blood lead levels after the phasing out of leaded gasoline in Shantou, China. *Arch. environ. Health*, **58**, 184–187

Lussenhop, D.H., Parker, D.L., Barklind, A. & McJilton, C. (1989) Lead exposure and radiator repair work. *Am. J. public Health*, **79**, 1558–1560

Lustberg, M. & Silbergeld, E. (2002) Blood lead levels and mortality. *Arch. intern. Med.*, **162**, 2443–2449

Luster, M.I., Faith, R.E. & Kimmel, C.A. (1978) Depression of humoral immunity in rats following chronic developmental lead exposure. *J. environ. Pathol. Toxicol.*, **1**, 397–402

Lynge, E., Kurppa, K., Kristofersen, L., Malker, H. & Sauli, H. (1986) Silica dust and lung cancer: Results from the Nordic occupational mortality and cancer incidence registers. *J. natl Cancer Inst.*, **77**, 883–889

Lyon, T.D.B., Patriarca, M., Howatson, A.G., Fleming, P.J., Blair, P.S. & Fell, G.S. (2002) Age dependence of potentially toxic elements (Sb, Cd, Pb, Ag) in human liver tissue from paediatric subjects. *J. environ. Monit.*, **4**, 1034–1039

Maddaloni, M., Lolacono, N., Manton, W., Blum, C., Drexler, J. & Graziano, J. (1998) Bioavailability of soilborne lead in adults, by stable isotope dilution. *Environ. Health Perspect.*, **106** (Suppl. 6), 1589–1594

Maenhaut, W., Zoller, W.H., Duce, R.A. & Hoffman, G.L. (1979) Concentration and size distribution of particulate trace elements in the south polar atmosphere. *J. geophys. Res.*, **84**, 2421–2431

Mahaffey, K.R. & Annest, J.L. (1986) Association of erythrocyte protoporphyrin with blood lead level and iron status in the second National Health and Nutrition Examination Survey, 1976–1980. *Environ. Res.*, **41**, 327–338

Maja, M., Penazzi, N., Baudino, M. & Ginatta, M.V. (1989) *Recycling of Lead-acid Batteries. The Ginatta Process. Proceedings of the International Conference on Lead/Acid Batteries (LABAT '89)*, Drujba, Varna, Bulgaria

Makino, S., Matsuno, K., Hisanaga, N., Seki, Y., Ortega, V.S.D., Villanueva, M.B., Cucueco, M.T., Yu-Sison, S. & Castro, F.T., II (1994) [Medical examination of workers exposed to lead in the Philippines.] *Jpn. J. ind. Health*, **36**, 114–123 (in Japanese)

Mäki-Paakkanen, J., Sorsa, M. & Vainio, H. (1981) Chromosome aberrations and sister chromatid exchanges in lead-exposed workers. *Hereditas*, **94**, 269–275

Malcolm, D. & Barnett, H.A.R. (1982) A mortality study of lead workers 1925–1976. *Br. J. ind. Med.*, **39**, 404–410

Maldonado-Vega, M., Cerbón-Solórzano, J., Albores-Medina, A., Hernández-Luna, C. & Calderon-Salinas, J.V. (1996) Lead: Intestinal absorption and bone mobilization during lactation. *Hum. exp. Toxicol.*, **15**, 872–877

Maldonado-Vega, M., Solórzano, J.C. & Salinas, J.V. (2002) The effects of dietary calcium during lactation on lead in bone mobilization: Implications for toxicology. *Hum. exp. Toxicol.*, **21**, 409–414

Malkin, R. (1993) Health Hazard Evaluation Report, HETA 93-0739-2364, Curcio Scrap Metal and Cirello Iron and Steel, Saddle Brook, NJ, USA, NIOSH

Mallin, K., Rubin, M. & Joo, E. (1989) Occupational cancer mortality in Illinois white and black males, 1979–1984, for seven cancer sites. *Am. J. ind. Med.*, **15**, 699–717

Maltoni, C. (1976) Predictive value of carcinogenesis bioassays. *Ann. N.Y. Acad. Sci.*, **271**, 431–443

Maltoni, C., Morisi, L. & Chieco, P. (1982) Experimental approach to the assessment of the carcinogenic risk of industrial inorganic pigments. *Adv. mod. environ. Toxicol.*, **2**, 77–92

Mameli, O., Caria, M.A., Melis, F., Solinas, A., Tavera, C., Ibba, A., Tocco, M., Flore, C. & Sanna Randaccio, F. (2001) Neurotoxic effect of lead at low concentrations. *Brain Res. Bull.*, **55**, 269–275

Manton, W.I. (1985) Total contribution of airborne lead to blood lead. *Br. J. ind. Med.*, **42**, 168–172

Manton, W.I. (1994) Lead poisoning from gunshots — A five century heritage. *Clin. Toxicol.*, **32**, 387–389

Manton, W.I. & Cook, J.D. (1984) High accuracy (stable isotope dilution) measurements of lead in serum and cerebrospinal fluid. *Br. J. ind. Med.*, **41**, 313–319

Manton, W.I., Angle, C.R., Stanek, K.L., Reese, Y.R. & Kuehnemann, T.J. (2000) Acquisition and retention of lead by young children. *Environ. Res.*, **82**, 60–80

Manton, W.I., Rothenberg, S.J. & Manalo, M. (2001) The lead content of blood serum. *Environ. Res.*, **86**, 263–273

Mao, P. & Molnar, J.J. (1967) The fine structure and histochemistry of lead-induced renal tumors in rats. *Am. J. Pathol.*, **50**, 571–603

Maranelli, G. & Apostoli, P. (1987) Assessment of renal function in lead-poisoned workers. In: Foà, V., Emmet, E.A., Maroni, M., Colombi, A., eds, *Occupational and Environmental Chemical Hazards: Cellular and Biochemical Indices for Monitoring Toxicity*, Chichester, Ellis Horwood Ltd, pp. 344–348

Marcus, A.H. (1985) Multicompartment kinetic model for lead III. Lead in blood plasma and erythrocytes. *Environ. Res.*, **36**, 473–489

Marcus, A.H. & Schwartz, J. (1987) Dose–response curves for erythrocyte protoporphyrin vs blood lead: Effects of iron status. *Environ. Res.*, **44**, 221–227

Maresky, L.S. & Grobler, S.R. (1993) Effect of the reduction of petrol lead on the blood lead levels of South Africans. *Sci. total Environ.*, **136**, 43–48

Markowitz, M.E. & Shen, X.M. (2001) Assessment of bone lead during pregnancy: A pilot study. *Environ. Res.*, **A85**, 83–89

Markowitz, M.E. & Weinberger, H.L. (1990) Immobilization-related lead toxicity in previously lead-poisoned children. *Pediatrics*, **86**, 455–457

Markowitz, S.B., Nunez, C.M., Klitzman, S., Munshi, A.A., Kim, W.S., Eisinger, J. & Landrigan, P.J. (1994) Lead poisoning due to *hai ge fen*: The porphyrin content of individual erythrocytes. *J. Am. med. Assoc.*, **271**, 932–934

Marshall, J.H. & Onkelinx, C. (1968) Radial diffusion and power function retention of alkaline earth radioisotopes in adult bone. *Nature*, **217**, 742–743

Maslat, A.O. & Haas, H.J. (1989) Mutagenic effects of lead (II) bromide. *J. trace Elem. Electrolytes Health Dis.*, **3**, 187–191

Mathee, A., von Schirnding, Y.E.R., Levin, J., Ismail, A., Huntley, R. & Cantrell, A. (2002) A survey of blood lead levels among young Johannesburg school children. *Environ. Res.*, **90**, 181–184

Matte, T.D. (2003) [Effects of lead exposure on children's health]. *Salud Publica Mex.*, **45** (Suppl. 2), 220–224 (in Spanish)

Matte, T.D. & Burr, G.A. (1989a) Health Hazard Evaluation Report, HETA 87-0371-1986, Technical Assistance to the Jamaican Ministry of Health, Kingston, Jamaica, NIOSH

Matte, T.D. & Burr, G.A. (1989b) Health Hazard Evaluation Report, HETA 87-0371-1989, Technical Assistance to the Jamaican Ministry of Health, Kingston, Jamaica, NIOSH

Mattorano, D.A. (1996) Health Hazard Evaluation Report, HETA 94-0273-2556, Bruce Mansfield Power Station, Shippingport, PA, USA, NIOSH

Maynard, E., Thomas, R., Simon, D., Phipps, C., Ward, C. & Calder, I. (2003) An evaluation of recent blood lead levels in Port Pirie, South Australia. *Sci. total Environ.*, **303**, 25–33

Mazess, R.B. (1982) On aging bone loss. *Clin. Orthoped. rel. Res.*, **165**, 239–252

Mazess, R.B., Barden, H.S., Ettinger, M., Johnston, C., Dawson-Hughes, B., Baran, D., Powell, M. & Notelovitz, M. (1987) Spine and femur density using dual-photon absorptiometry in US white women. *Bone Miner.*, **2**, 211–219

McCammon, C.S., Daniels, W.J., Hales, T.R. & Lee, S.A. (1991) Health Hazard Evaluation Report, HETA 91-0290-2131, New England Lead Burning Co. (NELCO), Eaton Metals, Salt Lake City, UT, USA, NIOSH

McCammon, C.S., Hales, T.R., Daniels, W.J. & Lee, S.A. (1992) Health Hazard Evaluation Report, HETA 91-0391-2174, New England Lead Burning Co. (NELCO), Eaton Metals, Salt Lake City, UT, USA, NIOSH

McClain, R.M. & Siekierka, J.J. (1975) The placental transfer of lead-chelate complexes in the rat. *Toxicol. appl. Pharmacol.*, **31**, 443–451

McDonald, J.A. & Potter, N.U. (1996) Lead's legacy? Early and late mortality of 454 lead-poisoned children. *Arch. environ. Health*, **51**, 116–121

McGivern, R.F., Sokol, R.Z. & Berman, N.G. (1991) Prenatal lead exposure in the rat during the third week of gestation: Long-term behavioral, physiological, and anatomical effects associated with reproduction. *Toxicol. appl. Pharmacol.*, **110**, 206–215

McGlothlin, J., Mattorano, D.A., Harney, J.M., Habes, D., Cook, C. & Roegner, K. (1999) Health Hazard Evaluation Report, HETA 97-0196-2755, Astoria Metal Corp., Hunters Point Naval Shipyard, San Francisco, CA, USA, NIOSH

McGregor, A.J. & Mason, H.J. (1990) Chronic occupational lead exposure and testicular endocrine function. *Hum. exp. Toxicol.*, **9**, 371–376

McIntosh, J.F., Möller, E. & Van Slyke, D.D. (1928) Studies of urea excretion III. The influence of body size on urea output. *J. clin. Invest.*, **6**, 467–483

McLaughlin, J.K., Thomas, T.L., Stone, B.J., Blot, W.J., Malker, H.S., Wiener, J.A., Ericsson, J.L. & Malker, B.K. (1987) Occupational risks for meningiomas of the CNS in Sweden. *J. occup. Med.*, **29**, 66–68

McManus, K.P. (1991) Health Hazard Evaluation Report, HETA 91-0376-2154, U.S. Customs Service, World Trade Center New York, NY, USA, NIOSH

McMichael, A.J. & Johnson, H.M. (1982) Long-term mortality profile of heavily-exposed lead smelter workers. *J. occup. Med.*, **24**, 375–378

McMichael, A.J., Baghurst, P.A., Robertson, E.F., Vimpani, G.V. & Wigg, N.R. (1985) The Port Pirie cohort study. Blood lead concentrations in early childhood. *Med. J. Aust.*, **143**, 499–503

McMichael, A.J., Vimpani, G.V., Robertson, E.F., Baghurst, P.A. & Clark, P.D. (1986) The Port Pirie cohort study: Maternal blood lead and pregnancy outcome. *J. Epidemiol. Community Health*, **40**, 18–25

McMichael, A.J., Baghurst, P.A., Wigg, N.R., Vimpani, G.V., Robertson, E.F. & Roberts, R.J. (1988) Port Pirie cohort study: Environmental exposure to lead and children's abilities at the age of four years. *N. Engl. J. Med.*, **319**, 468–475

McNeill, F.E., Laughlin, N.K., Todd, A.C., Sonawane, B.R., Van de Wal, K.M. & Fowler, B.A. (1997) Geriatric bone lead metabolism in a female nonhuman primate population. *Environ. Res.*, **72**, 131–139

McNutt, T.K., Chambers-Emerson, J., Dethlefsen, M. & Shah, R. (2001) Bite the bullet: Lead poisoning after ingestion of 206 lead bullets. *Vet. hum. Toxicol.*, **43**, 288–289

Mehdi, J.K., Al-Imarah, F.J.M. & Al-Suhail, A.A. (2000) Levels of some trace metals and related enzymes in workers at storage-battery factories in Iraq. *East mediterr. Health J.*, **6**, 66–82

Mehra, R.K. & Tripathi, R.D. (2000) Phytochelatins and metal tolerance. In: Agarwal, S.B. & Agarwal, M., eds, *Environmental Pollution and Plant Responses*, Boca Raton, FL, Lewis Publishers, pp. 367–382

Mencel, S.J. & Thorp, R.H. (1976) A study of blood lead levels in residents of the Sydney area. *Med. J. Aust.*, **1**, 423–426

Meredith, P.A., Moore, M.R. & Goldberg, A. (1977) The effect of calcium on lead absorption in rats. *Biochem. J.*, **166**, 531–537

Merzenich, H., Hartwig, A., Ahrens, W., Beyersmann, D., Schlepegrell, R., Scholze, M., Timm, J. & Jöckel, K.-H. (2001) Biomonitoring on carcinogenic metals and oxidative DNA damage in a cross-sectional study. *Cancer Epidemiol. Biomarkers Prev.*, **10**, 515–522

Mexico City Commission for Prevention and Control of Pollution (1993) [*Program to Control Atmospheric Pollution in Mexico City*], Mexico City (in Spanish)

Meyer, B.R., Fischbein, A., Rosenman, K., Lerman, Y., Drayer, D.E. & Reidenberg, M.M. (1984) Increased urinary enzyme excretion in workers exposed to nephrotoxic chemicals. *Am. J. Med.*, **76**, 989–998

Michaels, D., Zoloth, S.R. & Stern, F.B. (1991) Does low-level lead exposure increase risk of death? A mortality study of newspaper printers. *Int. J. Epidemiol.*, **20**, 978–983

Mielke, H.W. (1991) Lead in residential soils: Background and preliminary results of New Orleans. *Water Air Soil Pollut.*, **57–58**, 111–119

Mielke, H.W., Anderson, J.C., Berry, K.J., Mielke, P.W., Chaney, R.L. & Leech, M. (1983) Lead concentrations in inner-city soils as a factor in the child lead problem. *Am. J. public Health*, **73**, 1366–1369

Mielke, H.W., Adams, J.L., Reagan, P.L. & Mielke, P.W., Jr (1989) Soil-dust lead and childhood lead exposure as a function of city size and community traffic flow: The case for lead abatement in Minnesota. *Environ. Chem. Health*, **9** (Suppl.), 253–271

Mielke, H.W., Dugas, D., Mielke, P.W., Jr, Smith, K.S., Smith, S.L. & Gonzales, C.R. (1997a) Associations between soil lead and childhood blood lead in urban New Orleans and rural Lafourche Parish of Louisiana. *Environ. Health Perspect.*, **105**, 950–954

Mielke, H.W., Taylor, M.D., Gonzales, C.R., Smith, M.K., Daniels, P.V. & Buckner, A.V. (1997b) Lead-based hair coloring products: Too hazardous for household use. *J. Am. pharm. Assoc.*, **NS37**, 85–89

Miller, G.D., Massaro, T.F., Granlund, R.W. & Massaro, E.J. (1983) Tissue distribution of lead in the neonatal rat exposed to multiple doses of lead acetate. *J. Toxicol. environ. Health*, **11**, 121–128

Miller, M.B., Curry, S.C., Kunkel, D.B., Arreola, P., Arvizu, E., Schaller, K. & Salmen, D. (1996) Pool cue chalk: A source of environmental lead. *Pediatrics*, **97**, 916–917

Miller, T.E., Golemboski, K.A., Ha, R.S., Bunn, T., Sanders, F.S. & Dietert, R.R. (1998) Developmental exposure to lead causes persistent immunotoxicity in Fischer 344 rats. *Toxicol. Sci.*, **42**, 129–135

Milne, K.L., Sandler, D.P., Everson, R.B. & Brown, S.M. (1983) Lung cancer and occupation in Alameda county: A death certificate case–control study. *Am. J. ind. Med.*, **4**, 565–575

Ministry of Health, Brazil (2004) Portaria No. 518, de 25 de março de 2004 [http://www.sabesp.com/legislacao/Pdf/518_04.pdf; assessed 01/02/2005] (in Portugese)

Ministry of Health, Labour and Welfare (2001) [Database for quality of water supply] (in Japanese) [http://www.jwwa.or.jp/mizu/bunpu/bunpu1_D.asp; accessed 26/01/2004]

Ministry of Health, Labour and Welfare (2002) *The National Nutrition Survey in Japan, 2001*, Tokyo, Dai-ichi Shuppan Publishers (in Japanese)

Ministry of Health, Labour and Welfare (2003) *Journal of Health and Welfare Statistics, Health and Welfare Statistics Association*, p. 269

Minnesota Pollution Control Agency (1987) *Soil Lead Report to the Minnesota State Legislature*, Minneapolis, Minnesota, Minnesota Pollution Control Agency & Minnesota Department of Health

Mira, M., Bawden-Smith, J., Causer, J., Alperstein, G., Karr, M., Snitch, P., Waller, G. & Fett, M.J. (1996) Blood lead concentrations of preschool children in Central and Southern Sydney. *Med. J. Australia*, **164**, 399–402

Mishra, K.P., Singh, V.K., Rani, R., Yadav, V.S., Chandran, V., Srivastava, S.P. & Seth, P.K. (2003) Effect of lead exposure on the immune response of some occupationally exposed individuals. *Toxicology*, **188**, 251–259

Mistry, P., Lucier, G.W. & Fowler, B.A. (1985) High-affinity lead binding proteins in rat kidney cytosol mediate cell-free nuclear translocation of lead. *J. Pharmacol. exp. Ther.*, **232**, 462–469

Mistry, P., Mastri, C. & Fowler, B.A. (1986) Influence of metal ions on renal cytosolic lead-binding proteins and nuclear uptake of lead in the kidney. *Biochem. Pharmacol.*, **35**, 711–713

Modak, A.T., Weintraub, S.T. & Stavincha, W.B. (1975) Effect of chronic ingestion of lead on the central cholinergic system in rat brain regions. *Toxicol. appl. Pharmacol.*, **34**, 340–347

Modak, A.T., Purdy, R.H. & Stavinoha, W.B. (1978) Changes in acetylcholine concentration in mouse brain following ingestion of lead acetate in drinking water. *Drug chem. Toxicol.*, **1**, 373–389

Mokhtar, M.B., Awaluddin, A.B., Yusof, A.B.B.M. & Bakar, B.B. (2002) Lead in blood and hair of shipyard workers, Sabah, Malaysia. *Bull. environ. Contam. Toxicol.*, **69**, 8–14

Mombeshora, C., Osibanjo, O. & Ajayi, S.O. (1983) Pollution studies on Nigerian rivers: The onset of lead pollution of surface waters in Ibadan. *Environ. Int.*, **9**, 81–84

Momcilovic, B. (1978) The effect of maternal dose on lead retention in suckling rats. *Arch. environ. Health*, **33**, 115–117

Momcilovic, B. (1979) Lead metabolism in lactation. *Experientia*, **35**, 517–518

Momcilovic, B. & Kostial, K. (1974) Kinetics of lead retention and distribution in suckling and adult rats. *Environ. Res.*, **8**, 214–220

Monchaux, G., Morin, M., Morlier, J.P. & Olivier, M.F. (1997) Long-term effects of combined exposure to fission neutrons and inhaled lead oxide particles in rats. *Ann. occup. Hyg.*, **41** (Suppl. 1), 630–635

Montopoli, M., Seligman, P., O'Brien, D. & Zaebst, D. (1989) Health Hazard Evaluation Report, HETA 88-0244-1951, Orrville Bronze and Aluminum Co., Orrville, OH, USA, NIOSH

Moon, C.-S. & Ikeda, M. (1996) Pollutant levels in ambient air and blood in Korea. *Environ. Health prev. Med.*, **1**, 33–38

Moon, D.-H. & Lee, C.-U. (1992) [A study on the ambient air pollution by heavy metals in Pusan area.] *Inje. Med. J.*, **13**, 61–91 (in Korean with English abstract)

Moon, C.-S., Zhang, Z.-W., Shimbo, S., Watanabe, T., Moon, D.-H., Lee, C.-U., Lee, B.-K., Ahn, K.-D., Lee, S.-H. & Ikeda, M. (1995) Dietary intake of cadmium and lead among the general population in Korea. *Environ. Res.*, **71**, 46–54

Moore, M.R. (1988) Haematological effects of lead. *Sci. tot. Envir.*, **71**, 419–431

Moore, J.F. & Goyer, R.A. (1974) Lead-induced inclusion bodies: Composition and probable role in lead metabolism. *Environ. Health Perspect.*, **7**, 121–127

Moore, M.R., Beattie, A.D., Thompson, G.G. & Goldberg, A. (1971) Depression of δ-aminolaevulinic acid dehydrase activity by ethanol in man and rat. *Clin. Sci.*, **40**, 81–88

Moore, P.J., Pridmore, S.A. & Gill, G.F. (1976) Total blood lead levels in petrol vendors. *Med. J. Aust.*, **1**, 438–440

Moore, M.R., Meredith, P.A., Campbell, B.C. & Watson, W.S. (1979) The gastrointestinal absorption of lead 203 chloride in man. In: Hemphill, D.D., ed., *Trace Substances in Environmental Health*, Vol. XIII, Columbia, MO, University of Missouri, pp. 368–373

Moore, M.R., Meredith, P.A., Watson, W.S., Sumner, D.J., Taylor, M.K. & Goldberg, A. (1980a) The percutaneous absorption of lead-203 in humans from cosmetic preparations containing lead acetate, as assessed by whole-body counting and other techniques. *Food Cosmet. Toxicol.*, **18**, 399–405

Moore, M.R., Meredith, P.A. & Goldberg A. (1980b) Lead and heme biosynthesis. In: Singhal, R.L. & Thomas, J.A., eds, *Lead Toxicity*, Baltimore, Urban and Schwarzenberg, pp. 79–117

Moore, M.R., Goldberg, A., Pocock, S.J., Meredith, A., Stewart, I.M., MacAnespie, H., Lees, R. & Low, A. (1982) Some studies of maternal and infant lead exposure in Glasgow. *Scot. med. J.*, **27**, 113–121

Moorman, W.J., Skaggs, S.R., Clark, J.C., Turner, T.W., Sharpnack, D.D., Murrell, J.A., Simon, S.D., Chapin, R.E. & Schrader, S.M. (1998) Male reproductive effects of lead, including species extrapolation for the rabbit model. *Reprod. Toxicol.*, **12**, 333–346

Moreira, E.G., de Magalhaes Rosa, G.J., Barros, S.B.M., Vassilieff, V.S. & Vassillieff, I. (2001) Antioxidant defense in rat brain regions after developmental lead exposure. *Toxicology*, **169**, 145–151

Morgan, A. & Holmes, A. (1978) The fate of lead in petrol-engine exhaust particulates inhaled by the rat. *Environ. Res.*, **15**, 44–56

Morgan, A., Holmes, A. & Evans, J.C. (1977) Retention, distribution, and excretion of lead by the rat after intravenous injection. *Br. J. ind. Med.*, **34**, 37–42

Morgan, B.W., Todd, K.H. & Moore, B. (2001) Elevated blood lead levels in urban moonshine drinkers. *Ann. emerg. Med.*, **37**, 51–54

Morrison, J.N. & Quarterman, J. (1987) The relationship between iron status and lead absorption in rats. *Biol. trace Elem. Res.*, **14**, 115–126

Morrow, P.E., Beiter, H., Amato, F. & Gibb, F.R. (1980) Pulmonary retention of lead: An experimental study in man. *Environ. Res.*, **21**, 373–384

Moser, R., Oberley, T.D., Daggett, D.A., Friedman, A.L., Johnson, J.A. & Siegel, F.L. (1995) Effects of lead administration on developing rat kidney. I. Glutathione S-transferase isoenzymes. *Toxicol. appl. Pharmacol.*, **131**, 85–93

Mouradian, R.F. & Kinnes, G.M. (1991) Health Hazard Evaluation Report, HETA 90-0348-2135, Grosse Pointes-Clinton Refuse Disposal Authority, Mount Clemens, MI, USA, NIOSH

Muldoon, S.B., Cauley, J.A., Kuller, L.H., Scott, J. & Rohay, J. (1994) Lifestyle and sociodemographic factors as determinants of blood lead levels in elderly women. *Am. J. Epidemiol.*, **139**, 599–608

Mulligan, C.N., Yong, R.N. & Gibbs, B.F. (2001) Remediation technologies for metal-contaminated soils and groundwater: An evaluation. *Eng. Geol.*, **60**, 193–207

Murata, K., Araki, S. & Aono, H. (1987) Effects of lead, zinc, and coper absorption on peripheral nerve conduction in metal workers. *Int. Arch. occup. environ. Health*, **59**, 11–20

Murata, K., Araki, S., Yokoyama, K., Nomiyama, K., Nomiyama, H., Tao, Y.-X. & Liu, S.-J. (1995) Autonomic and central nervous system effects of lead in female glass workers in China. *Am. J. ind. Med.*, **28**, 233–244

Muro, L.A. & Goyer, R.A. (1969) Chromosome damage in experimental lead poisoning. *Arch. Path.*, **87**, 660–663

Murphy, M.J., Graziano, J.H., Popovac, D., Kline, J.K., Mehmeti, A., Factor-Litvak, P., Ahmedi, G., Shrout, P., Rajovic, B., Nenezic, D.U. & Stein, Z.A. (1990) Past pregnancy outcomes among women living in the vicinity of a lead smelter in Kosovo, Yugoslavia. *Am. J. pub. Health*, **80**, 33–35

Mushak, P. (1991) Gastro-intestinal absorption of lead in children and adults: Overview of biological and biophysico-chemical aspects. *Chem. Spec. Bioavail.*, **3**, 87–104

Muskett, C.J. & Caswell, R. (1980) An investigation into lead in two indoor small-bore rifle ranges. *Ann. occup. Hyg.*, **23**, 283–294

Mykkänen, H.M. & Wasserman, R.H. (1982) Effect of vitamin D on the intestinal absorption of ^{203}Pb and ^{47}Ca in chicks. *J. Nutr.*, **112**, 520–527

Mykkänen, H.M., Lancaster, M.C. & Dickerson, J.W.T. (1982) Concentrations of lead in the soft tissues of male rats during a long-term dietary exposure. *Environ. Res.*, **28**, 147–153

Mykkänen, H.M., Fullmer, C.S. & Wasserman, R.H. (1984) Effect of phosphate on the intestinal absorption of lead (^{203}Pb) in chicks. *J. Nutr.*, **114**, 68–74

Mylius, E.A. & Ophus, E.M. (1977) Pulmonary distributions of lead in human subjects. *Bull environ. Contam. Toxicol.*, **17**, 302–310

Nakaji, S., Fukuda, S., Sakamoto, J., Sugawara, K., Shimoyama, T., Umeda, T. & Baxter, D. (2001) Relationship between mineral and trace element concentrations in drinking water and gastric cancer mortality in Japan. *Nutr. Cancer*, **40**, 99–102

Nambi, K.S.V., Raghunath, R., Tripathi, R.M. & Khandekar, R.N. (1997) Scenario of 'Pb pollution and children' in Mumbai: Current air quality standard vindicated. *Energy Environ. Monitor.*, **13**, 53–60

Namihira, D., Saldivar, L., Pustilnik, N., Carreón, G.J. & Salinas, M.E. (1993) Lead in human blood and milk from nursing women living near a smelter in Mexico City. *J. Toxicol. environ. Health*, **38**, 225–232

Nathan, E., Huang, H.F.S., Pogach, L., Giglio, W., Bogden, J.D. & Seebode, J. (1992) Lead acetate does not impair secretion of Sertoli cell function marker proteins in the adult Sprague Dawley rat. *Arch. environ. Health*, **47**, 370–375

National Food Processors Association (1992) *Public Comment on the Toxicological Profile for Lead*. Submitted to the Academy for Toxic Substances and Disease Registry. Washington, DC, February 4, 1992

National Institute for Occupational Safety and Health (1994a) *Lead by GFAAS, Method 7105, Issue 2*, In: NIOSH Manual of Analytical Methods (NMAM), 4th Ed.

National Institute for Occupational Safety and Health (1994b) *Lead by Flame AAS, Method 7082, Issue 2*, In: NIOSH Manual of Analytical Methods (NMAM), 4th Ed.

National Institute for Occupational Safety and Health (1994c) *Tetraethyl Lead (as Pb), Method 2533, Issue 2*, In: NIOSH Manual of Analytical Methods (NMAM), 4th Ed.

National Institute for Occupational Safety and Health (1994d) *Tetramethyl Lead (as Pb), Method 2534, Issue 2*, In: NIOSH Manual of Analytical Methods (NMAM), 4th Ed.

National Institute for Occupational Safety and Health (1995) *Report to Congress on Workers' Home Contamination Study Conducted Under the Workers' Family Protection*, Cincinnati, OH, National Institute for Occupational Safety and Health

National Institute for Occupational Safety and Health (1998) *Lead by Field Portable XRF, Method 7702, Issue 1*, In: NIOSH Manual of Analytical Methods (NMAM), 4th Ed.

National Institute for Occupational Safety and Health (2001) *Health Hazard Evaluations: Occupational Exposure to Lead 1994 to 1999*, Research Triangle Park, NC, Centers for Disease Control and Prevention

National Institute for Occupational Safety and Health (2003a) *Elements by ICP (Nitric/Perchloric Acid Ashing), Method 7300, Issue 3*. In: NIOSH Manual of Analytical Methods (NMAM), 4th Ed.

National Institute for Occupational Safety and Health (2003b) *Lead by Portable Ultrasonic Extraction/ASV, Method 7701, Issue 2*. In: NIOSH Manual of Analytical Methods (NMAM), 4th Ed.

National Institute of Health Sciences, Japan (2000) [*Total Diet Survey in Japan (Estimation of Daily Dietary Intake of Food Contaminants)*, 1977–1999], National Institute of Health Sciences, Tokyo (in Japanese)

National Institute of Nutrition (1995–96) *Annual Report*, Hyderabad, National Institute of Nutrition, pp. 43–44

National Library of Medicine (2003) [http://chem.sis.nlm.nih.gov/chemidplus/chemidlite, jsp; accessed 01/02/2004]

National Oceanic and Atmospheric Administration (1998a) Sampling and analytical methods of the national status and trends program: 1993–1996 update. Method 140.0. In: *National Environmental Methods Index*

National Oceanic and Atmospheric Administration (1998b) Sampling and analytical methods of the national status and trends program: 1993–1996 update. Method 172.0. In: *National Environmental Methods Index*

National Oceanic and Atmospheric Administration (1998c) Sampling and analytical methods of the national status and trends program: 1993–1996 update. Method 160.0. In: *National Environmental Methods Index*

National Research Council (1993) *Measuring Lead Exposure in Infants, Children, and Other Sensitive Populations* (ISBN 030904927X), *Committee on Measuring Lead in Critical Populations*, NRC, Washington DC, National Academies Press

Navas-Acién, A., Pollán, M., Gustavsson, P. & Plato, N. (2002) Occupation, exposure to chemicals and risk of gliomas and meningiomas in Sweden. *Am. J. ind. Med.*, **42**, 214–227

Nawrot, T.S., Thijs, L., Den Hond, E.M., Roels, H.A. & Staessen, J.A. (2002) An epidemiological re-appraisal of the association between blood pressure and blood lead: A meta-analysis. *J. Human Hypert.*, **16**, 123–131

Nayak, B.N., Ray, M., Persaud, T.V.N. & Nigli, M. (1989) Relationship of embryotoxicity to genotoxicity of lead nitrate in mice. *Exp. Pathol.*, **36**, 65–73

Needleman, H.L., Gunnoe, C., Leviton, A., Reed, R., Peresie, H., Maher, C. & Barret, P. (1979) Deficits in psychologic and classroom performance of children with elevated dentine lead levels. *New Engl. J. Med.*, **300**, 689–695

Needleman, H.L., Leviton, A. & Bellinger, D. (1982) Lead-associated intellectual deficit. *New Engl. J. Med.*, **306**, 367

Needleman, H.L., Rabinowitz, M., Leviton, A., Linn, S. & Schoenbaum, S. (1984) The relationship between prenatal exposure to lead and congenital anomalies. *J. Am. med. Assoc.*, **251**, 2956–2959

Needleman, H.L., Schell, A., Bellinger, D., Leviton, A. & Allred, E.N. (1990) The long-term effects of exposure to low doses of lead in childhood. An 11-year follow-up report. *New Engl. J. Med.*, **322**, 83–88

Needleman, H.L., Riess, J.A., Tobin, M.J., Biesecker, G.E. & Greenhouse, J.B. (1996) Bone lead levels and delinquent behavior. *J. Am. med. Assoc.*, **275**, 363–369

Needleman, H.L., McFarland, C., Ness, R.B., Fienberg, S.E. & Tobin, M.J. (2002) Bone lead levels in adjudicated delinquents. A case control study. *Neurotoxicol. Teratol.*, **24**, 711–717

Nehéz, M., Lorencz, R. & Dési, I. (2000) Simultaneous action of cypermethrin and two environmental pollutant metals, cadmium and lead, on bone marrow cell chromosomes of rats in subchronic administration. *Ecotoxicol. environ. Safety*, **45**, 55–60

Neri, L.C., Hewitt, D. & Orser, B. (1988) Blood lead and blood pressure: Analysis of cross-sectional and longitudinal data from Canada. *Environ. Health Perspect.*, **78**, 123–126

Nestmann, E.R., Matula, T.I., Douglas, G.R., Bora, K.C. & Kowbel, D.J. (1979) Detection of the mutagenic activity of lead chromate using a battery of microbial tests. *Mutat. Res.*, **66**, 357–365

Neuberger, J.S. & Hollowell, J.G. (1982) Lung cancer excess in an abandoned lead-zinc mining and smelting area. *Sci. total Environ.*, **25**, 287–294

Neuman, D.R. & Dollhopf, D.J. (1992) Lead levels in blood from cattle residing near a lead smelter. *J. environ. Qual.*, **21**, 181–184

Nevin, R. (2000) How lead exposure relates to temporal changes in IQ, violent crime, and unwed pregnancy. *Environ. Res.*, **83**, 1–22

Newton, D., Pickford, C.J., Chamberlain, A.C., Sherlock, J.C. & Hislop, J.S. (1992) Elevation of lead in human blood from its controlled ingestion in beer. *Hum. exp. Toxicol.*, **11**, 3–9

Ng, R. & Martin, D.J. (1977) Lead poisoning from lead-soldered electric kettles. *Can. med. Assoc. J.*, **116**, 508–509, 512

Ng, T.P., Goh, H.H., Ng, Y.L., Ong, H.Y., Ong, C.N., Chia, K.S., Chia, S.E. & Jeyaratnam, J. (1991) Male endocrine functions in workers with moderate exposure to lead. *Br. J. ind. Med.*, **48**, 485–491

Nielsen, T., Jensen, K.A. & Grandjean, P. (1978) Organic lead in normal human brains. *Nature*, **274**, 602–603

Nielsen, C.J., Nielsen, V.K., Kirkby, H. & Gyntelberg, F. (1982) Absence of peripheral neuropathy in long-term lead-exposed subjects. *Acta. neurol. scand.*, **65**, 241–247

NIH (1994) Optimal calcium intake. Consensus development panel on optimal calcium uptake. *J. Am. med. Assoc.*, **272**, 1942–1948

Nilas, L. & Christiansen, C. (1988) Rates of bone loss in normal women: Evidence of accelerated trabecular bone loss after the menopause. *Eur. J. clin. Invest.*, **18**, 529–534

Nilsson, U., Attewell, R., Christoffersson, J.O., Schutz, A., Ahlgren, L., Skerfving, S. & Mattsson, S. (1991) Kinetics of lead in bone and blood after end of occupational exposure. *Pharmacol. Toxicol.*, **69**, 477–84

Nishii, K. (1993) A study of modulation by phosphate salts and potassium citrate on rat renal tumorigenesis. *J. Nara Med. Ass.*, **44**, 156–167

Nishioka, H. (1975) Mutagenic activities of metal compounds in bacteria. *Mutat. Res.*, **31**, 185–189

Nogueira, E. (1987) Rat renal carcinogenesis after chronic simultaneous exposure to lead acetate and N-nitrosodiethylamine. *Virchows Arch.*, **B53**, 365–374

Nolan, C.V. & Shaikh, Z.A. (1992) Lead nephrotoxicity and associated disorders: Biochemical mechanisms. *Toxicology*, **73**, 127–146

Nomiyama, K., Nomiyama, H., Liu, S.-J., Tao, Y-X., Nomiyama, T. & Omae, K. (2002) Lead induced increase of blood pressure in female lead workers. *Occup. environ. Med.*, **59**, 734–739

Noranda (2003) *Product Data Sheet: Lead*, Belledune, New Brunswick

Nordenson, I., Beckman, G., Beckman, L. & Nordström, S. (1978) Occupational and environmental risks in and around a smelter in northern Sweden. IV. Chromosomal aberrations in workers exposed to lead. *Hereditas*, **88**, 263–267

Nordström, S., Beckman, L. & Nordenson, I. (1978) Occupational and environmental risks in and around a smelter in northern Sweden. III. Frequencies of spontaneous abortion. *Hereditas*, **88**, 51–54

Nordström, S., Beckman, L. & Nordenson, L. (1979a) Occupational and environmental risks in and around a smelter in northern Sweden. VI. Congenital malformations. *Hereditas*, **90**, 297–302

Nordström, S., Beckman, L. & Nordenson, I. (1979b) Occupational and environmental risks in and around a smelter in northern Sweden. V. Spontaneous abortion among female employees and decreased birth weight in their offspring. *Hereditas*, **90**, 291–296

Norman, E.H., Hertz-Picciotto, I., Salmen, D.A. & Ward, T.H. (1997) Childhood lead poisoning and vinyl miniblind exposure. *Arch. pediatr. adoles. Med.*, **151**, 1033–1037

Novotny, T., Cook, M., Hughes, J. & Lee, S.A. (1987) Lead exposure in a firing range. *Am. J. Public Health*, **77**, 1225–1226

Nriagu, J.O. (1978) Lead in soils, sediments and major rock types. In: Nriagu, J.O., ed., *The Biogeochemistry of Lead in the Environment. Part A. Ecological Cycles*, New York, Elsevier/North-Holland Biomedical Press, pp. 15–72

Nriagu, J.O. (1992) Toxic metal pollution in Africa. *Science tot. Environ.*, **121**, 1–37

Nriagu, J.O. & Pacyna, J.M. (1988) Quantitative assessment of worldwide contamination of air, water and soils by trace metals. *Nature*, **333**, 134–139

Nriagu, J., Jinabhai, C., Naidoo, R. & Coutsoudis, A. (1996a) Atmospheric lead pollution in KwaZulu/Natal, South Africa. *Sci. total Environ.*, **191**, 69–76

Nriagu, J.O., Blankson, M.L. & Ocran, K. (1996b) Childhood lead poisoning in Africa: A growing public health problem. *Sci. total Environ.*, **181**, 93–100

Nriagu, J., Jinabhai, C.C., Naidoo, R. & Coutsoudis, A. (1997a) Lead poisoning of children in Africa, II. Kwazulu/Natal, South Africa. *Sci. total Environ.*, **197**, 1–11

Nriagu, J., Oleru, N.T., Cudjoe, C. & Chine, A. (1997b) Lead poisoning of children in Africa, III. Kaduna, Nigeria. *Sci. total Environ.*, **197**, 13–19

Nwankwo, J.N. & Elinder, C.G. (1979) Cadmium, lead and zinc concentrations in soils and in food grown near a zinc and lead smelter in Zambia. *Bull. environ. contam. Toxicol.*, **22**, 625–631

Oberto, A., Marks, N., Evans, H.L. & Guidotti, A. (1996) Lead (Pb^{2+}) promotes apoptosis in newborn rat cerebellar neurons: Pathological implications. *J. Pharmacol. exp. Ther.*, **279**, 435–442

Occupational Safety and Health Administration (2002a) *Metal and Metalloid Particulates in Workplace Atmospheres (Atomic Absorption), Method No. ID-121*, US Department of Labor, Division of Physical Measurements and Inorganic Analyses, Sandy, UT, USA

Occupational Safety and Health Administration (2002b) *Metal and Metalloid Particulates in Workplace Atmospheres (ICP Analysis), Method No. ID-125G*, US Department of Labor, Division of Physical Measurements and Inorganic Analyses, Sandy, UT, USA

Occupational Safety and Health Administration (2002c) *ICP Analysis of Metal/Metalloid Particulates from Solder Operations*, US Department of Labor, Division of Physical Measurements and Inorganic Analyses, Sandy, UT, USA

Occupational Safety and Health Administration (2003) *Lead (Pb) on Surfaces by a Portable X-Ray Fluorescence (XRF) Analyzer, Method No. OSS1*, US Department of Labor, Division of Physical Measurements and Inorganic Analyses, Sandy, UT, USA

Octel Ltd (1982) *World Wide Survey of Motor Gasoline Quality*, London

Octel Ltd (1988) *World Wide Survey of Motor Gasoline Quality 1987*, London

Octel Ltd (1990) *World Wide Survey of Motor Gasoline Quality*, London

OECD (1993) *Lead — Background And National Experience With Reducing Risk* (Risk Reduction Monograph No. 1; OCDE/GD(93)67), Paris, Organization for Economic Co-operation and Development

O'Flaherty, E.J. (1991a) Physiologically based lead kinetics. *Trace Subst. environ. Health*, **24**, 44–54

O'Flaherty, E.J. (1991b) Physiologically based models for bone-seeking elements. I. Rat skeletal and bone growth. *Toxicol. appl. Pharmacol.*, **111**, 299–312

O'Flaherty, E.J. (1991c) Physiologically based models for bone-seeking elements. II. Kinetics of lead disposition in rats. *Toxicol. appl. Pharmacol.*, **111**, 313–331

O'Flaherty, E.J. (1992) Modeling bone mineral metabolism, with special reference to calcium and lead. *Neurotoxicology*, **13**, 789–798

O'Flaherty, E.J. (1993) Physiologically based models for bone-seeking elements. IV. Kinetics of lead disposition in humans. *Toxicol. appl. Pharmacol.*, **118**, 16–29

O'Flaherty, E.J. (1995) Physiologically based models for bone-seeking elements. V. Lead absorption and disposition in childhood. *Toxicol. appl. Pharmacol.*, **131**, 297–308

O'Flaherty, E.J. (1998) A physiologically based kinetic model for lead in children and adults. *Environ. Health Perspect.*, **106** (Suppl. 6), 1495–1503

O'Flaherty, E.J. (2000) Modeling normal aging bone loss, with consideration of bone loss in osteoporosis. *Toxicol. Sci.*, **55**, 171–188

O'Flaherty, E.J., Hammond, P.B. & Lerner, S.I. (1982) Dependence of apparent blood lead half-life on the length of previous lead exposure in humans. *Fundam. appl. Toxicol.*, **2**, 49–54

O'Flaherty, E.J., Inskip, M.J., Yagminas, A.P. & Franklin, C.A. (1996) Plasma and blood lead concentrations, lead absorption, and lead excretion in nonhuman primates. *Toxicol. appl. Pharmacol.*, **138**, 121–130

O'Flaherty, E.J., Inskip, M.J., Franklin, C.A., Durbin, P.W., Manton, W.I. & Baccanale, C.L. (1998) Evaluation and modification of a physiologically based model of lead kinetics using data from a sequential isotope study in cynomolgus monkeys. *Toxicol. appl. Pharmacol.*, **149**, 1–16

Ogunsola, O.J., Oluwole, A.F., Asubiojo, O.I., Olaniyi, H.B., Akeredolu, F.A., Akanle, O.A., Spyrou, N.M., Ward, N.I. & Ruck, W. (1994a) Traffic pollution: Preliminary elemental characterisation of roadside dust in Lagos, Nigeria. *Sci. total Environ.*, **146/147**, 175–184

Ogunsola, O.J., Oluwole, A.F., Asubiojo, O.I., Durosinmi, M.A., Fatusi, A.O. & Ruck, W. (1994b) Environmental impact of vehicular traffic in Nigeria: Health aspects. *Sci. total Environ.*, **146–147**, 111–116

Oishi, H., Nomiyama, H., Nomiyama, K. & Tomokuni, K. (1996a) Comparison between males and females with respect to the porphyrin metabolic disorders found in workers occupationally exposed to lead. *Int. Arch. occup. environ. Health*, **68**, 298–304

Oishi, H., Nomiyama, H., Nomiyama, K. & Tomokuni, K. (1996b) Fluorometric HPLC determination of Δ-aminolevulinic acid (ALA) in the plasma and urine of lead workers: Biological indicators of lead exposure. *J. anal. Toxicol.*, **20**, 106–110

Okada, I.A., Sakuma, A.M., Maio, F.D., Dovidauskas, S. & Zenebon, O. (1997) [Evaluation of lead and cadmium levels in milk due to environmental contamination in the Paraiba Valley Region of southeastern Brazil.] *Rev. Saúde pública*, **31**, 140–143 (in Portuguese)

Okayama, A., Fujii, S. & Miura, R. (1990) Optimized fluorometric determination of urinary delta-aminolevulinic acid by using pre-column derivatization, and identification of the derivative. *Clin. Chem.*, **36**, 1494–1497

Olaiz, G., Fortoul, T.I., Rojas, R., Doyer, M., Palazuelos, E. & Tapia, C.R. (1996) Risk factors for high levels of lead in blood of schoolchildren in Mexico City. *Arch. environ. Health*, **51**, 122–126

Olejnik, D., Walkowska, A., Wisniewska, J. & Ziembinski, R. (1985) [Evaluation of the daily intake of mercury, lead and cadmium in the meals of some population groups.] *Roczn. Pzh.*, **XXXVI**, 9–21 (in Polish, with English abstract)

Olguín, A., Jauge, P. & Cebrián, M.E. (1982) Determinación del plomo en leches industrializadas. Resúmenes. II. Congreso sobre Problemas Ambientales de México, ENCB-IPN, México, p. 60

Oliveira, S., Aro, A., Sparrow, D. & Hu, H. (2002) Season modifies the relationship between bone and blood lead levels: The Normative Aging Study. *Arch. environ. Health*, **57**, 466–472

Olshan, A.F., Breslow, N.E., Daling, J.R., Falletta, J.M., Grufferman, S., Robison, L.L., Waskerwitz, M. & Hammond, G.D. (1990) Wilms' tumor and paternal occupation. *Cancer Res.*, **50**, 3212–3217

Omokhodion, F.O. (1994) Blood lead and tap water lead levels in Ibadan, Nigeria. *Sci. total Environ.*, **151**, 187–190

Omokhodion, F.O. & Crockford, G.W. (1991a) Sweat lead levels in persons with high blood lead levels: Experimental elevation of blood lead by ingestion of lead chloride. *Sci. total Environ.*, **108**, 235–242

Omokhodion, F.O. & Crockford, G.W. (1991b) Lead in sweat and its relationship to salivary and urinary levels in normal healthy subjects. *Sci. total Environ.*, **103**, 113–122

Omokhodion, F.O. & Howard, J.M. (1991) Sweat lead levels in persons with high blood lead levels: Lead in sweat of lead workers in the tropics. *Sci. total Environ.*, **103**, 123–128

Onalaja, A.O. & Claudio, L. (2000) Genetic susceptibility to lead poisoning. *Environ. Health Perspect.*, **108**, 23–28

O'Neil, M.J., ed. (2003) *The Merck Index*, 15th Ed., Whitehouse Station, NJ, Merck & Co., available on CD-Rom

Ong, C.N., Phoon, W.O., Law, H.Y., Tye, C.Y. & Lim, H.H. (1985) Concentrations of lead in maternal blood, cord blood, and breast milk. *Arch. Dis. Child.*, **60**, 756–759

Ong, C.N., Endo, G., Chia, K.S., Phoon, W.O. & Ong, H.Y. (1987) Evaluation of renal function in workers with low blood lead levels. In: Foà, V., Emmet, E.A., Maroni, M. & Colombi, A., eds, *Occupational and Environmental Chemical Hazards: Cellular and Biochemical Indices for Monitoring Toxicity*, Chichester, Ellis Horwood Ltd, pp. 327–333

Ong, C.N., Kong, Y.M., Ong, H.Y. & Teramoto, K. (1990) The *in vitro* and *in vivo* effects of lead on δ-aminolevulinic acid dehydratase and pyrimidine 5′-nucleotidase. *Pharmacol. Toxicol.*, **66**, 23–26

Onyari, J.M., Wandiga, S.O., Njenga, G.K. & Nyatebe, J.O. (1991) Lead contamination in street soils of Nairobi City and Mombasa Island, Kenya. *Bull. environ. Contam. Toxicol.*, **46**, 782–789

Ordóñez, B.R., Ruíz Romero, L. & Mora, R. (2003) [Epidemiological investigations on the lead levels of a childhood population and the home environment of Juarez City, Chihuahua, in relation to a smelter from El Paso, Texas.] *Salud pub. Mex.*, **45** (Suppl. 2), 281–295 (in Spanish)

O'Riordan, M.L. & Evans, H.J. (1974) Absence of significant chromosome damage in males occupationally exposed to lead. *Nature*, **247**, 50–53

Oskarsson, A., Squibb, K.S. & Fowler, B.A. (1982) Intracellular binding of lead in the kidney: The partial isolation and characterization of postmichondrial lead binding components. *Biochem. biophys. Res. Commun.*, **104**, 290–298

Oskarsson, A., Jorhem, L., Sundberg, J., Nilsson, N.G. & Albanus, L. (1992) Lead poisoning in cattle — Transfer of lead to milk. *Sci. total Environ.*, **111**, 83–94

Otto, D.A. & Fox, D.A. (1993) Auditory and visual dysfunction following lead exposure. *Neurotoxicology*, **142**, 191–203

Otto, D., Robinson, G., Baumann, S., Schroeder, S., Mushak, P., Kleinbaum, D. & Boone, L. (1985) 5-Year follow-up study of children with low to-moderate lead absorption: Electrophysiological evaluation. *Environ. Res.*, **38**, 168–186

Overmann, S.R. (1977) Behavioral effects of asymptomatic lead exposure during neonatal development in rats. *Toxicol. appl. Pharmacol.*, **41**, 459–471

Oyasu, R., Battifora, H.A., Clasen, R.A., McDonald, J.H. & Hass, G.M. (1970) Induction of cerebral gliomas in rats with dietary lead subacetate and 2-acetylaminofluorene. *Cancer Res.*, **30**, 1248–1261

Paglia, D.E. & Valentine, W.N. (1975) Characteristics of a pyrimidine-specific 5′-nucleotidase in human erythrocytes. *J. biol. Chem.*, **250**, 7973–7979

Paglia, D.E., Valentine, W.N. & Dahlgren, J.G. (1975) Effects of low-level lead exposure on pyrimidine 5′-nucleotidase and other erythrocyte enzymes: Possible role of pyrimidine 5′-nucleotidase in the pathogenesis of lead-induced anaemia. *J. clin. Invest.*, **56**, 1164–1169

Pagliuca, A., Mufti, G.J., Baldwin, D., Lestas, A.N., Wallis, R.M. & Bellingham, A.J. (1990) Lead poisoning: Clinical, biochemical, and haematological aspects of a recent outbreak. *Clin. Pathol.*, **43**, 277–281

Palminger Hallén, I. & Oskarsson, A. (1993) Dose dependent transfer of ^{203}lead to milk and tissue uptake in suckling offspring studied in rats and mice. *Pharmacol. Toxicol.*, **73**, 174–179

Palminger Hallén, I. & Oskarsson, A. (1995) Bioavailability of lead from various milk diets studied in a suckling rat model. *Biometals*, **8**, 231–236

Palminger Hallén, I., Jorhem, L., Lagerkvist, B.J. & Oskarsson, A. (1995a) Lead and cadmium levels in human milk and blood. *Sci. tot. Environ.*, **166**, 149–155

Palminger Hallén, I., Jorhem, L. & Oskarsson, A. (1995b) Placental and lactational transfer of lead in rats: A study on the lactational process and effects on offspring. *Arch. Toxicol.*, **69**, 596–602

Palminger Hallén, I., Jonsson, S., Karlsson, M.O. & Oskarsson, A. (1996a) Kinetic observations in neonatal mice exposed to lead via milk. *Toxicol. appl. Pharmacol.*, **140**, 13–18

Palminger Hallén, I., Jonsson, S., Karlsson, M.O. & Oskarsson, A. (1996b) Toxicokinetics of lead in lactating and nonlactating mice. *Toxicol. appl. Pharmacol.*, **136**, 342–347

Palus, J., Rydzynski, K., Dziubaltowska, E., Wyszynska, K., Natarajan, A.T. & Nilsson, R. (2003) Genotoxic effects of occupational exposure to lead and cadmium. *Mutat. Res.*, **540**, 19–28

P'an, A.Y.S. & Kennedy, C. (1989) Lead distribution in rats repeatedly treated with low doses of lead acetate. *Environ. Res.*, **48**, 238–247

Pan American Health Organization (1997) *Eliminating Lead in Gasoline in Latin America and the Caribbean. Report — 1996, Epidemiol. Bulletin*, **18**, 9–10

Parikh, D., Pandya, C.B. & Kashyap, S.K. (1999) Investigating environmental lead sources and pathways. In: *Lead Poisoning Prevention and Treatment: Implementing a National Programme in Developing Countries, February 8–10, Bangalore, India*, pp. 205–208 [http:/www.leadpoison.net/environment/investigating.htm; accessed 09/02/2004]

Parkinson, D.K., Hodgson, M.J., Bromet, E.J., Dew, M.A. & Connell, M.M. (1987) Occupational lead exposure and blood pressure. *Br. J. ind. Med.*, **44**, 744–748

Parkpian, P., Leong, S.T., Laortanakul, P. & Thunthaisong, N. (2003) Regional monitoring of lead and cadmium contamination in a tropical grazing land site, Thailand. *Environ. Monitor. Assess.*, **85**, 157–173

Parry, C. & Eaton, J. (1991) Kohl: A lead-hazardous eye makeup from the Third World to the First World. *Environ. Health Perspect.*, **94**, 121–123

Parsons, P.J., Reilly, A.A. & Esernio-Jenssen, D. (1997) Screening children exposed to lead: An assessment of the capillary blood lead fingerstick test. *Clin. Chem.*, **43**, 302–311

Parsons, P.J., Reilly, A.A., Esernio-Jenssen, D., Werk, L.N., Mofenson, H.C., Stanton, N.V. & Matte, T.D. (2001) Evaluation of blood lead proficiency testing: Comparison of open and blind paradigms. *Clin. Chem.*, **47**, 322–330

Partanen, T., Heikkila, P., Hernberg, S., Kauppinen, T., Moneta, G. & Ojajarvi, A. (1991) Renal cell cancer and occupational exposure to chemical agents. *Scand. J. Work. environ. Health*, **17**, 231–239

Pasminco Metals (1998) *Product Specification Sheet: 99.97% & 99.99% Lead Product*, Melbourne

Pasminco Metals (2000) *Product Specification Sheet: Pasminco Preferred Products (PPP): Oxide Lead*, Melbourne

Pasternack, B. & Ehrlich, L. (1972) Occupational exposure to an oil mist atmosphere. A 12-year mortality study. *Arch. environ. Health*, **25**, 286–294

Patel, A.B., Williams, S.V., Frumkin, H., Kondawar, V.K., Glick, H. & Ganju, A.K. (2001) Blood lead in children and its determinants in Nagpur, India. *Int. J. occup. environ. Health*, **7**, 119–126

Patierno, S.R. & Landolph, J.R. (1989) Soluble vs insoluble hexavalent chromate. Relationship of mutation to in vitro transformation and particle uptake. *Biol. trace Elem. Res.*, **21**, 469–474

Patierno, S.R., Banh, D. & Landolph, J.R. (1988) Transformation of C3H/10T1/2 mouse embryo cells to focus formation and anchorage independence by insoluble lead chromate but not soluble calcium chromate: Relationship to mutagenesis and internalization of lead chromate particles. *Cancer Res.*, **48**, 5280–5288

Patriarca, M., Menditto, A., Rossi, B., Lyon, T.D.B. & Fell, G.S. (2000) Environmental exposure to metals of newborns, infants and young children. *Microchem. J.*, **67**, 351–361

Patterson, C., Ericson, J., Manea-Krichten, M. & Shirahata, H. (1991) Natural skeletal levels of lead in *Homo sapiens sapiens* uncontaminated by technological lead. *Sci. total Environ.*, **107**, 205–236

Paul, R., White, F. & Luby, S. (2003) Trends in lead content of petrol in Pakinstan. *Bull. World Health Org.*, **81**, 468

Pawlik-Skowronska, B. (2001) Phytochelatin production in freshwater algae *Stigeoclonium* in response to heavy metals contained in mining water; effects of some environmental factors. *Aquat. Toxicol.*, **52**, 241–249

Pawlik-Skowronska, B., Sanità di Toppi, L., Favali, M.A., Fossati, F., Pirszel, J. & Skowronski, T. (2002) Lichens respond to heavy metals by phytochelatin synthesis. *New Phytol.*, **156**, 95–102

Penoles (2003) *Product Data Sheet: Lead*, Torreon, Coah

Peraino, C., Fry, R.J.M. & Staffeldt, E. (1971) Reduction and enhancement by phenobarbital of hepatocarcinogenesis induced in the rat by 2-acetylaminofluorene. *Cancer Res.*, **31**, 1506–1512

Pereira, L., Mañay, N., Cousillas, Z.A., Barregård, L., Sällsten, G. & Schütz, A. (1996) Occupational lead exposure in Montevideo, Uruguay. *Int. J. occup. environ. Health*, **2**, 328–330

Perino, J. & Ernhart, C.B. (1974) The relation of subclinical lead level to cognitive and sensorimotor impairment in black preschoolers. *J. learning Disord.*, **7**, 26–30

Perkins, K.C. & Oski, F.A. (1976) Elevated blood lead in a 6-month-old breast-fed infant: The role of newsprint logs. *Pediatrics*, **57**, 426–427

Pesch, B., Haerting, J., Ranft, U., Klimpel, A., Oelschlagel, B. & Schill, W. & the MURC Study Group (2000) Occupational risk factors for renal cell carcinoma: Agent-specific results from a case–control study in Germany. *Int. J. Epidemiol.*, **29**, 1014–1024

Petering, D.H., Huang, M., Moteki, S. & Shaw, C.F., III (2000) Cadmium and lead interactions with transcription factor IIIA from Xenopus laevis: A model for zinc finger protein reactions with toxic metal ions and metallothionein. *Mar. environ. Res.*, **50**, 89–92

Petrucci, R., Leonardi, A. & Battistuzzi, G. (1982) The genetic polymorphism of δ-aminolevulinate dehydrase in Italy. *Hum. Genet.*, **60**, 289–290

Phuapradit, W., Jetsawangsri, T., Chaturachinda, K. & Noinongyao, N. (1994) Maternal and umbilical cord blood lead levels in Ramathibodi Hospital, 1993. *J. med. Assoc. Thai.*, **77**, 368–372

Physical and Theoretical Chemistry Laboratory (2004) Chemistry resoures [http://physchem.ox.ac.uk/resources.html; accessed 01/02/2004]

Pickston, L., Brewerton, H.V., Drysdale, J.M., Hughes, J.T., Smith, J.M., Love, J.L., Sutcliffe, E.R. & Davidson, F. (1985) The New Zealand diet: A survey of elements, pesticides, colours, and preservatives. *N.Z. J. Technol.*, **1**, 81–89

Piechalak, A., Tomaszewska, B., Baralkiewicz, D. & Malecka, A. (2002) Accumulation and detoxification of lead ions in legumes. *Phytochemistry*, **60**, 153–162

Pinkerton, L.E., Biagini, R.E., Ward, E.M., Hull, R.D., Deddens, J.A., Boeniger, M.F., Schnorr, T.M., MacKenzie, B.A. & Luster, M.I. (1998) Immunologic findings among lead-exposed workers. *Am. J. ind. Med.*, **33**, 400–408

Pinon-Lataillade, G., Thoreux-Manlay, A., Coffigny, H., Monchaux, G., Masse, R. & Soufir, J.-C. (1993) Effect of ingestion and inhalation of lead on the reproductive system and fertility of adult male rats and their progeny. *Hum. exp. Toxicol.*, **12**, 165–172

Piomelli, S., Corash, L., Corash, M.B., Seaman, C., Mushak, P., Glover, B. & Padgett, R. (1980) Blood lead concentrations in a remote Himalayan population. *Science*, **210**, 1135–1137

Pirkle, J.L., Brody, D.J., Gunter, E.W., Kramer, R.A., Paschal, D.C., Flegal, K.M. & Matte, T.D. (1994) The decline in blood lead levels in the United States — The National Health and Nutrition Examination Surveys (NHANES). *J. Am. med. Assoc.*, **272**, 284–291

Pirkle, J.L., Kaufmann, R.B., Brody, D.J., Hickman, T., Gunter, E.W. & Paschal, D.C. (1998) Exposure of the US population to lead, 1991–1994. *Environ. Health Perspect.*, **106**, 745–750

Poirier, L.A., Theiss, J.C., Arnold, L.J. & Shimkin, M.B. (1984) Inhibition by magnesium and calcium acetates of lead subacetate- and nickel acetate-induced lung tumors in strain A mice. *Cancer Res.*, **44**, 1520–1522

Polák, J., O'Flaherty, E.J., Freeman, G.B., Johnson, J.D., Liao, S.C. & Bergstrom, P.D. (1996) Evaluating lead bioavailability data by means of a physiologically based lead kinetic model. *Fundam. appl. Toxicol.*, **29**, 63–70

Pollock, C.A. & Ibels, L.S. (1988) Lead nephropathy — A preventable cause of renal failure. *Int. J. artif. Organs*, **11**, 75–78

Pollution Control Department (1996) *Pollution Thailand, 1995*, Bangkok, Ministry of Science, Technology and Environment, the Government of Thailand, pp. 8–9

Pönkä, A. (1998) Lead in the ambient air and blood of children in Helsinki. *Sci. total Environ.*, **219**, 1–5

Pönkä, A., Salminen, E. & Ahonen, S. (1993) Lead in the ambient air and blood specimens of children in Helsinki. *Sci. total Environ.*, **138**, 301–308

Pontifex, A.H. & Garg, A.K. (1985) Lead poisoning from an Asian Indian folk remedy. *Can. med. Assoc. J.*, **133**, 1227–1228

Potula, V.L. & Hu, H. (1996a) Occupational and lifestyle determinants of blood lead levels among men in Madras, India. *Int. J. occup. environ. Health*, **2**, 1–4

Potula, V.L. & Hu, H. (1996b) Relationship of hemoglobin to occupational exposure to motor vehicle exhaust. *Toxicol. ind. Health*, **12**, 629–637

Pounds, J.G. & Leggett, R.W. (1998) The ICRP age-specific biokinetic model for lead: Validations, empirical comparisons, and explorations. *Environ. Health Perspect.*, **106** (Suppl. 6), 1505–1511

Pounds, J.G. & Rosen, J.F. (1986) Cellular metabolism of lead: A kinetic analysis in cultured osteoclastic bone cells. *Toxicol. appl. Pharmacol.*, **83**, 531–545

Pounds, J.G., Marlar, R.J. & Allen, J.R. (1978) Metabolism of lead-210 in juvenile and adult rhesus monkeys (*Macaca mulatta*). *Bull. environ. Contam. Toxicol.*, **19**, 684–691

Pounds, J.G., Wright, R. & Kodell, R.L. (1982) Cellular metabolism of lead: A kinetic analysis in the isolated rat hepatocyte. *Toxicol. appl. Pharmacol.*, **66**, 88–101

Prince, T.S. & Horstman, S.W. (1993) Case study at a college rifle range: The effect of a new ventilation system on air and blood lead levels. *Appl. Occup. Environ. Hyg.*, **8**, 909–911

Prpic-Majic, D., Pizent, A., Jurasovic, J., Pongracic, J. & Restek-Samarzija, N. (1996) Lead poisoning associated with the use of Ayurvedic metal-mineral tonics. *Clin. Toxicol.*, **34**, 417–423

Pulido, M.D. & Parrish, A.R. (2003) Metal-induced apoptosis: Mechanisms. *Mutat. Res.*, **533**, 227–241

Purser, D.A., Berrill, K.R. & Majeed, S.K. (1983) Effects of lead exposure on peripheral nerve in the cynomolgus monkey. *Br. J. ind. Med.*, **40**, 402–412

Quarterman, J. & Morrison, J.N. (1975) The effects of dietary calcium and phosphorus on the retention and excretion of lead in rats. *Br. J. Nutr.*, **34**, 351–362

Quarterman, J., Morrison, J.N. & Humphries, W.R. (1977) The role of phospholipids and bile in lead absorption. *Proc. Nutr. Soc.*, **36**, 103A

Quarterman, J., Morrison, J.N. & Humphries, W.R. (1978) The influence of high dietary calcium and phosphate on lead uptake and release. *Environ. Res.*, **17**, 60–67

Quarterman, J., Humphries, W.R., Morrison, J.N. & Morrison, E. (1980) The influence of dietary amino acids on lead absorption. *Environ. Res.*, **23**, 54–67

Queirolo, F., Stegen, S., Restovic, M., Paz, M., Ostapczuk, P., Schwuger, M.J. & Muñoz, L. (2000) Total arsenic, lead, and cadmium levels in vegetables cultivated at the Andean villages of northern Chile. *Sci. total Environ.*, **255**, 75–84

Queiroz, M.L., Perlingeiro, R.C., Bincoletto, C.,. Almeida, M., Cardoso, M.P. & Dantas, D.C. (1994a) Immunoglobulin levels and cellular immune function in lead exposed workers. *Immunopharmacol. Immunotoxicol.*, **16**, 115–128

Queiroz, M.L.S., Costa, F.F., Bincoletto, C., Perlingeiro, R.C.R., Dantas, D.C.M., Cardoso, M.P. & Almeida, M. (1994b) Engulfment and killing capabilities of neutrophils and phagocytic splenic function in persons occupationally exposed to lead. *Int. J. Immunopharmacol.*, **16**, 239–244

Quinn, M.J. (1985) Factors affecting blood lead concentrations in the UK: Results of the EEC blood lead surveys, 1979–1981. *Int. J. Epidemiol.*, **14**, 420–431

Quinn, M.J. & Delves, H.T. (1987) UK blood lead monitoring programme 1984–1987: Protocol and results for 1984. *Human Toxicol.*, **6**, 459–474

Quinn, M.J. & Delves, H.T. (1988) UK blood lead monitoring programme 1984–1987: Results for 1985. *Human Toxicol.*, **7**, 105–123

Quinn, M.J. & Delves, H.T. (1989) The UK blood lead monitoring programme 1984–1987: Results for 1986. *Human Toxicol.*, **8**, 205–220

Quintanilla-Vega, B., Hoover, D.J., Bal, W., Silbergeld, E.K., Waalkes, M.P. & Anderson, L.D. (2000) Lead interaction with human protamine (HP2) as a mechanism of male reproductive toxicity. *Chem. Res. Toxicol.*, **13**, 594–600

Rabinowitz, M.B. (1991) Toxicokinetics of bone lead. *Environ. Health Perspect.*, **91**, 33–37

Rabinowitz, M.B. (1995) Relating tooth and blood lead levels in children. *Bull. environ. Contam. Toxicol.*, **55**, 853–857

Rabinowitz, M. & Needleman, H.L. (1982) Temporal trends in the lead concentrations of umbilical cord blood. *Science*, **216**, 1429–1431

Rabinowitz, M.B., Wetherill, G.W. & Kopple, J.D. (1976) Kinetic analysis of lead metabolism in healthy humans. *J. clin. Invest.*, **58**, 260–270

Rabinowitz, M.B., Wetherill, G.W. & Kopple, J.D. (1977) Magnitude of lead intake from respiration by normal man. *J. Lab. clin. Med.*, **90**, 238–248

Rabinowitz, M.B., Kopple, J.D. & Wetherill, G.W. (1980) Effect of food intake and fasting on gastrointestinal lead absorption in humans. *Am. J. clin. Nutr.*, **33**, 1784–1788

Rabinowitz, M.B., Needleman, H., Burley, M., Finch, H. & Rees, J. (1984) Lead in umbilical blood, indoor air, tap water, and gasoline in Boston. *Arch. environ. Health*, **39**, 299–301

Rabinowitz, M., Leviton, A. & Needleman, H. (1985) Lead in milk and infant blood: A dose–response model. *Arch. environ. Health*, **40**, 283–286

Rader, J.I., Peeler, J.T. & Mahaffey, K.R. (1981) Comparative toxicity and tissue distribution of lead acetate in weanling and adult rats. *Environ. Health Perspect.*, **42**, 187–195

Ragan, H.A. (1977) Effects of iron deficiency on the absorption and distribution of lead and cadmium in rats. *J. Lab. clin. Med.*, **90**, 700–706

Raghavan, S.R.V., Culver, B.D. & Gonick, H.C. (1980) Erythrocyte lead-binding protein after occupational exposure. I. Relationship to lead toxicity. *Environ. Res.*, **22**, 264–270

Raghunath, R. & Nambi, K.S.V. (1998) Lead leaching from pressure cookers. *Sci. total Environ.*, **224**, 143–148

Raghunath, R., Tripathi, R.M., Khandekar, R.N. & Nambi, K.S.V. (1997) Retention time of Pb, Cd, Cu and Zn in children's blood. *Sci. total Environ.*, **207**, 133–139

Raghunath, R., Tripathi, R.M., Kumar, A.V., Sathe, A.P., Khandekar, R.N. & Nambi, K.S. (1999) Assessment of Pb, Cd, Cu and Zn exposures of 6 to 10 year old children in Mumbai. *Environ. Res.*, **80**, 215–221

Raghunath, R., Tripathi, R.M., Sastry, V.N. & Krishnamoorthy, T.M. (2000) Heavy metals in maternal and cord blood. *Sci. total Environ.*, **250**, 135–141

Rahbar, M.H., White, F., Agboatwalla, M., Hozhabri, S. & Luby, S. (2002) Factors associated with elevated blood lead concentrations in children in Karachi, Pakistan. *Bull. World Health Org.*, **80**, 769–775

Rahman, H., Al Khayat, A. & Menon, N. (1986) Lead poisoning in infancy — Unusual causes in the UAE. *Ann. trop. Paediatr.*, **6**, 213–217

Rahman, A., Maqbool, E. & Zuberi, H.S. (2002) Lead-associated deficits in stature, mental ability and behaviour in children in Karachi. *Ann. trop. Paediatr.*, **22**, 301–311

Rai, U.N. & Sinha, S. (2001) Distribution of metals in aquatic edible plants: *Trapa natans* (Roxb.) Makino and *Ipomoea aquatica* Forsk. *Environ. Monitor. Assess.*, **70**, 241–252

Rai, U.N., Sinha, S. & Chandra, P. (1996) Metal biomonitoring in water resources of Eastern Ghats, Koraput (Orissa), India by aquatic plants. *Environ. Monitor. Assess.*, **43**, 125–137

Rai, U.N., Tripathi, R.D., Vajpayee, P., Jha, V. & Ali, M.B. (2002) Bioaccumulation of toxic metals (Cr, Cd, Pb and Cu) by seeds of *Euryale ferox* Salisb. (Makhana). *Chemosphere*, **46**, 267–272

Rajah, T. & Ahuja, Y.R. (1995) In vivo genotoxic effects of smoking and occupational lead exposure in printing press workers. *Toxicol. Lett.*, **76**, 71–75

Ramel, C. & Magnusson, J. (1979) Chemical induction of nondisjunction in Drosophila. *Environ. Health Perspect.*, **31**, 59–66

Ramesh, G.T., Manna, S.K., Aggarwal, B.B. & Jadhav, A.L. (2001) Lead exposure activates nuclear factor kappa B, activator protein-1, c-Jun N-terminal kinase and caspases in the rat brain. *Toxicol. Lett.*, **123**, 195–207

Razmiafshari, M., Kao, J., d'Avignon, A. & Zawia, N.H. (2001) NMR identification of heavy metal-binding sites in a synthetic zinc finger peptide: Toxicological implications for the interactions of xenobiotic metals with zinc finger proteins. *Toxicol. appl. Pharmacol.*, **172**, 1–10

Rees, D.C., Duley, J.A. & Marinaki, A.M. (2003) Pyrimidine 5′ nucleotidase deficiency. *Br. J. Haematol.*, **120**, 375–383

Regional Environmental Center for Central and Eastern Europe (1998) *Sofia Initiative on Local Air Quality: Phase-out of Leaded Gasoline — Synthesis Report*, Szentendre, Hungary

Reh, C.M. & Klein, M.K. (1990) Health Hazard Evaluation Report, HETA 87-0376-2018, U.S. Dept. of Justice, U.S. Marshals Service, Washington, DC, USA, NIOSH

Rencher, A.C., Carter, M.W. & McKee, D.W. (1977) A retrospective epidemiological study of mortality at a large western copper smelter. *J. occup. Med.*, **19**, 754–758

Rendall, R.E.G., Baily, P. & Soskolne, C.L. (1975) The effect of particle size on absorption of inhaled lead. *Am. ind. Hyg. Assoc. J.*, **36**, 207–213

Revich, B.A., Bykov, A.A., Liapunov, S.M., Prikhozhan, A.M., Seregina, I.F. & Sobolev, M.B. (1998) [Experience in the study of the effects of lead on the health status of children in Belovo.] *Med. Tr. Prom. Ekol.*, **12**, 25–32 (in Russian)

Reynolds, S.J., Seem, R., Fourtes, L.J., Sprince, N.L., Johnson, J., Walkner, L., Clarke, W. & Whitten, P. (1999) Prevalence of elevated blood leads and exposure to lead in construction trades in Iowa and Illinois. *Am. J. ind. Med.*, **36**, 307–316

Rice, D.C. (1997) Effects of lifetime lead exposure in monkeys on detection of pure tones. *Fundam. appl. Toxicol.*, **36**, 112–118

Rice, D.C. & Hayward, S. (1999) Comparison of visual function at adulthood and during aging in monkeys exposed to lead or methylmercury. *NeuroToxicology*, **20**, 767–784

Richter, E.D., Yaffe, Y. & Gruener, N. (1979) Air and blood lead levels in a battery factory. *Environ. Res.*, **20**, 87–98

Richter, J., Hájek, Z., Pfeifer, I. & Šubrt, P. (1999) Relation between concentration of lead, zinc and lysozyme in placentas of women with intrauterine foetal growth retardation. *Cent. Eur. J. public Health*, **7**, 40–42

Rinehart, R. & Almaguer, D. (1992) Health Hazard Evaluation Report, HETA 90-084-2219, Kansas City Kansas Police Dept., Kansas City, KS, USA, NIOSH

Risch, H.A., Burch, J.D., Miller, A.B., Hill, G.B., Steele, R. & Howe, G.R. (1988) Occupational factors and the incidence of cancer of the bladder in Canada. *Br. J. ind. Med.*, **45**, 361–367

Robbiano, L., Carrozzino, R., Puglia, C.P., Corbu, C. & Brambilla, G. (1999) Correlation between induction of DNA fragmentation and micronuclei formation in kidney cells from rats and humans and tissue-specific carcinogenic activity. *Toxicol. appl. Pharmacol.*, **161**, 153–159

Robbins, S.K., Blehm, K.D. & Buchan, R.M. (1990) Controlling airborne lead in indoor firing ranges. *Appl. Occup. Environ. Hyg.*, **5**, 435–439

Roberts, H.J. (1983) Potential toxicity due to dolomite and bonemeal. *South. med. J.*, **76**, 556–559

Robertson, I.K. & Worwood, M. (1978) Lead and iron absorption from rat small intestine: The effect of dietary Fe deficiency. *Br. J. Nutr.*, **40**, 253–260

Robins, T.G., Bornman, M.S., Ehrlich, R.I., Cantrell, A.C., Pienaar, E., Vallabh, J. & Miller, S. (1997) Semen quality and fertility of men employed in a South African lead acid battery plant. *Am. J. ind. Med.*, **32**, 369–376

Robison, S.H., Cantoni, O. & Costa, M. (1984) Analysis of metal-induced DNA lesions and DNA-repair replication in mammalian cells. *Mutat. Res.*, **131**, 173–181

Rodamilans, M., Osaba, M.J.M., To-Figueras, J., Rivera Fillat, F., Marques, J.M., Perez, P. & Corbella, J. (1988) Lead toxicity on endocrine testicular function in an occupationally exposed population. *Hum. Toxicol.*, **7**, 125–128

Rodamilans, M., Torra, M., To-Figueras, J., Corbella, J., López, B., Sánchez, C. & Mazzara, R. (1996) Effect of the reduction of petrol lead on blood lead levels of the population of Barcelona (Spain). *Bull. environ. Contam. Toxicol.*, **56**, 717–721

Roe, F.J.C., Boyland, E., Dukes, C.E. & Mitchley, B.C.V. (1965) Failure of testosterone or xanthopterin to influence the induction of renal neoplasms by lead in rats. *Br. J. Cancer*, **ii**, 860–866

Roels, H.A., Hoet, P. & Lison, D. (1999) Usefulness of biomarkers of exposure to inorganic mercury, lead, or cadmium in controlling occupational and environmental risks of nephrotoxicity. *Ren. Fail.*, **21**, 251–262

Rogalla, T., Ehrnsperger, M., Preville, X., Kotlyarov, A., Lutsch, G., Ducasse, C., Paul, C., Wieske, M., Arrigo, A.-P., Buchner, J. & Gaestel, M. (1999) Regulation of Hsp27 oligomerization, chaperone function, and protective activity against oxidative stress/tumor necrosis factor alpha by phosphorylation. *J. biol. Chem.*, **274**, 18947–18956

Rogan, W.J., Ragan, N.B., Damokosh, A.L., Davoli, C., Shaffer, T.R., Jones, R.L., Wilkens, S., Heenehan, M.C., Ware, J.H. & Henretig, F. (1999) Recall of a lead-contaminated vitamin and mineral supplement in a clinical trial. *Pharmacoepidemiol. Drug Saf.*, **8**, 343–350

Roh, Y.-M., Kim, K. & Kim, H. (2000) Zinc protoporphyrin IX concentrations between normal adults and the lead-exposed workers measured by HPLC, spectrofluorometer, and hematofluorometer. *Ind. Health*, **38**, 372–379

Romero, A.J. (1996) The environmental impact of leaded gasoline in Venezuela. *J. environ. Dev.*, **5**, 434–438

Romieu, I. & Lacasana, M. (1996) Lead in the Americas. A call for action. In: Howson, C.P., Hernández-Avila, M. & Rall, D.P., eds, *Committee to Reduce Lead Exposure in the Americas*, Board on International Health Institute of Medicine, Washington, DC in collaboration with the National Institute of Public Health, Cuernavaca, Morelos, Mexico

Romieu, I., Lacasana, M., McConnell, R. & the Lead Research Group of the Pan-American Health Organization (1997) Lead exposure in Latin America and the Caribbean. *Environ. Health Perspect.*, **105**, 398–405

Ronis, M.J.J., Badger, T.M., Shema, S.J., Roberson, P.K. & Shaikh, F. (1996) Reproductive toxicity and growth effects in rats exposed to lead at different periods during development. *Toxicol. appl. Pharmacol.*, **136**, 361–371

Rosenkranz, H.S. & Poirier, L.A. (1979) Evaluation of the mutagenicity and DNA-modifying activity of carcinogens and noncarcinogens in microbial systems. *J. natl Cancer Inst.*, **62**, 873–891

Roses, O.E., Gonzalez, D.E., López, C.M., Piñeiro, A.E. & Villaamil, E.C. (1997) Lead levels in Argentine market wines. *Bull. environ. Contam. Toxicol.*, **59**, 210 215

Rosman, K.J.R., Chisholm, W., Boutron, C.F., Candelone, J.P. & Hong, S. (1994a) Isotopic evidence to account for changes in the concentration of lead in Greenland snow between 1960 and 1988. *Geochim. Cosmochim. Acta*, **58**, 3265–3269

Rosman, K.J.R., Chisholm, W., Boutron, C.F., Candelone, J.P. & Patterson, C.C. (1994b) Anthropogenic lead isotopes in Antarctica. *Geophys. Res. Lett.*, **21**, 2669–2672

Rothenberg, S.J., Karchmer, S., Schnaas, L., Perroni, E., Zea, F. & Fernandez Alba, J. (1994) Changes in serial blood lead levels during pregnancy. *Environ. Health Perspect.*, **102**, 876–880

Rothenberg, S.J., Schnaas, L., Perroni, E., Hernández, R.M. & Karchmer, S. (1998) Secular trend in blood lead levels in a cohort of Mexico City children. *Arch. environ. Health*, **53**, 231–235

Rothenberg, S.J., Manalo, M., Jiang, J., Khan, F., Cuellar, R., Reyes, S., Sanchez, M., Reynoso, B., Aguilar, A., Diaz, M., Acosta, S., Jauregui, M. & Johnson, C. (1999) Maternal blood lead level during pregnancy in South Central Los Angeles. *Arch. environ. Health*, **54**, 151–157

Rothenberg, S.J., Khan, F., Manalo, M., Jiang, J., Cuellar, R., Reyes, S., Acosta, S., Jauregui, M., Diaz, M., Sanchez, M., Todd, A.C. & Johnson, C. (2000) Maternal bone lead contribution to blood lead during and after pregnancy. *Environ. Res.*, **82**, 81–90

Rothenberg, S.J., Kondrashov, V., Manalo, M., Jiang, J., Cuellar, R., Garcia, M., Reynoso, B., Reyes, S., Diaz, M. & Todd, A.C. (2002) Increases in hypertension and blood pressure during pregnancy with increased bone lead levels. *Am. J. Epidemiol.*, **156**, 1079–1087

Roy, N.K. & Rossman, T.G. (1992) Mutagenesis and comutagenesis by lead compounds. *Mutat. Res.*, **298**, 97–103

Roy, M.M., Gordon, C.L., Beaumont, L.F., Chettle, D.R. & Webber, C.E. (1997) Further experience with bone lead content measurements in residents of southern Ontario. *Appl. Radiat. Isot.*, **48**, 391–396

Rudnick, R.L. & Fountain, D.M. (1995) Nature and composition of the continental crust: A lower crustal perspective. *Rev. Geophys.*, **33**, 267–309

Ruhe, R.L. (1982a) Health Hazard Evaluation Report, HETA 81-0426-1062, Xomox Corp., Cincinnati, OH, USA, NIOSH

Ruhe, R.L (1982b) Health Hazard Evaluation Report, HETA 81-0438-1090, Matryx Corp., Sharonville, OH, USA, NIOSH

Ruhe, R.L. & Thoburn, T.W. (1984) Health Hazard Evaluation Report, HETA 83-0459-1465, Stuart Manufacturing, Denver, CO, USA, NIOSH

Russell, J.C., Griffin, T.B., McChesney, E.W. & Coulston, F. (1978) Metabolism of airborne particulate lead in continuously exposed rats: Effect of penicillamine on mobilization. *Ecotoxicol. Environ. Saf.*, **2**, 49–53

Ryu, J.E., Ziegler, E.E. & Fomon, S.J. (1978) Maternal lead exposure and blood lead concentration in infancy. *J. Pediatrics*, **93**, 476–478

Ryu, J.E., Ziegler, E.E., Nelson, S.E. & Fomon, S.J. (1983) Dietary intake of lead and blood lead concentration in early infancy. *Am. J. Dis. Child*, **137**, 886–891

Ryu, J.E., Ziegler, E.E., Nelson, S.E. & Fomon, S.J. (1985) Dietary and environmental exposure to lead and blood lead during early infancy. In: Mahaffey, K.R., ed., *Chapter 7, Dietary and Environmental Lead: Human Health Effects*, Amsterdam, Elsevier Science Publishers, pp. 187–209

Sadasivan, S., Negi, B.S. & Mishra, U.C. (1987) Atmospheric lead levels in some cities in India. *Indian J. environ. Health*, **29**, 280–286

Saenger, P., Markowitz, M.E. & Rosen, J.F. (1984) Depressed excretion of 6-beta-hydroxycortisol in lead-toxic children. *J. clin. Endocrinol. Metab.*, **58**, 363–367

Sakai, T. (2000) Biomarkers of lead exposure. *Ind. Health*, **38**, 127–142

Sakai, T. & Ushio, K. (1986) A simplified method for determining erythrocyte pyrimidine 5′-nucleotidase (P5N) activity by HPLC and its value in monitoring lead exposure. *Br. J. ind. Med.*, **43**, 839–844

Sakai, T., Yanagihara, S. & Ushio, K. (1980) Restoration of lead-inhibited 5-aminolevulinate dehydratase activity in whole blood by heat, zinc ion, and (or) dithiothreitol. *Clin. Chem.*, **26**, 625–628

Sakai, K., Susuki, M., Yamane, Y., Takahashi, A. & Ide, G. (1990) Promoting effect of basic lead acetate administration on the tumorigenesis of lung in N-nitrosodimethylamine-treated mice. *Bull. environ. Contam. Toxicol.*, **44**, 707–714

Sallmén, M., Lindbohm, M.-L., Anttila, A., Taskinen, H. & Hemminki, K. (2000) Time to pregnancy among wives of men occupationally exposed lo lead. *Epidemiology*, **11**, 141–147

Salt, D.E., Blaylock, M., Kumar, N.P.B.A., Dushenkov, V., Ensley, B.D., Chet, I. & Raskin, I. (1995) Phytoremediation: A novel strategy for the removal of toxic metals from the environment using plants. *Bio/Technology*, **13**, 468–474

Salt, D.E., Smith, R.D. & Raskin, I. (1998) Phytoremediation. *Ann. Rev. Plant Physiol. Plant mol. Biol.*, **49**, 643–668

Sandhu, S.S., Ma, T.-H., Peng, Y. & Zhou, X.-D. (1989) Clastogenicity evaluation of seven chemicals commonly found at hazardous industrial waste sites. *Mutat. Res.*, **224**, 437–445

Sanín, L.H., Gonzalez-Cossio, T., Romieu, I., Peterson, K.E., Ruíz, S., Palazuelos, E., Hernandez-Avila, M. & Hu, H. (2001) Effect of maternal lead burden on infant weight and weight gain at one month of age among breastfed infants. *Pediatrics*, **107**, 1016–1023

Sankila, R., Karjalainen, S., Pukkala, E., Oksanen, H., Hakulinen, T., Teppo, L. & Hakama, M. (1990) Cancer risk among glass factory workers: An excess of lung cancer? *Br. J. ind. Med.*, **47**, 815–818

Sauerhoff, M.W. & Michaelson, I.A. (1973) Hyperactivity and brain catecholamines in lead-exposed developing rats. *Science*, **182**, 1022–1024

Savolainen, K.M., Loikkanen, J., Eerikainen, S. & Naarala, J. (1998) Glutamate-stimulated ROS production in neuronal cultures: Interactions with lead and the cholinergic system. *Neurotoxicology*, **19**, 669–674

Saxena, D.K., Srivastava, R.S., Lal, B. & Chandra, S.V. (1987) The effect of lead exposure on the testis of growing rats. *Exp. Pathol.*, **31**, 249–252

Saxena, D.K., Lal, B., Srivastava, R.S. & Chandra, S.V. (1990) Lead induced testicular hypersensitivity in stressed rats. *Exp. Pathol.*, **39**, 100–109

Saxena, D.K, Singh, C., Murthy, R.C., Mathur, N. & Chandra, S.V. (1994) Blood and placental lead levels in an Indian city: A preliminary report. *Arch. environ. Health*, **49**, 106–110

Scarano, G. & Morelli, E. (2002) Characterization of cadmium- and lead-phytochelatin complexes formed in a marine microalga in response to metal exposure. *Biomet.*, **15**, 145–151

Scelfo, G.M. & Flegal, A.R. (2000) Lead in calcium supplements. *Environ. Health Perspect.*, **108**, 309–313

Schaller, K.H., Angerer, J. & Drexler, H. (2002) Review. Quality assurance of biological monitoring in occupational and environmental medicine. *J. Chromatogr. B.*, **778**, 403–417

Schechtman, L.M., Hatch, G.G., Anderson, T.M., Putman, D.L., Kouri, R.E., Cameron, J.W., Nims, R.W., Spalding, J.W., Tennant, R.W. & Lubet, R.A. (1986) Analysis of the interlaboratory and intralaboratory reproducibility of the enhancement of simian adenovirus SA7 transformation of Syrian hamster embryo cells by model carcinogenic and noncarcinogenic compounds. *Environ. Mutag.*, **8**, 495–514

Schmid, E., Bauchinger, M., Pietruck, S. & Hall, G. (1972) [Cytogenetic action of lead in human peripheral lymphocytes *in vitro* and *in vivo*.] *Mutat. Res.*, **16**, 401–406 (in German)

Schmitt, C.J. & Brumbaugh, W.G. (1990) National contaminant biomonitoring program: Concentrations of arsenic, cadmium, cooper, lead, mercury, selenium, and zinc in U.S. freshwater fish, 1976–1984. *Arch. environ. Contam. Toxicol.*, **19**, 731–747

Schmitt, M.D.C., Trippler, D.J., Wachtler, J.N. & Lund, G.V. (1988) Soil lead concentrations in residential Minnesota as measured by ICP-AES. *Water Air Soil Pollut.*, **39**, 157–168

Schnaas, L., Rothenberg, S.J., Perroni, E., Martínez, S., Hernández, C. & Hernández, R.M. (2000) Temporal pattern in the effect of postnatal blood lead level on intellectual development of young children. *Neurotoxicol. Teratol.*, **22**, 805–810

Schroeder, H.A. & Mitchener, M. (1971) Toxic effects of trace elements on the reproduction of mice and rats. *Arch. environ. Health*, **23**, 102–106

Schroeder, H.A., Balassa, J.J. & Vinton, W.H., Jr (1965) Chromium, cadmium and lead in rats: Effects of life span, tumors and tissue levels. *J. Nutr.*, **86**, 51–66

Schroeder, H.A., Mitchener, M. & Nason, A.P. (1970) Zirconium, niobium, antimony, vanadium and lead in rats: Life term studies. *J. Nutr.*, **100**, 59–68

Schuhmacher, M., Bellés, M., Rico, A., Domingo, J.L. & Corbella, J. (1996a) Impact of reduction of lead in gasoline on the blood and hair lead levels in the population of Tarragona Province, Spain, 1990–1995. *Sci. total Environ.*, **184**, 203–209

Schuhmacher, M., Hernández, M., Domingo, J.L., Fernández-Ballart, J.D., Llobet, J.M. & Corbella, J. (1996b) A longitudinal study of lead mobilization during pregnancy: Concentrations in maternal and umbilical cord blood. *Trace Elem. Electrolytes*, **13**, 177–181

Schuhmacher, M., Paternain, J.L., Domingo, J.L. & Corbella, J. (1997) An assessment of some biomonitors indicative of occupational exposure to lead. *Trace elem. Electrolytes*, **14**, 145–149

Schütz, A., Skerfving, S., Ranstam, J. & Christoffersson, J.-O. (1987) Kinetics of lead in blood after the end of occupational exposure. *Scand. J. Work Environ. Health*, **13**, 221–231

Schütz, A., Attewell, R. & Skerfving, S. (1989) Decreasing blood lead in Swedish children, 1978–1988. *Arch. environ. Health*, **44**, 391–394

Schütz, A., Bergdahl, I.A., Ekholm, A. & Skerfving, S. (1996) Measurement by ICP-MS of lead in plasma and whole blood of lead workers and controls. *Occup. environ. Med.*, **53**, 736–740

Schütz, A., Barregård, L., Sällsten, G., Wilske, J., Manay, N., Pereira, L. & Cousillas, Z.A. (1997) Blood lead in Uruguayan children and possible sources of exposure. *Environ. Res.*, **74**, 17–23

Schwanitz, G., Lehnert, G. & Gebhart, E. (1970) [Chromosome damage after occupational exposure to lead.] *Dtsch. Med. Wochenschr.*, **95**, 1636–1641 (in German)

Schwanitz, G., Gebhart, E., Rott, H.-D., Schaller, K.-H., Essing, H.-G., Lauer, O. & Prestele, H. (1975) [Chromosome investigations in subjects with occupational lead exposure.] *Dtsch. med. Wochenschr.*, **100**, 1007–1011 (in German)

Schwartz, J. (1994) Low-level lead exposure and children's IQ: A meta-analysis and search for a threshold. *Environ. Res.*, **65**, 42–55

Schwartz, J. & Otto, D. (1987) Blood lead, hearing thresholds and neurobehavioral development in children and youth. *Arch. environ. Health*, **42**, 153–160

Schwartz, J., Landrigan, P.J., Feldman, R.G., Silbergeld, E.K., Baker, E.L., Jr & von Lindern, I.H. (1988) Threshold effect in lead-induced peripheral neuropathy. *J. Pediatr.*, **112**, 12–17

Schwartz, J., Landrigan, P.J., Baker, E.L., Jr, Orenstein, W.A. & von Lindern, I.H. (1990) Lead-induced anemia: Dose–response relationships and evidence for a threshold. *Am. J. pub. Health*, **80**, 165–168

Schwartz, B.S., Lee, B.-K., Stewart, W., Ahn, K.-D., Springer, K. & Kelsey, K. (1995) Associations of δ-aminolevulinic acid dehydratase genotype with plant, exposure duration, and blood lead and zinc protoporphyrin levels in Korean lead workers. *Am. J. Epidemiol.*, **142**, 738–745

Schwartz, B.S., Stewart, W.F., Todd, A.C. & Links, J.M. (1999) Predictors of dimercaptosuccinic acid chelatable lead and tibial lead in former organolead manufacturing workers. *Occup. environ. Med.*, **56**, 22–29

Schwartz, B.S., Stewart, W.F., Todd, A.C., Simon, D. & Links, J.M. (2000a) Different associations of blood lead, meso 2,3-dimercaptosuccinic acid (DMSA)-chelatable lead, and tibial lead levels with blood pressure in 543 former organolead manufacturing workers. *Arch. environ. Health*, **55**, 85–92

Schwartz, B.S., Lee, B.K., Lee, G.S., Stewart, W.F., Simon, D., Kelsey, K. & Todd, A.C. (2000b) Associations of blood lead, dimercaptosuccinic acid-chelatable lead, and tibia lead with polymorphisms in the vitamin D receptor and δ-aminolevulinic acid dehydratase genes. *Environ. Health Perspect.*, **108**, 949–954

Schwartz, B.S., Lee, B.-K., Lee, G.-S., Stewart, W.F., Lee. S.-S., Hwang, K.-Y., Ahn, K.-D., Kim, Y.-B., Bolla, K.L., Simon, D., Parsons, P.J. & Todd, A.C. (2001) Associations of blood lead, dimercaptosuccinic acid-chelatable lead, and tibia lead with neurobehavioral test scores in South Korean lead workers. *Am. J. Epidemiol.*, **153**, 453–464

Seidel, S., Kreutzer, R., Smith, D., McNeel, S. & Gilliss, D. (2001) Assessment of commercial laboratories performing hair mineral analysis. *J. Am. med. Assoc.*, **285**, 67–72

Selevan, S.G., Landrigan, P.J., Stern, F.B. & Jones, J.H. (1985) Mortality of lead smelter workers. *Am. J. Epidemiol.*, **122**, 673–683

Seppäläinen, A.M., Tola, S., Hernberg, S. & Kock, B. (1975) Subclinical neuropathy at 'safe' levels of lead exposure. *Arch. environ. Health*, **30**, 180–183

Seppäläinen, A.M., Hernberg, S. & Kock, B. (1979) Relationship between blood lead levels and nerve conduction velocities. *Neurotoxicology*, **1**, 313–332

Seppäläinen, A.M., Hernberg, S., Vesanto, R . & Kock, B. (1983) Early neurotoxic effects of lead exposure: A prospective study. *Neurotoxicology*, **4**, 181–192

Sepúlveda, V., Vega, J. & Delgado, I. (2000) [Severe exposure to environmental lead in a child population in Antofagasta, Chile.] *Rev. méd. Chile*, **128**, 221–232 (in Spanish)

Shaltout, A., Yaish, S.A. & Fernando, N. (1981) Lead encephalopathy in infants in Kuwait. *Ann. trop. Paediatr. (London)*, **1**, 209–215

Sharma, K. & Reutergardh, L.B. (2000) Exposure of preschoolers to lead in the Makati area of Metro Manila, the Phillippines. *Environ. Res.*, **A83**, 322–332

Sheffet, A., Thind, I., Miller, A.M. & Louria, D.B. (1982) Cancer mortality in a pigment plant utilizing lead and zinc chromates. *Arch. environ. Health*, **37**, 44–52

Shen, X.-M., Rosen, J.F., Guo, D. & Wu, S.-M. (1996) Childhood lead poisoning in China. *Sci. total Environ.*, **181**, 101–109

Shen, X., Yan, C., Zhang, Y., Wu, S., Jiang, F., He, J., Yin, J., Ao, L., Zhang, Y. & Li, R. (1999) [Comparison of children's blood lead levels in Shanghai before and after the introduction of lead free gasoline]. *Natl med. J. China*, **79**, 739–741 (in Chinese)

Sherlock, J.C., Smart, G.A., Walters, B., Evans, W.H., McWeeny, D.J. & Cassidy, W. (1983) Dietary surveys on a population at Shipham, Somerset, United Kingdom. *Sci. total Environ.*, **29**, 121–142

Sherlock, J.C., Pickford, C.J. & White, G.F. (1986) Lead in alcoholic beverages. *Food addit. Contam.*, **3**, 347–354

Shih, T.-M. & Hanin, I. (1978) Chronic lead exposure in immature animals: Neurochemical correlates. *Life Sci.*, **23**, 877–888

Shimbo, S., Zhang, Z.-W., Moon, C.-S., Watanabe, T., Nakatsuka, H., Matsuda-Inoguchi, N., Higashikawa, K. & Ikeda, M. (2000) Correlation between urine and blood concentrations, and dietary intake of cadmium and lead among women in the general population of Japan. *Int. Arch. occup. environ. Health*, **73**, 163–170

Shimbo, S., Zhang, Z.-W., Watanabe, T., Nakatsuka, H., Matsuda-Inoguchi, N., Higashikawa, K. & Ikeda, M. (2001) Cadmium and lead contents in rice and other cereal products in Japan in 1998-2000. *Sci. total Environ.*, **281**, 165–175

Shimkin, M.B., Stoner, G.D. & Theiss, J.C. (1977) Lung tumor response in mice to metals and metal salts. *Adv. exp. Med. Biol.*, **91**, 85–91

Shirai, T., Ohshima, M., Masuda, A., Tamano, S. & Ito, N. (1984) Promotion of 2-(ethylnitrosamino)ethanol-induced renal carcinogenesis in rats by nephrotoxic compounds: Positive responses with folic acid, basic lead acetate, and N-(3,5-dichlorophenyl)succinimide but not with 2,3-dibromo-1-propanol phosphate. *J. natl Cancer Inst.*, **72**, 477–482

Shukla, R., Bornschein, R.L., Dietrich, K.N., Buncher, C.R., Berger, O.G., Hammond, P.B. & Succop, P.A. (1989) Fetal and infant lead exposure: Effects on growth in stature. *Pediatrics*, **84**, 604–612

Shukla, R., Dietrich, K.N., Bornschein, R.L., Berger, O. & Hammond, P.B. (1991) Lead exposure and growth in the early preschool child: A follow-up report from the Cincinnati lead study. *Pediatrics*, **88**, 886–892

Shukla, V.K., Prakash, A., Tripathi, B.D., Reddy, D.C.S. & Singh, S. (1998) Biliary heavy metal concentrations in carcinoma of the gall bladder: Case–control study. *Br. med. J.*, **317**, 1288–1289

Siddiqui, M.K.J., Srivastava, S. & Mehrotra, P.K. (2002) Environmental exposure to lead as a risk for prostate cancer. *Biomed. environ. Sci.*, **15**, 298–305

Sidhu, M.K., Fernandez, C., Khan, M.Y. & Kumar, S. (1991) Induction of morphological transformation, anchorage-independent growth and plasminogen activators in non-tumorigenic human osteosarcoma cells by lead chromate. *Anticancer Res.*, **11**, 1045–1053

Siemiatycki, J. (1991) *Risk Factors for Cancer in the Workplace*, Boca Raton, FL, CRC Press

Silbergeld, E.K. (1991) Lead in bone: Implications for toxicology during pregnancy and lactation. *Environ. Health Perspect.*, **91**, 63–70

Silbergeld, E.K. & Chisholm, J.J., Jr (1976) Lead poisoning: Altered urinary catecholamine metabolites as indicators of intoxication in mice and children. *Science*, **192**, 153–155

Silbergeld, E.K. & Goldberg, A.M. (1975) Pharmacological and neurochemical investigations of lead-induced hyperactivity. *Neuropharmacology*, **14**, 431–444

Silbergeld, E.K., Schwartz, J. & Mahaffey, K. (1988) Lead and osteoporosis: Mobilization of lead from bone in postmenopausal women. *Environ. Res.*, **47**, 79–94

Silbergeld, E.K., Waalkes, M. & Rice, J.M. (2000) Lead as a carcinogen: Experimental evidence and mechanisms of action. *Am. J. ind. Med.*, **38**, 316–323

de Silva, P.E. & Donnan, M.B. (1977) Petrol vendors, capillary blood lead levels and contamination. *Med. J. Aust.*, **1**, 344–347

de Silva, P.E. & Donnan, M.B. (1980) Blood lead levels in Victorian children. *Med. J. Aust.*, **2**, 315–318

Silva, P.A., Hughes, P., Williams, S. & Faed, J.M. (1988) Blood lead, intelligence, reading attainment, and behaviour in eleven year old children in Dunedin, New Zealand. *J. Child Psychol. Psychiat.*, **29**, 43–52

Silvany Neto, A.M., Carvalho, F.M., Lima, M.E.C. & Tavares, T.M. (1985) [Social determination of lead intoxication in children from Santo Amaro-Bahia] *Ciê. Cultura*, **37**, 1614–1626 (in Portuguese)

Silvany-Neto, A.M., Carvalho, F.M., Chaves, M.E.C., Brandão, A.M. & Tavares, T.M. (1989) Repeated surveillance of lead poisoning among children. *Sci. total Environ.*, **78**, 179–186

Silvany-Neto, A.M., Carvalho, F.M., Tavares, T.M., Guimarães, G.C., Amorim, C.J.B., Peres, M.F.T., Lopes, R.S., Rocha, C.M. & Raña, M.C. (1996) Lead poisoning among children of Santo Amaro, Bahia, Brazil in 1980, 1985, and 1992. *Bull. PAHO*, **30**, 51–62

Silver, W. & Rodriguez-Torres, R. (1968) Electrocardiographic studies in children with lead poisoning. *Pediatrics*, **41**, 1124–1127

Simmon, V.F. (1979) In vitro assays for recombinogenic activity of chemical carcinogens and related compounds with *Saccharomyces cerevisiae* D3. *J. natl Cancer Inst.*, **62**, 901–909

Simmonds, P.L., Luckhurst, C.L. & Woods, J.S. (1995) Quantitative evaluation of heme biosynthetic pathway parameters as biomarkers of low-level lead exposure in rats. *J. Toxicol. environ. Health*, **44**, 351–367

Simon, J.A. & Hudes, E.S. (1999) Relationship of ascorbic acid to blood lead levels. *J. am. med. Assoc.*, **281**, 2289–2293

Simons, T.J.B. (1995) The affinity of human erythrocyte porphobilinogen synthase for Zn^{2+} and Pb^{2+}. *Eur. J. Biochem.*, **234**, 178–183

Singal, M., Zey, J.N. & Arnold, S.J. (1985) Health Hazard Evaluation Report, HETA 84-0041-1592, Johnson Controls, Inc., Owosso, MI, USA, NIOSH

Singh, K.P. (1996) *Monitoring and Assessment of the Gomti River Quality* (Project Report), Lucknow, Industrial Toxicology Research Centre

Singh, R.P., Tripathi, R.D., Sinha, S.K., Maheshwari, R. & Srivastava, H.S. (1997) Response of higher plants to lead contaminated environment. *Chemosphere*, **34**, 2467–2493

Singh, B., Chandran, V., Bandhu, H.K., Mittal, B.R., Bhattacharya, A., Jindal, S.K. & Varma, S. (2000) Impact of lead exposure on pituitary–thyroid axis in humans. *Biometals*, **13**, 187–192

Singh, V.K., Mishra, K.P., Rani, R., Yadav, V.S., Awasthi, S.K. & Garg, S.K. (2003) Immunomodulation by lead. *Immunol. Res.*, **28**, 151–166

Sithisarankul, P., Schwartz, B.S., Lee, B.-K., Kelsey, K.T. & Strickland, P.T. (1997) Aminolevulinic acid dehydratase genotype mediates plasma levels of the neurotoxin, 5-aminolevulinic acid, in lead-exposed workers. *Am. J. ind. Med.*, **32**, 15–20

Six, K.M. & Goyer, R.A. (1970) Experimental enhancement of lead toxicity by low dietary calcium. *J. Lab. clin. Med.*, **76**, 933–942

Six, K.M. & Goyer, R.A. (1972) The influence of iron deficiency on tissue content and toxicity of ingested lead in the rat. *J. Lab. clin. Med.*, **76**, 128–136

Skerfving, S., Schütz, A. & Ranstam, J. (1986) Decreasing lead exposure in Swedish children, 1978–84. *Sci. total Environ.*, **58**, 225–229

Skreb, Y. & Habazin-Novak, V. (1977) Lead induces modifications of the response to X-rays in human cells in culture. *Stud. biophys.*, **63**, 97–104

Slorach, S., Gustafsson, I.-B., Jorhem, L. & Mattsson, P. (1983) Intake of lead, cadmium and certain other metals via a typical Swedish weekly diet. *Vår Föda*, **35** (Suppl. 1), 3–16

Slovin, D.L. & Albrecht, W.N. (1982) Health Hazard Evaluation Report, HETA 81-0356-1183, Sherwin Williams Co., Coffeyville, KS, USA, NIOSH

Smith, D.L. (1976) Lead absorption in police small-arms instructors. *J. Soc. occup. Med.*, **26**, 139–140

Smith, G.R. (1999) *Lead*, Reston, VA, US Geological Survey

Smith, G.R. (2002) *2002 Minerals Yearbook: Lead*, Reston, VA, US Geological Survey

Smith, C.M., DeLuca, H.F., Tanaka, Y. & Mahaffey, K.R. (1978) Stimulation of lead absorption by vitamin D administration. *J. Nutr.*, **108**, 843–847

Smith, M., Delves, T., Lansdown, R., Clayton, B. & Graham, P. (1983) The effects of lead exposure on urban children: The institute of child health/Southampton Study. *Dev. Med. Child Neurol.*, **25** (Suppl.), 1–54

Smith, D.R., Markowitz, M.E., Crick, J., Rosen, J.F. & Flegal, A.R. (1994) The effects of succimer on the absorption of lead in adults determined by using the stable isotope ^{204}Pb. *Environ. Res.*, **67**, 39–53

Smith, C.M., Wang, X., Hu, H. & Kelsy, K.T. (1995) A polymorphism in the δ-aminolevulinic acid dehydratase gene may modify the pharmacokinetics and toxicity of lead. *Environ. Health Perspect.*, **103**, 248–253

Smith, D.R., Osterloh, J.D. & Flegal, A.R. (1996) Use of endogenous, stable lead isotopes to determine release of lead from the skeleton. *Environ. Health Perspect.*, **104**, 60–66

Smith, D.R., Ilustre, R.P. & Osterloh, J.D. (1998) Methodological considerations for the accurate determination of lead in human plasma and serum. *Am. J. ind. Med.*, **33**, 430–438

Smith, D., Hernandez-Avila, M., Téllez-Rojo, M.M., Mercado, A. & Hu, H. (2002) The relationship between lead in plasma and whole blood in women. *Environ. Health Perspect.*, **110**, 263–268

Smitherman, J. & Harber, P. (1991) A case of mistaken identity: Herbal medicine as a cause of lead toxicity. *Am. J. ind. Med.*, **20**, 795–798

Smolders, A.J.P., Lock, R.A.C., Van der Velde, G., Medina Hoyos, R.I. & Roelofs, J.G.M. (2003) Effects of mining activities on heavy metal concentrations in water, sediment, and macroinvertebrates in different reaches of the Pilcomayo River, South America. *Arch. environ. Contam. Toxicol.*, **44**, 314–323

Snyder, R.D., Davis, G.F. & Lachmann, P.J. (1989) Inhibition by metals of X-ray and ultraviolet-induced DNA repair in human cells. *Biol. trace Elem. Res.*, **21**, 389–398

Sobel, A.E. & Burger, M. (1955) Calcification. XIII. The influence of calcium, phosphorus, and vitamin D on the removal of lead from blood and bone. *J. biol. Chem.*, **212**, 105–110

Sobotka, T.J. & Cook, M.P. (1974) Postnatal lead acetate exposure in rats: Possible relationship to minimal brain dysfunction. *Am. J. ment. Defic.*, **79**, 5–9

Sokol, R.Z. & Berman, N. (1991) The effect of age of exposure on lead-induced testicular toxicity. *Toxicology*, **69**, 269–278

Sokol, R.Z., Madding, C.E. & Swerdloff, R.S. (1985) Lead toxicity and the hypothalamic–pituitary–testicular axis. *Biol. Reprod.*, **33**, 722–728

Solliway, B.M., Schaffer, A., Pratt, H., Mittelman, N. & Yannai, S. (1995) Visual evoked potentials N75 and P100 latencies correlate with urinary δ-aminolevulinic acid, suggesting γ-aminobutyric acid involvement in their generation. *J. neurol. Sci.*, **134**, 89–94

Solt, B. & Farber, E. (1976) New principle for the analysis of chemical carcinogenesis. *Nature*, **263**, 701–703

Somervaille, L.J., Chettle, D.R., Scott, M.C., Aufderheide, A.C., Wallgren, J.E., Wittmers, L.E., Jr & Rapp, G.R., Jr (1986) Comparison of two *in vitro* methods of bone lead analysis and the implications for *in vivo* measurements. *Phys. Med. Biol.*, **31**, 1267–1274

Southpolymetal (2003) *Product Data Sheet: Lead*, Shymkent

Spanò, M., Bonde, J.P., Hjøllund, H.I., Kolstad, H.A., Cordelli, E., Leter, G. & The Danish First Pregnancy Planner Study Team (2000) Sperm chromatin damage impairs human fertility. *Fertil. Steril.*, **73**, 43–50

Spickett, J.T., Bell, R.R., Stawell, J. & Polan, S. (1984) The influence of dietary citrate on the absorption and retention of orally ingested lead. *Agents Actions*, **15**, 459–462

Spivey, G.H., Baloh, R.W., Brown, C.P., Browdy, B.L., Campion, D.S., Valentine, J.L., Morgan, D.E. & Culver, B.D. (1980) Subclincal effects of chronic increased lead absorption — A prospective study. III. Neurological findings at follow-up examination. *J. occup. Med.*, **22**, 607–612

Sprinkle, R.V. (1995) Leaded eye cosmetics: A cultural cause of elevated lead levels in children. *J. fam. Pract.*, **40**, 358–362

Srianujata, S. (1998) Lead — The toxic metal to stay with human. *J. toxicol. Sci.*, **23** (Suppl. 2), 237–240

Srikanth, R., Madhumohan Rao, A., Shravan Kumar, C. & Khanum, A. (1993) Lead, cadmium, nickel, and zinc contamination of ground water around Hussain Sagar Lake, Hyderabad, India. *Bull. environ. Contam. Toxicol.*, **50**, 138–143

Srikanth, R., Ramana, D. & Rao, V. (1995a) Lead uptake from beer in India. *Bull. environ. Contam. Toxicol.*, **54**, 783–786

Srikanth, R., Ramana, D. & Rao, V. (1995b) Role of rice and cereal products in dietary cadmium and lead intake among different socio-economic groups in south India. *Food Addit. Contam.*, **12**, 695–701

Srivastava, S., Mehrotra, P.K., Srivastava, S.P., Tandon, I. & Siddiqui, M.K.J. (2001) Blood lead and zinc in pregnant women and their offpring in intrauterine growth retardation cases. *J. anal. Toxicol.*, **25**, 461–465

Staessen, J., Yeoman, W.B., Fletcher, A.E., Markowe, H.L.J., Marmot, M.G., Rose, G., Semmence, A., Shipley, M.J. & Bulpitt, C.J. (1990) Blood lead concentration, renal function, and blood pressure in London civil servants. *Br. J. ind. Med.*, **47**, 442–447

Staessen, J.A., Lauwerys, R.R., Buchet, J.-P., Bulpitt, C.J., Rondia, D., Vanrenterghem, Y., Amery, A. & the Cadmibel Study Group (1992) Impairment of renal function with increasing blood lead concentrations in the general population. *New Engl. J. Med.*, **327**, 151–156

Staessen, J.A., Bulpitt, C.J., Fagard, R., Lauwerys, R.R., Roels, H., Thijs, L. & Amery, A. (1994) Hypertension caused by low-level lead exposure: Myth or fact? *J. cardiovasc. Risk*, **1**, 87–97

Staessen, J.A., Roels, H., Lauwerys, R.R. & Amery, A. (1995) Low-level lead exposure and blood pressure. *J. hum. Hypertens.*, **9**, 303–328

Stauber, J.L. & Florence, T.M. (1988) A comparative study of copper, lead, cadmium and zinc in human sweat and blood. *Sci. total Environ.*, **74**, 235–247

Stauber, J.L., Florence, T.M., Gulson, B.L. & Dale, L.S. (1994) Percutaneous absorption of inorganic lead compounds. *Sci. total Environ.*, **145**, 55–70

Steenland, K. & Boffetta, P. (2000) Lead and cancer in humans: Where are we now? *Am. J. ind. Med.*, **38**, 295–99

Steenland, K., Selevan, S. & Landrigan, P. (1992) The mortality of lead smelter workers: An update. *Am. J. public Health*, **82**, 1641–1644

Steenland, K., Loomis, D., Shy, C. & Simonsen, N. (1996) Review of occupational carcinogens. *Am. J. ind. Med.*, **29**, 474–490

Steffee, C.H. & Baetjer, A.M. (1965) Histopathologic effects of chromate chemicals. *Arch. environ. Health*, **11**, 66–75

Stephenson, R.L. & Burt, S. (1992) Health Hazard Evaluation Report, HETA 89-0252,0293-2178, Chempower Inc., Combustion Engineering Inc., Albright Power Station, Albright, WV, USA, NIOSH

Sternowsky, H.J. & Wessolowski, R. (1985) Lead and cadmium in breast milk. *Arch. Toxicol.*, **57**, 41–45

Stevenson, A.J., Kacew, S. & Singhal, R.L. (1977) Reappraisal of the use of a single dose of lead for the study of cell proliferation in kidney, liver and lung. *J. Toxicol. environ. Health*, **2**, 1125–1134

Stewart, W.F., Schwartz, B.S., Simon, D., Kelsey, K. & Todd, A.C. (2002) *ApoE* genotype, past adult lead exposure and neurobehavioral function. *Environ. Health Perspect.*, **110**, 501–505

STN International (2003) Registry file [http://stuweb.cas.org; latest update 25/11/2003]

Stockholm Municipal Environment and Health Administration (1983) *Undersokningar av Fordonstrafikens Luftfororeningar under 1982* [Investigations of air pollution from the traffic during 1982], Stockholm (in Swedish)

Stoner, G.D., Shimkin, M.B., Troxell, M.C., Thompson, T.L. & Terry, L.S. (1976) Test for carcinogenicity of metallic compounds by the pulmonary tumor response in strain A mice. *Cancer Res.*, **36**, 1744–1747

Stoner, G.D., Conran, P.B., Greisiger, E.A., Stober, J., Morgan, M. & Pereira, M.A. (1986) Comparison of two routes of chemical administration on the lung adenoma response in strain A/J mice. *Toxicol. appl. Pharmacol.*, **82**, 19–31

Stowe, H.D., Goyer, R.A., Krigman, M.M., Wilson, M. & Cates, M. (1973) Experimental oral lead toxicity in young dogs. Clinical and morphologic effects. *Arch. Pathol.*, **95**, 106–116

Stretesky, P.B. & Lynch, M.J. (2001) The relationship between lead exposure and homicide. *Arch. pediat. adol. Med.*, **155**, 579–582

Strömberg, U., Schütz, A. & Skerfving, S. (1995) Substantial decrease of blood lead in Swedish children, 1978–94, associated with petrol lead. *Occup. environ. Med.*, **52**, 764–769

Subramanian, K.S. (1989) Determination of lead in blood by graphite furnace atomic absorption spectrometry — A critique. *Sci. total Environ.*, **89**, 237–250

Sun, C.-C., Wong, T.-T., Hwang, Y.-H., Chao, K.-Y., Jee, S.-H. & Wang, J.-D. (2002) Percutaneous absorption of inorganic lead compounds. *Am. ind. Hyg. Assoc. J.*, **63**, 641–646

Sundström, R. & Karlsson, B. (1987) Myelin basic protein in brains of rats with low dose lead encephalopathy. *Arch. Toxicol.*, **59**, 341–345

Suplido, M.L. & Ong, C.N. (2000) Lead exposure among small-scale battery recyclers, automobile radiator mechanics, and their children in Manila, the Philippines. *Environ. Res.*, **82**, 231–238

Sussell, A.L. & Piacitelli, G.M. (1999) Health Hazard Evaluation Report, HETA 98-0283, Illinois Historic Preservation Agency, Springfield, IL, USA, NIOSH

Sussell, A.L. & Piacitelli, G.M. (2001) Health Hazard Evaluation Report, HETA 99-0113-2853, University of California-Berkeley, Berkeley, CA, USA, NIOSH

Sussell, A.L., Montopoli, M. & Tubbs, R. (1992a) Health Hazard Evaluation Report, HETA 91-0006-2193, M & J Painting Company, Covington, KY, USA, NIOSH

Sussell, A.L., Elliott, L.J., Wild, D. & Freund, E. (1992b) Health Hazard Evaluation Report, HETA 90-0070-2181, HUD Lead-Based Paint Abatement Demonstration Project

Sussell, A.L., Mickelsen, R.L. & Rubin, C. (1992c) Health Hazard Evaluation Report, HETA 91-0209-2249, Seaway Painting, Inc., Annapolis, MD, USA, NIOSH

Sussell, A.L., Weber, A., Wild, D., Ashley, K. & Wall, D. (1993) Health Hazard Evaluation Report, HETA 92-0095-2317, Ohio University, Athens, OH, USA, NIOSH

Sussell, A.L., Gittleman, J. & Singal, M. (1997) Health Hazard Evaluation Report, HETA 93-0818-2646, People Working Cooperatively, Cincinnati, OH, USA, NIOSH

Sussell, A.L., Piacitelli, G.M. & Trout, D. (2000) Health Hazard Evaluation Report, HETA 96-0200-2799, Rhode Island Department of Health, Providence, RI, USA, NIOSH

Sussell, A.L., Piacitelli, G.M., Chaudre, Z. & Ashley, K. (2002) Health Hazard Evaluation Report, HETA 99-0305-2878, Lead Safe Services, Inc., Neenah, WI, USA, NIOSH

Suwansaksri, J. & Wiwanitkit, V. (2001) Monitoring of lead exposure among mechanics in Bangkok. *Southeast Asian J. trop. Med. public Health*, **32**, 661–663

Suwansaksri, J., Teerasart, N., Wiwanitkit, V. & Chaiyaset, T. (2002) High blood lead level among garage workers in Bangkok, public concern is necessary. *Biometals*, **15**, 367–370

Süzen, H.S., Duydu, Y., Aydin, A., Isimer, A. & Vural, N. (2003) Influence of the delta-aminolevulinic acid dehydratase (ALAD) polymorphism on biomarkers of lead exposure in Turkish storage battery manufacturing workers. *Am. J. ind. Med.*, **43**, 165–171

Suzuki, S. (1990) Health effects of lead pollution due to automobile exhaust: Findings from field surveys in Japan and Indonesia. *J. hum. Ergol.*, **19**, 113–122

Svensson, B.G., Schütz, A., Nilsson, A. & Skerfving, S. (1992) Lead exposure in indoor firing ranges. *Int. Arch. Occup. Environ. Health*, **64**, 219–221

Sweeney, M.H., Beaumont, J.J., Waxweiler, R.J. & Halperin, W.E. (1986) An investigation of mortality from cancer and other causes of death among workers employed at an east Texas chemical plant. *Arch. environ. Health*, **41**, 23–28

Sylvain, D.C. (1996) Health Hazard Evaluation Report, HETA 94-0122-2578, Bath Iron Works Corp., Bath, ME, USA, NIOSH

Symanski, E. & Hertz-Picciotto, I. (1995) Blood lead levels in relation to menopause, smoking, and pregnancy history. *Am. J. Epidemiol.*, **141**, 1047–1058

Tabuchi, T., Okayama, A., Ogawa, Y., Miyajima, K., Hirata, M., Yoshida, T., Sugimoto, K. & Morimoto, K. (1989) A new HPLC fluorimetric method to monitor urinary delta-aminolevulinic acid (ALA-U) levels in workers exposed to lead. *Int. Arch. occup. environ. Health*, **61**, 297–302

Tachi, K., Nishimae, S. & Saito, K.(1985) Cytogenetic effects of lead acetate on rat bone marrow cells. *Arch. environ. Health*, **40**, 144–147

Tait, P.A., Vora, A., James, S., Fitzgerald, D.J. & Pester, B.A. (2002) Severe congenital lead poisoning in a preterm infant due to a herbal remedy. *Med. J. Aust.*, **177**, 193–195

Tamayo, L., Liceaga, C., Sánchez, P. & Herce, J.L. (1984) Estudio comparativo de envases de frutas y jugos. *Rev. Soc. Quím. Méx.*, **28**, 359–362

Tanner, D.C. & Lipsky, M.M. (1984) Effect of lead acetate on N-(4′-fluoro-4-biphenyl)acetamide-induced renal carcinogenesis in the rat. *Carcinogenesis*, **5**, 1109–1113

Tantanasrikul, S., Chaivisuth, B., Siriratanapreuk, S., Padungtod, C., Pleubreukan, R., Boonnark, T., Worahan, S., Bhumiratanarak, P. & Chomchai, C. (2002) The management of environmental lead exposure in the pediatric population: Lessons from Clitty Creek, Thailand. *J. med. Assoc. Thai.*, **85** (Suppl. 2), S762–S768

Taskinen, H., Nordman, H., Hernberg, S. & Engström, K. (1981) Blood lead levels in Finnish preschool children. *Sci. total Environ.*, **20**, 117–129

Taupeau, C., Poupon, J., Treton, D., Brosse, A., Richard, Y. & Machelon, V. (2003) Lead reduces messenger RNA and protein levels of cytochrome p450 aromatase and estrogen receptor beta in human ovarian granulosa cells. *Biol. Reprod.*, **68**, 1982–1988

Tavares, T.M. (1990) *Avaliação de Efeitos das Emissões de Cádmio e Chumbo em Santo Amaro, Bahia*, PhD Thesis, São Paulo, University of São Paulo

Tavares, T.M. (1991) Ecological studies of the Recôncavo, Bahia, Brazil (1976 until 1990). *Rev. int. Contam. ambient.*, **7**, 33–50

Tavares, T.M. (1992) The role of lead and cadium reference samples in an epidemiological case study at Santo Amaro, Bahia, Brazil. In: Rossbach, M., Schladot, J.D. & Ostapczuk, P., eds, *Specimen Banking: Environmental Monitoring and Modern Analytical Approaches*, Berlin, Springer Verlag, pp. 89–98

Tavares, T.M. (1996a) *Distribuição Espacial de Poluentes Atmosféricos no entorno da RLAM in Programa de Monitoramento dos Ecossistemas ao Norte da Baía de Todos os Santos, 1994–1995*, Tomo 8, Vol. II, Salvador, Bahia, Petrobrás

Tavares, T.M. (1996b) *Distribuição Espacial de Metais Pesados e Hidrocarbonetos ao Norte da Baía de Todos os Santos em Programa de Monitoramento dos Ecossistemas ao Norte da Baía de Todos os Santos, 1994–1995*, Tomo 8, Vol. I, Salvador, Bahia, Petrobrás

Taylor, S.R. & McLennan, S.M. (1995) The geochemical evolution of the continental crust. *Rev. Geophys.*, **33**, 241–265

Taylor, R., Bazelmans, J., Golec, R. & Oakes, S. (1995) Declining blood lead levels in Victorian children. *Aust. J. public Health*, **19**, 455–459

Teck Cominco (2003) *Product Data Sheet: Lead*, Vancouver, BC

Telisman, S., Cvitkovic, P., Jurasovic, J., Pizent, A., Gavella, M. & Rocic, B. (2000) Semen quality and reproductive endocrine function in relation to biomarkers of lead, cadmium, zinc, and copper in men. *Environ. Health Perspect.*, **108**, 45–53

Téllez-Rojo, M.M., Hernández-Avila, M., González-Cossio, T., Romieu, I., Aro, A., Palazuelos, E., Schwartz, J. & Hu, H. (2002) Impact of breastfeeding on the mobilization of lead from bone. *Am. J. Epidemiol.*, **155**, 420–428

Teraki, Y. & Uchiumi, A. (1990) Inorganic elements in the tooth and bone tissues of rats bearing nickel acetate- and lead acetate-induced tumors. *Shigaku*, **78**, 269–273

Tharr, D. (1993) Lead contamination in radiator repair shops. *Appl. occup. environ. Hyg.*, **8**, 434–438

Tharr, D. (1997) Lead exposure during custodial activities. *Appl. occup. environ. Hyg.*, **12**, 395–399

Thier, R., Bonacker, D., Stoiber, T., Bohm, K.J., Wang, M., Unger, E., Bolt, H.M. & Degen, G. (2003) Interaction of metal salts with cytoskeletal motor protein systems. *Toxicol. Lett.*, **140–141**, 75–81

Thomas, V.M., Socolow, R.H., Fanelli, J.J. & Spiro, T.G. (1999) Effects of reducing lead in gasoline: An analysis of the international experience. *Environ. Sci. Technol.*, **33**, 3942–3948

Thoreux-Manlay, A., Vélez de la Calle, J.F., Olivier, M.F., Soufir, J.C., Masse, R. & Pinon-Lataillade, G. (1995) Impairment of testicular endocrine function after lead intoxication in the adult rat. *Toxicology*, **100**, 101–109

Threlfall, T., Kent, N., Garcia-Webb, P., Byrnes, E. & Psaila-Savona, P. (1993) Blood lead levels in children in Perth, Western Australia. *Aust. J. public Health*, **17**, 379–381

Todd, A.C. & Chettle, D.R. (1994) *In vivo* X-ray fluorescence of lead in bone: Review and current issues. *Environ. Health Perspect.*, **102**, 172–177

Todd, A.C., Carroll, S., Godbold, J.H., Moshier, E.L. & Khan, F.A. (2000a) Variability in XRF-measured tibia lead levels. *Phys. Med. Biol.*, **45**, 3737–3748

Todd, A.C., Ehrlich, R.I., Selby, P. & Jordaan, E. (2000b) Repeatability of tibia lead measurement by X-Ray fluorescence in a battery-making workforce. *Environ. Res.*, **84**, 282–289

Todd, A.C., Lee, B.-K., Lee, G.-S., Ahn, K.-D., Moshier, E. & Schwartz, B.S. (2001a) Predictors of DMSA chelatable lead, tibial lead, and blood lead in 802 Korean lead workers. *Occup. environ. Med.*, **58**, 73–80

Todd, A.C., Buchanan, R., Carroll, S., Moshier, E.L., Popovac, D., Slavkovich, V. & Graziano, J.H. (2001b) Tibia lead levels and methodological uncertainty in 12-year-old children. *Environ. Res.*, **A86**, 60–65

Todd, A.C., Carroll, S., Godbold, J.H., Moshier, E.L. & Khan, F.A. (2001c) The effect of measurement location on tibia lead XRF measurement results and uncertainty. *Phys. Med. Biol.*, **46**, 29–40

Todd, A.C., Parsons, P.J., Tang, S. & Moshier, E.L. (2001d) Individual variability in human tibia lead concentration. *Environ. Health Perspect.*, **109**, 1139–1143

Todd, A.C., Parsons, P.J., Carroll, S., Geraghty, C., Khan, F.A., Tang, S. & Moshier, E.L. (2002) Measurements of lead in human tibiae. A comparison between K-shell x-ray fluorescence and electrothermal atomic absorption spectrometry. *Phys. Med. Biol.*, **47**, 673–687

Toews, A.D., Kolber, A., Hayward, J., Krigman, M.R. & Morell, P. (1978) Experimental lead encephalopathy in the suckling rat: Concentration of lead in cellular fractions enriched in brain capillaries. *Brain Res.*, **147**, 131–138

Toffaletti, J. & Savory, J. (1976) An overview of the laboratory diagnosis of lead poisoning. *Ann. clin. Lab. Sci.*, **6**, 529–536

Tola, S., Hernberg, S., Asp, S. & Nikkanen, J. (1973) Parameters indicative of absorption and biological effect in new lead exposure: A prospective study. *Br. J. ind. Med.*, **30**, 134–141

Tomokuni, K. & Ichiba, M. (1988a) A simple method for colorimetric determination of urinary delta-aminolevulinic acid in workers exposed to lead. *Jpn J. ind. Health*, **30**, 52–53

Tomokuni, K. & Ichiba, M. (1988b) Comparison of inhibition of erythrocyte pyrimidine 5′-nucleotidase and delta-aminolevulinic acid dehydratase by lead. *Toxicol. Lett.*, **40**, 159–163

Tomokuni, K. & Ogata, M. (1976) Relationship between lead concentration in blood and biological response for porphyrin metabolism in workers occupationally exposed to lead. *Arch. Toxicol.*, **35**, 239–246

Tomokuni, K., Ichiba, M., Hirai, Y., Sugimoto, K., Yoshida, T. & Hirata, M. (1988) Comparison between the fluorimetric HPLC method and the conventional method for determining urinary δ-aminolevulinic acid and coproporphyrin as indices of lead exposure. *Int. Arch. occup. environ. Health*, **61**, 153–156

Tomokuni, K., Ichiba, M. & Mori, K. (1992) Relation between urinary β-aminoisobutyric acid excretion and concentration of lead in the blood of workers occupationally exposed to lead. *Br. J. ind. Med.*, **49**, 365–368

Tomsig, J.L. & Suszkiw, J.B. (1996) Metal selectivity of exocytosis in alpha-toxin-permeabilized bovine chromaffin cells. *J. Neurochem.*, **66**, 644–650

Tong, S., Baghurst, P., McMichael, A., Sawyer, M. & Mudge, J. (1996) Lifetime exposure to environmental lead and children's intelligence at 11–13 years: The Port Pirie cohort study. *Br. med. J.*, **312**, 1569–1575

Tönz, O. (1957) [Changes in the kidney of rats after chronic experimental exposure to lead.] *Z. ges. exp. Med.*, **128**, 361–377 (in German)

Torelli, G. (1930) L'influenza dell'avvelenamento cronico da piombo (saturnismo) sulla discendenza. *La Medicina del Lavoro*, **3**, 110–121

Torrance, J.D., Mills, W., Kilroe-Smith, T.A. & Smith, A.N. (1985) Erythrocyte pyrimidine-5′-nucleotidase activity as a sensitive indicator of lead exposure. *S. Afr. med. J.*, **67**, 850–852

Torvik, E., Pfitzer, E., Kereiakes, J.G. & Blanchard, R. (1974) Long term effective half-lives for lead-210 and polonium-210 in selected organs of the male rat. *Health Phys.*, **26**, 81–87

Treble, R.G. & Thompson, T.S. (1997) Preliminary results of a survey of lead levels in human liver tissue. *Bull. environ. Contam. Toxicol.*, **59**, 688–695

Treble, R.G. & Thompson, T.S. (2002) Elevated blood lead levels resulting from the ingestion of air rifle pellets. *J. anal. Toxicol.*, **26**, 370–373

Triebig, G., Weltle, D. & Valentin, H. (1984) Investigations on neurotoxicity of chemical substances at the workplace. V. Determination of the motor and sensory nerve conduction velocity in persons occupationally exposed to lead. *Int. Arch. occup. environ. Health*, **53**, 189–203

Tripathi, R.K., Sherertz, P.C., Llewellyn, G.C., Armstrong, C.W. & Ramsey, S.L. (1989) Overexposures to lead at a covered outdoor firing range. *J. Am. College Toxicol.*, **8**, 1189–1195

Tripathi, R.K., Sherertz, P.C., Llewellyn, G.C., Armstrong, C.W. & Ramsey, S.L. (1990) Reducing exposures to airborne lead in a covered, outdoor firing range by using totally copper-jacketed bullets. *Am. Ind. Hyg. Assoc. J.*, **51**, 28–31

Tripathi, R.K., Sherertz, P.C., Llewellyn, G.C. & Armstrong, C.W. (1991) Lead exposure in outdoor firearm instructors. *Am. J. publ. Health*, **81**, 753–755

Tripathi, R.M., Raghunath, R., Kumar, A.V., Sastry, V.N. & Sadasivan, S. (2001) Atmospheric and children's blood lead as indicators of vehicular traffic and other emission sources in Mumbai, India. *Sci. total Environ.*, **267**, 101–108

Trotter, R.T. (1990) The cultural parameters of lead poisoning: A medical anthropologist's view of intervention in environmental lead exposure. *Environ. Health Perspect.*, **89**, 79–84

Tsaih, S.W., Schwartz, J., Lee, M.-L., Amarasiriwardena, C., Aro, A., Sparrow, D. & Hu, H. (1999) The independent contribution of bone and erythrocyte lead to urinary lead among middle-aged and elderly men: The Normative Aging Study. *Environ. Health Perspect.*, **107**, 391–396

Tubbs, R.L., Moss, C.E. & Fleeger, A. (1992) Health Hazard Evaluation Report, HETA 89-0364-2202, ARMCO Advanced Materials Corp., Butler, PA, USA, NIOSH

Turlakiewicz, Z. & Chmielnicka, J. (1985) Diethyllead as a specific indicator of occupational exposure to tetraethyllead. *Br. J. ind. Med.*, **42**, 682–685

Tuthill, R.W. (1996) Hair lead levels related to children's classroom attention-deficit behavior. *Arch. environ. Health*, **51**, 214–220

Ukhun, M.E., Nwazota, J. & Nkwocha, F.O. (1990) Levels of toxic mineral elements in selected foods marketed in Nigeria. *Bull. environ. contam. Toxicol.*, **44**, 325–330

Umicore Precious Metals (2002) *Technical Data Sheet: Lead*, Hoboken

Ündeger, Ü., Basaran, N., Canpinar, H. & Kansu, E. (1996) Immune alterations in lead-exposed workers. *Toxicology*, **109**, 167–172

US Department of Housing and Urban Development (US DHUD) (1987) *Code Fed. Regul.*, **24 CFR 35, 510, 511, 570, 590**

US Department of the Treasury (1991) *Report of Analyses of Wines and Related Products to Determine Lead Content*, Washington, DC, US Department of the Treasury, Bureau of Alcohol, Tobacco and Firearms

US Environmental Protection Agency (US EPA) (1978) *Lead (AA, Direct Aspiration), Method No. 239.1*

US Environmental Protection Agency (1982) *An Exposure and Risk Assessment for Lead* (EPA/440/4-85/010, NTIS PB85-220606), Washington DC, Office of Water Regulations and Standards, Monitoring and Data Support Division

US Environmental Protection Agency (1985) *National Air Quality and Emissions Trends Report 1983* (EPA-450/4-84-029), Bethesda, MD

US Environmental Protection Agency (1986a) *Air Quality Criteria for Lead* (EPA 600/8-83-028F), Research Triangle Park, NC, Office of Research and Development, Office of Health and Environmental Assessment, Environmental Criteria and Assessment Office

US Environmental Protection Agency (1986b) *Lead (AA, Direct Aspiration), Method No. 7420*

US Environmental Protection Agency (1986c) *Lead (AA, Furnace Technique), Method No. 7421*

US Environmental Protection Agency (1989) *Evaluation of the Potential Carcinogenicity of Lead and Lead Compounds (EPA/600/8-89/045A)*, Washington, DC, US Environmental Protection Agency, Office of Health and Environmental Assessment

US Environmental Protection Agency (1991) Maximum contaminant level goals and national primary drinking water regulations for lead and copper. *Fed. Reg.*, **56**, 26461–26564

US Environmental Protection Agency (1992) *National Air Quality and Emissions Trends Report 1991 (EPA 450-R-92-001)*, Bethesda, MD

US Environmental Protection Agency (1994) *Guidance Manual for the Integrated Exposure Uptake Biokinetic Model for Lead in Children* (EPA/540/R-93/081; PB93-963510), Research Triangle Park, NC, US Environmental Protection Agency, DC 20460

US Environmental Protection Agency (1996a) *National Air Quality and Emissions Trends Report 1995*, Washington DC, Office of Air Quality Planning and Standards

US Environmental Protection Agency (1996b) *Urban Soil Lead Abatement Demonstration Project* (EPA/600/P-93/001aF), Washington DC, Office of Research and Development

US Environmental Protection Agency (1996c) *Determination of Trace Elements in Ambient Waters by Off-Line Chelation, Preconcentration and Stabilized Temperature Graphite Furnace Atomic Absorption, Method 1637*, Washington, DC, Office of Water

US Environmental Protection Agency (1996d) *Determination of Trace Elements in Ambient Waters by Inductively Coupled Plasma Mass Spectrometry, Method 1638*, Washington, DC, Office of Water

US Environmental Protection Agency (1997a) *Determination of Trace Elements in Water by Preconcentration and Inductively Coupled Plasma–Mass Spectrometry, Method 1640*, Washington, DC, Office of Water

US Environmental Protection Agency (1997b) *Determination of Trace Elements in Marine Waters by Stabilized Temperature Graphite Furnace Atomic Absorption, Method 200.12*, Cincinnati, OH, National Exposure Research Laboratory, Office of Research and Development

US Environmental Protection Agency (1997c) *Determination of Trace Elements in Marine Waters by On-Line Chelation Preconcentration and Inductively Coupled Plasma–Mass Spectrometry, Method 200.10*, Cincinnati, OH, National Exposure Research Laboratory, Office of Research and Development

US Environmental Protection Agency (2000) *Inductively Coupled Plasma–Atomic Emission Spectrometry, Method 6010C*

US Food and Drug Administration (1994) *Action Levels for Poisonous or Deleterious Substances in Human Food and Animal Feed*, Department of Health and Human Services, Public Health Service

US Food and Drug Administration (2000a) Flame atomic absorption spectrometric determination of lead and cadmium extracted from ceramic foodware. In: *FDA Elemental Analysis Manual For Food and Related Products*

US Food and Drug Administration (2000b) Graphite furnace atomic absorption spectrometric determination of lead and cadmium extracted from ceramic foodware. In: *FDA Elemental Analysis Manual For Food and Related Products*

Vaglenov, A.K., Laltchev, S.G., Nosko, M.S. & Pavlova, S.P. (1997) Cytogenetic monitoring of workers exposed to lead. *Cent. Eur. J. occup. environ. Med.*, **3**, 298–308

Vaglenov, A., Carbonell, E. & Marcos, R. (1998) Biomonitoring of workers exposed to lead. Genotoxic effects, its modulation by polyvitamin treatment and evaluation of the induced radioresistance. *Mutat. Res.*, **418**, 79–92

Vaglenov, A., Creus, A., Laltchev, S., Petkova, V., Pavlova, S. & Marcos, R. (2001) Occupational exposure to lead and induction of genetic damage. *Environ. Health Perspect.*, **109**, 295–298

Vahter, M., Berglund, M., Slorach, S., Friberg, L., Šaric, M., Xingquan, Z. & Fujita, M. (1991a) Methods for integrated exposure monitoring of lead and cadmium. *Environ. Res.*, **56**, 78–89

Vahter, M., Berglund, M., Lind, B., Jorhem, L., Slorach, S. & Friberg, L. (1991b) Personal monitoring of lead and cadmium exposure — A Swedish study with special reference to methodological aspects. *Scand. J. Work environ. Health*, **17**, 65–74

Vahter, M., Counter, S.A., Laurell, G., Buchanan, L.H., Ortega, F., Schütz, A. & Skerfving, S. (1997) Extensive lead exposure in children living in an area with production of lead-glazed tiles in the Ecuadorian Andes. *Int. Arch. occup. environ. Health*, **70**, 282–286

Valverde, M., Fortoul, T.I., Díaz-Barriga, F., Mejía, J. & Rojas del Castillo, E. (2002) Genotoxicity induced in CD-1 mice by inhaled lead: Differential organ response. *Mutagenesis*, **17**, 55–61

Valway, S.E., Martyny, J.W., Miller, J.R., Cook, M. & Mangione, E.J. (1989) Lead absorption in indoor firing range users. *Am. J. Public Health*, **79**, 1029–1032

Van Barneveld, A.A. & Van den Hamer, C.J.A. (1985) Influence of Ca and Mg on the uptake and deposition of Pb and Cd in mice. *Toxicol. appl Pharmacol.*, **79**, 1–10

Vander, A.J., Taylor, D.L., Kalitis, K., Mouw, D.R. & Victery, W. (1977) Renal handling of lead in dogs: Clearance studies. *Am. J. Physiol.*, **233**, F532–F538

Van Esch, G.J. & Kroes, R. (1969) The induction of renal tumours by feeding basic lead acetate to mice and hamsters. *Br. J. Cancer*, **23**, 765–771

Van Esch, G.J., Van Genderen, H. & Vink, H.H. (1962) The induction of renal tumours by feeding of basic lead acetate to rats. *Cancer*, **16**, 289–297

Varnai, V.M., Piasek, M., Blanuša, M., Saric, M.M., Šimic, D. & Kostial, K. (2001) Calcium supplementation efficiently reduces lead absorption in suckling rats. *Pharmacol. Toxicol.*, **89**, 326–330

Varo, P. & Koivistoinen, P. (1983) Mineral element composition of Finnish foods. XII. General discussion and nutritional evaluation. *Acta agric. Scand.*, **22**, 165–171

Vassil, A.D., Kapulnik, Y., Raskin, I. & Salt, D.E. (1998) The role of EDTA in lead transport and accumulation by Indian mustard. *Plant Physiol.*, **117**, 447–453

Vatsala, S. & Ramakrishna, T. (1985) 'Tinning' of brass ustensils: Possibility of lead poisoning. *Indian J. environ. Health*, **27**, 140–141

Vena, J.E. (1983) Lung cancer incidence and air pollution in Erie County, New York. *Arch. environ. Health*, **38**, 229–236

Venable, H.L., Moss, C.E., Connon, C.L., Kinnes, G.M., Freund, E., Seitz, T.A. & Kaiser, E.A. (1993) Health Hazard Evaluation Report, HETA 90-0075-2298, Boston Edison Co., Boston, MA, USA, NIOSH

Verberk, M.M., Willems, T.E.P., Verplanke, A.J.W. & De Wolff, F.A. (1996) Environmental lead and renal effects in children. *Arch. environ. Health*, **51**, 83–87

Verity, M.A. (1990) Comparative observations on inorganic and organic lead neurotoxicity. *Environ. Health Perspect.*, **89**, 43–48

Verrengia Guerrero, N.R. & Kesten, E.M. (1994) Levels of heavy metals in waters from the La Plata River, Argentina: An approach to assess bioavailability. *Bull. environ. Contam. Toxicol.*, **52**, 254–260

Verschoor, M., Wibowo, A., Herber, R., van Hemmen, J. & Zielhuis, R. (1987) Influence of occupational low-level lead exposure on renal parameters. *Am. J. ind. Med.*, **12**, 341–351

Victery, W. (1988) Evidence for effects of chronic lead exposure on blood pressure in experimental animals: An overview. *Environ. Health Perspect.*, **78**, 71–76

Victery, W., Vander, A.J., Shulak, J.M., Schoeps, P. & Julius, S. (1982) Lead, hypertension, and the renin-angiotensin system in rats. *J. Lab. clin. Med.*, **99**, 354–362

Vig, E.K. & Hu, H. (2000) Lead toxicity in older adults. *J. Am. Geriatr. Soc.*, **48**, 1501–1506

Viskum, S., Rabjerg, L., Jørgensen, P.J. & Grandjean, P. (1999) Improvement in semen quality associated with decreasing occupational lead exposure. *Am. J. ind. Med.*, **35**, 257–263

Von Schirnding, Y.E.R. & Fuggle, R.F. (1984) A study of the relationship between low level lead exposure and classroom performance in South African children. *Int. J. Biol. Sci.*, **6**, 97–106

Von Schirnding, Y., Bradshaw, D., Fuggle, R. & Stokol, M. (1991a) Blood lead levels in South African inner-city children. *Environ. Health Perspect.*, **94**, 125–130

Von Schirnding, Y.E.R., Fuggle, R.F. & Bradshaw, D. (1991b) Factors associated with elevated blood lead levels in inner city Cape Town children. *S. Afr. Med. J.*, **79**, 454–456

Vural, N. & Duydu, Y. (1995) Biological monitoring of lead in workers exposed to tetraethyllead. *Sci. total Environ.*, **171**, 183–187

Waalkes, M.P., Diwan, B.A., Ward, J.M., Devor, D.E. & Goyer, R.A. (1995) Renal tubular tumors and atypical hyperplasias in B6C3F1 mice exposed to lead acetate during gestation and lactation occur with minimal chronic nephropathy. *Cancer Res.*, **55**, 5265–5271

Waalkes, M.P., Fox, D.A., States, J.C., Patierno, S.R. & McCabe, M.J., Jr (2000) Metals and disorders of cell accumulation: Modulation of apoptosis and cell proliferation. *Toxicol. Sci.*, **56**, 255–261

Wadge, A. & Hutton, M. (1987) The leachability and chemical speciation of selected trace elements in fly ash from coal combustion and refuse incineration. *Environ. Pollut.*, **48**, 85–99

Wahid, A., Koul, P.A., Shah, S.U., Khan, A.R., Bhat, M.S. & Malik, M.A. (1997) Lead exposure in papier mâché workers. *Hum. exp. Toxicol.*, **16**, 281–283

Wai, C.M., Knowles, C.R. & Keely, J.F. (1979) Lead caps on wine bottles and their potential problems. *Bull. environ. Contam. Toxicol.*, **21**, 4–6

Wallace, D.M., Kalman, D.A. & Bird, T.D. (1985) Hazardous lead release from glazed dinnerware: A cautionary note. *Sci. total Environ.*, **44**, 289–292

Walmsley, T.A., Sise, J.A. & Hinton, D. (1988) *Blood Lead Levels — Population Data Base. Trace Elements in New Zealand: Environmental, Human and Animal. Proceedings of the New Zealand Trace Elements Group Conference, 30 November to 2 December 1988*, Canterbury, Lincoln College, pp. 125–131

Walmsley, T., Grant, S. & George, P. (1995) Trends in adult blood lead levels in New Zealand, 1974–1994. *N.Z. public Health Rep.*, **2**, 81–82

Walsh, C.T. & Ryden, E.B. (1984) The effect of chronic ingestion of lead on gastrointestinal transit in rats. *Toxicol. appl. Pharmacol.*, **75**, 485–495

Walsh, T.J. & Tilson, H.A. (1984) Neurobehavioral toxicology of the organoleads. *Neurotoxicology*, **5**, 67–86

Wananukul, W., Sirivarasai, J., Sriapha, C., Chanatara, V., Chunvimaluang, N., Keanpoompuang, A., Boriboon, W., Pumala, K. & Kaojarern, S. (1998) Lead exposure and accumulation in healthy Thais: Assessed by lead levels, EDTA mobilization and heme synthesis-related parameters. *J. med. Assoc. Thai.*, **81**, 110–116

Wang, Y.-L. (1984) Industrial lead poisoning in China over the past 33 years. *Ecotoxicol. environ. Saf.*, **8**, 526–530

Wang, L. (1988) Blood lead levels of children with different degree of lead exposures. *Environ. Health*, **5**, 1–4

Wang, L., Xu, S., Zhang, G.-D. & Wang, W.-Y. (1989) Study of lead absorption and its effect on children's development. *Biomed. environ. Sci.*, **2**, 325–330

Wang, J.-D., Soong, W.-T., Chao, K.-Y., Hwang, Y.-H. & Jang, C.-S. (1998) Occupational and environmental lead poisoning: Case study of a battery recycling smelter in Taiwan. *J. toxicol. Sci.*, **23** (Suppl. 2), 241–245

Wang, C., Huang, L., Xu, G. & Xin, Y. (2000) [Dynamic study on blood and milk lead levels of pregnant women in three districts of Hubei.] *J. Hyg. Res.*, **29**, 149–150, 153 (in Chinese)

Wang, C.-L., Chuang, H.-Y., Ho, C.-K., Yang, C.-Y., Tsai, J.-L., Wu, T.-S. & Wu, T.N. (2002a) Relationship between blood lead concentrations and learning achievement among primary school children in Taiwan. *Environ. Res.*, **89**, 12–18

Wang, V.-S., Lee, M.-T., Chiou, J.-Y., Guu, C.-F., Wu, C.-C., Wu, T.-N. & Lai, J.-X. (2002b) Relationship between blood lead levels and renal function in lead battery workers. *Int. Arch. occup. environ. Health*, **75**, 569–575

Wasserman, G.A., Liu, X., Popovac, D., Factor-Litvak, P., Kline, J., Waternaux, C., LoIacono, N. & Graziano, J.H. (2000) The Yugoslavia prospective lead study: Contributions of prenatal and postnatal lead exposure to early intelligence. *Neurotoxicol. Teratol.*, **22**, 811–818

Waszynski, E. (1977) Nonneoplastic and neoplastic changes in the kidneys and other organs in rodents fed lead acetate and sulfathiazole chronically. *Pathol. pol.*, **28**, 101–111

Watanabe, T., Fujita, H., Koizumi, A., Chiba, K., Miyasaka, M. & Ikeda, M. (1985) Baseline level of blood lead concentration among Japanese farmers. *Arch. environ. Health*, **40**, 170–176

Watanabe, T., Nakatsuka, H. & Ikeda, M. (1989) Cadmium and lead contents in rice available in various areas of Asia. *Sci. total Environ.*, **80**, 175–184

Watanabe, T., Nakatsuka, H., Shimbo, S., Iwami, O., Imai, Y., Moon, C.-S., Zhang, Z.-W., Iguchi, H. & Ikeda, M. (1996) Reduced cadmium and lead burden in Japan in the past 10 years. *Int. Arch. occup. environ. Health*, **68**, 305–314

Watanabe, T., Zhang, Z.-W., Qu, J.-B., Gao, W.-P., Jian, Z.-K., Shimbo, S., Nakatsuka, H., Matsuda-Inoguchi, N., Higashikawa, K. & Ikeda, M. (2000) Background lead and cadmium exposure of adult women in Xian city and two farming villages in Shaanxi Province, China. *Sci. total Environ.*, **247**, 1–13

Watson, D.S. (1985) The use of ultrasound scanning by Aboriginal health workers in antenatal care in a remote area of Australia. *Med. J. Austr.*, **143**, S61–S62

Watson, W.S., Hume, R. & Moore, M.R. (1980) Oral absorption of lead and iron. *Lancet*, **ii**, 236–237

Watson, W.S., Morrison, J., Bethel, M.I.F., Baldwin, N.M., Lyon, D.T.B., Dobson, H., Moore, M.R. & Hume, R. (1986) Food iron and lead absorption in humans. *Am. J. clin. Nutr.*, **44**, 248–256

Weaver, V.M., Schwartz, B.S., Ahn, K.-D., Stewart, W.F., Kelsey, K.T., Todd, A.C., Wen, J., Simon, D.J., Lustberg, M.E., Parsons, P.J., Silbergeld, E.K. & Lee, B.-K. (2003) Associations of renal function with polymorphisms in the δ-aminolevulinic acid dehydratase, vitamin D receptor, and nitric oxide synthase genes in Korean lead workers. *Environ. Health Perspect.*, **111**, 1613–1619

Webber, C.E., Chettle, D.R., Bowins, R.J., Beaumont, L.F., Gordon, C.L., Song, X., Blake, J.M. & McNutt, R.H. (1995) Hormone replacement therapy may reduce the return of endogenous lead from bone to the circulation. *Environ. Health Perspect.*, **103**, 1150–1153

Wedeen, R.P., Mallik, D.K. & Batuman, V. (1979) Detection and treatment of occupational lead nephropathy. *Arch. intern. Med.*, **139**, 53–57

Weitzman, M., Aschengrau, A., Bellinger, D., Jones, R., Hamlin, J.S. & Beiser, A. (1993) Lead-contaminated soil abatement and urban children's blood lead levels. *J. Am. med. Assoc.*, **269**, 1647–1654

Wesseling, C., Pukkala, E., Neuvonen, K., Kauppinen, T., Boffetta, P. & Partanen, T. (2002) Cancer of the brain and nervous system and occupational exposures in Finnish women. *J. occup. environ. Med.*, **44**, 663–668

West, R. (1998) Vinyl miniblinds and childhood lead poisoning. *Arch. pediatr. adolesc. Med.*, **152**, 512–513

West, W.L., Knight, E.M., Edwards, C.H., Manning, M., Spurlock, B., James, H., Johnson, A.A., Oyemade, U.J., Cole, O.J., Westney, O.E., Laryea, H., Jones, S. & Westney, L.S. (1994) Maternal low level lead and pregnancy outcomes. *J. Nutr.*, **124**, 981S–986S

Wetmur, J.G., Kaya, A.H., Plewinska, M. & Desnick, R.J. (1991a) Molecular characterization of the human δ-aminolevulinate dehydratase 2 ($ALAD_2$) allele: Implications for molecular screening of individuals for genetic susceptibility to lead poisoning. *Am. J. hum. Genet.*, **49**, 757–763

Wetmur, J.G., Lehnert, G. & Desnick, R.J. (1991b) The δ-aminolevulinic dehydratase polymorphism: Higher blood lead levels in lead workers and environmentally exposed children with the 1-2 and 2-2 isozymes. *Environ. Res.*, **56**, 109–119

Weyermann, M. & Brenner, H. (1998) Factors affecting bone demineralization and blood lead levels of postmenopausal women — A population-based study from Germany. *Environ. Res.*, **76**, 19–25

WHO (1977) *Lead* (Environmental Health Criteria 3), Geneva, World Health Organization

WHO (1980) *WHO Study Group Recommended Health-based Limits in Occupational Exposure to Heavy Metals* (Tech. Rep. Ser. 647), Geneva, pp. 36–80

WHO (1985) *Inorganic Lead* (Environmental Health Criteria 165), Geneva, International Programme on Chemical Safety

WHO (1989) Lead — Environmental Aspects (Environmental Health Criteria 85), Geneva, World Health Organization

WHO (1995) *Inorganic Lead* (Environmental Health Criteria 165), Geneva, International Programme on Chemical Safety, World Health Organization

WHO (1996) *Biological Monitoring of Chemical Exposure in the Workplace. Guidelines*, Vol. 1, Geneva, International Programme on Chemical Safety, World Health Organization, pp. 20–51

WHO (2000a) *Air Quality Guidelines for Europe* (European Series, No. 91), Copenhagen, World Health Organization, Regional Office for Europe, pp. 149–153

WHO (2000b) *Safety Evaluation of Certain Food Additives and Contaminant — Lead* (WHO Food Additives Series 44), Geneva, International Programme on Chemical Safety, World Health Organization

Wibberley, D.G., Khera, A.K., Edwards, J.H. & Rushton, D.I. (1977) Lead levels in human placentae from normal and malformed births. *J. med. Gen.*, **14**, 339–345

Wiebe, J.P., Barr, K.J. & Buckingham, K.D. (1982) Lead administration during pregnancy and lactation affects steroidogenesis and hormone receptors in testes of offspring. *J. Toxicol. environ. Health*, **10**, 653–666

Wiebe, R.A., Anderson, B.S., Lehman, C.W. & Fu, D.J. (1991) Lead poisoning in Hawaii: 1990. *Hawaiian Med. J.*, **50**, 89–95

Wietlisbach, V., Rickenbach, M., Berode, M. & Guillemin, M. (1995) Time trend and determinants of blood lead levels in a Swiss population over a transition period (1984–1993) from leaded to unleaded gasoline use. *Environ. Res.*, **68**, 82–90

Wilkins, J.R., 3rd & Sinks, T.H., Jr (1984a) Occupational exposures among fathers of children with Wilms' tumor. *J. occup. Med.*, **26**, 427–435

Wilkins, J.R., 3rd & Sinks, T.H., Jr (1984b) Paternal occupation and Wilms' tumour in offspring. *J. Epidemiol. Community Health*, **38**, 7–11

Willems, M.I., de Schepper, G.G., Wibowo, A.A.E., Immel, H.R., Dietrich, A.J.J. & Zielhuis, R.L. (1982) Absence of an effect of lead acetate on sperm morphology, sister chromatid exchanges or on micronuclei formation in rabbits. *Arch. Toxicol.*, **50**, 149–157

Willes, R.F., Lok, E., Truelove, J.F. & Sundaram, A. (1977) Retention and tissue distribution of $^{210}Pb(NO_3)_2$ administered orally to infant and adult monkeys. *J. Toxicol. environ. Health*, **3**, 395–406

Williams, M.K., King, E. & Walford, J. (1969) An investigation of lead absorption in an electric accumulator factory with the use of personal samplers. *Br. J. ind. Med.*, **26**, 202–216

Wilson, D., Esterman, A., Lewis, M., Roder, D. & Calder, I. (1986) Children's blood lead levels in the lead smelting town of Port Pirie, South Australia. *Arch. environ. Health*, **41**, 245–250

Wingren, G. & Axelson, O. (1985) Mortality pattern in a glass producing area in SE Sweden. *Br. J. ind. Med.*, **42**, 411–414

Wingren, G. & Axelson, O. (1987) Mortality in the Swedish glassworks industry. *Scand. J. Work Environ. Health*, **13**, 412–416

Wingren, G. & Axelson, O. (1993) Epidemiologic studies of occupational cancer as related to complex mixtures of trace elements in the art glass industry. *Scand. J. Work Environ. Health*, **19**, 95–100

Wingren, G. & Englander, V. (1990) Mortality and cancer morbidity in a cohort of Swedish glassworkers. *Int. Arch. occup. environ. Health*, **62**, 253–257

Winneke, G., Hrdina, K.G. & Brockhaus, A. (1982) Neuropsychological studies in children with elevated tooth-lead concentrations. I. Pilot study. *Int. Arch. occup. environ. Health*, **51**, 169–183

Winneke, G., Kramer, U., Brockhaus, A., Ewers, U., Kujanek, G., Lechner, H. & Janke, W. (1983) Neuropsychological studies in children with elevated tooth-lead concentrations. II. Extended study. *Int. Arch. occup. environ. Health*, **51**, 231–252

Wise, J.P., Leonard, J.C. & Patierno, S.R. (1992) Clastogenicity of lead chromate particles in hamster and human cells. *Mutat. Res.*, **278**, 69–79

Wise, J.P., Sr, Stearns, D.M., Wetterhahn, K.E. & Patierno, S.R. (1994) Cell-enhanced dissolution of carcinogenic lead chromate particles: The role of individual dissolution products in clastogenesis. *Carcinogenesis*, **15**, 2249–2254

Wittmers, L.E., Jr, Aufderheide, A.C., Wallgren, J., Rapp, G., Jr & Alich, A. (1988) Lead in bone. IV. Distribution of lead in the human skeleton. *Arch. environ. Health*, **43**, 381-391

Wong, O. & Harris, F. (2000) Cancer mortality study of employees at lead battery plants and lead smelters, 1947–1995. *Am. J. ind. Med.*, **38**, 255–270

Wozniak, K. & Blasiak, J. (2003) In vitro genotoxicity of lead acetate: Induction of single and double DNA strand breaks and DNA–protein cross-links. *Mutat. Res.*, **535**, 127–139

Wright, R.O., Tsaih, S.W., Schwartz, J., Wright, R.J. & Hu, H. (2003) Association between iron deficiency and blood lead level in a longitudinal analysis of children followed in an urban primary care clinic. *J. Pediatr.*, **142**, 9–14

Wu, J., Hsu, F.C. & Cunningham, S.D. (1999) Chelate-assisted Pb phytoextraction: Pb availability, uptake, and translocation constraints. *Environ. Sci. Technol.*, **33,** 1898–1904

Wu, T.-N., Yang, K.-C., Wang, C.-M., Lai, J.S., Ko, K.N., Chang, P.Y. & Liou, S.H. (1996) Lead poisoning caused by contaminated Cordyceps, a Chinese herbal medicine: Two case reports. *Sci. total Environ.*, **182**, 193–195

Wu, F.-Y., Chang, P.-W., Wu, C.-C. & Kuo, H.-W. (2002) Correlations of blood lead with DNA–protein cross-links and sister chromatid exchanges in lead workers. *Cancer Epidemiol. Biomarkers Prev.*, **11**, 287–290

Wu, Y., Huang, Q., Zhou, X., Hu, G., Wang, Z., Li, H., Bao, R., Yan, H., Li, C., Wu, L. & He, F. (2002) Study on the effects of lead from small industry of battery recycling on environment and children's health. *Chin. J. Epidemiol.*, **23**, 167–171

Wulff, M., Högberg, U. & Sandström, A. (1996) Cancer incidence for children born in a smelting community. *Acta Oncol.*, **35**, 179–183

Xu, J., Wise, J.P. & Patierno, S.R. (1992) DNA damage induced by carcinogenic lead chromate particles in cultured mammalian cells. *Mutat. Res.*, **280**, 129–136

Yamamura, K., Kishi, R., Maehara, N., Sadamoto, T. & Uchino, E. (1984) An experimental study of the effects of lead acetate on hearing. Cochlear microphonics and action potential of the guinea pig. *Toxicol. Lett.*, **21**, 41–47

Yáñez, L., García-Nieto, E., Rojas, E., Carrizales, L., Mejía, J., Calderón, J., Razo, I. & Díaz-Barriga, F. (2003) DNA damage in blood cells from children exposed to arsenic and lead in a mining area. *Environ. Res.*, **93**, 231–240

Yang, J.J. & Ma, Y.P. (1997) [The characteristics of metal elements in airborne particle in Taiyuan.] *J. Hyg. Res.*, **26**, 87–89 (in Chinese)

Yang, J.-L., Yeh, S.-C. & Chang, C.-Y. (1996) Lead acetate mutagenicity and mutational spectrum in the hypoxanthine guanine phosphoribosyltransferase gene of Chinese hamster ovary K1 cells. *Mol. Carcinog.*, **17**, 181–191

Yang, J.-L., Wang, L.-C., Chang, C.-Y. & Liu, T.-Y. (1999) Singlet oxygen is the major species participating in the induction of DNA strand breakage and 8-hydroxydeoxyguanosine adduct by lead acetate. *Environ. mol. Mutag.*, **33**, 194–201

Ye, X.-B., Fu, H., Zhu, J.-L., Ni, W.-M., Lu, Y.-W., Kuang, X.-Y., Yang, S.-L. & Shu, B.-X. (1999) A study on oxidative stress in lead-exposed workers. *J. Toxicol. environ. Health*, **A56**, 161–172

Yokoyama, K., Araki, S., Murata, K., Morita, Y., Katsuno, N., Tanigawa, T., Mori, N., Yokota, J., Ito, A. & Sakata, E. (1997) Subclinical vestibulo-cerebellar, anterior cerebellar lobe and spino-cerebellar effects in lead workers in relation to concurrent and past exposure. *Neurotoxicology*, **18**, 371–380

Yuan, X. & Tang, C. (2001) The accumulation effect of lead on DNA damage in mice blood cells of three generations and the protection of selenium. *J. environ. Sci. Health*, **A36**, 501–508

Yule, W., Lansdown, R., Millar, I.B. & Urbanowicz, M.A. (1981) The relationship between blood lead concentrations, intelligence and attainment in a school population: A pilot study. *Dev. Med. Child Neurol.*, **23**, 567–576

Yule, W., Urbanowicz, M.A., Lansdown, R. & Millar, I. (1984) Teachers ratings of children's behavior in relation to blood lead levels. *Br. J. dev. Psychol.*, **2**, 295–305

Yusof, M., Yildiz, D. & Ercal, N. (1999) N-Acetyl-L-cysteine protects against δ-aminolevulinic acid-induced 8-hydroxydeoxyguanosine formation. *Toxicol. Lett.*, **106**, 41–47

Zawia, N.H., Crumpton, T., Brydie, M., Reddy, G.R. & Razmiafshari, M. (2000) Disruption of the zinc finger domain: A common target that underlies many of the effects of lead. *Neurotoxicology*, **21**, 1069–1080

Zawirska, B. (1981) The role of the kidneys in disorders of porphyrin metabolism during carcinogenesis induced with lead acetate. *Environ. Res.*, **24**, 391–408

Zawirska, B. & Medras, K. (1968) [Tumors and disorders of porphyrin metabolism in rats with chronic experimental lead poisoning. I. Morphological studies]. *Zdrav. Prac.*, **111**, 1–12 (in German)

Zawirska, B. & Medras, K. (1972) The role of the kidneys in disorders of porphyrin metabolism during carcinogenesis induced with lead acetate. *Arch. immunol. Ther. exp.*, **20**, 257–272

Zejda, J.E., Sokal, A., Grabecki, J., Panasiuk, Z., Jarkowski, M. & Skiba, M. (1995) Blood lead concentrations in school children of Upper Silesian Industrial Zone, Poland. *Cent. Eur. J. Public Health*, **3**, 92–96

Zelikoff, J.T., Li, J.H., Hartwig, A., Wang, X.W., Costa, M. & Rossman, T.G. (1988) Genetic toxicology of lead compounds. *Carcinogenesis*, **9**, 1727–1732

Zeng, J. & Kagi, J.H.R. (1995) Zinc fingers and metallothionein in gene expression. In: Goyer, R.A. & Cherian, M.G., eds, *Toxicology of Metals*, Heidelberg, Springer Verlag, pp. 333–335

Zey, J.N. & Cone, J.E. (1982) Health Hazard Evaluation Report, HETA 81-0039-1104, Modine Manufacturing Co., Bloomington, IL, USA, NIOSH

Zhang, J., Ichiba, M., Wang, Y., Yukitake, S. & Tomokuni K. (1998) Relation between polymorphism of δ-aminolevulinic acid dehydratase and some parameters in lead workers. *J. occup. Health*, **40**, 77–78

Zhang, Z.-W., Moon, C.-S., Watanabe, T., Shimbo, S. & Ikeda, M. (1996) Lead content of rice collected from various areas in the world. *Sci. total Environ.*, **191**, 169–175

Zhang, Z.-W., Moon, C.-S., Watanabe, T., Shimbo, S., He, F.-S., Wu, Y.-Q., Zhou, S.-F., Su, D.-M., Qu, J.-B. & Ikeda, M. (1997a) Background exposure of urban populations to lead and cadmium: Comparison between China and Japan. *Int. Arch. occup. environ. Health*, **69**, 273–281

Zhang, Z.-W., Qu, J.-B., Xu, G.-F., Song, L.-H., Wang, J.-J., Shimbo, S., Watanabe, T., Nakatsuka, H., Higashikawa, K. & Ikeda, M. (1997b) Maize and foxtail millet as substantial sources of dietary lead intake. *Sci. total Environ.*, **208**, 81–88

Zhang, Z.W., Shimbo, S., Ochi, N., Eguchi, M., Watanabe, T., Moon, C.S. & Ikeda, M. (1997c) Determination of lead and cadmium in food and blood by inductively coupled plasma mass spectrometry: A comparison with graphite furnace atomic absorption spectrometry. *Sci. total Environ.*, **205**, 179–187

Zhang, Z.-W., Qu, J.-B. & Ikeda, M. (1998) Lead and cadmium levels in the atmosphere in mainland China: A review. *J. occup. Health*, **40**, 257–263

Zhang, Z.-W., Qu, J.-B., Watanabe, T., Shimbo, S., Moon, C.-S. & Ikeda, M. (1999) Exposure of citizens in China and in Japan to lead and cadmium: A comparative study. *Toxicol. Lett.*, **108**, 167–172

Zhang, Z.-W., Moon, C.-S., Shimbo, S., Watanabe, T., Nakatsuka, H., Matsuda-Inoguchi, N., Higashikawa, K. & Ikeda, M. (2000) Further reduction in lead exposure in women in general populations in Japan in the 1990s, and comparison with levels in east and south-east Asia. *Int. Arch. occup. environ. Health.*, **73**, 91–97

Zheng, X.Q., Liu, J.R. & Song, H.Q. (1993) Blood lead levels of children and their relationship with blood lead levels of adults. *Public Health Res.*, **23** (Suppl.), 29–33

Zheng, Y., Leng, S., Song, W., Wang, Y., Niu, Y., Zhang, W., Yan, H., Liu, Y., Huang, Q. & Wu, Y. (2002) [A molecular epidemiological study of childhood lead poisoning in lead-polluted environment.] *Chin. J. Epidemiol.*, **23**, 175–78 (in Chinese)

Zhou, W.X. & Chen, J.Z. (1988) Health effects of lead exposure in children. *Environ. Health*, **5**,18–22

Zhou, W., Yuan, D., Ye, S., Qi, P., Fu, C. & Christiani, D.C. (2001) Health effects of occupational exposures to vehicle emissions in Shanghai. *Int. J. occup. environ. Health*, **7**, 23–30

Zhu, B.G., Su, D.Q., Qin, M. & Jian, C.P. (1984) [Study of chronic lead-poisoning from using tin-kettles.] *Chinese J. Prevent. Med.*, **18**, 328–330 (in Chinese)

Ziegler, E.E., Edwards, B.B., Jensen, R.L., Mahaffey, K.R. & Fomon, S.J. (1978) Absorption and retention of lead by infants. *Pediatr. Res.*, **12**, 29–34

Zollinger, H.U. (1953) [Renal adenomas and carcinomas induced in rats after chronic lead exposure, and their relationship with corresponding neoplasia in humans.] *Virchows Arch.*, **323**, 697–710 (in German)

Zuckerman, M.A. (1991) Lead exposure from lead crystal. *Lancet*, **337**, 550

LIST OF ABBREVIATIONS USED IN THIS VOLUME

1,25-$(OH)_2$D: 1,25-dihydroxycholecalciferol
2-AAF: 2-acetylaminofluorene
6βOHF: 6β-hydroxycortisol
8-OH-dG: 8-OH-deoxyguanosine
AAS: atomic absorption spectrometry
ABEP: auditory brainstem evoked potential
ACGIH: American Conference of Governmental Industrial Hygienists
ALA: ∂-aminolevulinic acid
ALAD: ∂-aminolevulinate dehydratase
ALT: alanine aminotransferase
AOAC: Association of Official Analytical Chemists
AST: aspartate aminotransferase
ASTM: American Society for Testing and Materials
ASV: anode-stripping voltammetry
ATP: Adenosine triphosphate
AUC: area-under-the-curve
BEI: biological exposure index
bw: body weight
CaBP: calcium-binding proteins
CAT: computerized axial tomography
CBLI: cumulative blood lead index
CDC: US Centers for Disease Control and Prevention
CI: confidence interval
CNS: central nervous system
CRP: C-reactive protein
DMSA: dimercaptosuccinic acid
DMT: divalent cation metal transporter
DNA: deoxyribonucleic acid
DTH: delayed-type hypersensitivity
EDTA: ethylenediaminetetracetic acid
EHEN: *N*-ethyl-*N*-hydroxyethylnitrosamine
EP: erythrocyte protoporphyrin
EPA: Environmental Protection Agency (USA)
FBPA: *N*-(4′-fluoro-4-biphenyl) acetamide
Fpg: formamidopyrimidine-DNA glycosylase

FSH: follicle-stimulating hormone
GABA: γ-aminobutyric acid
GC: gas chromatography
GF–AAS: graphite furnace–atomic absorption spectrometry
GFR: glomerular filtration rate
GSH: reduced glutathione
GST: glutathione *S*-transferase
HOME: home observation for measurement of the environment
HP2: human protamine 2
HPG: hypothalamic–pituitary–gonadal
HPLC: high-performance liquid chromatography
Hsp: heat-shock protein
ICD-8: international classification of diseases 8th revision
ICD-9: international classification of diseases 9th revision
ICP-AES: inductively coupled plasma–atomic emission spectrometry
ICP-MS: inductively coupled plasma–mass spectrometry
IFN: interferon
IL: interleukin
IQ: intelligence quotient
IUGR: intrauterine growth retardation
IUPAC: International Union of Pure and Applied Chemistry
JECFA: Joint FAO/WHO Expert Committee on Food Additives
KαXRF: X-ray fluorescence, using K-alpha line excitation
LH: luteinizing hormone
MAPK: mitogen-activated protein kinase
MEK: MAP kinase kinase
MMAD: mass median aerodynamic diameter
MMD: mass median diameter
MNNG: *N*-methyl-*N*-nitro-*N*-nitrosoguanidine
NAG: *N*-acetyl-β-D-glucosaminidase
NBBN: *N*-butyl-*N*(4-hydroxybutyl) nitrosamine
NDEA: *N*-nitrosodiethylamine
NDMA: *N*-nitrosodimethylamine
NHANES II: National Health and Nutrition Examination Survey II
NIOSH: National Institute for Occupational Safety and Health (USA)
NK: natural killer
NO: nitric oxide
NOAA: National Oceanic and Atmospheric Administration
OECD: Organisation for Economic Co-operation and Development
OR: odds ratio
OSHA: Occupational Safety and Health Administration (USA)
P5′N: pyrimidine 5′-nucleotidase

PbBP: lead-binding protein
PBGS: porphobilinogen synthase
PBMC: peripheral blood mononuclear cell
PBPK: physiologically based pharmacokinetic model
PBZ: personal breathing zone
PHA: phytohaemagglutinin
PID: photoionization detection
PKC: protein kinase C
PMOR: proportional mortality odds ratio
PVC: polyvinyl chloride
ROS: reactive oxygen species
SBG: steroid binding globulin
SBIS: Stanford-Binet Intelligence Scale
SCGE: single-cell gel electophoresis
SIR: standardized incidence ratio
SMR: standardized mortality ratio
SOD: superoxide dismutase
SPMR: standardized proportional mortality rate
T3: triiodothyronine
T4: thyroxine
TFIIIA: transcription factor IIIA
TH: tyrosine hydrolase
TIMS: thermal ionization–mass spectrometry
TNF: tumor necrosis factor
TPA: 12-*O*-tetradecanoyl phorbol-13-acetate
TSH: thyroid-stimulating hormone
US DHUD: United States Department of Housing and Urban Development
US EPA: United States Environmental Protection Agency
US FDA: United States Food and Drug Administration
UV: ultraviolet
VDR: vitamin D receptor
VEP: visual-evoked potential
WISC-R: Wechsler revised intelligence scale for children
XRF: X-ray fluorescence
ZPP: zinc protoporphyrin
βNF: 5,6-benzoflavone
γGT: γ-glutamyl transpeptidase

CUMULATIVE CROSS INDEX TO *IARC MONOGRAPHS ON THE EVALUATION OF CARCINOGENIC RISKS TO HUMANS*

The volume, page and year of publication are given. References to corrigenda are given in parentheses.

A

B

E

F

G

H

K

L

M

N

O

Q

R

S

T

List of IARC Monographs on the Evaluation of Carcinogenic Risks to Humans*

Volume 1
Some Inorganic Substances, Chlorinated Hydrocarbons, Aromatic Amines, *N*-Nitroso Compounds, and Natural Products
1972; 184 pages (out-of-print)

Volume 2
Some Inorganic and Organometallic Compounds
1973; 181 pages (out-of-print)

Volume 3
Certain Polycyclic Aromatic Hydrocarbons and Heterocyclic Compounds
1973; 271 pages (out-of-print)

Volume 4
Some Aromatic Amines, Hydrazine and Related Substances, *N*-Nitroso Compounds and Miscellaneous Alkylating Agents
1974; 286 pages (out-of-print)

Volume 5
Some Organochlorine Pesticides
1974; 241 pages (out-of-print)

Volume 6
Sex Hormones
1974; 243 pages (out-of-print)

Volume 7
Some Anti-Thyroid and Related Substances, Nitrofurans and Industrial Chemicals
1974; 326 pages (out-of-print)

Volume 8
Some Aromatic Azo Compounds
1975; 357 pages (out-of-print)

Volume 9
Some Aziridines, *N*-, *S*- and *O*-Mustards and Selenium
1975; 268 pages (out-of-print)

Volume 10
Some Naturally Occurring Substances
1976; 353 pages (out-of-print)

Volume 11
Cadmium, Nickel, Some Epoxides, Miscellaneous Industrial Chemicals and General Considerations on Volatile Anaesthetics
1976; 306 pages (out-of-print)

Volume 12
Some Carbamates, Thiocarbamates and Carbazides
1976; 282 pages (out-of-print)

Volume 13
Some Miscellaneous Pharmaceutical Substances
1977; 255 pages

Volume 14
Asbestos
1977; 106 pages (out-of-print)

Volume 15
Some Fumigants, the Herbicides 2,4-D and 2,4,5-T, Chlorinated Dibenzodioxins and Miscellaneous Industrial Chemicals
1977; 354 pages (out-of-print)

Volume 16
Some Aromatic Amines and Related Nitro Compounds—Hair Dyes, Colouring Agents and Miscellaneous Industrial Chemicals
1978; 400 pages

Volume 17
Some *N*-Nitroso Compounds
1978; 365 pages

Volume 18
Polychlorinated Biphenyls and Polybrominated Biphenyls
1978; 140 pages (out-of-print)

Volume 19
Some Monomers, Plastics and Synthetic Elastomers, and Acrolein
1979; 513 pages (out-of-print)

Volume 20
Some Halogenated Hydrocarbons
1979; 609 pages (out-of-print)

Volume 21
Sex Hormones (II)
1979; 583 pages

Volume 22
Some Non-Nutritive Sweetening Agents
1980; 208 pages

Volume 23
Some Metals and Metallic Compounds
1980; 438 pages (out-of-print)

Volume 24
Some Pharmaceutical Drugs
1980; 337 pages

Volume 25
Wood, Leather and Some Associated Industries
1981; 412 pages

Volume 26
Some Antineoplastic and Immunosuppressive Agents
1981; 411 pages (out-of-print)

Volume 27
Some Aromatic Amines, Anthraquinones and Nitroso Compounds, and Inorganic Fluorides Used in Drinking-water and Dental Preparations
1982; 341 pages (out-of-print)

Volume 28
The Rubber Industry
1982; 486 pages (out-of-print)

Volume 29
Some Industrial Chemicals and Dyestuffs
1982; 416 pages (out-of-print)

Volume 30
Miscellaneous Pesticides
1983; 424 pages (out-of-print)

---

*High-quality photocopies of all out-of-print volumes may be purchased from University Microfilms International, 300 North Zeeb Road, Ann Arbor, MI 48106-1346, USA (Tel.: +1 313-761-4700, +1 800-521-0600).

Volume 31
Some Food Additives, Feed Additives and Naturally Occurring Substances
1983; 314 pages (out-of-print)

Volume 32
Polynuclear Aromatic Compounds, Part 1: Chemical, Environmental and Experimental Data
1983; 477 pages (out-of-print)

Volume 33
Polynuclear Aromatic Compounds, Part 2: Carbon Blacks, Mineral Oils and Some Nitroarenes
1984; 245 pages (out-of-print)

Volume 34
Polynuclear Aromatic Compounds, Part 3: Industrial Exposures in Aluminium Production, Coal Gasification, Coke Production, and Iron and Steel Founding
1984; 219 pages (out-of-print)

Volume 35
Polynuclear Aromatic Compounds, Part 4: Bitumens, Coal-tars and Derived Products, Shale-oils and Soots
1985; 271 pages

Volume 36
Allyl Compounds, Aldehydes, Epoxides and Peroxides
1985; 369 pages

Volume 37
Tobacco Habits Other than Smoking; Betel-Quid and Areca-Nut Chewing; and Some Related Nitrosamines
1985; 291 pages (out-of-print)

Volume 38
Tobacco Smoking
1986; 421 pages

Volume 39
Some Chemicals Used in Plastics and Elastomers
1986; 403 pages (out-of-print)

Volume 40
Some Naturally Occurring and Synthetic Food Components, Furocoumarins and Ultraviolet Radiation
1986; 444 pages (out-of-print)

Volume 41
Some Halogenated Hydrocarbons and Pesticide Exposures
1986; 434 pages (out-of-print)

Volume 42
Silica and Some Silicates
1987; 289 pages

Volume 43
Man-Made Mineral Fibres and Radon
1988; 300 pages (out-of-print)

Volume 44
Alcohol Drinking
1988; 416 pages

Volume 45
Occupational Exposures in Petroleum Refining; Crude Oil and Major Petroleum Fuels
1989; 322 pages

Volume 46
Diesel and Gasoline Engine Exhausts and Some Nitroarenes
1989; 458 pages

Volume 47
Some Organic Solvents, Resin Monomers and Related Compounds, Pigments and Occupational Exposures in Paint Manufacture and Painting
1989; 535 pages (out-of-print)

Volume 48
Some Flame Retardants and Textile Chemicals, and Exposures in the Textile Manufacturing Industry
1990; 345 pages

Volume 49
Chromium, Nickel and Welding
1990; 677 pages

Volume 50
Pharmaceutical Drugs
1990; 415 pages

Volume 51
Coffee, Tea, Mate, Methyl-xanthines and Methylglyoxal
1991; 513 pages

Volume 52
Chlorinated Drinking-water; Chlorination By-products; Some Other Halogenated Compounds; Cobalt and Cobalt Compounds
1991; 544 pages

Volume 53
Occupational Exposures in Insecticide Application, and Some Pesticides
1991; 612 pages

Volume 54
Occupational Exposures to Mists and Vapours from Strong Inorganic Acids; and Other Industrial Chemicals
1992; 336 pages

Volume 55
Solar and Ultraviolet Radiation
1992; 316 pages

Volume 56
Some Naturally Occurring Substances: Food Items and Constituents, Heterocyclic Aromatic Amines and Mycotoxins
1993; 599 pages

Volume 57
Occupational Exposures of Hairdressers and Barbers and Personal Use of Hair Colourants; Some Hair Dyes, Cosmetic Colourants, Industrial Dyestuffs and Aromatic Amines
1993; 428 pages

Volume 58
Beryllium, Cadmium, Mercury, and Exposures in the Glass Manufacturing Industry
1993; 444 pages

Volume 59
Hepatitis Viruses
1994; 286 pages

Volume 60
Some Industrial Chemicals
1994; 560 pages

Volume 61
Schistosomes, Liver Flukes and *Helicobacter pylori*
1994; 270 pages

Volume 62
Wood Dust and Formaldehyde
1995; 405 pages

Volume 63
Dry Cleaning, Some Chlorinated Solvents and Other Industrial Chemicals
1995; 551 pages

Volume 64
Human Papillomaviruses
1995; 409 pages

Volume 65
Printing Processes and Printing Inks, Carbon Black and Some Nitro Compounds
1996; 578 pages

Volume 66
Some Pharmaceutical Drugs
1996; 514 pages

Volume 67
Human Immunodeficiency Viruses and Human T-Cell Lymphotropic Viruses
1996; 424 pages

Volume 68
Silica, Some Silicates, Coal Dust and *para*-Aramid Fibrils
1997; 506 pages

Volume 69
Polychlorinated Dibenzo-*para*-Dioxins and Polychlorinated Dibenzofurans
1997; 666 pages

Volume 70
Epstein-Barr Virus and Kaposi's Sarcoma Herpesvirus/Human Herpesvirus 8
1997; 524 pages

Volume 71
Re-evaluation of Some Organic Chemicals, Hydrazine and Hydrogen Peroxide
1999; 1586 pages

Volume 72
Hormonal Contraception and Post-menopausal Hormonal Therapy
1999; 660 pages

Volume 73
Some Chemicals that Cause Tumours of the Kidney or Urinary Bladder in Rodents and Some Other Substances
1999; 674 pages

Volume 74
Surgical Implants and Other Foreign Bodies
1999; 409 pages

Volume 75
Ionizing Radiation, Part 1, X-Radiation and γ-Radiation, and Neutrons
2000; 492 pages

Volume 76
Some Antiviral and Anti-neoplastic Drugs, and Other Pharmaceutical Agents
2000; 522 pages

Volume 77
Some Industrial Chemicals
2000; 563 pages

Volume 78
Ionizing Radiation, Part 2, Some Internally Deposited Radionuclides
2001; 595 pages

Volume 79
Some Thyrotropic Agents
2001; 763 pages

Volume 80
Non-Ionizing Radiation, Part 1: Static and Extremely Low-Frequency (ELF) Electric and Magnetic Fields
2002; 429 pages

Volume 81
Man-made Vitreous Fibres
2002; 418 pages

Volume 82
Some Traditional Herbal Medicines, Some Mycotoxins, Naphthalene and Styrene
2002; 590 pages

Volume 83
Tobacco Smoke and Involuntary Smoking
2004; 1452 pages

Volume 84
Some Drinking-Water Disinfectants and Contaminants, including Arsenic
2004; 512 pages

Volume 85
Betel-quid and Areca-nut Chewing and Some Areca-nut-derived Nitrosamines
2004; 334 pages

Volume 86
Cobalt in Hard Metals and Cobalt Sulfate, Gallium Arsenide, Indium Phosphide and Vanadium Pentoxide
2006; 330 pages

Volume 87
Inorganic and Organic Lead Compounds
2006; 506 pages

Supplement No. 1
Chemicals and Industrial Processes Associated with Cancer in Humans (*IARC Monographs*, Volumes 1 to 20)
1979; 71 pages (out-of-print)

Supplement No. 2
Long-term and Short-term Screening Assays for Carcinogens: A Critical Appraisal
1980; 426 pages (out-of-print)
(updated as IARC Scientific Publications No. 83, 1986)

Supplement No. 3
Cross Index of Synonyms and Trade Names in Volumes 1 to 26 of the *IARC Monographs*
1982; 199 pages (out-of-print)

Supplement No. 4
Chemicals, Industrial Processes and Industries Associated with Cancer in Humans (*IARC Monographs*, Volumes 1 to 29)
1982; 292 pages (out-of-print)

Supplement No. 5
Cross Index of Synonyms and Trade Names in Volumes 1 to 36 of the *IARC Monographs*
1985; 259 pages (out-of-print)

Supplement No. 6
Genetic and Related Effects: An Updating of Selected *IARC Monographs* from Volumes 1 to 42
1987; 729 pages (out-of-print)

Supplement No. 7
Overall Evaluations of Carcinogenicity: An Updating of *IARC Monographs* Volumes 1–42
1987; 440 pages (out-of-print)

Supplement No. 8
Cross Index of Synonyms and Trade Names in Volumes 1 to 46 of the *IARC Monographs*
1990; 346 pages (out-of-print)

Achevé d'imprimer sur rotative par l'Imprimerie Darantiere
à Dijon-Quetigny en août 2006

Dépôt légal : août 2006 - N° d'impression : 26-1273

Imprimé en France

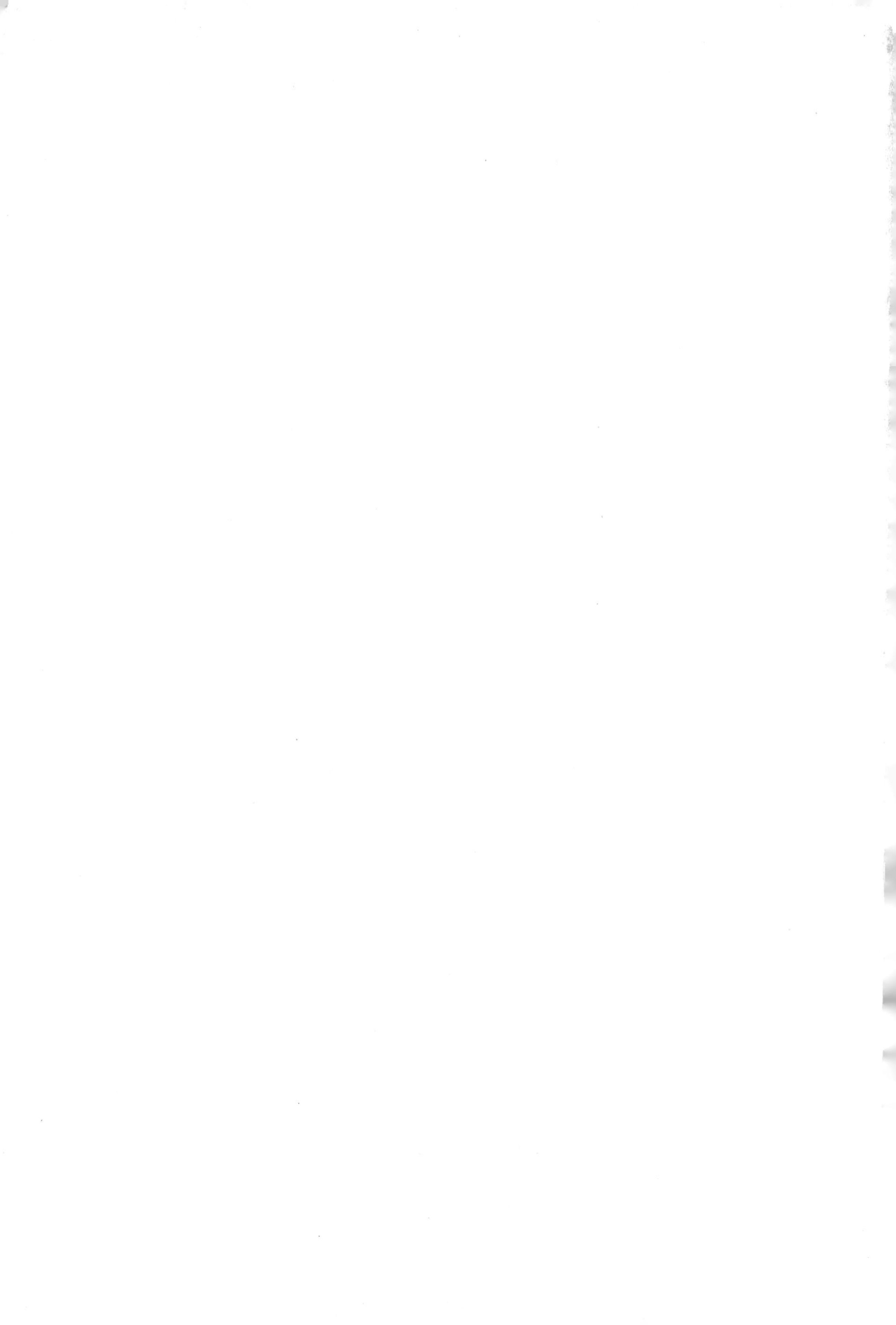